Aromatherapy for Health Professionals

For Elsevier

Commissioning Editor: Karen Morley
Development Editor: Louise Allsop
Project Manager: Elouise Ball
Design: Andrew Chapman
Illustrator: Hardlines Studio
Illustration Buyer: Gillian Murray

Aromatherapy for Health Professionals

THIRD EDITION

Edited by

Shirley Price Cert Ed FISPA MIFA FIAM Hon. Member IFPA
Author Practitioner and Lecturer in Aromatherapy, Hinckley, Leicestershire

Len Price Cert Ed MIT FISPA FIAM Hon. Member IFPA
Author and Lecturer in Aromatherapy, Hinckley, Leicestershire

Foreword by
HRH The Prince of Wales

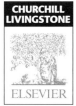

CHURCHILL
LIVINGSTONE

ELSEVIER

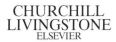

CHURCHILL
LIVINGSTONE
ELSEVIER

First Edition 1995
Second Edition 1999
Third Edition 2007

ISBN 10: 0-443-10134-5
ISBN 13: 9780443101342

British Library Cataloguing in Publication Data
A catalogue record for this book is available from the British Library

Library of Congress Cataloging in Publication Data
A catalog record for this book is available from the Library of Congress

Notice
Knowledge and best practice in this field are constantly changing. As new research and experience broaden our knowledge, changes in practice, treatment and drug therapy may become necessary or appropriate. Readers are advised to check the most current information provided (i) on procedures featured or (ii) by the manufacturer of each product to be administered, to verify the recommended dose or formula, the method and duration of administration, and contraindications. It is the responsibility of the practitioner, relying on their own experience and knowledge of the patient, to make diagnoses, to determine dosages and the best treatment for each individual patient, and to take all appropriate safety precautions. To the fullest extent of the law, neither the Publisher nor the Authors assume any liability for any injury and/or damage to persons or property arising out of or related to any use of the material contained in this book.

The Publisher

Working together to grow
libraries in developing countries

www.elsevier.com | www.bookaid.org | www.sabre.org

ELSEVIER   BOOK AID International   Sabre Foundation

ELSEVIER your source for books, journals and multimedia in the health sciences

www.elsevierhealth.com

The publisher's policy is to use **paper manufactured from sustainable forests**

Printed in China

Contents

Contributors

Angela Avis MBE MA RGN DN Cert PG Dip Ed
PG Dip Advanced Health Care Practice
Senior lecturer, Oxford Brookes University

Elaine Cooper MIFPA LIAM
Lead complementary therapist for Walsall NHS;
aromatologist; teacher Primary Care Trust

Jane Cummins RGN MIFPA LDCA
Nurse; aromatherapist

Jenny Henry Dip Cot MSROT MIFPA
Occupational therapist; aromatherapy
practitioner

Dr William E Morden CChem MRSC
Consultant specializing in analysis, quality
control and chemistry of essential oils

Penny Price M Ed MIFPA MIFA FIAM
Lecturer; Principal, Penny Price Academy;
aromatologist

Christine Stacey MA Dip HE BSc (Hons)
Complementary Therapies RSCN RN
Senior lecturer/programme leader,
Complementary Therapies, University of
Greenwich

The Rev. Dr. Robert Stephen BA BD MTh
(Oxon) FSA Scot FIAM Dip Clin Arom
Teacher; priest; aromatologist

Denise Tiran MSc RM RGN ADM PGCEA
Director, Expectancy Ltd; honorary lecturer,
University of Greenwich, London

Elizabeth Walsh RN (LD) Dip Couns BSc (Hons)
Complementary Therapies
Medway NHS Trust community nurse – post
diagnostic support

Sue Whyte RGN RM Cert Ed FE MIFPA
Macmillan lecturer practitioner (retired);
aromatherapy practitioner – Oncology Unit,
Walsgrave Hospital, Coventry

Foreword

CLARENCE HOUSE

This book presents one of the key holistic approaches to health care that I have sought to promote through my Foundation for Integrated Health and I am, therefore, delighted to see that the purpose is not only to broaden the knowledge of those within Aromatherapy itself, but also to educate and inform all practising health professionals who are interested and committed to integrated healthcare.

The publication offers an explanation of the science and principles underlying the practice of aromatherapy and in doing so raises awareness of a therapy that is growing and maturing, taking its place alongside more established treatments. Significant progress has been made since the first edition in adopting a more scientific approach and, within the profession itself, moving towards self-regulation.

The advantages of aromatherapy are self evident; it is simple and effective in use and can be delivered at low cost. It may be used in conjunction with most other complementary therapies and, equally, can be used to complement and supplement allopathic medicine, often with remarkable effects (when aromatherapy is used in hospitals the oils used may be the only non-synthetic materials in the building). With aromatherapy, which respects the individual person, the approach is holistic and so it can be used not only for healing but also as a preventative measure, strengthening the immune system, promoting relaxation and reducing stress.

The contributors to this book are drawn from a wide spectrum of those involved in aromatherapy as practitioners, educators and researchers. Some, working within the National Health Service, have had experience of allopathic medicine; others base their writing on their experience of practising aromatherapy and/or aromatic medicine. The synergy created in the partnership of these authors is in itself powerful.

I commend this book – in its third edition – as an important contribution to all who have concern for the future of aromatherapy, and towards further establishing its role and place within integrated healthcare in the UK.

Preface

Thirty years ago aromatherapy was little known, being regarded merely as a pleasant adjunct to a beauty treatment, or at best a 'rejuvenating' skin treatment; however, the health promoting aspect has been in the ascendant and has progressed considerably during the last 10 years. There still exists inadequate training in some sectors, but the situation for would-be professionals has been addressed and minimum training standards set by the major professional associations. Aromatherapy involves and necessitates knowledge of a wide range of topics from botany, organic chemistry, and essential oil understanding to massage, client care, mind effects, safety factors, etc. therefore it is difficult for there to be a unique, omniscient, undoubted authority. While aromatherapy as a complement to conventional medical treatment has recently made remarkable and significant progress, especially in hospitals, there still remains much to be discovered through research and experience. A multitude of books on the subject have been written in the past for the lay public (not all of them completely reliable), each containing more or less the same information. It is only in the last dozen years that books have been written specifically as an aid for those health professionals wishing to practise *therapeutic* aromatherapy safely and effectively. For this reason it is advisable to say a few words on the quality of the information contained in this book.

The Aromatherapy Workbook (first edition 1993) was one of the first aimed at helping student aromatherapists acquire in-depth knowledge of the physiological and psychological effects of essential oils. The importance of accurately specifying the essential oils employed was stressed, by using the botanical name and part of the plant in preference to the common plant name only.

However, because professionals such as physiotherapists, occupational therapists and nurses have become increasingly aware of the possibilities of using essential oils in many areas (e.g. hospices, hospitals, clinics, day care, residential and community care work) the Editors felt that the time was ripe for a book aimed specifically at health professionals. This feeling was confirmed at lectures and workshops given at many hospitals throughout the UK, S. Ireland, N. Ireland and Switzerland as early as 1992 to 1995, where it became clear that many nurses were introducing essential oils into their hospitals without attending an accredited training course. This problem may have arisen because so much aromatherapy course time is concerned with full-body massage, something that is seldom utilized by professionals in health-care situations, who rarely have the time to carry this out. In response to this, we devised an advanced, comprehensive course on aromatic medicine (= aromatology), which has been extremely successful – in fact, it is our opinion that this is the only way forward for professional aromatherapists. We also felt that a book which emphasizes the need to obtain extensive knowledge of essential oils before using them on sick people will discourage the incorrect application of these powerful agents, which in some unfortunate instances has led to their use being limited, discouraged or forbidden in some health-care settings.

To be able to put together such a book it has been necessary to look at the hundreds of existing references on the properties and actions of essential oils researched in the past – carried out principally for the perfume and food industries. There is a large body of information available on some of the antiseptic, antibacterial, antiparasitic and even anti-viral properties of some essential oils, and their effects on the skin, but the information is by no means complete and much more research needs to be done with aromatherapy and health problems in mind. Progress is being made however; thus it was thought desirable to bring out a third edition of 'Aromatherapy for health professionals' to:

- update information on some aspects of essential oils and carrier oils
- add a small amount on hydrolats as an introduction to the authors' book 'Understanding Hydrolats', published in 2004
- expand the information on aromatherapy worldwide. In addition, the chapters in Section 3 (Aromatherapy in context) have been written by practising nurses with aromatherapy training using essential oils in their own particular field, thus giving the most up-to-date information
- include two additional chapters, one on the aspect of aromatic medicine and the second looking at aromatherapy as practised by private therapists outside the NHS.

Unreferenced consumer books on aromatherapy have not been used at all for this book, except for the writings of eminent practitioners, for without evidence of this kind this book would be quite slim and of little use. Trial and pilot studies, anecdotal evidence and single case studies are almost all that aromatherapy has to rely on at this time, and we have thought it better to give this information rather than the usual copying of properties from herbal books – the properties of the essential oil and a given plant are not necessarily the same.

The bulk of research done in the past has been *in vitro* or on animals and it can be difficult – and often impossible – to extrapolate such results to humans. There is a dearth of information on aspects such as (for example) analgesic and diuretic effects of essential oils, and when it comes to the effects of essential oils on conditions such as bronchitis, arthritis, headaches, etc there is realistically only anecdotal evidence available. Properly constructed and conducted trials are desperately needed, but aromatherapists have neither the appropriate training nor the necessary finances to carry out this work, although this situation is now changing. The Research Council for Complementary Medicine has an increasing data bank of research trials using aromatherapy, as have one or two private companies such as Essential Oil Resource Consultants, who provide research information in the field of essential oils. As for double-blind tests, new thinking will have to be adopted – it is not possible to do this type of test using an aromatic substance, as the presence or absence of an aroma is immediately obvious to the participants. Double-blind studies, though desirable, can usually be achieved only by internal use, a rarely used method in aromatherapy.

Thus, while there is a great deal of information in this book, anecdotal evidence has been used where 'scientific' evidence is not available. In our opinion it is of good quality, having been carefully selected – where it is in accord with our own experience obtained over three decades of practice and teaching – from acknowledged sources (many French) some of whom are medical doctors.

We must be receptive to possibilities that science has not yet grasped. It is absurd not to use treatments that work, just because we do not yet understand them.

Siegel (1988)

It is the moral duty of aromatherapists to carry out such investigations as far as they are able to determine how and whether or not essential oils work in particular circumstances, and to have a unified system of reporting and sharing information: at the present time this is not in place. Many more trials, projects and single case studies are needed to demonstrate unequivocally the efficacy of these holistic medicines before they can be generally accepted. Professionals in the 'orthodox' field generally fall into two categories: either they help to design protocols for such studies, or they stand back and criticize our lack of proper research, of which we are already painfully aware, not needing it to be drawn to our attention.

It is realized that the value of anecdotal evidence is questionable due to various factors:

- many illnesses are self-limiting and sponta- neously disappear
- some are only in the mind of the sufferer and such people are usually open to suggestion
- with some illnesses the sufferer has phases of feeling poorly alternating with phases of feel- ing well.

There are also the unexplained 'miraculous' cures which do occasionally happen. Obviously false good results can appear to occur, but it is against common sense to dismiss all anecdotal evidence gathered over the years.

This book contains guidelines on the prep- aration of a professionally based policy and protocol to present to hospital management when applying for permission to use essential oils in a health-care setting. In those hospitals where the use of essential oils has already been introduced on a correct footing, many trials and projects have been carried out. Although not constituting research in the accepted scientific sense of the word, such studies are extremely valuable for the future acceptance of aromatic medicine. It is hoped that by publicizing some of them here, more health professionals will be encouraged to continue the good work.

We would like to express our thanks to the many therapists from far and wide who have contacted us with information on the result of their own treatments. This sort of information is most helpful and such courteous cooperation between therapists, authors and the professional societies is greatly to be encouraged. A volume of anecdotal evidence properly classified and collated can be stimulus which leads to a research study; the sharing of information is vital to the advancement of our fascinating profession of aromatherapy.

Should doctors bother with this strange therapy? We hope that this book will convince the doubters that there is something of substance to be looked into, something which can be used alongside orthodox treatments, especially in hospitals where, in addition, there may be sub- stantial cash savings to be made. Most general practitioners discuss alternative (complementary) treatments with their patients and over half of them refer patients to alternative practitioners (Anderson & Anderson 1987, Borkan et al 1994).

There is an excellent case for having orthodox doctors take a long, hard look at the manner in which their complementary competitors operate, with a view to adopting those features of their approach which are of such patent value to their clients – empathy, demonstrable concern, making an effort to reassure, simple courtesy, and, above all, treating the person as more important than the disease (Gould 1985).

As long ago as 1995 many general practitioners believed that alternative medicine had ideas and methods from which conventional medicine could benefit (Verhoef & Sutherland 1995a), and in a questionnaire 73% of physicians felt that they should have some knowledge of the most import- ant alternative treatments (Verhoef & Sutherland 1995b). These beliefs and feelings have definitely augmented in number over the last 10 years! And even earlier, Wharton and Lewith (1986) found that although most general practitioners knew little of the techniques of complementary medi- cine, a majority found that the complementary techniques being assessed had been useful to their patients. Most had referred patients for this type of treatment during the previous year not only to their medical colleagues but also to comp- lementary practitioners, even though they felt that complementary practitioners needed statutory regulation. Harmonization of training and regu- lation of practitioners is the urgent requirement in the immediate future (Fisher & Ward 1994). Happily the situation has improved in this respect over the past years, and is currently being addressed (see Chapter 16 (Part I) on Aroma- therapy in the UK).

Albeit that the editors are not themselves either doctors or nurses, they are health professionals with over three decades of experience in the field. However, as in all written texts compiled in a changing world, this book undoubtedly falls short of its goals. Nevertheless, we offer this text in the hope that it will lead those with a genuine interest in essential oils to a better understanding of their properties and possible uses and trust that this book will prove to be of value to all health pro- fessionals and their associates.

Shirley and Len Price
Hinckley 2006

References

Anderson E, Anderson P 1987 General practitioners and alternative medicine. Journal of Royal College of General Practitioners Feb 37(295): 52–55

Borkan J, Neher J O, Anson O, Smoker B 1994 Referrals for alternative therapies. Journal of Family Practice 39(6): 545–550

Fisher P, Ward A 1994 Complementary medicine in Europe. British Medical Journal 309(6947): 107–111

Gould D 1985 The black and white medicine show: how doctors serve and fail their customers. Hamish Hamilton, London, pp. 228–229

Siegel B S 1988 Love, medicine and miracles. Arrow Books, London, p. 37

Verhoef M J, Sutherland L R 1995a Alternative medicine and general practitioners. Opinions and behaviour. Canadian Family Physician 41: 1005–1011

Verhoef M J, Sutherland L R 1995b General practitioners' assessment of and interest in alternative medicine in Canada. Social Science and Medicine 41(4): 511–515

Wharton R, Lewith G 1986 Complementary medicine and the general practitioner. British Medical Journal (Clinical Research) June 7 292(6533): 1498–1500

Acknowledgements

The authors wish to thank not only Karen Morley, Louise Allsop and Elouise Ball for their understanding and help with this third edition of their book, but also Katherine Vaughan, for her exciting phone call to tell us that Prince Charles would be delighted to write the foreword. We offer our sincere appreciation to him.

Our thanks and gratitude go to Dr Bill Morden, for his expert help and advice on the chemistry aspects of essential oils.

We are indebted to all those enthusiastic people who supplied the text for the chapter on aromatherapy worldwide – it was a mammoth task to find contacts in each country. We would also like to thank those who supplied the text for the different applications of aromatherapy in context, in Section 3.

Further thanks are due to those aromatherapists who provided new case studies. I trust they will understand – and forgive – the fact that their cases have been abbreviated and put into a standard format, without always mentioning nutrition, etc. and the holistic relationship between client and patient (so necessary in complementary therapies). It was done simply so that the aromatherapy interventions could be read more easily; no-one is more aware than the authors that treatments should always aim to rebalance clients at a physical, mental and emotional level.

Introduction

INTRODUCTION

There is some discussion as to the exact meaning of the word aromatherapy and therefore on how the essential oils should be used. Aroma is from Latin *aroma* = sweet odour, spice which is in turn from Greek *aroma* = spice, and therapy from Latin *therapia* Greek *therapeia* = curing, healing. The purists maintain that the word intends the oils to be used only in ways which conform to the meaning of therapy through aroma, that is not by massage or other ways of application but only by inhalation. Of course, this is quite correct if the true sense of the word is rigidly adhered to. Some support is given by Schulz et al (1998) who write that aromatic herbs are effective only when the molecules of their volatile oils come in contact with the nasal mucosa through inhalation: the classic prototype is smelling salts – a preparation no longer manufactured, but a home-made version is prepared by putting 1–4 drops essential oil on a tissue and inhaling from it. A tradition of using the oils in many different ways has, however, built up over the course of time to such an extent that it is now (almost) universally accepted that the word aromatherapy encompasses all methods of applying essential oils, but note that this always includes inhalation.

There is also some difference of opinion about the use of the word essential – 'the traditional term "essential oil" still persists even though the essence of the plant is a poorly defined concept of medieval pharmacy' (Guenther 1948) therefore Hay & Waterman (1993 p. 1) prefer the term 'volatile oil' because it refers to the fact that most components of the oils have low boiling points and can be removed from the plant by steam distillation. Nevertheless, we in aromatherapy continue to use the words 'essential oil' and understand the meaning, even though it is acknowledged that 'plant volatile oil' is a more accurate term.

The subject of aromatherapy involves pharmacy and farming, botany and bodies, medicine and chemistry, toxicity and safety, all so intertwined and interconnected that it is scarcely possible to disentangle the ramifications for the purpose of setting them down without some repetition and much cross-referral.

HISTORICAL USE OF ESSENTIAL OILS

Plants and their extracts have been used since time immemorial to relieve pain, aid healing, kill bacteria and thus revitalize and maintain good health. Most books on aromatherapy include its history in more or less detail. Suffice it to say here that although the word itself was not coined until this century, the distilled extracts from plants – the essential oils – have been employed by mankind for countless years in religious rites, perfumery and hygiene. Cedarwood oil, known to have been used by the Egyptians for embalming and for hygienic purposes 5000 years ago, was probably the first 'distilled' oil to have been produced although the process used is open to speculation (Ch. 2). Both the plant and the essential oil of lavender were used by the Abbess Hildegard of Bingen as early as the 12th century and by the 15th century it is thought that essential oils of turpentine, cinnamon, frankincense, juniper, rose and sage were also known and used (Pignatelli 1991). About 60 oils were known and used in perfumes and medicines by the beginning of the 17th century (Valnet 1980 p. 28).

MODERN EVIDENCE FOR THE ANTISEPTIC POWERS OF ESSENTIAL OILS

Towards the end of the 19th century, the action of turpentine (terebinth) oil was observed by Koch in 1881 against the anthrax bacillus, soon to be followed by research by Chamberland (1887) which proved the antiseptic properties of essential oils and then early in the 20th century by Cavel's research into the individual effects of 35 essential oils on microbial cultures in sewage. The most effective oil required to render inactive 1000 ml of culture was found to be thyme (0.7 ml). Two other well-known oils showing high efficacy were sweet orange (1.2 ml, 3rd) and peppermint (2.5 ml, 9th) (Cavel 1918). The antiseptic power of several oils has now been proved to be many times greater than that of phenol. Certain essential oils have also been shown to be effective against different bacteria, e.g. lemon, which is one of the best in its antiseptic and bactericidal properties, neutralizing both the typhus bacillus and *Staphylococcus aureus* in a matter of minutes. Cinnamon kills the typhus bacillus when diluted 1 part in 300 (Valnet 1980 p. 36). Professor Griffon, a member of the French Academy of Pharmacy, made up a blend of seven essential oils (cinnamon, clove, lavender, peppermint, pine, rosemary and thyme), to study their antiseptic effect on the surrounding air when sprayed from an aerosol; all the staphylococci and moulds present were destroyed after 30 minutes (Valnet 1980 p. 37). See Chapter 4 for more recent studies on the antiseptic properties of essential oils.

The bacteriological approach of aromatherapy is an extremely complex field of the utmost interest, opening the way to the ecological understanding and management of the different colonies and floras that live in cohabitations – or at war – within us. Allopathic medicine has begun to realize that the misuse of antibiotics leads to numerous side-effects and sometimes results in chronic disastrous conditions (i.e. systemic candidosis) that could have been avoided if medical aromatherapy had been implemented in due time (Pénoël 1993 personal communication).

Today, the properties of herb volatile oils are researched in many centres throughout the world, assessing antibacterial and antifungal properties of essential oils and their constituents.

ESSENTIAL OIL USE IN INDUSTRY AND AROMATHERAPY

Tens of thousands of tonnes of essential oils are used by the food industry and a large but declining amount by the perfume industry (Verlet 1993) due to the increased use of synthetic copies; because they are antioxidants, essential oils are used to protect food from spoilage and the quantities used for toothpastes and mouthwashes have grown spectacularly (Hay & Waterman 1993 p. 3). The total amount of essential oils used by the aromatherapy profession, although increasing, is nevertheless extremely small by comparison, which contributes to the difficulties of obtaining high quality, pure, natural oils (Ch. 2). Some beneficial oils used not to be supplied by distillers because they are not required by the giant users who are more concerned with quantity and cost rather than quality but fortunately, in latter years, the number of independent distillers producing essential oils solely for aromatherapy use has increased, although such products naturally tend to be more expensive.

DEFINITION OF ESSENTIAL OIL FOR AROMATHERAPEUTIC PURPOSES

There are only two plant extracts which should be given this name for aromatherapy purposes:

- **Essential oils:** these are plant extracts which have been achieved by steam distillation of plant material from a single botanical source; nothing is involved in this process save water, heat and the plant material. The essential oil is separated from the condensed steam and nothing is added and nothing is taken away.
- **Expressed oils:** these are the product of citrus fruits, and they are achieved by simple pressing (expression) of the citrus peel, without heat or aid of solvents. Nothing is added and nothing is taken away.

Care is needed in the way essential oils are sold to protect both the lay public and aromatherapists. The oils for therapeutic use must be whole and unadulterated, accurately identified and labelled, and must have been correctly stored.

N.B. Not all plants yield an essential oil and some yield so little that the oil would be too expensive; oils such as hyacinth, lilac, lime blossom, honeysuckle and jasmine do not exist in a distilled form; their fragrance is extracted by other means and it is incorrect for anyone to name extracts from these plants as essential oils in the context of aromatherapeutic use.

AROMATHERAPY OILS

This term is widely used in the marketplace, but is a vague, almost meaningless term, which does not adequately describe the product. Products labelled thus usually consist of a 2% maximum dilution of essential oil(s) in a fixed oil. Often these inexpensive products are sold in small bottles having an integral dropper, which is misleading as droppers are not necessary for diluted oils and their presence can give the impression (sometimes intentional) that they are neat essential oils – they are often sold at the pure essential oil price, thus yielding an excessive profit. Oils sold under this heading usually contain standardized oils of low quality, more suited to industries other than complementary medicine. Other ways of extracting plant components follow, none of which should be classed as essential oils for aromatherapy purposes.

ABSOLUTES

These are aromatic liquids – not essential oils – which are extracted from plant material using solvents such as hexane, butane, etc., then subjected to alcohol extraction. It is a complex process, yielding a liquid substance called an absolute, which is totally soluble in alcohol and important in the perfume industry, although still containing traces of solvent.

MACERATED OILS

Macerated oils are made by putting plant material into a fixed vegetable oil, when those plant molecules soluble in the oil are taken up by the vegetable oil used. Examples are *Calendula officinalis* [marigold] and *Hypericum perforatum* [St John's wort]. These should not be sold in small bottles and passed off as essential oils, although they are important carriers of essential oils and for use on the skin (Ch. 7).

IGNORANCE IS BLISS?

Much of the misnaming of oils for aromatherapy comes through ignorance on the part of the suppliers. Occasionally a supplier sells an expensive fixed oil, such as *Oenothera biennis* [evening primrose], as an essential oil, putting it into a small bottle with an integral dropper and within an essential oil price range. Unfortunately, aromatherapy is a popular bandwagon to jump on, and the very word aromatherapy has selling power, used by the unscrupulous, sometimes at the expense of the unwary honest dealer. Standardized oils are cheap and easy to obtain, unlike the genuine essential oils necessary for aromatherapy.

WIDE-RANGING APPLICATION

Genuine essential oils can be put to a multitude of uses both in general practice and in hospitals, as this quotation from Dr J Valnet illustrates:

> The doctor who is familiar with essential oils can use them to treat a whole range of infections – pulmonary, hepatic, intestinal, urinary, uterine, rhinopharyngeal and cutaneous (infected wounds and suppurating dermatoses). The use of these oils usually produces satisfactory results, provided they have been prescribed wisely and that, in the case of certain long-standing complaints, the treatment is followed for a long enough period. Aromatic therapy can neutralize enteritis, colitis and putrid fermentations, and can relieve chronic bronchitis and pulmonary tuberculosis. The colon bacillus cannot resist essential oils.

Valnet (1980 p. 41)

Orthodox medicine currently uses plant material to help cure diseases which previously had a high death rate. Twenty years ago, four out of every five children with leukaemia lost their lives; now, four out of five are returned to health with the aid of vincristine and vinblastine, derivatives of the rosy periwinkle – a plant used for hundreds of years by tribal healers as a medicine (Craker 1990). The snakeroot plant from India is now used in the western world to treat hypertension; digitalis, for heart conditions, is produced from the humble foxglove and the well-known rhododendron is used in the treatment of fatigue.

> Plants are an intrinsic part of natural medicine, and not even the most orthodox doctor can get by without them; indeed they represent the link between the natural and the orthodox, the traditional and the ultra-new.

Pahlow (1980)

Phytotherapy (Chs 4 and 17) is the name given to the use of the whole, or part, of the plant for medicinal purposes. Aromatherapy and aromatic medicine (Ch. 9) are branches of this, but use only distilled essential oils, expressed citrus oils and hydrolats (Ch. 6). Plant oils are simple to use and administer, yet can compete with the steroids and antibiotics used in allopathic medicine today without the body's defence mechanism becoming exhausted or developing tolerance to them. The day will surely come when orthodox doctors will regard plant volatile oils as a necessary and easily administered part of everyday medicine, effective but inexpensive.

- The basic reason which accounts for the diversity of conception and application of aromatherapy lies in the very nature of the aromatic substance. Essential oils have many properties which make them highly suitable therapeutic substances:
  - The capacity to effect cutaneous penetration quickly and easily.
  - Being endowed with the capacity to influence the mind through their powerful impact on the human olfactory system (Ch. 8): they were traditionally used in analeptics (an old term denoting a restorative remedy for states of weakness frequently accompanied by faintness and dizziness (Aschner 1986)) to stimulate the olfactory nerve and the sensory trigeminal nerve endings causing a reflex stimulation of respiration and circulation (Schulz, Hänsel & Tyler 1998 p. 105).
  - Having multiple pharmacological properties due to their highly active molecular compounds.

Thus it was perhaps inevitable for aromatic substances to find healing application in so many areas.

POWERFUL HEALING AGENTS

Many plant extracts used in the production of conventional medicines are, like the foxglove, poisonous and therefore exceptionally low doses are employed. Some essential oils are also toxic when used incorrectly and the most powerful of these are not normally available to aromatherapists (Chs 3 and 4). Essential oils are concentrated and intensely energetic in their effects, so very little is needed for successful treatment (even of those in general use) – dilutions generally being in the range 0.05–3%, occasionally up to 10%, depending on the oil(s) used, but their use undiluted may be suitable under certain circumstances. Apart from the difference in the intensity of the aroma, no apparent benefit is gained from higher concentrations, particularly where the problem is an emotional one, although more concentrated solutions are used in certain medical conditions in aromatic medicine (aromatology) (Ch. 9).

It cannot yet be proved exactly *how* essential oils work, but research and extensive anecdotal evidence exists to prove that they *do* work. In the distant past, essences have been used to heal wounds, inhibit the decay of flesh (as in mummification) and reduce the spread of infection (as in the time of the Black Death) – all without anyone knowing how they worked, just as the humble aspirin was in use for many years before anyone knew its mode of action.

USER-FRIENDLY

Bios is the Greek word for life and essential oils may be classed as probiotic (for life), as opposed to antibiotic (against life). To illustrate this point, antibiotics kill not only harmful bacteria, but also the beneficial flora needed to keep us healthy, leaving the body in a weakened state. Carefully selected essential oils kill only the bacteria inimical to the successful functioning of the body (Valnet 1980 p. 45). 'A serious condition obviously authorizes the use of antibiotics, and in high doses; but one should be aware that the price of a cure may be a permanent disability' (Valnet 1980 p. 54).

Many essential oils possess antiviral and fungicidal qualities and natural, whole essential oils can be used on living tissue with minimal unwanted effects (unlike some synthetic drugs, however successful against their intended targets). Also, the human body accustoms itself to the effects of chemical synthetics, leading to escalating doses. This has not been found to be the case with essential oils, which retain their effectiveness in repeated applications and can in fact strengthen the living tissue while killing off the unwanted bacteria (Valnet 1980 p. 48). This may be due to the fact that essential oils are natural products and their composition is not fixed but tends to vary from season to season.

Compared to the very high price of drugs (perhaps due to tremendous research and development costs) essential oils are extremely inexpensive – a factor which should interest those in charge of public health funds. Not only that, they are pleasant to use for both patient and carer. In many hospitals and hospices they are used not only to improve the quality of a patient's life but in waiting rooms to relieve the anxiety of relatives and friends. More specifically, they can be used in place of secondary drugs, which might be prescribed to counteract the iatrogenic effects of primary drugs.

AREAS OF USE

Essential oils have been found to aid relaxation effectively, both pre- and postoperatively, to regenerate tissue in cases of severe burns and inflammation, and to relieve pain in cases of rheumatoid arthritis. They have helped to improve the quality of life for the terminally ill (Ch. 15) and have also found important uses in maternity care (Ch. 12). They are used more and more to help people with learning disabilities (Ch. 13) and in elderly care, particularly with regard to dementia (Ch. 14) as well as being used extensively to improve or uplift a patient's state of mind (Ch. 8). The effect of attitude of mind on a person's health is being recognized more and more – Florence Nightingale said 'what nursing has to do . . . is to put the patient in the best condition for nature to act upon him', reinforcing the ancient tag *medicus cura, natura sanat* – the doctor treats, nature cures.

By far the majority of essential oil users are outside the medical profession, some people using them merely on instruction from one of the many books written for the general public on the subject. They are simple to use and it should come as a relief to GPs that minor everyday ailments such as a sore throat or a winter cold, and also some chronic disorders like bronchitis, sinusitis and rheumatism can be treated in the home easily and successfully, leaving the doctor more time for his patients.

All this is achievable by anyone, without professional medical skills. However, in France (from where aromatherapy was introduced to the UK) medical doctors prescribe essential oils for internal use in capsules, diluted in alcohol or in suppositories and pessaries (Ch. 17) as well as using them externally in dressings, inhalations, ointments and in foot, hand or whole body baths although massage is not used. The original concept of aromatherapy in England was to use

the essential oils in massage only – suitably diluted in a fixed vegetable oil, which unfortunately led to the belief that that is all there is to it – and the authors are actively trying to correct this image. UK training now includes inhalation, baths, compresses and in some schools, the use of pessaries and suppositories – which is also taught on an aromatic medicine (aromatology) course.

Since the second edition of this book 7 years ago essential oil therapy has been introduced into many hospitals, hospices and clinics, but more progress must be made and it needs the medical profession not only to take a greater interest in essential oils and demand research studies but also to use its professional skills to use these precious commodities to their fullest capabilities in order to bring the benefits of this aromatic therapy to all hospitals throughout the world in the 21st century.

References

Aschner B 1986 Lehrbuch der Konstitutionstherapie. Hippokrates, Stuttgart, p. 107

Cavel L 1918 Sur la valeur antiseptique de quelques huiles essentielles. Comptes Rendus (Académie des Sciences) 166: 827

Chamberland M 1887 Les essences au point du vue de leurs propriétés antiseptiques. Annales Institut Pasteur 1: 153–154

Craker L E 1990 News and commentary. The Herb, Spice and Medicinal Plant Digest 8(4): 5

Guenther E 1948 The essential oils. Van Nostrand, New York, pp. 3–4

Hay R K M, Waterman P G 1993 Volatile oil crops: their biology, biochemistry and production. Longman Scientific & Technical, Harlow

Pahlow M 1980 Living medicine. Thorsons, Wellingborough, p. 9

Pignatelli M F 1991 Viaggio nel mondo della essenze. Muzzio, Padora

Schulz V, Hänsel R, Tyler V E 1998 Rational phytotherapy: a physicians' guide to herbal medicine. Springer, Berlin, p. 105

Valnet J 1980 The practice of aromatherapy. Daniel, Saffron Walden

Verlet N 1993 Commercial aspects. In: Hay R K M, Waterman P G (eds) Volatile oil crops. Longman, Harlow, pp. 138, 145–146

SECTION 1

Essential oil science

Chapter 1

The genesis of essential oils

Len Price

INTRODUCTION

Aromatherapy involves the use of essential oils, all of which are derived from plants. Anyone wishing to practise aromatherapy must gain as full an understanding of the plants concerned as possible, so that the oils can be used knowledgeably to their best effect. This chapter enables the practitioner to do this, looking beyond the oil in the little glass bottle to the plant from which it was extracted, its growing environment and the family to which it belongs.

BOTANY FOR AROMATHERAPISTS

What has botany to do with aromatherapy?

Everyone agrees with the quotation from Shakespeare (Romeo and Juliet) 'What's in a name? That which we call a rose by any other name would smell as sweet.' – so why do therapists need to bother themselves about botany? After all, what's in a name?

The answer when dealing with essential oils is – *everything!*

To be an effective aromatherapist it is crucial to a good outcome that aromatherapeutic quality essential oils pertinent to the particular client be employed, and to be able to do this the therapist must be able to discriminate between therapeutic quality oils and those produced for other industries, which is the overwhelming bulk of essential oils produced. To be able to select such oils is not possible unless the therapist has a basic knowledge of some aspects of botany and in particular the nomenclature used.

> *That botany is a useful study is plain; because it is in vain that we know betony is good for headaches, or self-heal for wounds unless we can distinguish betony and self-heal from one another.*

> John Hill, The Family Herbal (1808)

PRE-LINNAEAN CHAOS

In the early 18th century the identification of plants was in a chaotic state, for example John Tradescant brought spiderworts to England from North America and named it – including his own name after the fashion of the time – *Phalangum Ephenerum Virginianum Johannis Tradescanti.*

There was an obvious need for better naming of plants, names that were accurate, unambiguous, concise and part of a universally acknowledged and accepted system.

> *A good name is rather to be chosen than great riches.*

> The Bible, Proverbs 22:1

TAXONOMY

Then along came the Swedish naturalist Carl von Linné or Linnaeus (1707–1778) and changed everything. He devised the binomial system and applied it universally, making the precise nominal identification of plants possible; (the spiderworts mentioned above are now known as *Tradescantia andersoniana*, a simple binomial title which is recognized the world over). Binomial means a two name system; millions of people are differentiated by a family name and an individual personal name; in similar fashion plant names are made up of a generic name and an individual specific descriptive name. Binomials are written in italics and may be followed by the name (perhaps abbreviated) of one or more persons. *Panax quinquefolius* L; the L stands for Carl Linnaeus, the author of this name for American ginseng. Sometimes there is a double citation (a second

botanist) and this means that the plant has been reclassified, the original author being put first, in parentheses: although not essential, it does give an abbreviated bibliographical reference. Over the years the Linnaean system of classifying organisms in groups according to their similarities has been subject to much modification but is still at the core of the international taxonomic system used today.

What is taxonomy? – a study devoted to producing a system of classification of organisms which best reflects the totality of their similarities and differences (Cronquist 1968 p. 3) The word taxonomy comes from two Greek words (*taxis* – arrangement and *-nomia* – method). Major taxonomic groups of the plant kingdom include categories as follows, and several subgroups:

Kingdom: Plantae
Division: Tracheophyta
Subdivision: Spermatophyta
Class: Dicotyledons
Subclass: Asteridae
Order: Lamiales
Family: Lamiaceae
Genus: *Lavandula*
Species: *angustifolia*

In aromatherapy it is sufficient for identification purposes to know:

- **The family** that the plant belongs to (all family names end in -aceae).
- **The genus**; generic names are based on structural characteristics and are always written in italics with an initial capital letter and can be used alone.
- **The species**; these are adjectival describing the genus and are never written with a capital letter, even when it is after a person e.g. *smithii* the whole word is in lower-case italics and cannot be used by itself.

Lavender must therefore be referred to by the genus name *Lavandula* and the descriptive adjective *angustifolia* to identify the particular plant (and its essential oil).

However, there are further divisions below this level, such as:

- **Subspecies:** often denotes a geographic variation of a species.
- **Variety:** indicates a rank between subspecies and forma. They are named by adding 'var.' in

Roman font and the italicized variety name, e.g. *Citrus aurantium* var. *amara*. The label 'var.' is used to indicate a major subdivision of a species, or a variant of horticultural origin or importance (although these are now labelled cultivar). Many names of horticultural origin reflect the historical use of the variety rank.

- **Forma:** denotes trivial differences.
- **Cultivar:** indicates a cultivated variety, and a rank known only in horticultural cultivation. These names are non-Latinized and in living languages (usually the name of, or chosen by, the originator, in the following case Monsieur Maillette). They are not italicized, and appear within quotation marks, e.g. *Lavandula angustifolia* 'Maillette'.
- **Chemotype:** indicates visually identical plants but having different, perhaps significantly so, chemical components, resulting in different therapeutic properties. Chemotypes occur naturally in plants grown in the wild, some species throwing up many chemical variations; they can be propagated by cuttings for cultivation and they are named by the abbreviation 'ct.' followed by the chemical constituent, e.g. *Thymus vulgaris* ct. thujanol-4, *T. vulgaris* ct. geraniol, *T. vulgaris* ct. carvacrol, etc. Chemotypes are plants that look the same from the outside, but have different chemical constituents inside; by contrast **phenotypes** are plants that look different on the outside but are chemically similar inside.
- **Hybrid:** indicates natural or artificially produced crosses between species. The name contains 'x' (in Roman font) which means the plant is a hybrid produced by sexual crossing e.g. *Mentha* x *piperita*, which is a cross between *Mentha aquatica* and *Mentha spicata*.

When procuring and prescribing essential oils therapists must take care to identify precisely the plants from which they are derived, and this means giving not only the generic and specific names but also specifying, where necessary, the chemotype, variety, cultivar, etc. as well.

Note on pronunciation: aromatherapists are sometimes worried about how to pronounce the Latinized names, but there are no strict rules and almost anything goes! The same names are used throughout the world but there is a wide variation in pronunciation from country to country, and indeed by individuals within a country.

METABOLISM

Each plant is a vibrant chemical factory capable of transforming the electromagnetic rays from the sun into energetic substances which are then available for the plant's use. The plant takes up water and minerals from the soil through its roots and carbon dioxide from the air mainly through its leaves. These supplies are then converted by the energy absorbed from the sun into a simple six-carbon sugar, glucose, which provides food for the plant's growth. The waste product of this chemical change is oxygen. The metabolic changes in plants are made possible by the action of protein catalysts known as enzymes. Enzymes are highly specific and assist in only one particular reaction (as they do in humans). To function they need manganese or iron combined with a tiny amount of energy that is to be found stored in phosphate bonds in the plant chemicals. The whole process is called photosynthesis, and because it is essential to the life of the plant it is termed primary metabolism.

Chemicals produced by plants that do not have an obvious value to the producer plant are known as secondary metabolites; the array of secondary metabolites, which of course includes volatile oils, is enormous (Waterman 1993 p. 31). Secondary metabolism products include alkaloids, bitters, glycosides, gums, mucilages, saponins, steroids, tannins and essential oils, which are not necessary for the vital functions of the plant (see Fig. 1.1) and of these secondary metabolites it is the essential oils that have the greatest commercial significance, being used in many industries (Verlet 1993). Volatile oil secondary metabolites vary widely in chemical structure and their purpose and function in the plant is little understood.

WHY DOES A PLANT CONTAIN ESSENTIAL OIL?

Before seeing how an essential oil comes into being, it is worth reflecting on what value essential oils have for plants. This has been debated for many years and there is as yet no definitive answer. Perhaps there never will be, given that science is much better at answering the question 'how?' than the question 'why?', and that there is no obvious commercial advantage in this knowledge. Most commercial research effort is put into investigating the properties and effects of the oils themselves, and it is left to disinterested investigators at universities to look into what possible use the essential oils may be to the plant. However, conjecture on the subject has thrown up many possible reasons:

- To prevent attack by herbivores: both mono- and sesquiterpenes are involved in various ways, such as acting as insect hormones to interfere with the development of the feeding insects, or having a straightforward repellent action. Essential oils and other secondary metabolites can render plant tissue bitter and unpalatable.
- To prevent attack from insects: it has been shown that the number of oil glands in a plant increases when it is under attack by insects (Carlton 1990, Carlton, Gray & Waterman 1992).
- To prevent attack by bacteria, fungi and other microorganisms: there is ample proof available from studies done *in vitro* on the antifungal and bactericidal properties of herb volatile oils (see section on aromatograms in Ch. 4).
- To aid pollination by attracting bees and other insects such as moths and bats (Harborne 1988).
- To help in the healing of wounds inflicted on the plant itself.
- To act as an energy reserve.
- To help survival in difficult growth conditions: for instance by the production of allelopathic compounds, such as 1,8-cineole and camphor, which are freely given off from the plant and find their way to the soil where they prevent other plants from growing (Deans & Waterman 1993).
- To prevent dehydration and afford some degree of protection in hot dry climates by surrounding the plant with a haze of volatile oil, thus helping to prevent water loss from its foliage. Leaves with a dense covering of glandular hairs can help trap the water molecules that evaporate through the stomata. One of the oldest plants in the world, the leaves of which can be as much as 10% oil by weight, is the eucalyptus. Living

root stock of this plant has been found dating back thousands of years to the Ice Age (Dr Mike Crisp, Australian National Botanic Gardens unpublished information 1986). The free oil vapour emanating from other ancient plants, e.g. pine trees, can be smelt easily when walking in pine forests on a sunny day.

Whatever else they may do, they do give the plant its aroma and flavour and often have a significant physiological effect on people.

Secretory structures

Essential oils and their mixtures with resins and gums are commonly found in special secretory structures. Secretory structures in plants are divided into two main types: those occurring on the plant surfaces, which usually secrete substances directly to the outside of the plant (exogenous secretion), and those which occur within the plant body and secrete substances into specialized intercellular spaces (endogenous secretion) (Svoboda 2003).

Essential oils are synthesized and stored in different sites; oils may be found, for instance, in the leaves, seeds, petals, roots, bark, etc. Sometimes different oils occur in more than one site in a plant; for example two different oils are produced by the cinnamon tree (bark, leaf), and three different oils by the orange tree (leaf, blossom, peel). The type of structure is one of the characteristics of a plant family and, based on detailed observations and description, it is possible to divide the secretory structures into the following categories:

- Oil cells and resin cells
  Lauraceae (e.g. cinnamon)
  Zingiberaceae (e.g. cardamom, ginger, turmeric)
  Piperaceae (e.g. black pepper)
  Myristicaceae (e.g. nutmeg)
  Illiciaceae (e.g. star anise)
- Cavities, sacs, oil reservoirs (schizolysigenous)
  Rutaceae (e.g. orange)
  Myrtaceae (e.g. clove, eucalyptus)
- Oil or resin canals, ducts
  Apiaceae (e.g. dill)
  Pinaceae (e.g. pine, cedarwood)
  Burseraceae (e.g. myrrh)
- Glandular hairs, trichomes
  Lamiaceae (e.g. lavender, rosemary)

Asteraceae (e.g. elecampane)

Geraniaceae (e.g. geranium)

■ Internal hairs

Orchidaceae (e.g. vanilla)

■ Epidermal cells

Essential oils obtained from flowers such as roses are usually not secreted by glandular hairs, but by the actual epidermal cells of the petals. The amount of essential oil in flowers *(Rose, Acacia, Jasminum* sp.) is very low, usually between 0.02 and 0.08% (v/w).

■ Isodiametric cells

Orchid flower epidermal tissues called osmophores secrete the volatile substances.

■ Stigmata

Many flowering plants also secrete volatile oils, lipids, sugars and amino acids.

■ Tree buds

Such as horse chestnut, alder, poplar, cherry, and buckthorn, secrete sticky substances (mucilages); similar tissues also occur on the stipules and the edges of their young leaves (Svoboda 2003).

THE GENESIS OF ESSENTIAL OILS

Plants produce a tremendous variety of chemicals, including a major group of compounds, the terpenes. According to Harborne (1988) more than 1000 monoterpenes and possibly 3000 sesquiterpenes have presently been identified. The phenylpropenes constitute another much smaller but significant group: they always consist of a 3-carbon side chain having a double bond attached to an aromatic ring. In essential oils most of the components belong either to the terpene group, based on the mevalonic acid pathway, or to the phenylpropene group, formed through the shikimic acid pathway.

Synthesis of volatile oils

Photosynthesis is the process by which green plants use the electro-magnetic energy of sunlight, absorbed by the chlorophyll in the plant, to drive a series of chemical reactions leading to the formation of carbohydrates. All animals, including humans, depend on photosynthesis because it is the method by which the basic food, sugar, is created.

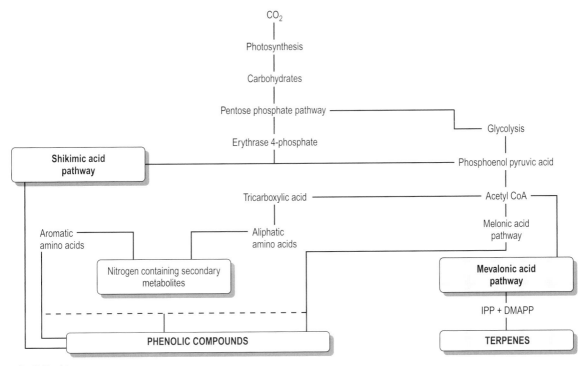

after S. Turnidge

Figure 1.1 Secondary metabolite synthesis within the plant.

During the complex reactions of the first, *light reaction* stage of photosynthesis, light energy is used to split water (H_2O) into oxygen (O_2), protons (hydrogen ions H^+) and electrons; the oxidation of water gives rise to free oxygen. In the second, *dark reaction* stage, no light is required and the protons and electrons are used to reduce carbon dioxide, which enters the plant through the stomata, to carbohydrates in the form of simple sugars. A complex series of chemical changes occurs, which can be represented by the equation

$$6CO_2 + 12H_2O \rightarrow C_6H_{12}O_6 + 6O_2 + 6H_2O$$

(in this example the formation of glucose).

Simple sugars that provide energy for the plant are stored as starch; glucose is released from starch as and when energy is required.

The elements in sugar (carbon, hydrogen and oxygen) are the same as those in essential oils, but differently grouped, and hundreds of chemicals are produced by the decomposition/glycolysis of sugars with aid of enzymes. Mevalonic acid goes through phosphorylization, decarboxylation and dehydration to become five-carbon isoprene units that are the basic building blocks for the terpenes found in essential oils (Fig. 1.1). The phenols are derived via a different route – the shikimic acid pathway.

Biochemical experiments have proved that essential oils are synthesized in the glands of the plant. Various enzymes specific for essential oil biosynthesis were shown to be located exclusively in trichomes. By employing specialized techniques, it is possible to isolate secretory cells and to investigate their content. Thus biosynthetic pathways have been elucidated, along with their complete sets of enzymes, and it is possible to purify these enzymes and use them in further experiments.

Plants can be considered as biochemical factories that have been evolving their programmes over the last 400 million years! With genetic techniques, it is now possible to intervene in these pathways and change both the quality and quantity of essential oils – a prospect which brings new dimensions into the natural balance (Svoboda 2003).

CHEMICAL VARIATION WITHIN SPECIES

Chemotype is a term applied to plants of the same genus and species, which have the same external appearance but differ, sometimes considerably, in their internal chemical composition. These chemotypes usually occur naturally in plants growing in the wild, and can result partly from cross-pollination. The place and manner of a plant's growing will also promote internal changes; many essential-oil-bearing plants, e.g. rosemary and thyme, are prone to this kind of change owing to genetic and environmental factors. They become resistant to local pests and diseases and have adapted to make the best use of the soil and other surrounding conditions. Such plants are termed 'landrace', and strains which yield specified chemical constituents are sought and selected for propagation by cloning: that is to say, cuttings are taken and then cultivated to produce the specific oils required. Included in this category are the thymes and lavenders flourishing wild on the sunny dry hills of Provence which are extensively cloned and then grown commercially.

THYME CHEMOTYPES

The thyme plant is particularly prolific in spontaneously producing strains bearing essential oils of different compositions. Some of these are described below:

- *Thymus vulgaris* ct. thymol. The thymol-bearing thyme is strongly antiseptic and aggressive to the skin owing to the presence of the phenol thymol. Cut in the spring the essential oil contains 30% thymol (Fig. 1.2) plus para-cymene (also written *p*-cymene) (a monoterpene hydrocarbon). When the same plant is cut in the autumn the essential oil may be found on analysis to contain 60–70% thymol and less *p*-cymene (Table 1.1).

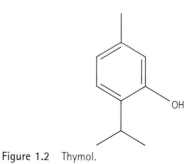

Figure 1.2 Thymol.

Table 1.1 *Thymus vulgaris* chemotypes – variation with season

Chemotype	Spring	Autumn
Thymol	γ-Terpinene + *p*-cymene	Thymol
Carvacrol	γ-Terpinene + *p*-cymene	Carvacrol
Geraniol	Geranyl acetate	Geraniol

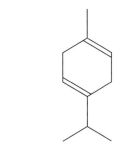

Figure 1.4   γ-Terpinene

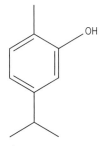

Figure 1.3   Carvacrol.

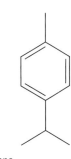

Figure 1.5   *p*-Cymene.

- *Thymus vulgaris* ct. carvacrol. This variant behaves in the same way as the thymol chemotype of thyme, but the phenol involved is carvacrol (Fig. 1.3). In the spring the essential oil contains 30% carvacrol, which increases to 60–80% in the autumn (Table 1.1).
- The thymol and carvacrol chemotypes do not flourish at high altitudes but are cultivated in the valleys. Both of these phenolic chemotypes are often, although inaccurately, referred to as red thymes (because the now obsolete iron stills imparted a red colour to the oil) and they are major antiinfective agents with a wide range of action (Belaiche 1979). For the thyme chemotypes, the harvesting time is crucial in order to obtain the required composition of an essential oil, as the internal chemistry of the plant changes with the seasons (see also Fig. 1.11). Concerning the thymol and carvacrol chemotypes, *p*-cymene is the precursor of both thymol and carvacrol (see Table 1.2); at the beginning of the season, in the spring, the plants contain γ-terpinene (Fig. 1.4) and *p*-cymene (Fig. 1.5), but as the season progresses these precursors are transformed into either carvacrol or thymol, so that plants harvested in the autumn yield essential oils containing phenols.

Table 1.2 *Thymus vulgaris* chemotypes – variation with stage of growth

	Stage of growth		
	Bud	Flower	End of flowering
Carvacrol	22.8	35.9	53.7
Thymol	5	10.7	13.7
p-Cymene	32.1	22.4	17.8
γ-Terpinene	13.5	7.4	0.9

- The alcohol-containing chemotypes below are commonly referred to as yellow or sweet thymes. These chemotypes do not have the aggressive effects of the red thymes (thymol and carvacrol) and can be used safely on children, sensitive skins and mucous surfaces (Roulier 1990 p. 305).
- *Thymus vulgaris* ct. linalool. The linalool-bearing thyme has a herbaceous smell and (like the thujanol and terpineol thymes) is grown at high altitudes. It contains the alcohol linalool (Fig. 1.6) and the ester linalyl acetate, therefore the essential oil from the linalool thyme is gentle in

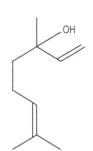

Figure 1.6   Linalool.

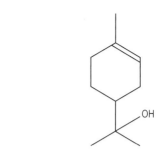

Figure 1.8   α-Terpineol.

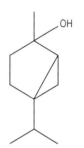

Figure 1.7   Thujanol-4.

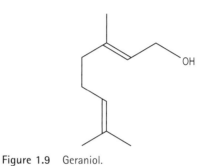

Figure 1.9   Geraniol.

action. This chemotype is antibacterial, fungicidal (e.g. against *Candida albicans*), viricidal, parasiticidal and vermifugal, also neurotonic and uterotonic (Franchomme & Pénoël 1990 p. 403).

■ *Thymus vulgaris* ct. thujanol-4. In contrast to all the other chemotypes of thyme, the thujanol-4 type does not show seasonal variation in the constitution of the essential oil, but is the same all year round with a content of 50% of the alcohol *trans*-thujanol-4 (Fig. 1.7), 15% approximately of terpinen-4-ol and 15% approximately of *cis*-myrcenol-8. It is found only in the wild because it has so far resisted all attempts to cultivate it – cloning has not yet been successful, except on a very small scale. It has a floral smell. The oil is antiinfectious, bactericidal (against *Chlamydia*), and a powerful viricide. It stimulates the immune system (by augmenting IgA) and the circulation. It is described as neurotonic, balancing to the nervous system, hormonelike and antidiabetic (Franchomme & Pénoël 1990 p. 403). According to Roulier (1990 p. 305) this oil is a notable hepatic regenerator and is non-irritant.

■ *Thymus vulgaris* ct. α-terpineol. The oil from this chemotype contains the ester terpenyl acetate (more so in the spring) and the alcohol α-terpineol (Fig. 1.8) (80–90% free and esterified). The smell is slightly peppery.

■ *Thymus vulgaris* ct. geraniol. The geraniol thyme grows at high altitude and the oil contains the ester geranyl acetate and the alcohol geraniol (80–90% in free and esterified forms) (Fig. 1.9); again there is a seasonal variation, the thyme chemotype which produces geraniol in the autumn contains geranyl acetate in the spring and geraniol in the autumn (see Table 1.1). This thyme is very assertive and when grown in a field of mixed thymes it gradually comes to predominate. It has a lemony smell. (It is interesting to note that the creeping wild thyme (*Thymus serpyllum*), which is found everywhere in the hills, also has a somewhat lemony smell because the geraniol chemotype is dominant and is gradually taking over.) The properties are antiviral, antifungal and antibacterial, also uterotonic, neurotonic and cardiotonic (Franchomme & Pénoël 1990 p. 402). Other *Thymus vulgaris* chemotypes also exist. The cineole-bearing plant has 80–90% 1,8-cineole. According to Franchomme and Pénoël (1990

p. 403), the *p*-cymene chemotype is analgesic when applied to the skin, a notable anti-infectious agent and useful for rheumatism and arthritis.

Altitude and light

The lower the altitude at which the thyme plant is grown the more pronounced are the following effects:

- The essential oil becomes more aggressive – more phenolic and antiseptic.
- The colour of the essential oil also changes, from a light straw to a deeper hue.
- The structure of the main component molecule changes from an open chain to a monocyclic chain to an aromatic ring base.

These effects are due in part to the quality of light available to the plant. At high altitudes (above 1000 metres) there is a relatively high amount of free ultraviolet, while at low altitudes there is less ultraviolet and a proportional increase in the more penetrating infrared frequencies. The plant responds to the quality of light falling on it (and to other growing conditions) and produces different chemicals accordingly. Another influencing factor is the latitude of the country of origin. The further north the plant grows, the more phenols are produced – for instance *Thymus vulgaris* grown in Finland produces up to 89% phenol (von Schantz et al 1987).

More changes may be expected in oil-bearing plants in the future because of chlorofluorocarbon damage to the ozone layer. Higher levels of ultraviolet radiation are expected to reach the surface of the earth, and research carried out to test the possible effects of this on plant growth suggests that alpine species will be least affected by increased ultraviolet radiation. These tests involved *Aquilegia canadensis* and *A. caerulea*. The first normally grows at low altitude, and showed less growth during the test, but the second, alpine, plant was not affected in this way: it even grew extra leaves (Gates 1991).

ROSEMARY CHEMOTYPES

Rosemary has three chemotypes, all of which are used in aromatherapy.

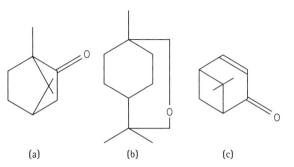

Figure 1.10 (a) Camphor; (b) 1,8-cineole; (c) verbenone.

- *Rosmarinus officinalis* ct. camphor (camphor 30%) (Fig. 1.10a) with the properties: mucolytic, cholagogic, diuretic, circulatory decongestant/stimulant (vein), emmenagogic (non-hormonal), muscle relaxant.
- *Rosmarinus officinalis* ct. cineole (1,8-cineole 40–55%) (Fig. 1.10b) whose properties are anticatarrhal, mucolytic, expectorant, fungicidal (e.g. *Candida albicans*), bactericidal (*Staphylococcus aureus* and *S. alba*).
- *Rosmarinus officinalis* ct. verbenone (Fig. 1.10c) (verbenone 15–40%, α-pinene 15–35%). It is anticatarrhal, expectorant, mucolytic (Roulier 1990 p. 298) and antispasmodic (which Roulier attributes to the cineole and camphor chemotypes – this has been our experience also), cicatrizant and an endocrine system regulator (Franchomme & Pénoël 1990 p. 393).

Roulier (1990) classes the camphor and cineole chemotypes together as having similar effects, as the authors have done in this book, because more often than not rosemary oil contains similar quantities of cineole and camphor.

OTHER CHEMOTYPES

Some further examples of plants with different chemotype forms are:

- *Artemisia dracunculus* [tarragon] ct. estragole, ct. sabinene (Tucker & Maciarello 1987).
- *Ocimum basilicum* [basil] ct. linalool, ct. estragole, ct. eugenol (Sobti et al 1978).
- *Salvia officinalis* [sage] ct. thujone, ct. cineole (there is also a thujone-free chemotype) (Tegel 1984, Tucker & Maciarello 1990).

- *Valeriana officinalis* [valerian] ct. valeranone, ct. valeranal, ct. cryptofuranol (Bos, van Putten & Hendricks 1986).
- *Melissa officinalis* [lemon balm] ct. citral, ct. citronellal (Lawrence 1989).

LAVENDER

Three lavenders are described below:

- *Lavandula angustifolia* contains mainly alcohols and esters. It is a calming oil recommended to induce sleep. However, an overdose has the opposite effect – another pointer to the importance of using these potent oils correctly. It has been recommended for respiratory ailments, asthma, spasmodic cough (whooping cough), influenza, bronchitis, tuberculosis and pneumonia (Valnet 1980) on account of its anti-inflammatory properties.
- *Lavandula latifolia* [spike lavender] (syn. *L. spica*) is a much bigger plant, with larger florets than true lavender. It contains very few esters and is slightly lower in alcohol content also, containing instead about 30% of the oxide 1,8-cineole and about 15% of the ketone camphor. It is an efficient expectorant and is also indicated for severe burns (Franchomme & Pénoël 1990 p. 365) because it is well tolerated on all parts of the skin surface. It is especially useful in chest and throat infections, whether for children or adults (Roulier 1990 p. 276).
- *Lavandula stoechas* contains about 75% ketones, of which almost two-thirds is fenchone. It shares some properties with the previous two, being anticatarrhal, antiinflammatory and cicatrizant. This plant, sometimes known as Spanish lavender, sometimes as French lavender, is believed to be the one used by the Romans in their baths and gave rise to the name lavender but has never been cultivated commercially (Meunier 1985). It is not easily available, which is perhaps fortunate because it is sometimes confused with true lavender (*L. angustifolia*) which is almost free of ketones. The effects of *L. stoechas* can be found in many other, safer oils.

CLONES OF LAVENDER AND LAVANDIN

True lavender grown from seed is properly called *Lavandula angustifolia* Miller (syn. *L. officinalis*, *L. vera*). When grown from seed it is described as 'population'. Many cultivated lavender plants are cloned, i.e. not grown from seed but grown from cuttings selected from the hardiest, healthiest, most colourful and biggest plants with a high yield of good quality oil, the name of probably the most popular clone nearest to true lavender being *L. angustifolia* 'Maillette'.

Unlike population plants, which being grown from seed are much richer in their array of constituents, clones contain only the constituents found in the source plant, and this lack of complexity of composition renders them more liable to disease. For aromatherapy purposes the volatile oil is of a lesser quality although perhaps the oil from cloned plants is of a more consistent quality from year to year.

Lavandins

Lavandin is the natural hybrid between *L. angustifolia* Miller and *L. latifolia* Medicus. The resulting plant has been given many taxonomical classifications, such as *Lavandula x burnatii* 'Briq.', *Lavandula spica-latifolia* 'Albert', *Lavandula x hortensis* 'Hy', *Lavandula x leptostachya* 'Pau', etc. All these are in common use along with other names – Duraffourd (1982 p. 77) calls it *Lavandula fragrans*. This confused state of affairs prompted Tucker (1981) to research the situation and he reported that the correct name for lavandin is *Lavandula x intermedia* 'Emeric' ex 'Loiseleur', which covers all the lavandin cultivars, and *Lavandula x intermedia* is the name used in this book. The 'x' in the names above indicates that the plant is a hybrid or cross-pollinated plant and should not be mistaken for a variety of true lavender. Lavandin plants occur naturally, but cultivators have attempted for many years to find a plant that combines the oil yield of *L. latifolia* with the aromatic quality of *L. angustifolia*. As a result hundreds of lavandins have been created, many with little or no benefit, and there are numerous cultivars currently grown, including *L. x intermedia* 'Abrialis', *L. x intermedia* 'Super', *L. x intermedia* 'Grosso' and *L. x intermedia* 'Reydovan'. Although the Abrialis clone is deteriorating after long use, other cultivars are now producing large quantities of lavandin oil. All cultivated lavandin plants are grown from cuttings – they are all clones.

When lavandin is used, especially in clinical trials, it is imperative to specify the particular clone. The two clones of lavandin most used in aromatherapy are:

- *L.* x *intermedia* 'Reydovan': principally antibacterial, antifungal and antiviral, it is also a nerve tonic and expectorant.
- *L.* x *intermedia* 'Super' (sometimes known under other names): this is calming, sedative and antiinflammatory. It seems to display many of the properties of true lavender (Franchomme & Pénoël 1990 p. 364), and production is on the increase. It was this oil which was used by Buckle (1993) along with true lavender in tests on cardiac patients; the oil from this cultivar of lavandin was found to be more effective than oil of lavender in this instance.

HUMAN FACTORS IN PLANT CHANGE

It is not only nature which brings about changes in the chemicals produced in a plant: farmers have an influence too. The use of chemicals in the form of artificial fertilizers influences some of the plant's secondary metabolites, but has little effect on the essential oils. These are composed in the main of carbon, hydrogen and oxygen, whereas fertilizers are made up of nitrogen, phosphates and potassium. However, as fertilizers cause an increase in plant growth, there may be an overall gain in the yield of essential oil.

Herbicides, pesticides and heavy metals are absorbed by the plant, and the more pesticides are absorbed, the more they appear as residue. A safe level of residue may be regarded as 2 mg (per) 1 kg of dry material. Some safe herbicides are decomposed in the plant, but still add to the residue levels. In Europe, toxic pesticides are prohibited, but unfortunately they are still manufactured and sent to developing countries (Wabner 1993). Although heavy metals do not pass over in the steam distillation process many herbicide and pesticide molecules are similar in size to volatile oil molecules and can end up in essential oils, because although many pesticides contain volatile molecules it is not clear how many of these are taken into a distilled oil. Toxic residues are easily transferred to expressed oils, absolutes and vegetable oils, which makes it necessary to know the source and the manner of growing of such oils before using them therapeutically.

Wabner (1993) concludes that 'aromatherapy is much safer than eating' because 'no clear-cut correlation has been established between pesticide residues in oils and detrimental effects on the human organism' and 'essential oils are used in much smaller quantities and much less frequently than food products'. This article emphasizes the fact that health professionals should purchase their oils for therapeutic use from a trusted supplier, who knows where to procure high quality, pesticide-free, unadulterated essential oils and fixed vegetable oils, especially the latter, as they normally make up 95% or more of any oil prepared for application to the skin.

YIELD OF ESSENTIAL OILS

Many factors affect the yield, in terms of both quantity and quality, of an essential oil. Some are under the control of the farmer, e.g. time of harvest, chemicals used and plant selection, and others are more or less beyond control, e.g. available light, altitude, temperature and rain (although drought can be remedied by use of a watering system).

Essential oils are not spread equally throughout all parts of the plant, and the quantity of essential oil varies throughout the growing season to such a degree that the time of harvesting, even to the time of day, can have a critical effect on the quantity and quality of the essential oil derived (Fig. 1.11).

The farmer may have to face the fact that the time of maximum yield of essential oil may not coincide with the quality required. This is especially so when the oils are intended for therapeutic use, when compromise on quantity against quality cannot be accepted.

PLANT FAMILIES WHICH PRODUCE ESSENTIAL OILS

Plants are divided into families, and it is generally recognized that familial therapeutic characteristics may be ascribed to many of the individual plants in a particular family, e.g. the beneficial influence

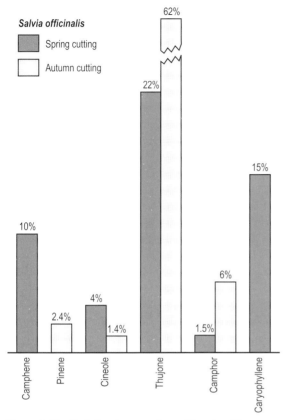

Figure 1.11 Variation in sage oil constituents with season.

on the digestive system of the citrus oils or the warming action of oils from the ginger family. There can also be toxic familial effects, as with the Solanaceae and Apiaceae. Several hundred plant essential oils have been identified worldwide. Many are not commercially available, either because the yield of distilled oil is so small that the cost is prohibitive (as in the case of lime blossom oil) or because there is no commercial demand for them. Between 40 and 60 essential oils are normally used by the professional aromatherapist, and most suppliers offer in the region of 70–80. These oils generally belong to just a few of the many plant families, and the families dealt with below include the majority of plants harvested for the production of essential oils.

In the text below, the common names have been used, since to name each species or variety is not necessary when giving general familial characteristics. The botanical name will be used when talking about a specific essential oil. Where only one oil from a family is used in aromatherapy, no family characteristics will be given, only the therapeutic properties of that individual oil. Where there are several oils in a family, only the family properties will be given. The list is not comprehensive – the main purpose in this book is to make health professionals aware of the principal beneficial essential oils. Specific individual properties, indications and composition of about 100 essential oils can be found in Appendix A.

Reference sources for the properties and effects of the essential oils mentioned below are as follows: Bardeau (1976), Bernadet (1983), Duraffourd (1982), Franchomme & Pénoël (1990), Lautié & Passebecq (1984), Mailhebiau (1989), Roulier (1990). Other references are mentioned individually.

ANGIOSPERMAE

Because they bear seeds, all the plants used to obtain essential oils belong to the Spermatophyta subdivision. The vast majority also belong to the class Angiospermae, or flowering plants.

Anonaceae

This family consists of only one species, *Cananga odorata*, with two varieties, of which ylang ylang is one (*C. odorata* forma *genuina*). Distillation is carried out in several stages, and the resulting oils (superior, extra and grades one, two and three) each have a slightly different make up and aroma and consequently a variation in effect. It is not easy to procure the complete oil, which would be preferable for the holistic aspect of aromatherapy (Price 2000). *C. odorata* is antiinflammatory, antispasmodic, hypotensive, sedative and a tonic to the pancreas.

Apiaceae

Examples include aniseed, caraway, coriander, dill and fennel. In this family the oils are usually extracted from the seeds, which are renowned for their digestive properties. They have been used in digestive and aperitif drinks and consumed for centuries with bread, and as an accompaniment to cheeses such as Munster. Apiaceae therapeutic qualities are aromatic, carminative, stimulating, tonic and warming when grown naturally in dry regions. It should be noted that this family is also known as the hemlocks. If grown in the shade or humid regions a narcotic principle can develop (particularly so for green anise), and many of the oils in this family are neurotoxic because of the presence of particular ketones or phenolic ethers.

Asteraceae

Examples include *Calendula officinalis* (only available macerated in a fixed oil), the chamomiles, tagetes and tarragon. The essential oils from plants in the Asteraceae are taken from the flower heads. In the case of calendula they are macerated in a fixed oil – not distilled, so the fixed oil also contains larger non-volatile plant molecules, including some coloured molecules. Two of the main characteristics of essential oils in this family are their antiinflammatory and antiseptic action on the skin and digestive tract, notably oils from the chamomiles. Many toxic oils come from this family, e.g. the artemisias, which contain a high percentage of ketones or phenolic ethers. *Tagetes glandulifera* also contains a ketone (tagetone) at 50% and should be used with caution.

Burseraceae

Examples include frankincense (olibanum) and myrrh. These two are available as distilled oils and as resinoids, but the distilled oils are required for therapeutic use. The family has cicatrizant properties, indicating their use for scar tissue, ulcers and wounds. They are also expectorant, and useful in catarrhal conditions. *Boswellia carteri* [frankincense] is also indicated in the treatment of depression, immune system deficiency and perhaps cancer (Franchomme & Pénoël 1990 p. 328).

Cupressaceae and Pinaceae

Examples include cypress, juniper (Cupressaceae), pine and cedar (Abietaceae). The chief common characteristics of essential oils derived from plants in these two families of the conifer order are their good general hygienic qualities, particularly in the air and on the skin. Cedar, cypress and juniper also have specific individual properties for urinary tract infections, the circulatory system and

scalp maladies (Rouvière & Meyer 1983 p. 7). Thuja belongs to the Pinaceae, but is not used in aromatherapy because of its toxic high ketone content. These two families are noted for their beneficial effects on the respiratory system.

Geraniaceae

The oil utilized from this small family comes from one or two species belonging to the Pelargonium genus. The essential oil of *Pelargonium graveolens* [geranium] has antiinflammatory, astringent, cicatrizant and haemostatic properties and is anti-diabetic (Valnet 1980 p. 133).

GYMNOSPERMAE

The Gymnospermae display their seeds directly, rather than hiding them within a structure of petals. The important oil-bearing plants of this class belong to the order Coniferae (cone-bearing plants).

Lamiaceae

This is by far the biggest family from which essential oils are gained; examples include basil, clary, hyssop, lavandin, lavender, marjoram, melissa, origanum, patchouli, peppermint, rosemary, sage, savory and thyme. Of all the families in the plant kingdom none offers a greater array of healing aromatic plants than the Lamiaceae. These plants are strongly aromatic owing to the volatile essence stored in special glandular trichomes, which are found principally on the leaves. In general the Lamiaceae produce both relaxing and stimulating essential oils, which bring vigour and energy to the whole body (or sometimes to just one system in particular, e.g. the respiratory system). They have remarkable antiseptic and antispasmodic properties and some are also emmenagogic and sudorific. Oils derived from the Lamiaceae are generally safe, with one or two possible exceptions such as *Salvia officinalis* [sage] and *Hyssopus officinalis* [hyssop], both of which contain ketones (thujone and pinocamphone respectively) and could theoretically be neurotoxic in overdose. Ingestion of large quantities of these two oils can lead to serious disorders, as pointed out by the Centre Anti-poisons de Marseille (Rouvière & Meyer 1983 p. 6).

Many of the plants in this family have been in constant culinary use for thousands of years, not only to add flavour but for their preservative and health-giving properties as well. The use and ingestion of herbs and their essential oils in small doses over such a long period of time proves their fundamental safety.

Lauraceae

Examples include cinnamon and camphor. Members of this family generally have a pleasant aroma, sometimes strong and penetrating, a warm pungency, and are sometimes bitter. All the oils are considered to be uplifting in their effects (Rouvière & Meyer 1983 p. 7). However, the majority of the family are highly toxic (e.g. cassia, laurel and sassafras), and they will not be recommended in this book because similar therapeutic properties can be found in other safer oils. Even when they are not actually dangerous, these oils all need expertise and extra care in use.

Myrtaceae

Examples include cajuput, eucalyptus, niaouli, clove and tea tree. The essential oils from this family are contained in cells in the body of the leaf. They are powerful antiseptics (especially to the respiratory system) as well as being antiviral, astringent, stimulant and tonic.

It is advisable to use them with caution as they can be irritant. This is particularly so of clove and adulterated niaouli. It is worth mentioning that the latter oil is adulterated more often than not and will not have the desired therapeutic effect unless effort has been made to obtain a genuine oil. Rectified *Eucalyptus globulus* [Tasmanian blue gum] is irritant because the natural balance has been destroyed. It can be identified because the rectification process renders it clear and unfortunately very little of the eucalyptus oil harvest escapes this fate.

Oleaceae

Jasminum officinale is a well-loved oil, but a steam-distilled essential oil does not exist and the absolute is subject to the most deplorable adulteration. 'A large number of synthetic materials, some of them chemically related to the jasmones . . . are of great help . . . to reproduce the much

wanted jasmine effect at a much lower cost. . . . Jasmine absolute is frequently adulterated. Its high cost seems to tempt certain suppliers and producers beyond their moral resistance' (Arctander 1960 pp. 310–311). This makes jasmine absolute unsuitable for use on the skin and if it is to be used therapeutically at all (it is sometimes used as a relaxant on account of its aroma) then only the finest quality should be procured. Jasmine extracts are not used by the authors.

Piperaceae

Examples include black pepper and cubeb. *Piper nigrum* is the most used of the two oils and possesses analgesic, anticatarrhal, expectorant, stimulant and tonic properties.

Poaceae

Examples include citronella, lemongrass, palmarosa and vetiver. Most of this family have anti-inflammatory and tonic properties, *Vetivera zizanioides* [vetiver] also being stimulating to the immune system (Franchomme & Pénoël 1990 p. 405). Oils from this family, together with lemon and/or grapefruit oil, are used to make a cheap 'melissa' oil.

Rosaceae

The only essential oil utilized from this family is rose otto, whose aroma is less sweet than the absolute oil obtained by solvent extraction. Strictly speaking, only the distilled oil should be used by health professionals (see *J. officinale* above). Rose otto has astringent, antihaemorrhagic, cicatrizant, hormonal and neurotonic properties.

Rutaceae

Citrus oils are derived from three different sites in the plant. These are:

- **Peel:** bergamot, grapefruit, lemon, mandarin and orange; to obtain citrus peel oils for aromatherapy the rinds are not distilled, but mechanically expressed. They are therefore not strictly essential oils and are more properly described as essences. They contain large molecules which would not come over in distillation, including colour and waxes, and the latter can precipitate if the oils are stored incorrectly or kept for a long time; the waxes do no harm and may be removed by filtration. Citrus essences are especially susceptible to oxidation and the precious active aldehydes may degrade into acids; to help prevent this nitrogen gas is used to displace the air as the oil is decanted. For small bottles, the air can be displaced with tiny glass beads as the level of the oil goes down with use. Expressed oils from the citrus family have a refreshing aroma and are antiseptic, stimulating and tonic, having significant effects on the whole of the digestive tract. This is especially true of bergamot and bitter orange, which are stomach antispasmodics. These two are also sedative to the nervous system.

- **Leaf:** petitgrain essential oils, mainly from the bitter orange, but occasionally from other citrus trees. Petitgrain bigarade from the bitter orange tree (bigarade means 'bitter') is indicated for infected acne, whereas neroli bigarade is indicated for varicose veins and haemorrhoids, and is also a hypotensor.
- **Flower:** neroli, mainly from the bitter orange tree for therapeutic purposes.

Both leaf and flower oils from *Citrus aurantium* [orange] are obtained by distillation and their aroma is sweeter and more floral than that of the peel oils. The best leaf and flower oils are obtained from the bitter orange, *C. aurantium* var. *amara*: both of these oils are effective on the nervous system, relieving irritability and promoting sleep (Mailhebiau 1989 pp. 269–270).

Styracaceae

The only extracts from this family which are of interest to aromatherapists are the resinoids from *Styrax tonkinensis* and *S. benzoin* (both have the common name benzoin). This resinoid is anti-catarrhal and expectorant. It is also cicatrizant, promoting healing on cracked and dry skin. Care should be taken when purchasing this oil: some sources abroad still use benzene as a solvent (forbidden in Europe), and a high proportion of benzene may remain in the final product.

Valerianaceae

Examples include valerian and spikenard. The general family effects are calming and sedative, and they are helpful in the reduction of varicose veins and haemorrhoids. The true oil is very difficult to obtain.

Verbenaceae

Aloysia triphylla (= *Lippia citriodora*) [lemon verbena] is rarely obtainable; like jasmine it is frequently grossly adulterated and *Thymus hiemalis* is often sold in its place as Spanish verbena (Arctander 1960 pp. 648–649).

SUMMARY

Traditionally, plants have been the main source of materials to maintain health and prevent ill health, and it is only comparatively recently that they have been replaced by synthetics. The study of plant structure and function should not be regarded simply as an interesting but inessential requirement for aromatherapy. The more knowledgeable therapists are about the exact botanical derivation of the oils used, the more effective they can be in practice.

References

Arctander S 1960 Perfume and flavour materials of natural origin. Published by the author, Elizabeth, New Jersey

Bardeau F 1976 La médecine aromatique. Laffont, Paris

Belaiche P 1979 Traité de phytothérapie et d'aromathérapie, vol 1. Maloine, Paris, p. 93

Bernadet M 1983 La phyto-aromathérapie pratique. Dangles, St-Jean-de-Braye

Bos R, van Putten F M S, Hendriks H 1986 Variations in the essential oil content and composition in individual plants obtained after breeding experiments with a *Valeriana officinalis* strain. In: Brunke E J (ed) Progress in essential oil research. W de Gruyter, Hamburg, pp. 223–230

Buckle J 1993 Does it matter which lavender essential oil is used? Nursing Times 89(20): 32–35

Carlton R R 1990 An investigation into the rapidly induced responses of *Myrica gale* to insect herbivory. Unpublished PhD Thesis, University of Strathclyde

Carlton R R, Gray A I, Waterman P G 1992 The

antifungal activity of the leaf gland oil of sweet gale (*Myrica gale*). Chemecology 3: 55–59

Craker L E 1990 Herbs and volatile oils. Herb, Spice and Medicinal Plant Digest 8(4): 1–5

Deans S G, Waterman P G 1993 Biological activity of volatile oils. In: Hay R K M, Waterman P G (eds) Volatile oil crops. Longman, Harlow, pp. 100–101

Duraffourd P 1982 En forme tous les jours. La Vie Claire, Périgny

Franchomme P, Pénoël D 1990 L'aromathérapie exactement. Jollois, Limoges

Gates P 1991 Gardening in tomorrow's world. Gardener's World July: 4

Harborne J B 1988 Introduction to ecological biochemistry. Academic Press, London

Hill J 1808 The family herbal. Brightly & Kinnersley

Lamy J 1985 De la culture à la distilleries. Quelques facteurs influant sur la composition des huiles essentielles. Chambre d'Agriculture de la Drôme, Valence

Lamy J 1988 Présentation de 30 huiles essentielles typées produites dans la Drôme. Congress des Parfumeurs Allemandes, pp. 23–25

Lautié R, Passebecq A 1984 Aromatherapy. Thorsons, Wellingborough

Lawrence B M 1989 Progress in essential oils. Perfumer and Flavorist 14(3): 71

Mailhebiau P 1989 La nouvelle aromathérapie. Vie Nouvelle, Toulouse

Meunier C 1985 Lavandes et lavandins. Edisud, Aix-en-Provence

Price S 2000 The aromatherapy workbook. Thorsons, London, pp. 119–120

Roulier G 1990 Les huiles essentielles pour votre santé. Dangles, St-Jean-de-Braye

Rouvière A, Meyer M C 1983 La santé par les huiles essentielles. M A Editions, Paris

Sobti S N, Pushpangadan P, Thapa R K, Aggarwal S G, Vashist V N, Atal C K 1978 Chemical and genetic investigations in essential oils of some *Ocimum* species, their F1 hybrids and synthesised allopolyploids. Lloydia 41: 50–55

Svoboda K 2003 Secrets of plant life. In Essence, Autumn 2(2): 6–11

Tegel C 1984 Morphologische und chemische Variabilität sowie Anbau und Verwendung von *Salvia* sp (Salbei). Unpublished MSc Thesis, Technical University of Munich

Tucker A O 1981 The correct name of lavandin and its cultivars (Labiatae). Baileya 21: 131–133

Tucker A O, Maciarello M J 1987 Plant identification. In: Simon J E, Grant L (eds) Proceedings of the first national herb growing and marketing conference. Purdue University Press, West Lafayette, pp. 341–372

Tucker A O, Maciarello M J 1990 Essential oils of cultivars of Dalmatian sage (*Salvia officinalis* L). Journal of Essential Oil Research 2: 139–144

Valnet J 1980 The practice of aromatherapy. Daniel, Saffron Walden

Verlet N 1993 Commercial aspects. In: Hay R K M, Waterman P G (eds) Volatile oil crops. Longman, Harlow, Ch. 8, p. 144

von Schantz M, Holm Y, Hiltunen R, Galambosi B 1987 Arznei- und Gewürzpflanzenversuche zum Anbau in Finnland. Deutsche Apotheke Zeitung 127: 2543–2548

Wabner D 1993 Purity and pesticides. International Journal of Aromatherapy 5(2): 27–29

Waterman P G 1993 The chemistry of volatile oils. In: Hay R K M, Waterman P G (eds) Volatile oil crops; their biology, biochemistry and production. Longman Scientific, Harlow

Bibliography

Bailey LH 1963 How plants get their names. Dover, New York

Foster S 1979 Latin binomials: learning to live with the system. Well-Being 48 (Dec): 41–42

Foster S (ed) 1992 Herbs of commerce. American Herbal Products Association, Austin

Foster S 1993 Herbal renaissance. Gibbs Smith, Salt Lake City

International Code of Botanical Nomenclature

Jeffrey C 1977 Biological nomenclature. Crane Russack, New York

Stern WT 1983 Botanical Latin. David & Charles, Newton Abbot

Tippo O, Stern WL 1977 Humanistic botany. Norton, New York

Chapter 2

Chemistry of essential oils

Len Price

INTRODUCTION

For the safe practice of aromatherapy it is essential to have at least a basic understanding of the chemistry of the essential oils before being able to use them in a meaningful, caring and effective way – not at random, or indiscriminately. Such understanding makes it evident that certain chemicals may have certain effects – 'may' because there is no direct link between even the major components of an essential oil and the effects of the complete oil. These complex relationships are little understood at present because hundreds of different chemical compounds are involved, and many of them are unknown. Suffice it to say that knowledge of the basic composition of each oil contributes to the overall background knowledge of aromatherapy, thus promoting confidence and aiding selection of the oils to be used, until such time as more is discovered about the interaction of the plant chemicals within the human body.

   The list of the physiological and pharmacological properties of aromatic molecules encompasses almost all the organs and all the functions of the organism, from skin conditions to psychological disturbances. Chemists have identified more than 3000 different molecules found in essential oils, and new ones are continually being discovered. Fortunately, these molecules are gathered in main groups, with a general relationship between the chemical function and the pharmacological activities. Although we use whole essential oils and not isolated molecules, it is necessary to undertake the study not only of the classes of molecules but also of a few important individual molecules and possible actions.

ESSENTIAL OIL COMPONENTS

It is not the intention to give a lesson in organic chemistry in this book, but a brief explanation of the building blocks which go to make up essential oils will be helpful. Carbon, hydrogen, oxygen are essential to life itself, and these three atoms are contained in every essential oil. They combine naturally in countless numbers of ways to make up terpenic and terpenoid compounds such as hydrocarbons, alcohols, aldehydes, ketones, acids, phenols, esters, coumarins and furanocoumarins. The name terpene here conveys the meaning of a compound made up entirely of carbon and hydrogen atoms and the name terpenoid means a molecule which includes the oxygen atom in addition.

TERPENE COMPOUNDS

All terpenes are hydrocarbons consisting only of carbon and hydrogen atoms and they are almost always easily recognizable from their name: all end in -ene. Terpenes are hydrocarbons arranged in a chain, which can be either straight, perhaps with branches, or cyclic. Within the plant, the starting point for the terpenes is acetyl coenzyme A (acetyl coA) from which is formed six-carbon mevalonic acid. This is then modified to the five-carbon unit commonly known as the isoprene unit (Fig. 2.1), which occurs in two unsaturated forms: IPP (isopentenyl pyrophosphate) (Fig. 2.1a) and DMAPP (dimethylallyl pyrophosphate) (Fig. 2.1b). This isoprene unit comprised of five carbon atoms does not exist on its own but is the basic building block for terpenes and is shown diagrammatically as a saturated chain (Fig. 2.1c) for the sake of simplicity, as used later in the book, but it must be borne in mind that it is in fact unsaturated.

Monoterpenes

Two isoprene units joined together head to tail form the basis of all monoterpenes (therefore monoterpene hydrocarbons have 10 carbon atoms

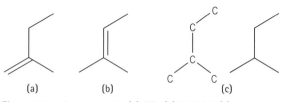

Figure 2.1   Isoprene unit. (a) IPP; (b) DMAPP; (c) isoprene carbon skeleton.

arranged in a chain) (Fig. 2.2a). Sometimes a chain can, as it were, loop round on itself (Fig. 2.2b) and give the appearance of a ring, although it is still a 10-carbon chain. When this looping occurs, the terpene is said to be monocyclic, because one circle has been created, and therefore the complete description is monocyclic monoterpene. More than one circle can arise in a chain, so that it is possible to have bicyclic and tricyclic monoterpenes. If they do not form a circle at all (i.e. if they form a straight chain) they are said to be acyclic (as in Fig. 2.2a). Not enough is yet understood about the pharmacological effects of these compounds in essential oils in order to know how these variations in structure may modify the effect. Further complexity arises when double bonds are added (by oxidation) or subtracted (by reduction).

Monoterpenes constitute the most commonly occurring kind of terpene in plant volatile oils and are formed, as stated above, from two isoprene units and so contain 10 carbon atoms, sesquiterpenes are formed from three isoprene units and have 15 carbon atoms, and diterpenes are made up of four isoprene units with 20 carbon atoms.

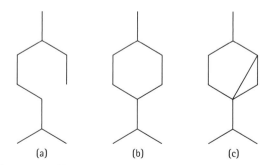

Figure 2.2   Monoterpenes: two isoprene units join to form a monoterpene. (a) An acyclic monoterpene; (b) a monocyclic monoterpene; (c) a bicyclic monoterpene (thujane).

Molecules larger than this do not occur in essential oils because the molecular weight exceeds the limit imposed by the distillation process.

Generally speaking, terpenes are the least active, albeit the most numerous, of all components which occur to a lesser or greater (usually) degree in all in essential oils and they tend to be regarded by some as being merely inert fillers. While it is true that the effects of terpenes on the human system are not very great, that is not to say that specific molecules do not have their uses, and a few examples are given below.

Effects of monoterpenes

They are all slightly antiseptic, bactericidal and they may also be analgesic, expectorant and stimulating (Franchomme & Pénoël 2001 pp. 239–244, Roulier 1990 p. 51) and they may also play an important part in the quenching effect mentioned earlier, thus making fragrance quality oils which have had the terpenes partially or totally removed (deterpenated oils) unsuitable for aromatherapeutic purposes.

The limonene found in citrus oils quenches the skin irritant properties of the citrals, as can readily be seen by the fact that deterpenized lemon oil is four or five times as irritant to the skin as whole lemon oil; others are recently thought to be possible antitumour agents, some stimulate the circulation, etc. and it is undeniable that pine oils with their rich content of terpenes are good as air antiseptics, etc.; moreover pine oils, rich in terpenes, appear to have a hormonelike effect on the suprarenal glands. The aromatic monoterpene *p*-cymene occurs in numerous essential oils and is known to be analgesic on the skin. The essential oil of *Cupressus sempervirens*, which may be up to 70% monoterpenes, is an antiinflammatory agent by immunomodulating action (Franchomme & Pénoël 2001 p. 243).

Sesquiterpenes

Three isoprene units provide the basic structure for the larger molecules known as sesquiterpenes (sesquiterpene hydrocarbons have 15 carbon atoms) (Fig. 2.3).

As well as the antiseptic and bactericidal properties mentioned above, the sesquiterpenes as a class are said to be antiinflammatory, calming

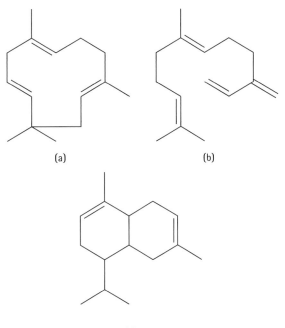

Figure 2.3   Sesquiterpenes: three isoprene units join to form a sesquiterpene. (a) An acyclic sesquiterpene (α-humulene); (b) a monocyclic sesquiterpene (*trans*-β-farnesene); (c) a bicyclic sesquiterpene (α-cadinene).

and slight hypotensors; some are analgesic (e.g. germacrene) and/or spasmolytic.

Diterpenes

Four isoprene units joined together are called diterpenes (diterpenic hydrocarbons have 20 carbon atoms) (Fig. 2.4), and are not often met with in steam-distilled oils because they are

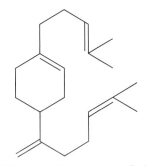

Figure 2.4   Diterpenes: four isoprene units join to form a diterpene. This figure shows a monocyclic diterpene (α-camphorene).

almost too heavy to come over in the distillation process – only a very few manage it.

Diterpenes are believed to have the further properties of being expectorant and purgative and some are antifungal and antiviral.

Terpenes have a reputation for causing skin irritation (perhaps this is unjust, as so many oils are adulterated with turpentine, polyethylene glycol, white spirit, isolated terpenes, etc., and not everyone is as careful as they should be when procuring their essential oils), but if irritation does occur then application of a fixed oil brings swift relief.

Terpenoids

When hydrocarbons, molecules consisting of only carbon and hydrogen, have oxygen added they are described as being terpenoid. With the addition of various oxygen-containing active groups to a compound, numerous alcohols, ketones, aldehydes and esters are formed and the effects produced in aromatherapy use are much more evident.

Nomenclature

The naming of molecules for a precise definition can be difficult and here the terms used above may be used for a full description, i.e. the type of chain, kind of terpene or the term 'aromatic' (ring-based) should be included when describing a particular chemical constituent of an essential oil. Here are some examples:

- myrcene – an acyclic monoterpene
- limonene – a monocyclic monoterpene
- cadinene – a bicyclic sesquiterpene
- patchoulol – a tricyclic sesquiterpenic alcohol
- citronellal – an acyclic monoterpenic aldehyde
- cinnamic aldehyde – an aromatic aldehyde
- geranic acid – an acyclic monoterpenic acid
- cinnamic acid – an aromatic acid.

THERAPEUTIC EFFECTS

In the chemical 'families' discussed below, some of the general therapeutic properties attributed to each of the families are based on a theory (set out in detail in Franchomme & Pénoël 2001 pp. 107–131) which associates certain properties

with the esters, alcohols, etc., taking into account the electronegative/positive nature of the molecules coupled with their polar/apolar properties. Although this information is a useful general guide to the probable properties of the chemical families discussed, the information given does not hold true for each and every compound (e.g. alcohols are given the familial characteristic of being stimulating, but the alcohol linalool shows as a sedative – see Table 4.11 – when tested on mice, although the results obtained in animal testing do not necessarily extrapolate directly to humans). In any case, aromatherapists do not use isolated compounds, but whole essential oils, and while it is both important and interesting to study the effects of single compounds it is worth repeating the statement made above that there is not necessarily any simple direct relationship between the therapeutic effect of any one constituent and that of the whole essential oil.

ALCOHOLS

When a hydroxyl group (or hydroxyl radical as it is sometimes called), consisting of one oxygen atom and one hydrogen atom (–OH) joins on to one of the carbons in a chain by displacing one of the hydrogen molecules, an alcohol (Figs 2.5, 2.6, 2.7) is formed: a monoterpenic alcohol, sesquiterpenic alcohol or diterpenic alcohol, depending on whether the chain to which it attaches itself has two, three or four isoprene units. The name of the alcohol so formed always ends in -ol, e.g. geraniol. There are alternative names which are in current use for these alcohols: monoterpenic alcohol is also called monoterpenol, sesquiterpenic alcohol is known also as sesquiterpenol and diterpenic alcohol as diterpenol and also diol.

Effects of alcohols

Alcohols as a group are antiinfectious, strongly bactericidal, antiviral while they are stimulating to the immune system; they are generally non-toxic in use and do not cause skin irritation (Roulier 1990 p. 53). The thujanol-4 molecule is a liver stimulant, as is menthol. Some of the heavier alcohols appear to have a balancing effect on the hormonal system, e.g. the diterpenic alcohol sclareol in *Salvia sclarea* [clary], as does the sesquiterpenic alcohol viridiflorol in *Melaleuca viridiflora*

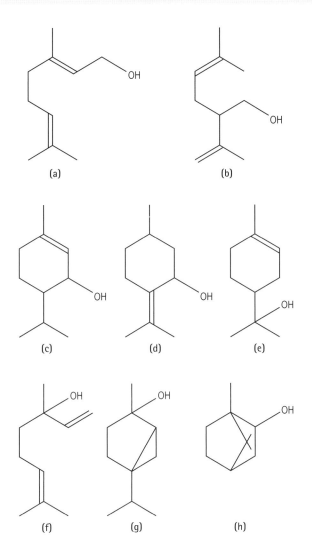

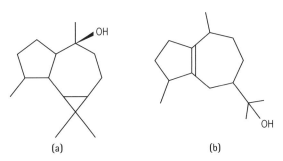

Figure 2.6   Alcohols – sesquiterpenols (15 C). (a) A bicyclic sesquiterpenol (viridiflorol); (b) a bicyclic sesquiterpenol (guaiol).

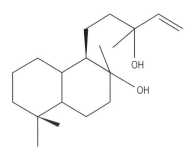

Figure 2.7   Alcohols – diols (20 C). This figure shows a bicyclic diol (sclareol).

Figure 2.5   Alcohols – monoterpenols (10 C). (a) An acyclic monoterpenol (geraniol); (b) an acyclic monoterpenol (lavandulol); (c) a monocyclic monoterpenol (piperitol); (d) a monocyclic monoterpenol (pulegol); (e) a monocyclic monoterpenol (α-terpineol); (f) an acyclic monoterpenol (linalool); (g) a bicyclic monoterpenol (thujanol-4); (h) a bicyclic monoterpenol (borneol).

[niaouli]: borneol is given as a cholagogue and analgesic, cedrol is phlebotonic and spathulenol is fungicidal – as is sclareol (Beckstrom-Sternberg & Duke 1996 pp. 384, 416, Franchomme & Pénoël 2001 pp. 133, 135).

The aromatic ring

The second building block for the volatile molecules found in distilled plant oils occurs when six carbon atoms join together in the form of a ring, which is not formed from isoprene units, giving a completely different structure from that of the terpenes. Energy transference across the aromatic ring is much greater (due to conjugation) than in the terpenes making them much more reactive, thus the effects of aromatic compounds on the body can be quite remarkable, making care in use essential. Note that the term 'ring' is reserved for this six-carbon unit C_6H_6 which has three names in common use:

1. Aromatic ring, because many of the substances based on it are pleasant smelling.
2. Benzene ring, because the basic ring of six carbon atoms and six hydrogen atoms is known as benzene.
3. Phenyl ring, because phenols are formed from this base.

As seen above, when the hydroxyl group –OH is attached to a chain it is an alcohol (Fig. 2.8a); but when the same group is attached to a benzene ring (see below) it is a phenol (Fig. 2.8b). Thus both

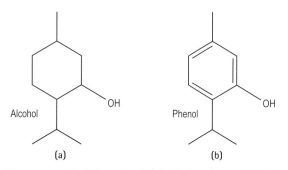

Figure 2.8   Alcohol vs phenol. (a) A hydroxyl group (–OH) attached to a chain gives an alcohol (menthol); (b) a hydroxyl group (–OH) attached to a benzene ring gives a phenol (thymol).

aliphatic and aromatic aldehydes, ketones and organic acids (involving both chain and ring building blocks) are to be found occurring naturally in essential oils.

PHENOLS – THE OTHER ALCOHOLS

When the hydroxyl group attaches itself to a carbon in an aromatic (also phenyl also benzene) ring, the resulting molecule is known as a phenol (Fig. 2.9), which may also be termed an aromatic alcohol, and has strong effects. Phenols also have names which end in 'ol', e.g. carvacrol; to discriminate between the two classes it is necessary to learn the names of the most important members in each group.

Phenols, like alcohols, are antiseptic and bactericidal and because they stimulate both the nervous system (making them effective against depressive illness) and the immune system, they

activate the body's own healing process. However, because the –OH is attached to a ring rather than to a chain molecule, aromatic phenols, unlike the aliphatic alcohols, can be toxic to the liver and irritant to the skin if used in substantial amounts or for too long a time (Roulier 1990 pp. 51–52). 'Some oils – for example, thyme and origanum – owe their value in the pharmaceutical field almost entirely to the antiseptic and germicidal properties of their phenolic content' (Guenther 1949). Eugenol is an effective antispasmodic (Franchomme & Pénoël 2001 p. 134).

METHYL ETHERS

These generally are more complicated structures than the phenols: precursors (phenylalanine, tyrosine, cinnamic acid) of these molecules act to form compounds that include a six-carbon benzene ring attached to a short (three-carbon) chain. Even though this type of molecule occurs much less frequently in essential oils than do terpenes, they can have a great impact on the aroma, flavour and therapeutic effect. They have various forms of name, as seen in the following examples: safrole, methyl chavicol, eugenol methyl ether and asarone (which may cause confusion owing to the similarity to the ketone name ending); other examples are estragole in tarragon oil, cinnamaldehyde in cinnamon bark oil, anethole (Fig. 2.10a) in aniseed oil and apiole (Fig. 2.10b) in fennel seed oil.

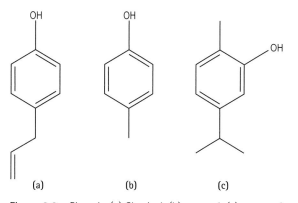

Figure 2.9   Phenols. (a) Chavicol; (b) p-cresol; (c) carvacrol.

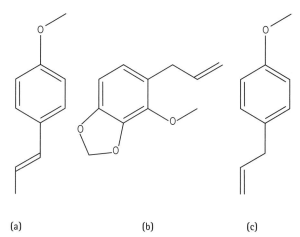

Figure 2.10   Methyl ethers. (a) trans-Anethole; (b) apiole; (c) chavicol methyl ether.

Some occur in two forms, as in *trans*-anethole and *cis*-anethole, the latter being the more toxic of the two (Witty 1993 personal communication).

Effects

These molecules have powerful effects on the body and essential oils containing them should always be used with great care. Several of them are amphetamine-like and may be neurotoxic if present in large amounts in an essential oil, thus such oils should be used only in the short term and in low concentration. Whereas the phenols are aggressive to the skin and mucous surfaces, in the phenyl methyl ethers it seems that the methylation of the phenol function negates this aggressive aspect and these compounds are well-tolerated on the skin. They are, as a class, strong antispasmodics: anethole (*para*-anol methyl ether) is oestrogen-like (see also Hormone-like, Ch. 4) and β-asarone (asarol trimethyl ether) is sedative; safrole relieves pain and myristicin has anaesthetic and hallucinogenic properties (Beckstrom-Sternberg & Duke 1996 p. 406).

Ethers rarely, if ever, occur alone in essential oils but their relationship to phenyl methyl ethers is close, and their antidepressant, antispasmodic and sedative properties echo those of the phenolic ethers, as do those of esters (see below) (Roulier 1990 p. 53).

ALDEHYDES

An aldehyde is formed when the carbonyl radical (=O) together with a hydrogen atom (–H) attaches itself to one of the carbon atoms in the basic structure, forming a –CHO group (Fig. 2.11). It is easy to recognize an aldehyde from its name, as either aldehydes end in -al, e.g. citral, or the name aldehyde is stated, as in cinnamic aldehyde (may be shortened to cinnamal). Benzaldehyde is one of the three constituents of vitamin B_{17}. They usually have powerful aromas, making them important to the perfumer, and are very reactive, which means that they must be used with care in aromatherapy.

Effects

The beneficial properties of aldehydes are that they are antiviral, antiinflammatory, calming to the nervous system, hypotensors, vasodilators,

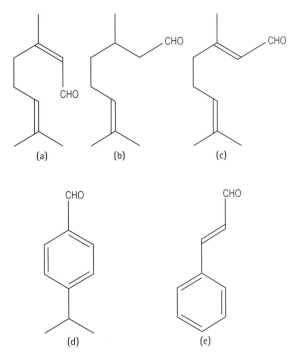

Figure 2.11 Aldehydes. (a) An acyclic monoterpenal (neral); (b) an acyclic monoterpenal (citronellal); (c) an acyclic monoterpenal (geranial); (d) an aromatic aldehyde (cuminal); (e) an aromatic aldehyde (cinnamal).

air antiseptics and antipyretic; their negative properties – when used incorrectly or ill advisedly – include skin irritation and skin sensitivity (Franchomme & Pénoël 2001 pp. 231–236, Roulier 1990 p. 53). Aldehydes, with their lemon-like aroma, are reputed to calm the tension following nicotine withdrawal in those who are giving up smoking. Cinnamaldehyde is a general tonic and stimulates peristalsis and uterine contractions; cuminal, on the other hand, is sedative and calming.

KETONES

When the carbonyl group (=O) attaches itself (without a hydrogen atom this time) to a carbon on a chain structure, an aliphatic ketone (Fig. 2.12) is formed; aromatic ketones hardly ever occur in essential oils. The ketone names normally end in -one, but look out for false friends like asarone, mentioned above, which is a phenolic ether and not a ketone.

As with all molecules, the ketone molecules are not flat, two-dimensional structures but occupy

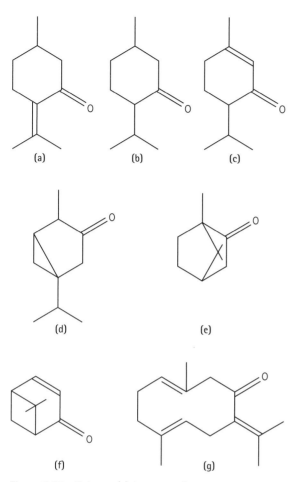

Figure 2.12 Ketones. (a) A monocyclic monoterpenone (pulegone); (b) a monocyclic monoterpenone (menthone); (c) a monocyclic monoterpenone (piperitone); (d) a bicyclic monoterpenone (thujone); (e) a bicyclic monoterpenone (camphor); (f) a bicyclic monoterpenone (verbenone); (g) a monocyclic sesquiterpenone (germacrone).

space in three dimensions. This means that changes in molecular spatial shape can take place. Hence differently shaped molecules made up of the same atoms do occur and their seemingly insignificant differences can alter the effect that these molecules have on the body. For example, (–)-carvone and (+)-carvone are two examples, one being less toxic than the other. Opdyke (1973, 1978) suggests that α-thujone and β-thujone may have differing effects on the body, but research along these lines is yet to be carried out.

Effects

Generally speaking, ketones are cicatrizant, lipolytic, mucolytic and sedative; some are also analgesic, anticoagulant, antiinflammatory, digestive, expectorant or stimulant. They need to be used with care, particularly by pregnant women (Franchomme & Pénoël 2001 p. 212, Roulier 1990 p. 53).

ORGANIC ACIDS AND ESTERS

Unlike the above there is no active radical group whose presence creates an ester. This type of compound is formed by the joining together of an organic acid (Fig. 2.13) with an alcohol, the formula being:

organic acid + alcohol = ester + water

It has been suggested that this chemical reaction may be capable, *in vivo*, of flowing the other way too, which could result in interchanges from acids to esters and back again. Perhaps this is why esters (Fig. 2.14) are useful for normalizing

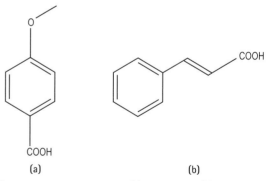

Figure 2.13 Organic acids. (a) Anisic acid; (b) cinnamic acid.

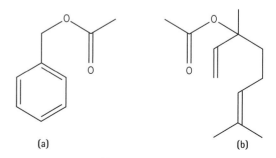

Figure 2.14 Esters. (a) Benzyl acetate; (b) linalyl acetate.

some emotional and bodily conditions which are out of balance. To recognize an ester from its name is not difficult: it usually ends with -ate, e.g. linalyl acetate, or else the word ester is included.

Effects

Esters generally are believed to be antifungal, antiinflammatory, antispasmodic, cicatrizant and both calming and tonic (adaptogenic), especially to the nervous system (Buchbauer, Jirovetz & Jäger 1992, Buchbauer et al 1993) (see Ch. 4). Like alcohols, they are gentle in action, and being free from toxicity they are 'user friendly'. The exception is methyl salicylate, which comprises over 90% of wintergreen and birch oils (neither of which is used in the present British style of aromatherapy).

OXIDES

The only oxide (Fig. 2.15) known well in aromatherapy is 1,8-cineole, which is otherwise known as eucalyptol; it may also be regarded as a bicyclic ether (Buchbauer 1993).

Effects

Eucalyptol is stimulant to mucous glands and is expectorant and mucolytic, its unwanted effect being skin irritation, especially on young children. Another oxide, ascaridole, is an anthelmintic and linalyloxide and piperitonoxide have antiviral properties ascribed to them.

LACTONES

Important members of this family occurring in essences are the coumarins and their derivatives (Fig. 2.16). They occur only in the expressed oils and some absolutes, e.g. jasmine, because the molecular weight is too great to allow distillation. They are sometimes called circular esters because the ester group is incorporated in the structure.

Effects

Lactones are reputed to be mucolytic, expectorant and temperature reducing, their negative aspects being skin sensitization and phototoxicity (Franchomme & Pénoël 2001 p. 222). Lactones are neurotoxic when ingested and some oils containing lactones are toxic on the skin, but the risk is slight as there is usually a very low content of lactones in an essential oil.

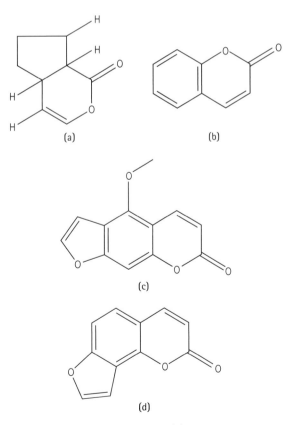

Figure 2.16   Lactones, coumarins. (a) Nepetalactone; (b) coumarin; (c) bergapten; (d) angelicin.

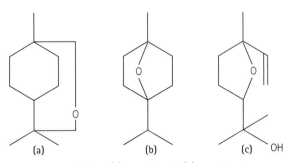

Figure 2.15   Oxides. (a) 1,8-cineole; (b) 1,4-cineole; (c) linalool oxide.

COUMARINS

Coumarins, which number probably almost a thousand, are present only in very low concentration in essential oils, but their presence has an undoubted effect.

Effects

Coumarins are anticoagulant hypotensors; they are uplifting and yet at the same time sedative (Buchbauer, Jirovetz & Jäger 1992, Franchomme & Pénoël 2001 p. 225). Lavender is known for its sedative properties and this is partly due to the synergistic presence of coumarins, albeit very low; unfortunately the coumarins appear only after longer distillation than is usually commercially viable, so unless the lavender has been distilled especially for aromatherapy then the full sedative potential is not realized.

Furanocoumarins are known mainly for their phototoxicity, and oils containing these should not be used immediately prior to sunbathing (or sunbeds) owing to their ability to increase the sensitivity of the skin to the sun, the main culprits in aromatherapy being psoralen and bergapten, found in the citrus essences. Some are antiviral and antifungal.

There are too many individual essential oil components (several thousand) to name here, but knowledge of the different chemical families will aid recognition of new constituents if they are encountered in a listing from a gas chromatograph report (see below).

STEREOCHEMISTRY

The word 'stereo' comes from the Greek meaning solid, and here refers to the spatial arrangement of atoms within a molecule. The same kinds and number of atoms in different molecules can occupy different relative positions, giving the molecules variations in shape which has an influence – perhaps slight, perhaps significant – on the chemical activity.

ISOMERS

In essential oils many compounds share the same molecular formula and thus are made up of precisely the same number and kind of atoms, but occupy different spatial arrangements: these are known as isomers. For example, many monoterpene hydrocarbons are made up of 10 carbon atoms and 16 hydrogen atoms, having the same molecular formula $C_{10}H_{16}$ but many different structures are made from these same atoms, each having differing properties. The difference between these structural isomers may lead to slight or great variations in characteristics.

Optical isomers

Some molecules are able to rotate plane-polarized light and are classed as either dextrorotatory (+) or laevorotatory (–), indicating their capability to rotate light in a particular direction. Molecules that divert the light to the right are known as dextrorotatory, written as (+)-, and molecules that turn the light to the left are known as laevorotatory, written as (–)-.

Carvone, a ketone, is one such molecule and exists in two forms, (–)-carvone (Fig. 2.17a) being present in spearmint, where it has the aroma of spearmint, and (+)-carvone (Fig. 2.17b) in caraway, where it has the aroma of caraway, showing that quite a small change in the spatial arrangement of atoms within the molecules can have a significant effect on the perceived aroma; Craker (1990) says that the stereochemical form of the molecule will determine the odour and flavour attributes of the oil.

Menthol, $C_{10}H_{20}O$, is also optically active but only the (–) form is found in nature, particularly in peppermint oils.

These optical isomers, sometimes called 'mirror molecules' are mirror images of each other, rather

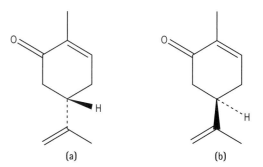

Figure 2.17 Isomers – molecules in the mirror.
(a) (–)-carvone; (b) (+)-carvone.

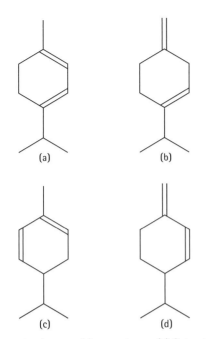

Figure 2.18   Isomers. (a) α-terpinene; (b) β-terpinene; (c) α-phellandrene; (d) β-phellandrene.

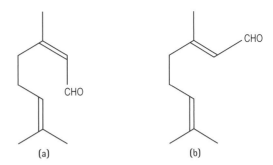

Figure 2.19   Geometric isomers. (a) *cis*-citral (neral); (b) *trans*-citral (geranial).

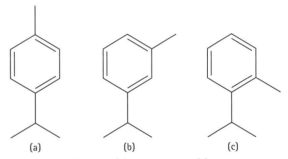

Figure 2.20   Isomers. (a) *para*-cymene; (b) *meta*-cymene; (c) *ortho*-cymene.

like a pair of hands which appear to be the same but in fact are different (gloves cannot be exchanged) and this is known as chirality (from the Greek word for hand). The majority of both mono- and sesquiterpenic compounds in any given essential oil are to be found in one stereochemical form. A mixture of dextrorotatory and laevorotatory forms of a molecule is termed racemic.

The terpene pinene occurs in two slightly different forms (distinguished nominally by the Greek letters α and β), with only a change in the position of the double bond (Fig. 2.18).

Geometric isomers

The aldehydes geranial and neral are very similar in structure and are said to be geometric isomers (Fig. 2.19). The prefixes *cis*- and *trans*- are used to describe the positioning of groups on either side of a double bond. Neral is a *cis*- isomer and geranial the *trans*- isomer and, because they often occur together and it is difficult to discriminate between the two during analysis, the mixture of these two isomers is called citral.

The aromatic terpene cymene is an example of a molecule that has three isomers, *para*-, *meta*- and *ortho*- respectively, denoting the positions of side groups attached to the benzene ring (Fig. 2.20).

Functional isomers

Both molecules shown here have the same molecular formula, C_2H_6O, but because of their arrangement have different functional groups. One is an ether and the other is an alcohol and so they have quite different characteristics despite being composed of the same atoms.

$$CH_3\text{-}O\text{-}CH_3 \qquad CH_3\text{-}CH_2OH$$
Ether   Alcohol

Since the different physical structures of isomers can give widely different physical properties such as boiling point, relative density, etc., then it is probable that the structural shape of the molecules also has an influence on therapeutic properties, as was the case with the drug thalidomide (see also Hormonal, Ch. 4).

CHEMICAL VARIABILITY

It is important to recognize that, because of the variability of both climate and soil, no natural chemical will be present in any essential oil in exactly the same proportion at each distillation. Further variations are produced according to the time the plant is harvested. For instance, sage plants cut early in the season contain a much lower percentage of ketones than do those harvested late (Lamy 1985). Constituents can vary sometimes from 20–70% in a genuine oil and suppliers must have obtained an oil from a specific plant grown in the right place and harvested at the right time to ensure the correct proportion of whatever component is required. If this is not the case then the oils may have been adulterated before they reach the buyer, unless bought from source. Even a gas–liquid chromatograph carried out by an independent authority cannot always be relied upon completely. More than one test is needed when checking the purity of an oil, and not all distributors are able to afford such an expensive procedure as this for each batch. A certificate showing that an oil is of a required standard is no guarantee unless it refers specifically to the batch currently being traded.

TESTING OILS FOR QUALITY

GAS CHROMATOGRAPHY (GC)

This is sometimes called gas–liquid chromatography (GLC). The gas chromatograph consists of a coiled, temperature-controlled, tubular column into which a minute amount (say 1 micro litre) of essential oil is injected and volatilized. It then passes through the column, which may be 10 to 50 m long and contains a liquid phase and a gas phase. At the other end is a flame ionization detector and a pen recorder, which plots a trace (Fig. 2.21) of each component of the essential oil as it exits the column. The smaller, lighter molecules have the shortest retention time and they appear after the shortest time, and so are recorded first on the trace. These are followed by successively larger molecules, the heaviest having the longest retention time and being recorded last. From the resulting trace the percentage of each constituent

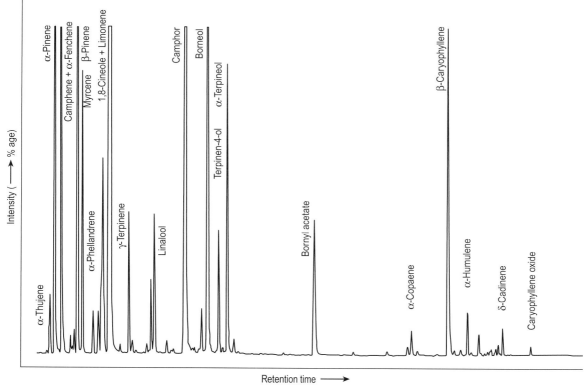

Figure 2.21   Gas chromatograph trace (rosemary).

present in the oil being tested can be calculated. As the reading will always differ for each batch of any one essential oil, a trace for each named essential oil is retained as a standard, to which all future batches are compared. It can be seen that this test is comparative rather than absolute, and although the GC does not directly identify the constituents present, this can be done by comparing the results obtained with known standards.

MASS SPECTROMETRY

The GC is a valuable test, but is not the only one. At the forefront of modern technology is the gas chromatography–mass spectrometry (GC–MS), a more expensive process that is capable of analysing and identifying the individual components of essential oils. The mass spectrometer is interfaced to the gas chromatograph apparatus described above and as the molecules emerge from the GC column they are bombarded with high energy electrons, which fragment them. There is a characteristic fragmentation pattern for each molecule, and for identification it is compared by computer with patterns held in a library. Using this technique it is possible to identify each component in a complex mixture such as an essential oil.

OPTICAL ROTATION

Some molecules are optically active and have the capacity to rotate plane-polarized light; the sense and degree of rotation is measured by an instrument called a polarimeter. This optical activity is measured using a polarimeter and the angle through which the light is rotated is an important physical characteristic by which an essential oil may be recognized.

The optical rotation of a whole essential oil is dependent on the mix of molecules within it and this results in the oils being what is termed 'optically active', with the ability to bend plane-polarized light. When plane polarized light is passed through a sample of the essential oil the direction and degree of rotation, as measured by a polarimeter, is an indication as to whether or not an essential oil has been adulterated. Table 2.1 gives some physical characteristics of essential oils by which the quality of oils may be judged.

REFRACTIVE INDEX

When light passes through a liquid it is refracted, and this refraction is easily measured to give consistent figures for a particular oil. This refractive index (Table 2.1) is quite consistent for a given oil and is another aid in the authentication of that oil.

Essential oils also undergo other checks on their physical characteristics, which must be within the accepted tolerances for the given oil. These checks include specific gravity, solubility in alcohol, colour, ester content and so on.

Table 2.1 Physical characteristics of some essential oils

Essential oil	Family	Optical rotation	Refractive index	Specific gravity
Cananga odorata (flos) [ylang ylang]	Annonaceae	−23.44 to −31.45	1.5041–1.5065	0.960–0.986 (20°)
Carum carvi (fruct.) [caraway]	Apiaceae	+74 to +80	1.485–1.492	0.902–0.912 (20°)
Cedrus atlantica (lig.) [Atlas cedarwood]	Pinaceae	+34 to +53.8	1.515–1.523	0.953–0.9756 (20°)
Cinnamomum zeylanicum (cort.) [cinnamon bark]	Lauraceae	0 to −2	1.573–1.500	1.000–1.040 (20°)
Citrus aurantium var. *amara* (per.) [orange bigarade]	Rutaceae	+94 to +99	1.472–1.476	0.842–0.848 (20°)
Citrus bergamia (per.) [bergamot]	Rutaceae	+8 to +24	1.465–1.4675	0.875–0.880 (20°)
Citrus limon (per.) [lemon]	Rutaceae	+57 to +65	1.474–1.476	0.849–0.858 (20°)
Citrus reticulata (per.) [mandarin]	Rutaceae	+65 to +75	1.475–1.478	0.854–0.859 (15°)

Table 2.1 Physical characteristics of some essential oils (*cont'd*)

Essential oil	Family	Optical rotation	Refractive index	Specific gravity
Coriandrum sativum (fruct.) [coriander]	Apiaceae	+8 to +12	1.462–1.472	0.863–0.870 (20°)
Cymbopogon flexuosus (fol.) [lemongrass]	Poaceae	–3 to +1	1.485–1.4899	0.889–0.911 (25°)
Eucalyptus globulus (fol.) [Tasmanian blue gum]	Myrtaceae	0 to +10	1.458–1.470	0.905–0.925 (20°)
Foeniculum vulgare var. *dulce* (fruct.) [fennel]	Apiaceae	+5 to +16.30	1.5500–1.5519	0.971–0.980 (20°)
Juniperus communis (fruct.) [juniper berry]	Cupressaceae	–15 to 0	1.4740–1.4840	0.854–0.871 (20°)
Lavandula angustifolia [lavender]	Lamiaceae	–5 to –12	1.457–1.464	0.878–0.892 (20°)
Melaleuca alternifolia (fol.) [tea tree]	Myrtaceae	+6.48 to +9.48	1.4760–1.4810	0.895–0.905 (15°)
Melaleuca leucadendron (fol.) [cajuput]	Myrtaceae	+1 to –4	1.464–1.472	0.910–0.923 (20°)
Mentha x piperita (fol.) [peppermint]	Lamiaceae	–16 to –30	1.460–1.467	0.900–0.912 (20°)
Myristica fragrans (sem.) [nutmeg EI]*	Myristicaceae	+8 to +25	1.475–1.488	0.883–0.917 (20°)
Myristica fragrans (sem.) [nutmeg WI]*	Myristicaceae	+25 to +45	1.467–1.477	0.854–0.880 (20°)
Nardostachys jatamansi (rad.) [spikenard]	Valerianaceae	–20	1.5078	0.9649–0.9732 (17°)
Ocimum basilicum (fol.) [basil]	Lamiaceae	–7.24 to –10.36	1.4821–1.4939	0.912–0.935 (20°)
Origanum majorana (fol.) [sweet marjoram]	Lamiaceae	+14.2 to +19.4	1.4700–1.4750	0.890–0.906 (25°)
Pelargonium graveolens (fol.) [geranium]	Geraniaceae	–7.0 to +13.15	1.461–1.472	0.888–0.896 (20°)
Piper nigrum (fruct.) [black pepper]	Piperaceae	–7.2 to +4	1.480–1.492	0.864–0.907 (20°)
Pogostemon patchouli (fol.) [patchouli]	Lamiaceae	–47 to –70	1.506–1.513	0.955–0.986 (20°)
Santalum album (lig.) [sandalwood]	Santalaceae	–15.58 to –20	1.505–1.510	0.971–0.983 (20°)
Syzygium aromaticum (flos) [clove bud]	Myrtaceae	–1.5	1.528–1.537	1.041–1.054 (20°)
Vetiveria zizanioides (rad.) [vetiver]	Poaceae	+19 to +30	1.514–1.519	0.9882–1.0219 (30°)
Zingiber officinale (rad.) [ginger]	Zingiberaceae	–28 to –45	1.4880–1.440	0.871–0.882 (20°)

*EI = East Indies; WI = West Indies.

INFRARED TEST

When electromagnetic radiation in the infrared region is passed through a sample of essential oil, the spectrum produced (Fig. 2.22) is a fingerprint from which the level of some of the components can be estimated. Some forms of adulteration can readily be seen by this method, depending to some extent on the skill and knowledge of the person who has carried out the adulteration.

THE NOSE

In addition to all this, possibly the finest tool for some purposes is a well-trained 'nose' (an expert perfumer, perhaps 20 years in the training) who can make an organoleptic assessment of the oil. The trained nose can identify the presence of certain molecules at extremely low levels that would be almost impossible for a mechanical device, although 'sniffing' technology is available (but expensive).

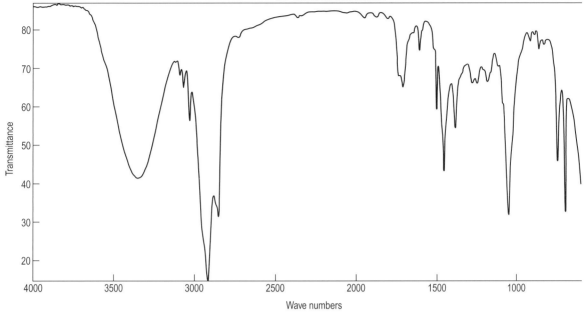

Figure 2.22   Example of an infrared spectrum (rose absolute).

THE DISTILLATION PROCESS

Distilling as we know it today can involve efficient cooling systems, electronic control gear to regulate the temperature and pressure of the process, energy-saving steam generators and so on. Some thousands of years ago, to obtain the essential oil, the plant material, cedarwood pieces (for example), was placed with water in a clay vessel with a lid made of woollen fibres. The vessel was heated over a wood fire, and as the volatile molecules from the water and the cedarwood escaped they were trapped in the wool. Later they were squeezed out by hand, and the aromatic water and essential oil, being of different densities, separated and so could be collected. Over the centuries methods of distillation gradually improved, and 4th century Chinese and 10th century Islamic scientists developed methods of obtaining the distillate. Since then, apart from minor improvements, distillation has remained very much the same in principle up to the present day. The availability of modern materials and resources, such as stainless steel and electricity, has permitted much greater control over the whole process and there is a dramatic increase in the quality of the essential oils produced today compared with that in former times. Oils produced in previous centuries, and even during the middle of the last century, cannot be compared with some of the very high quality products we have available for aromatherapy today (assuming they are not adulterated after distillation).

RECTIFICATION

Some essential oils are put through a rectification process; rectification means to put right, and this process is carried out to clean up an essential oil which has been contaminated with undesirable volatile plant products produced through careless distillation procedure. These undesirable products may be due to the decomposition of plant constituents, and although they occur mainly in the water, giving a smell which is rather 'off', they can also appear in the essential oil itself as, for example, unwanted aldehydes or bad smelling sulphur compounds. Sometimes a dark colour appears in the oil due to non-volatiles such as plant dust and rectification separates out any such material.

Rectified essential oils are not normally suitable for aromatherapy use.

FRACTIONAL DISTILLATION

This is a process which separates the volatile oil into its various fractions having different boiling points. This process is usually carried out under vacuum to keep temperatures involved at a low temperature and hence prevent degradation of the essential oil; it is a dry distillation; this means that no water or steam is used.

Fractionated essential oils are not normally suitable for aromatherapy use.

PERCOLATION

This is a fairly recent method of extraction; it is like usual distillation (but upside down!) in that the steam enters the alembic from the top and percolates down through the plant material. This percolation has been used on a small scale in France and when successful excellent oils are produced at a much lower cost, because the time of extraction with some plants is only a few minutes, saving man hours and fuel. The drawback is that sometimes an inseparable emulsion is produced which cannot be forecast and so this method of extraction has been put in abeyance until further work is carried out.

CARBON DIOXIDE

This is a new solvent extraction method using supercritical CO_2, by which a wider range of molecules can be extracted from the plant material than is possible by distillation. The CO_2 process is a selective method of extraction without distillation, yielding chemicals which are pure and stable: the solvent, CO_2, is colourless, odourless, tasteless and, unlike other solvents, is easily and completely removed. The whole process is performed without heat, which means that molecules are not degraded, thus producing a material which is new, and there is no doubt that CO_2 extracted oils will be of use to aromatherapists in the future. The oils produced by this newer method contain a different molecular mix and until more is known about them, and research carried out on their possibly different therapeutic (and possible toxic) effects, aromatherapists may be best advised for the time being to use only steam-distilled essential oils and expressed essences. These have been proven by tradition over a long period of time, as well as by supporting scientific research carried out over the last century, to be therapeutically effective.

COMPLEXITY OF ESSENTIAL OILS

During the 19th century the first analyses were carried out on essential oils, and attempts made to isolate and identify the various components, some of the terpenes, alcohols and aldehydes being among the first to be named. This was followed by successful attempts to synthesize the individual components; for example, eugenol found naturally in clove bud oil was synthesized in 1822 (Valnet 1980 p. 28).

The complexity of essential oils should be borne in mind when referring to the therapeutic qualities of a given oil; it helps to explain why one oil (lavender) can be listed as being at the same time 'analgesic, anticonvulsive, antidepressant, antimicrobial, antirheumatic, antiseptic, antispasmodic, antitoxic, carminative, cholagogic, choleretic, cicatrizant, cordial, cytophylactic, deodorant, diuretic, emmenagogic, hypotensive, insecticidal, nervine, parasiticidal, rubefacient, sedative, stimulant, sudorific, tonic, vermifuge, vulnerary'. This staggering array of properties (Lawless 1992) perhaps overstates the case, but demonstrates what the author describes as the 'shotgun' holistic approach which sprays all sorts of benefits (wanted side effects) in contrast to the 'single synthetic bullet' symptomatic approach aimed at a particular site, mostly with unwanted side effects.

This complexity underlines the fact that only genuine essential oils should be used therapeutically, even though there is natural variation in the oils. It needs to be emphasized that for perfectly valid reasons the fragrance industry requires essential oils which are standardized by one means or another and that most (if not all) essential oils in the general market place may have synthetic or natural additions or fractions removed. As well as these already-mentioned cautions, it is also true that some oils are not obtained from natural plants at all, for stainless steel plants do play their part! These laboratory creations are known as reconstructed oils (RCO) and lack many tiny and as yet unidentified components which could well be important to the overall effect of the natural oil.

SUMMARY

The requirements of the food and perfume industries differ dramatically from those of aromatherapy. Essential oils are very complex by nature, and careful selection and extensive testing are needed to obtain oils of therapeutic quality. When altered in any way essential oils will probably not be of a quality suitable for aromatherapy, since the synergy of the natural mix of components in the whole oil will have been destroyed. It goes without saying that they should be obtained only from a reliable and knowledgeable source. The therapist must have at least a basic knowledge of the chemistry of the molecules found in essential oils to:

- be able to appreciate fully the nature of plant volatile oils;
- increase their understanding of how essential oils may be used to best therapeutic advantage;
- be able to communicate with other health professionals;
- increase confidence in their own ability to treat clients.

References

Beckstrom-Sternberg S, Duke J A 1996 CRC handbook of medicinal mints. CRC Press, Boca Raton

Buchbauer G 1993 Biological effects of fragrances and essential oils. Perfumer & Flavorist 18: 22

Buchbauer G, Jirovetz L, Jäger W 1992 Passiflora and lime blossoms: motility effects after inhalation of the essential oils and some of the main constituents in animal experiments. Archiva Pharmaceutica (Weinheim) 325: 247–248

Buchbauer G, Jirovetz L, Jäger W, Plank C, Dietrich H 1993 Fragrance compounds and essential oils with sedative effects upon inhalation. Journal of Pharmaceutical Sciences 82(6): 660–664

Craker L E 1990 Herbs and volatile oils. Herb, Spice and Medicinal Digest 8(4): 1–5

Franchomme P, Pénoël D 2001 L 'aromathérapie exactement. Jollois, Limoges

Guenther E 1949 The essential oils, vol 2. Van Nostrand, New York, p. 499

Lamy J 1985 De la culture à la distillerie: quelques facteurs influant sur la composition des huiles essentielles. Chambre d'Agriculture de la Drôme, Valence, p. 5

Lautié R, Passebecq A 1984 Aromatherapy. Thorsons, Wellingborough

Lawless J 1992 The encyclopaedia of essential oils. Element, Shaftesbury, p. 118

Opdyke D L J 1973 Monographs on fragrance raw materials: laevo-carvone. Food and cosmetics toxicology, vol 11. Pergamon Press, Oxford, p. 1057

Opdyke D L J 1978 Monographs on fragrance raw materials: dextro-carvone. Food and cosmetics toxicology, vol. 16. Pergamon Press, Oxford, p. 673

Price S 2000 The aromatherapy workbook, 2nd edn Thorsons, London, pp. 31–36

Roulier G 1990 Les huiles essentielles pour votre santé. Dangles, St-Jean-de-Braye

Valnet J 1980 The practice of aromatherapy. Daniel, Saffron Walden

Chapter **3** **(Part I)**

Quality and safety

Len Price

INTRODUCTION

The dangers of essential oils have often been exaggerated, usually based on insufficient evidence and inappropriate comparisons. This chapter shows that these powerful substances, used knowledgeably and with due caution, pose no threat to health. The highest possible quality of medicament is always required in therapy and this chapter shows that aromatherapy is no exception to the rule. The main chemical groups found in essential oils are outlined, along with an account of methods of testing for quality.

To begin this chapter on the safe use of essential oils, three statements have to be made:

- Firstly, there is no doubt that essential oils are powerful mixtures and have physiological, psychological and pharmacological effects, both desirable and undesirable, when applied to the body.
- Secondly, in most countries, including the UK, these oils are freely available and there is no restriction on their sale and use.
- Thirdly, the majority of people who buy essential oils are members of the general public, who cannot be expected to have expert knowledge of their nature and use.

It is remarkable then that their safety record is as good as it undoubtedly is. Despite this record, statements are sometimes made which sensationalize aromatherapy or exaggerate unwanted effects of the oils. More to the point would be to educate both the supplier and the general user in the appropriate and safe use of essential oils. That way lies a safe and sound future for the popular use of aromatherapy.

ESSENTIAL OIL QUALITY

GENUINE AROMATHERAPEUTIC ESSENTIAL OILS

For therapeutic purposes the quality and wholeness of any essential oils used are of paramount importance, irrespective of the cost, whereas when used in flavours and fragrances, the taste and the aroma respectively are the most important considerations. For the food and perfume industries, the two major users, essential oils may be adjusted or changed to suit the particular need of the purchaser or the vendor. In these commercial enterprises price is an important consideration, and standardized essential oils are necessary to ensure repeatability and a consistent quality.

Throughout this chapter the term therapeutic essential oil will be used to indicate oils which are suitable for aromatherapy use, i.e. not adulterated, not 'ennobled', not redistilled, not fractionated, no parts removed or added, but which have been distilled specifically for aromatherapy from known plant material.

QUALITY VARIATION

Variation in the quality of an essential oil may be natural or due to human intervention. Wine is a commodity which is expected to have a different taste and character from year to year although harvested, processed and bottled at the same vineyard and from the same vines. These differences are even welcomed and certainly make for conversational one-upmanship! Plants, whether grown to make wine or essential oils, are subject to varying amounts of sunshine, frost, rain, heat or cold each year and it is these factors, plus the composition of the soil, which are responsible for the variations in quality and composition (and therefore aroma) of the plant extracts, occurring naturally from year to year. In that part of the essential oil world connected to perfumery and flavouring, this natural variation cannot be tolerated.

Synthetic materials

It is tacitly accepted that traders in essential oils add other cheaper oils or synthetics to the genuine oils, in order to maintain the same standard taste, aroma and price level for successive repeat deliveries to the same customer. Müller et al (1984) outline some contributory factors that lead essential oil merchants to modify the natural product: 'bad harvests, political conflicts, exhaustion of the soil or transportation difficulties are imponderables which make it impossible for the perfumer to rely entirely on Nature's raw materials. Against that background, synthetic fragrance substances appear as *economically indispensable substitutes for Nature's originals*' (author's italics). A good example is (–)-menthol (the chief compound in mint oil) where the synthetic product matches the natural exactly and is used world wide in pharmaceuticals, chewing gum, cigarettes, toothpastes, pills, paper handkerchiefs, foods, etc. The needs of the flavour and food industries are today so great that there are not enough natural products in the world to meet the demand, and even where available many products are just too expensive for their purposes compared with the synthetics currently used. 'Nature identical' products are manufactured in a laboratory and are simply synthetic copies of ingredients found in nature.

Most aromatherapy suppliers purchase their essential oils from importers who mainly supply the perfume and food industries, but this is not always a good and reliable source of unadulterated oils for therapeutic use. As Steffen Arctander explains in his book:

The author has nothing in principle against the addition of foreign or 'unnatural' materials to essential oils etc. as long as the intention and the result is an indisputable improvement in respect of perfumery performance and effect. However, the above philosophy should not indicate that the author approves of adulteration of natural perfume materials: quite the contrary. But the meaning of the term adulteration should be taken literally: with the intention of acquiring the business (order) through a devaluation of the oil in relation to the labelling of its container. The consumers of perfume oils are buying odor, not physico-chemical data. If the odor and the perfumery (or flavor) effect is in agreement with the customer's standards, there is no reason to talk about adulteration: the oil is then worth the full price of a true, natural oil and the 'adulteration', if any, has not been a means of direct economical gains.

Arctander (1960)

In contradistinction to the above, the aromatherapist is buying not merely an odour, but wishes above all to acquire the natural physicochemical characteristics, however these may vary from harvest to harvest.

Essential oils are made up of a vast array of distinct natural chemicals, many of which are found in more than one oil. It is a fairly simple matter for the chemist to remove a desired constituent from a cheap oil and add it to an expensive oil in order to lower the price for a customer, or to sell a modified 'pure' oil to an unsuspecting customer for a high price. Adulteration also takes place when a synthetic isolate is added, especially to one of the costly oils such as rose otto, when synthetic phenyl ethyl alcohol (occurring naturally in rose otto) is used as the adulterant. Alcohol, and occasionally a small amount of vegetable oil, which are both good solvents for essential oils, are also used to adulterate, stretch, or cut Nature's gifts, and many descriptive words are used to justify the standardization sometimes necessary in the fragrance and food industries. 'Certain suppliers with highly developed imagination will even use the term "ennobling" for the disfiguration of an essential oil' (Arctander 1960). With some oils it is almost standard practice to adulterate, e.g. the use of PEG (polyethylene glycol) to extend lavender essential oil.

Imitations

Genuine, expensive essential oils such as *Melissa officinalis* [melissa] and *Aloysia triphylla* [lemon verbena] are often imitated by the perfume industry by using blends of cheaper oils to simulate the aroma; to the perfumer, the aroma is the most important asset of an 'essential oil', not whether it is natural, adulterated or synthetic. Tisserand & Balacs (1995 p. 177) say that *Aloysia triphylla* should not be used in therapy, but this advice is based on tests carried out at 12% using fragrance quality oils (Opdyke 1992). Most oils named lemon verbena are blends of lemon, citronella, lemongrass, etc. as the genuine oil is very expensive; these 'made up' verbena oils are likely to be phototoxic and also skin sensitizers because of the high citral content in the oils from which they have been constructed. However, the genuine oil, which has a similar concentration of citral to the above oils, does not irritate the skin (Schnaubelt 1998 p.117) – a good point in favour of not buying perfume quality essential oils!

Deterpenized oils

Essential oils used in the fragrance industry often have their terpenes partly or wholly removed on account of their insolubility in alcohol, which would result in cloudiness – a distinct commercial and aesthetic disadvantage in a perfume! To the therapist, however, a deterpenized oil is incomplete. It then contains a higher percentage of the remaining constituents of the oil. For example, the deterpenization of peppermint increases the content of the possibly hazardous ketone menthone. 'In perfumery, certain essential oils are deterpenized, because too high a degree of terpenes reduces their solubility in alcohol. In aromatherapy, there is no necessity for this, and it is preferable to avoid interfering with the natural balance of the essence' (Lautié & Passebecq 1984 p. 15). Some therapists purchase bergapten-free bergamot oil, as this constituent (a furanocoumarin) can be responsible for phototoxicity of the skin in sunlight, but this is unnecessary and perhaps inadvisable (see Ch. 3 Part II).

Not everyone recommends the well-known book 'Essential Oil Safety' (Tisserand & Balacs 1995), because most of the information contained in it is based on information gained from tests carried out using perfume grade oils.

This book is not recommended for use by people who use good quality therapeutic grade oils because it does not contain any information relevant to such oils . . . it is a book on commercial grade oils. . . . If you are using cheap perfume grade oils, such as those in most retail stores, then you may need to read and heed this book.

Stewart (2004 p. 21).

The essential oils used in the tests were those suitable for the perfumery and food industries, not those specifically produced for therapeutic use. Such commercial quality oils are used in candles, soaps, shampoos, toothpaste, fragrancers etc and this is recreational aromatherapy, not therapeutic aromatherapy.

Stewart (2004 p. 11)

The book is about essential oil safety and is an excellent guide in itself, although the authors themselves say that 'this text is largely an extrapolation of toxicological reports from the Research Institute for Fragrant Materials' (RIFM). Nevertheless, in the absence of specific information on therapeutic oils, there is a useful body of knowledge on essential oils as used on the skin by the perfume industry, thanks to impressive work carried out by RIFM which was established in 1966. RIFM has published over 1000 monographs on fragrance materials and almost 200 of these concern aromatic materials derived from plants, including essential oils, absolutes and resins. The International Fragrance Association (IFRA) makes recommendations to the perfume industry for the safe use of such materials based on the published findings of RIFM, and these can be useful guides to aromatherapists when applying essential oils to the skin.

Contaminants

It is a fact that the majority of essential oils are produced for use by the food and fragrance industries that, generally speaking, are not concerned whether or not fertilizers, pesticides or herbicides may be present in the oil. Battaglia (2003 p. 49) tells us that contamination and adulteration may potentiate the toxicity of an otherwise safe essential oil and Stewart (2004 p.10) says that herbicides, fungicides and pesticides are intrinsically toxic and inevitably end up as contaminants in the oils, directly affecting their efficacy and safety.

To sum up, commercial grade oils can present their own toxic effects on account of the adulteration, folding, stretching, etc. to which they are subjected in order to have:

- a standardized product which can be repeated at any time, which is impossible with naturally grown plants

- a product at a price compatible with their marketing strategy (often meaning cheap).

PROCUREMENT OF GENUINE, AUTHENTIC ESSENTIAL OILS

Of the many factors involved in the safe use of therapeutic essential oils, not least is the specification of the oil itself. Knowledge of factors such as where it is grown, whether it is cloned by cuttings or grown from seed, the plant variety, how it is produced (wild, organic or with chemicals), the part of the plant used and the chemotype; all these are important for safe usage.

The need for the use of genuine essential oils in therapeutic treatments is illustrated perfectly by the following case cited by Valnet:

A patient being treated for a fistula of the anus by the instillation of pure and natural drops of lavender and who was beginning to recover had to go on a journey. Having forgotten his essential oil, he purchased a further supply from a chemist. Unfortunately, this essence was neither pure nor natural; one single instillation resulted in such severe inflammation that the patient was unable to sit down for over two weeks.

Valnet (1980 p. 27)

The overriding consideration must be consumer safety and to this end genuine, authentic essential oils must be procured, genuine in this case meaning of plant origin and authentic meaning not standardized: note that natural does not necessarily imply unadulterated.

It is not easy to procure such oils, for many and varied reasons, some of which follow:

1. High quality at the time of harvesting can diminish due to distillation, rectification, fractionation, adulteration, transportation, storage and time.
2. About 60 different standards exist for the chemical composition of essential oils, yet there are only 16 essential oils listed in the New European Pharmacopoeia (Dürbeck 2003).
3. The bulk of essential oils comes from faraway countries, only 3–5% coming from Europe.
4. Availability is influenced by various factors including war (vetiver, patchouli) and changing climate (ambrette seed).

5. The trade has very limited knowledge of Latin names and it is vitally necessary for aromatherapy to use the botanic, scientific name because the use of all sorts of local names for the oil-bearing plants does lead to confusion. More than one name may be given to the same plant or the same common name can be given to different plants (such as marjoram, which might be *Origanum majorana* or *Thymus mastichina*). An extreme example is cedarwood oil, which may be any one of the following, since all are traded as cedarwood:
    Cedrus atlantica [Atlas cedarwood]
    Cedrus deodora [deodar or Himalayan cedarwood]
    Cedrus libani [cedar of Lebanon]
    Chamaecyparis lawsoniana [western white cedar]
    Cryptomeria japonica [Japanese cedar]
    Juniperus procera [east African cedarwood]
    Juniperus mexicana [Texas cedarwood]
    Juniperus virginiana [red cedarwood]
    Thuja occidentalis [white cedar]
    Thuja plicata [western red cedar].
6. A supply problem exists because the market for herbal medicines is ever increasing and more oils are being introduced into aromatherapy, so it is necessary to seek them outside Europe and aromatherapy companies are not used to dealing with distant countries.
7. Wild plants are sometimes collected unsupervised by an unskilled labour force resulting in indiscriminate harvesting.

Proper identification of the essential oil

The importance of knowing what material is being used in a treatment is obvious, therefore it is imperative that the oil is precisely identified. This fact escapes the attention of many people treating others and even of some of those carrying out trials. Before embarking on a trial using essential oils it is of primary importance that a specified oil from a known source is used, and to have as a minimum a GC analysis of the oil actually used in the test. The scientific botanical name of the plant should be used and oil from the same harvest batch should be used throughout the test(s) for the reasons stated above.

In many cases it is not sufficient merely to specify in Latin the genus and species (and the variety if applicable); it is also necessary to designate the chemotype (explained in Ch. 1) and the part of the plant used for extraction. An example is the cinnamon tree where the oil from the bark consists principally of an aldehyde, while the oil from the leaf is mainly a phenol with different effects and uses. The oil from the thuja or white cedar tree, *Thuja occidentalis* (responsible for the restriction on cedarwood oils in France), is taken from the leaves, but other 'cedarwoods' are taken from the wood. In the Apiaceae family, the seed oils can be significantly different from oils extracted from other parts of the same plant, e.g. in the case of *Angelica archangelica* the root oil is phototoxic while that from the seed is not. Therapists need to be aware of this and it is their responsibility to ensure that inappropriate treatment is not given.

Some oils that are sold do not exist and they are called phantom oils by Dürbeck (2003); some examples are:

- Peru balsam from El Salvador and tolu balsam are both standardized or synthesized in Europe.
- Sandalwood from S. India is not available but still sold.
- Rosewood oil from the Amazon is not available because the industry is now finished.
- The same situation exists with *Copaiba balsam*.
- Tea tree – there is three times more sold in the world than is produced in Australia; tea tree oil is a comparatively simple essential oil comprising only about 30 compounds (cf ylang ylang with about 1200) and so is easy to reconstruct; also the 'natural' oil is often 'regulated' at source.
- Sumatran *Patchouli* may be relabelled Malaysian *Patchouli*.
- Barrème lavender (a lavender high in linalyl acetate) has not been produced for several years but still appears on some sales lists.

BRITISH PHARMACOPOEIA

Mabey (1988 p. 190) points out that no fewer than 80% of the medicines in the BP were plant based at one time (e.g. aspirin) – and even today 30% are still plant based (e.g. digitalis). Current pharmaceutical formulae demonstrate that essential oils and oleoresins derived from spices and herbs are valued not only as flavouring agents but also for other properties they posess; for instance, they:

- stimulate the appetite by increasing salivation
- act as carminatives to relieve gastric discomfort and flatulence
- counteract the griping action of purgatives
- contributes as mild expectorants in cough mixtures and pastilles
- check profuse secretion and relieve congestion of the bronchioles when used in inhalants
- act as counterirritants and rubefacients, for the chest in bronchitis and pleurisy, and for the relief of rheumatic pain, when formulated as ointments, creams and liniments.

As flavouring agents, essential oils are acceptable for repeated dosage, e.g. in tablets to be chewed and for repeated usage in such products as toothpaste. As perfumes they are present in a variety of cosmetics which are used daily over long periods of time.

A survey of the European pharmacopoeia (Bischof et al 1992) shows that only a few oils are common to the major pharmacopoeia – caraway, lemon, peppermint. Surprisingly, lavender is not one of them, but the Pharmacopoeia Helvetica does allow synthetic lavender: the Formulaire National de France has three monographs on lavender.

Ambiguous BP standards

Some essential oils listed in the British Pharmacopoeia (BP) are stocked in hospital pharmacies, but oils prepared to BP standards may not be suitable for use in aromatherapy. One reason for this is that many plants, for example thyme, *Thymus vulgaris*, exist in the wild as many different chemotypes, some of which are propagated and grown from cutting, each chemotype producing quite a different essential oil in make-up and therapeutic action (see Ch. 1), but these differences are not reflected in the pharmacopoeia. A critical commentary on the BP monograph for peppermint oil can be found in Hay & Waterman (1993 pp. 175–176).

The essential oils as specified in the BP may be suitable for use in aromatherapy/aromatic medicine because the specification is too broad or does not reflect the materials currently available. A request for lavender may produce *Lavandula angustifolia*, *L. x intermedia* or perhaps *L. spica*, all of which have different properties and indi-

cations: 'the analytical figures for the present English lavender oil do not correspond with the existing BP standards' (Trease & Evans 1983).

Similarly there are many different varieties of eucalyptus used in aromatherapy, each with its own characteristics, but many are lumped together in the BP where eucalyptus essential oil is given as *E. globulus* Labill, *E. fruticetorum* F von Muell, *E. polybractea* R T Baker, or *E. smithii* R T Baker. Each of these indeed has 1,8-cineole as its major component but the other constituents modify the effects of the whole oil. The BP gives the results of thin layer chromatography on some of the oils listed, but for some there is not even this specification.

According to the BP (1993) eucalyptus essential oil may be any one of four different species, which when unrectified may have different properties and indications, even though the principal constituent in each case is the oxide 1,8-cineole (eucalyptol). The same source states that it is not always the whole oil which is used therapeutically; it may be an incomplete oil (e.g. with some or all of the terpenes removed), an isolated active constituent, or even prepared synthetically.

Lemon is listed as *Citrus limon* (L.) Burm. with not less than 2.2% w/w and not more than 4.5% w/w of carbonyl components (calculated as citral) $C_{10}H_{16}O$. Also listed as *C. limon* is a folded (terpenes reduced) lemon oil containing not less than 40% w/w of aldehydes (calculated as citral) $C_{10}H_{16}O$: this oil would be a skin irritant and a folded essence is not used in aromatherapy or aromatic medicine: only unadulterated and unrectified oils may be used.

Some of the oils mentioned in the BP lack any complete specification: anise, caraway, cardamon, cedarwood, cinnamon, clove, coriander, dill, eucalyptus, lemon, nutmeg, orange, peppermint, spearmint and turpentine.

SAFETY

TRADITION AND EXPERIENCE

On the positive side, centuries of experience of many essential oils worldwide have proved them to be effective and safe when used knowledgeably and with care:

- The Egyptians proved the antiseptic powers of aromatics in the mummification process.
- Hippocrates fought the plague in Athens by using aromatic essences for fumigation.
- St Hildegard of Bingen was using lavender oil in the 12th century.
- Hungary water (a lotion scented with rosemary) began its 600-year life in the 14th century.
- By the year 1500, oils of benzoin, calamus, cedarwood, cinnamon, frankincense, myrrh, rose, rosemary, sage, spikenard and turpentine were known to and used by pharmacists.

Essential oils were first mentioned in an official pharmacopoeia around the year 1600 in Germany (Price 2000 p. 6). Borneo camphor (an alcohol) was mentioned in Schröder's pharmacopoeia of 1689 as a 'prodigious alexipharmic' or antidote to poison. For other oils there is little historical evidence, and for almost all essential oils, while there is ample proof of their antiseptic powers *in vitro*, clinical trials are lacking. While this may be due in part to shortage of research funds, it is also attributable to the difficulty (even impossibility) of conducting blind trials with aromatic substances.

ANIMAL TESTING

Although some tests have been performed on humans, aromatherapists should be aware that the majority of toxicological tests have almost always been carried out on animals – normally rabbits for dermal toxicity and rats for oral toxicity. To discover the unwanted effects, or toxicity, of essential oils, scientists have almost always carried out their tests on animals, but:

- Physiology cannot be compared with that of a human being.
- Absorption in any case is usually higher through animal skin than human skin (Hotchkiss 1994).
- Many tests were carried out using isolated components, which is not a valid test relevant to genuine whole oils used in the practice of aromatherapy.
- RIFM administered relatively massive overdoses to determine lethal toxicity.

Huge sums are spent on research, clinical trials and licensing for each orthodox medicine, pill or tablet which appears on the market. This is done

with the best will in the world – to help alleviate suffering and disease – but medical science is now faced with the situation, despite all the care and time spent on research, that there are still many serious side-effects. Essential oils have not been clinically tested in this way because it would cost billions, not millions, of pounds to test each oil and synergistic mix for each therapeutic effect of which it is capable. In the absence of scientific proof, orthodoxy finds it difficult to accept a discipline such as aromatherapy, which is still more art than science. Nevertheless essential oils have been used traditionally for hundreds of years to good effect. Had they manifested serious side-effects their use would certainly not have survived to the present day; yet in the recent past clinical tests on animals (which have a different physiology from humans) have allowed the creation of drugs which have had disastrous effects on humans; thalidomide and opren passed such recognized tests.

Apart from animal testing being abhorrent to the whole philosophy of natural holistic medicine, it has often proved impossible to extrapolate the results of animal testing to the human physiology. The enormous beneficial advances made in the field of orthodox medicine should not be underestimated, but appreciation and inclusion of the available natural ways are needed too – there is room for more than one approach in the healing arena. The relevance of animal testing to humans is debatable. For instance, basil and tarragon oils may contain estragole (methyl chavicol) in high amounts and this compound has been implicated by research on animals as being a strong carcinogen. By inference, the use of these oils in aromatherapy might be considered hazardous, but research at St Mary's Hospital in London indicates that the results of animal tests cannot be extended directly to humans. The carcinogenicity is due to the metabolite 1-hydroxyestragole, and the conclusion of the above study was that estragole presented little hazard to humans at normal food usage levels of 1 µg/kg per day (Howes, Chan & Caldwell 1990). The case for skin application of essential oils with a high content of estragole is still undecided. When applied to the skin, not all of the essential oil enters the body, but caution is advisable nevertheless, pending investigation of the metabolization of estragole in the transdermal route. It has been found that absorption of chemicals is usually higher through animal skin than through human, but for the aromatic amines the reverse is true: 13% of MDA (methylenedioxy-amphetamine) permeated the skin in rats compared with 33% in human skin, while for MbOCA (methylene bis[orthochloroaniline]) the figures were 2% and 6% respectively; for (+)-limonene the figures are 6% (rat) and 3% (human) (Hotchkiss 1994). All this underlines the inadvisability and uncertainty of extrapolating animal experiment results to humans.

EFFECTS OF MOLECULAR SHAPE

Carvone appears in laevo (–) and dextro (+) forms (see Ch. 2, Fig. 2.17) in different oils (for example (+)-carvone is present at 48–58% in caraway oil and (–)-carvone is the main constituent of spearmint oil). *Carum carvi* [caraway] is considered to be a safe oil in all respects by Tisserand (1985 p. 19) and by Tisserand & Balacs (1995 p. 204) (who also note that it is a mucous membrane irritant); Winter (1984 pp. 62–63) states that both (+)- and (–)-carvone are non-toxic; (–)-carvone has an LD_{50} of 1640 mg/kg in rats (Jenner et al 1964) and (+)-carvone one of 3.71 mg/kg in rats (Levenstein 1976).

Tyman (1990) has suggested that there are probably differences in effect between α- and β-thujone, and others have suggested that the same is true for *cis*- and *trans*-anethole. One frequently repeated statement is that all forms of ketones are neurotoxic, but this is not so (Tisserand 1985 p. 61). Thujone is not to be treated lightly whenever and wherever it occurs; however, the thujone molecule has four possible shapes, and it is not known whether they all have the same toxic potential and whether or not they ought all to be avoided (Tyman 1990). The seed oil of *Anethum graveolens* [dill] contains 40–60% of ketones, with a minimum of 28% (+)-carvone, and is considered neurotoxic by Franchomme & Pénoël (2001 p. 351). On the other hand, Tisserand (1985 p. 62) considers that 'carvone, which occurs in oils of caraway, dill, spearmint . . . is not present in sufficient quantity in the essential oils to present any risk'. There are many other anomalies such as this to be found in books on aromatherapy, which underlines the complexity of the

individual chemicals and the wide variation in percentages present in essential oils and therefore in the overall effect on human organisms.

Toxicity depends not only on the nature of the main component, but also on the relationships and synergy (see below) between this and some of the smaller (perhaps as yet unidentified) constituents, which are known to lessen or nullify undesirable effects in some cases. This may illustrate why certain oils high in ketones are not considered toxic, or even why a few oils, considered toxic by some people, do not appear to be so (see Synergism below).

Essential oils are very complex substances, and there is no simple direct relationship between the effects of any single component of an essential oil and the effects of the complete natural essential oil – essential oils are synergistic mixes.

Price (1990b)

The study of essential oils can be a minefield, and to understand them completely would take a lifetime. For the present, it may be preferable in the current state of knowledge to continue to regard aromatherapy as much an art as a science. Nevertheless, it should be remembered that a great deal of good has been done (and no serious harm has so far been recorded) by qualified aromatherapists since the 1960s in the UK.

SYNERGISM

Single oils

It is important to preserve the wholeness of an essential oil in order to guard its natural synergistic power. The full meaning of synergism is difficult to convey as it is used in the sense of extra energy; in other words, the combined action of disparate individual molecules within an essential oil has a greater total effect than the sum of their individual effects. The word itself is derived from the Greek syn = together, ergon = work.

As discussed in Chapter 2, essential oils are complex mixtures, some containing from a few dozen to several hundreds of different molecules and they act in synergy to produce their healing effect, but if these are altered in any way, the natural synergism is upset. When even a single active component is removed, not only is the synergy of the remaining constituents diminished or destroyed, but the isolated component generally needs much greater care when used alone – it may produce unwanted side-effects with continued use. However, when that same constituent is present in the whole oil, other constituents seem to act as 'quenchers' of these unwanted effects (see Quenching below) often enabling the oil to be used without harmful effect. Whole (or complete) essential oils have been found in practice to be more effective than their isolated principal constituent(s) and without side-effects (when used properly) on account of the synergistic effect (Hall 1904). Isolates, when tested individually, may behave differently than when in the presence of the other naturally occurring molecules within the make-up of the oil.

An essential oil is a synergy in itself, therefore it can be difficult to assess the contribution made by any one component to the total therapeutic effect of an essential oil; the therapeutic effects of an essential oil are not easy to ascribe to any one particular component. Very rarely an oil consists virtually of only one component and then the effects of the oil can be closely correlated with that of the main component, so that the effect of the oil and that of the main component are the same (e.g. wintergreen oil is almost wholly methyl salicylate, 98% or 99%). Usually however the essential oil consists of dozens or even hundreds of components producing a synergy and then it is not possible to ascribe the effects of the whole oil to one particular component, even if that component is a major part of the oil compared with the other components. It is possible that some quite minor component of the oil could have an effect out of all proportion to its size, as happens when the odour effect of an oil is being considered. 'It is this principle (synergism) which allows the achievement of strong effects from infinitely small doses of non-toxic products, but judiciously combined by nature herself' (Duraffourd 1982 p. 16). Constituents present in very small amounts (e.g. furanocoumarins) are often found to be as active as, or even more active than, the principal constituent.

The synergism of many essentials oils of commerce is destroyed during the production process, e.g. rectification and fractionation, as illustrated by the case of eucalyptus. Most eucalyptus products generally found commercially have routinely been redistilled, rectified and refined, which means that some molecules have been left behind in the redistillation process following the rectification of the crude oil, e.g. the rare phenol australol (Pénoël 1993 personal communication). Even if the proportion of a particular molecule seems low, it works in synergy with the main components and should be kept in order for the essential oil to express its full healing potential. The principle of synergy allows the achievement of strong effects from infinitely small doses (Duraffourd 1982).

Antimicrobial activity

Tests carried out on individual components from *Eucalyptus citriodora* revealed that they were relatively inactive; however, a combination of the three isolated major components in the same ratio as found in the natural oil produced a fourfold increase in antimicrobial activity against *S. aureus* (Low, Rawal & Griffin 1974).

Antioxidant activity

In tests to measure the antioxidant activity of essential oils, nutmeg, pepper and thyme oils, among others, were found to be effective and found to have beneficial effects on lipid metabolism (Simpson 1994). Thyme oils are known to be biologically active in the antibacterial, antifungal and antioxidant areas. Nine of the constituent components of thyme oil were shown to have antioxidant properties (linalool, thujone, camphene, thymol, carvacrol, γ-terpinene, β-caryophyllene, borneol, myrcene, listed in descending order of activity), but it was noted that antioxidant activity for the whole oil was greater than that of the most active single component linalool (Deans et al 1993).

ENHANCED EFFECT OF BLENDS

Apart from the synergy produced by the components of a single oil, there is also an enhancement of effect when two or more whole oils are mixed together. For example, the combined bactericidal effect of several oils together is greater than the effect of any of the individual oils which is why the authors have always recommended using a blend of two or three oils in a treatment.

The situation is the same with other herbal remedies; research has been done into the chemical constituents of *Echinacea* and these have been isolated and subjected to exhaustive clinical trials to try to determine the active principle within the plant. This has proved illusive; no individual constituent of the plant can, in isolation, produce the healing effect of the combined, complete plant medicine. The conclusion drawn from this has been that the medicinal effect is most likely to be as a result of the unique interplay of the naturally occurring substances within the living plant (Raynor 1999).

QUENCHING

Quenching is an important aspect of synergism and essential oils display a quenching effect whereby the potential unwanted side-effects of one component are nullified by the presence of other component(s). Just because an oil contains one or more components which are thought to be hazardous in some way it does not automatically follow that the oil is unsafe, although caution must be observed. A good illustration of this is found by comparing the effects of two eucalyptus oils, *Eucalyptus globulus* [Tasmanian blue gum] and *E. smithii* [gully gum]; both contain around 65% of 1,8-cineole (an oxide which is a skin irritant), yet the former is contraindicated for use on young children and the latter is not (Pénoël 1992/93). This quenching effect is well known in the perfumery industry, which turns it to advantage by adding quenching components to its perfumes to prevent skin irritation. This feature can also be made use of when mixing oils. The peel oils from *Citrus paradisi* [grapefruit] or *Citrus sinensis* [sweet orange] when added to *Cymbopogon citratus* in a 50–50 mix successfully quench the irritant properties of the latter (Witty 1992 personal communication).

Isolates

Isolates are sometimes used in pharmaceutical preparations and by the medical profession in France, but they need to be used sparingly, with knowledge, and should not be used in aromatherapy as practised in this country. Individual components in essential oils are known to have certain toxic effects, but in the whole oil, these effects are often quenched by one of the others present in the oil. For example, although citral on its own is a severe skin irritant, *whole* lemon oil, which contains citral in its complete 'recipe' of constituents, is not – thanks to the presence of (+)-limonene and its synergistic quenching effect. Also, although citral produces sensitization reactions in humans when applied alone, it produces no such reactions when applied as a mixture with other compounds (Opdyke 1976b). Whole, or complete, essential oils have also been found to more effective than their isolated principal component(s) – and certainly have fewer side-effects – on account of the synergistic effect (Hall 1904).

Phenol is a well known antiseptic which used to be used in hospitals, but the phenol in *Thymus vulgaris* ct. thymol, although it is 20 times stronger (more effective) than phenol, exhibits far less the mucosal irritating properties of the group (Mills 1991 p. 282). Schnaubelt (1998 p. 25) echoes this when he says that pure phenol is toxic, but natural plant phenols, such as thymol, 'have additional side chains that transform them into non-toxic, effective antiseptics'.

Tests carried out employing the isolates phenyl acetaldehyde, citral and cinnamic aldehyde – found in *Citrus aurantium* (flos) [neroli bigarade], *Cymbopogon citratus*, *C. flexuosus* [lemongrass] and *Cinnamomum zeylanicum* (cort.) [cinnamon] oils respectively – showed them to be skin sensitizers. However, the whole essential oils in which the aldehydes are present (at up to 85%) were found not to provoke sensitizing reactions.

It appeared that some other component(s) of the natural oil inhibited the induction or expression of sensitization (Opdyke 1976b). As a test of this hypothesis, several terpenes and alcohols found along with the particular aldehyde in the natural composition were combined with each of the aldehydes in question. It appears now to be a consistent finding that each of these aldehydes, although producing sensitization reactions when applied alone, produces no sensitization reactions in selected simple mixtures with other compounds

Table 3.1 Results of quenching tests on mixtures of cinnamic aldehyde with other essential oil components

Second test material	Relative proportions*	Results of sensitization test
Dipropylene glycol	1:1	+
Phenylethyl alcohol	1:1	+
Eugenol	1:1	−
Eugenol	1:1[†]	−
Eugenol	2.5:1[†]	+
Cinnamic alcohol	1:1	+
Benzyl salicylate	1:1	+
(+)-limonene	1:1	−

*Ratio (w/w) of cinnamic aldehyde to second test material. Each mixture was tested at an overall concentration of 6% in petrolatum by the maximization procedure (Kligman 1966, Kligman & Epstein 1975).
[†]Duplicate tests.
Reprinted from Opdyke 1979 p. 255, with kind permission from Elsevier Ltd.

(Opdyke 1979) (see Table 3.1). The irritant quality of oils with a high citral content (even 70%) can be quenched by adding an oil containing an equal amount of (+)-limonene (a terpene present in some citrus oils to around 80–90%). Similarly, the aldehyde citral is a constituent of *Citrus limon* [lemon] (5%) which, on its own, is irritating to the skin yet the whole oil is not.

These findings point to the difference between using a single compound and the use of a natural synergistic mix with inbuilt quenching action. The above-mentioned tests contrast with two earlier tests carried out by Kligman in 1971 and 1972 on 25 volunteers using cinnamon bark oil at 8% concentration and producing 18 and 20 sensitization reactions respectively (Kligman & Epstein 1975). Cinnamic aldehyde is not the only component in *C. zeylanicum* (cort.) [cinnamon bark] oil acting as a sensitizer, so perhaps this may be a case of synergy enhancing the unwanted effect. IFRA recommend that this oil is used at a maximum 1% concentration in a fragrance compound (IFRA 1992), equivalent to 0.2% in an aromatherapy massage oil (i.e. one drop in 25 ml carrier oil), although a lower level of use of 0.1% for the skin has been recommended (Tisserand & Balacs 1995 p. 130).

It is extremely difficult to judge the probable effects of an essential oil solely by knowing its principal chemical constituent(s), important though this knowledge is. The whole oil has to be considered in all its complexity, with the mixture of possibly hundreds of different types of molecules, their molecular energy and the overall synergy. It is worth repeating the statement made earlier: there is no simple direct relationship between any one of the chemical constituents and the therapeutic effect – or even the hazard – of the whole essential oil (Price 1990).

To recapitulate, such interaction of components takes place between the constituents within one oil and also between two or more essential oils, thus potentially toxic elements may be altered, enhanced or counteracted by other constituents present. It is for this reason that aromatherapists use the whole natural oil rather than an active isolate, e.g. eucalyptol from eucalyptus, thought to be responsible for the antiseptic, expectorant and contra-antigen action.

Gattefossé, chemist and perfumer, the man who coined the term aromatherapy, wrote that eucalyptole is 'a substance with no apparent activity' and is 'only an excipient' (Gattefossé 1937 pp. 41, 88).

Hindsight makes wise men of us all: Jürgens et al (1998) and his later work in 2003 regarding the steroid-saving and antiinflammatory effect of 1,8-cineole, isolated from *E. globulus*. This suggested an antiinflammatory activity of 1.8-cineole in asthma and a new rationale for its use as a mucolytic agent in upper and lower airway diseases.

SAFE QUANTITIES

Essential oils may be applied to the body in a variety of ways, and these are discussed in Chapter 5, but usually their use involves inhalation, application to the skin or ingestion. Essential oils are powerful, otherwise they would be of no use therapeutically, and this means that they must be employed with care and knowledge to achieve beneficial results. Inappropriate use in whatever way can bring about undesired effects. Dosage, in terms of both quantity and time, is all important since too little may mean little or no result, while too much may (depending on the oils used) either have a beneficial effect or create a serious problem. The majority of essential oils may be considered less toxic than the over-the-counter medicines aspirin and paracetamol, and aromatherapy is a safe therapy provided the therapist is suitably trained. If this requirement is observed, there need be no hesitation in introducing these natural aromatic products into a hospital environment. Many substances in common use are toxic in overdose, e.g. carrots are beneficial in moderation, although a surfeit will produce illness, and this is true of many other everyday foods such as tomatoes, saffron and mustard. Valnet (1980 p. 11) cites the loss of eyebrows and headaches in workers handling vanilla, but vanilla ice cream is produced, eaten and enjoyed without ill effect. An essential oil may be both safe and toxic depending on the amount administered – it all depends on the knowledge, skill and experience of the therapist. For example, we have observed that while lavender is sedative in low dose, a high dose can cause insomnia.

INGESTION OF ESSENTIAL OILS

Only therapeutic essential oils should be employed for internal use although, as we have seen, it is difficult for anyone to guarantee the purity of an essential oil, given the current state of the market. The ingestion of essential oils should be left in the hands of a competent aromatologist (e.g. a licentiate of the Institute of Aromatic Medicine), or an aromatherapist working under the direction of a doctor; such a therapist should exercise great care and discretion in advising both the use and the procurement of essential oils. Any national legal requirements and any rules of the hospital management board would have to be observed, as also will the ethical considerations of any professional body to which the aromatherapist may belong. Nevertheless, some conditions such as enteritis, irritable bowel syndrome and diverticulitis can scarcely be treated in any other way than by ingestion.

Essential oils should always be correctly diluted for internal use; the best medium, if a dispersant is not readily available, being a fixed oil because the essential oils will dissolve easily and completely in it (Collin P 1994 personal communication). Runny honey is also a good diluent, with the addition of a little water. Factors to be taken into account are age, body weight, general state of health, any current medication and the essential oils to be used. N.B. This method of using essential oils is not advised in the case of pregnant women and very young children.

INGESTION/OVERDOSE

When it comes to testing the toxic effects of swallowing essential oils, all studies have been carried out on animals. There is currently no viable alternative because testing on humans is considered too hazardous. Occasionally some knowledge is derived from an accident involving a child or a deliberate overdose by an adult. Therefore, many of the opinions offered on this subject in the aromatherapy literature must be regarded as speculative.

The ingestion of a large quantity of neat essential oil is unlikely as it would produce a burning sensation in the mouth and throat, and in some serious cases cause nausea, vomiting and diarrhoea. If the overdose is extreme there may follow lethargy, ataxia and coma or perhaps irritability and convulsions (e.g. pennyroyal). The pupils may be dilated (e.g. camphor) or constricted (e.g. eucalyptus). Table 3.2 shows the lethal dose (LD_{50} is the dose at which 50% of the test subjects die) of some representative oils for a typical adult and a small child. These figures have been extrapolated from figures derived from animal testing and as previously stated metabolization in humans is not always the same as in animals so their accuracy cannot be guaranteed (as seen above). In the absence of other information we must rely on these figures as a guide.

The quantities used in aromatherapy are very small, so there is normally an extremely high safety factor when comparing the lethal dose with the effective dose. The effective dose (ED_{50}) is the term used when some sort of response is being monitored in the experimental animal other than the death of the animal. The median effective dose is the dose at which 50% of the test subjects achieve the desired benefit.

Toxicity figures given in aromatherapy literature do not always make it clear that these doses are per kilogram of body weight. This could lead to the misunderstanding that the figures given are the effective or lethal doses for a person. They are not; it is dependent on their weight. For example

Table 3.2   Lethal dose (LD_{50})

Essential oil			LD_{50} g/kg (animal)	Lethal dose* 15 kg child	Lethal dose* 70 kg adult
Latin name	Common name			(mL)	(mL)
Aniba rosaeodora (lig)	rosewood		4.3	72	334
Boswellia carteri (resin)	frankincense		5	83	389
Cananga odorata (flos)	ylang ylang	more than	5	83	389
Cedrus atlantica (lig)	atlas cedarwood	more than	5	83	389
Chamaemelum nobile (flos)	Roman chamomile		8.56	143	666
Chamomilla recutita (flos)	German chamomile	more than	5	83	389
Cinnamomum zeylanicum (cort)	cinnamon bark		3.4	57	264
Cinnamomum zeylanicum (fol)	cinnamon leaf		2.65	44	206
Citrus aurantium var. amara (flos)	neroli	more than	5	83	389
Citrus aurantium var. amara (fol)	petitgrain orange	more than	5	83	389
Citrus bergamia (per)	bergamot	more than	10	167	778
Citrus reticulata (per)	mandarin	more than	5	83	389
Commiphora myrrha	myrrh		1.65	28	128
Coriandrum sativum (fruct)	coriander		4.13	69	321
Cupressus sempervirens (fol)	cypress	more than	5	83	389
Eucalyptus citriodora (fol)	eucalyptus	more than	5	83	389
Eucalyptus globulus (fol)	eucalyptus		4.44	74	345
Foeniculum vulgare var. dulce (fruct)	sweet fennel		3.8	63	296
Hyssopus officinalis	hyssop		1.4	23	109
Juniperus communis (fruct)	juniper berry		8	133	622
Lavandula angustifolia	lavender	more than	5	83	389
Lavandula x intermedia 'Super'	lavandin	more than	5	83	389
Melaleuca alternifolia (fol)	tea tree		1.9	32	148
Melaleuca leucadendron (fol)	cajuput		3.87	65	301
Mentha x piperita	peppermint		4.5	75	350
Myristica fragrans (sem)	nutmeg		2.6	43	202
Ocimum basilicum	basil		1.4	23	109
Origanum majorana	marjoram		2.24	37	174
Pelargonium graveolens (fol)	geranium	more than	5	83	389
Pimpinella anisum (fruct)	aniseed		2.25	38	175

*The human lethal doses are extrapolated from animal test results

Table 3.2 Lethal dose (LD_{50}) (*cont'd*)

Essential oil			LD_{50} g/kg (animal)	Lethal dose* 15 kg child	Lethal dose* 70 kg adult
Latin name	*Common name*			*(mL)*	*(mL)*
Pinus sylvestris (fol)	pine		6.88	115	535
Piper nigrum (fruct)	black pepper	more than	5	83	389
Pogostemon patchouli (fol)	patchouli	more than	5	83	389
Rosa damascena, R. centifolia (flos)	rose otto	more than	5	83	389
Rosmarinus officinalis	rosemary		5	83	389
Salvia officinalis	sage		2.52	42	196
Salvia sclarea	clary		5.6	93	436
Santalum album (lig)	sandalwood		5.58	93	434
Satureia hortensis	savory		1.37	23	107
Syzygium aromaticum (flos)	clove bud		2.65	44	206
Thymus mastichina	Spanish marjoram	more than	5	83	389
Thymus vulgaris ct. thymol	thyme		4.7	78	366
Vetiveria zizanioides (rad)	vetiver	more than	5	83	389
Zingiber officinale (rad)	ginger		5	83	389
Compound	1, 8-cineole		2.48	41	193
Compound	carvacrol		0.81	14	63
Compound	carvone		1.64	27	128
Compound	linalool		2.79	47	217
Compound	*p*-cymene		4.75	79	369
Compound	pulegone		0.4	7	31
Compound	safrole		1.95	33	152
Compound	terpinen-4-ol		4.3	72	334
Compound	thymol		0.98	16	76
Compound	camphor		0.9	15	70
Compound	borneol		2	33	156

*The human lethal doses are extrapolated from animal test results the LD_{50} value for the oil from *Salvia officinalis* [sage] is 2.6 g/kg, which equates to a fatal dose of approximately 170 ml for a 60 kg person; the equivalent figure for *Chamaemelum nobile* [Roman chamomile] is 570 ml for a 60 kg person. The quantities involved are so great that anyone in their right mind would jib at taking them; however, illness may be caused at a much lower dose.

Only steam-distilled oils and the expressed citrus essences should be employed for ingestion. The following classes of oils should never be administered internally:

- Oils obtained from gums (other than by distillation).
- Resins (because of the solvent residue).
- Absolutes (because of the solvent residue).
- Commercial quality oils (i.e. standardized) used by the perfume, food and pharmaceutical industries.

Ingestion of eucalyptus essential oil

Eucalyptus oil poisoning

There have been many cases of eucalyptus oil poisoning and it is puzzling why eucalyptus oil is so frequently taken by mouth, especially in Australia. A difficulty arises because there are very many kinds eucalyptus oil of varying composition and in none of the incidents referred to below is the botanical source specified: this may explain the sometimes conflicting recommendations for treatment given below. Ingestion of eucalyptus oil lead to coma in about 50% of 34 cases examined by Gurr & Scroggie (1965), which lasted from 30 minutes to 8 hours, usually with complete recovery after 24 hours after ingesting up to 25 ml: even after ingestion of 60 ml recovery has been noted. Another case of complete recovery was that of a 3-year-old boy who had ingested 10 ml of eucalyptus oil and was soon deeply comatose with shallow, irregular respiration. Gastric lavage was given, he regained consciousness after 5 hours and was normal after 24 hours (Patel & Wiggins 1980). Spoerke et al (1989) reviewed 14 cases of accidental exposure to eucalyptus oil of which nine were ingestion. They concluded that small amounts seemed to be comparatively harmless and for larger amounts gastrointestinal symptoms were the most common followed by central nervous system depression: amounts ingested ranged from 5 to 30 ml and patient age varied from 7 months to 20 plus years. Inhalation and skin exposure produced no or minimal symptoms.

A review of 41 child cases of eucalyptus poisoning in South East Queensland showed that 80% were completely asymptomatic, including four children who had swallowed more than 30 ml (maximum 45 ml). Two children were dizzy or ataxic, four had mildly depressed conscious levels, one child had an itchy rash and another had pruritus. A 4-month-old baby who had ingested 30 ml was the only one to display meiosis, hypertonia and hyperflexia. Presence and severity of symptoms was not related to the amounts ingested (Webb & Pitt 1993): it was suggested that children should not undergo gastrointestinal decontamination unless symptomatic on arrival at hospital. Tibbals (1995) looked at 109 cases of child eucalyptus oil poisoning and recommended that children should receive medical attention regardless of the amount ingested.

Action to be taken

Traditional treatment in the event of an overdose is quite rigorous involving gastric lavage or emesis and dilution with milk or fixed oil. Temple et al (1991) re-evaluated this protocol after reviewing five cases of child poisoning following ingestion of citronella essential oil. One of these five cases included a 16-month-old child who had ingested 25 ml of the oil but in all five cases there was little medical intervention and all patients recovered with no ill effects. They concluded that advice given in standard texts based on cases managed with outmoded techniques should be evaluated as the risks of evacuative and pharmacological interventions were considered greater than the risk of severe poisoning.

An example not to be followed

A nurse practising aromatherapy in a hospice some years ago was concerned to prove the safety of the oils she was administering to patients and took 5 ml of each of about 40 essential oils by mouth (one per week). In a personal communication she stated that she suffered no ill effects apart from sometimes dreaming more vividly than usual. The 40 oils included some that are potentially hazardous and it is advisable not to follow this extreme example. Individuals vary greatly in their reaction to different substances and such actions may produce a disastrous result. There is a large safety factor when using the oils in normal aromatherapy quantities, i.e. two or three drops compared with approximately 100 drops that a 5 ml teaspoon would hold.

Oils in the eye

Undiluted essential oils are never placed in the ear nor on ano-genital mucous surfaces and especially not in the eye, even diluted. If by accident essential oil does get into the eye then the advice given as to what to do varies slightly. One course of action is first to flush the eye under a running tap to expel most of essential oil and then secondly to apply a fixed vegetable oil (Baudoux 2000 p. 35). Zhiri (2002 p. 21) agrees that neat essential oils should never be applied to the eyes, ears and ano-genital mucous areas and also adds the nose; in case of accidental instillation or ingestion, either ingest or apply as appropriate a vegetable oil (e.g. olive, sunflower) to dissolve the essential oil, then seek medical aid. The authors have had experience of cases of mal use of essential oils in the eyes and on genital areas and have found the vegetable oil method to be effective, with minimum discomfort: essential oils are immediately soluble in vegetable oils which gives a dissolving/flushing action but hardly at all in water which gives only the flushing. For the eyes, the vegetable oil may be flooded in and for the genital area a piece of cloth soaked in a vegetable oil immediately reduces the painful sensation and usually there are no after effects.

Health professionals working in hospitals and similar establishments should secure the approval of a consultant or other suitably qualified and responsible person before giving oils by mouth (including gargles), or by the rectal and vaginal routes into the body. No carer without accredited training should administer oils in these ways unless under the supervision of an aromatologist or doctor. It is also important to preserve procedural safety; the prescriber, dispenser and administrator should be separate persons to guard against error.

UNDESIRED EFFECTS

While no doubt a synthetic modern drug can have a positive effect on a diseased organ or part of the body, it can also have an adverse effect on a previously healthy part of the body, resulting in a second drug having to be administered. This in turn can give another adverse side-effect, which will call for the administration of yet another drug. This cumulative effect of side-effects eventually killed the author's mother, who, at the time of her death, was on 22 different tablets a day, only one pertaining to her original problem.

In general, aromatherapists do not use the expression 'side-effects', because of its undesirable connotations. As can be seen from the list of properties given for lavender oil, most (but not all) of the side-effects of essential oils are desirable. For example, lavender oil may be used as part of a treatment for depression and if, as a result, there are other beneficial results such as the alleviation of insomnia and relief from rheumatic pain, this is to be welcomed. In orthodox medicine a single molecule 'bullet' is aimed at the symptom (see Ch. 4). In aromatherapy we point a shotgun at the problem, which sprays all sorts of beneficial shot, together with the very occasional unwanted effect. Many essential oils contain constituents which when isolated are found to be toxic, but many items normally regarded as quite safe also contain substances which, when isolated, could be shown to be toxic – tea, almonds, apples, pears, radishes, mustard, sage and hops, to name but a few (Griggs 1977).

Undesired side-effects occur usually as a result of the misuse of the oils, e.g. in the attempt to produce an abortion, or by accidental overdose – typically a toddler swallowing essential oils from a bottle. If essential oils are sold only in bottles with integral droppers and sensible precautions are taken to prevent access by children to the essential oils then this can be considered an extremely low risk therapy.

In normal aromatherapy or aromatology usage the dose is usually very low but, as with any form of treatment, idiosyncratic reaction is a rare possibility. Such a case was reported by Vilaplana, Romaguera & Grimalt (1991) of a middle-aged woman who used a cologne and developed itching which on testing was found to be due to

Bulgarian rose oil and geraniol. This was the first time a person had tested positive to Bulgarian rose oil in 326 cases of dermatitis and there were no other reported cases of dermatitis to the damask rose family, which prompts the question of quality of this particular rose oil.

HAZARDOUS OILS

Some oils are rarely or never used in aromatherapy because of possible harmful effects (see Appendix B.4). Some examples are *Juniperus sabina* [savin], *Gaultheria procumbens* [wintergreen], *Peumus boldus* [boldo leaf], *Sassafras officinale* [sassafras] and *Thuja occidentalis* [thuja].

Some other essential oils have a general prohibition on their use but without just cause. *Mentha pulegium* [pennyroyal] is alleged to be an abortifacient, but it may be used on men who are never likely to be pregnant! Those who are not pregnant may use this oil, albeit with care because of its high content of the ketone pulegone.

Hyssopus officinalis [hyssop] is an excellent oil for respiratory disorders but it is generally listed as toxic, as are *Pimpinella anisum* [aniseed] and several more.

Adding to the confusion, authors and companies give different warnings for different oils! One company, for example, gives only *Cedrus atlanticus* [cedarwood], *Helichrysum italicum* [helichrysum] and *Mentha x piperita* [peppermint] as the oils to be avoided during pregnancy!

Salvia officinalis [sage] contains the ketone thujone (up to around 47%) and though nothing has been proven against the ketone in whole sage oil, it would be prudent nevertheless to use it with care. The thujone in the whole essential oil of *Thuja occidentalis* (up to around 80%) is definitely toxic; however, the ketone content of essential oils such as eucalyptus (*E. globulus*) or rosemary (*Rosmarinus officinalis* ct. verbenone) is relatively unproblematic (Schnaubelt 1998 p. 27). Some ketones are neurotoxic, but not all. In some circumstances the so-called 'toxic' constituents are the very ones that are needed for beneficial results such as the phenol thymol in *Thymus vulgaris* ct. thymol, an extremely effective antiseptic and antifungal agent (Mills 1991).

Such oils may not be suitable for all health problems and may have contraindications making their use not suitable for certain people in certain circumstances, but if the therapist has had proper training and possesses common sense, it is possible to use effectively the so-called hazardous or 'toxic' oils to the greater advantage of their clients.

EPILEPSY

It is generally taught that *Hyssopus officinalis* used on a person will inevitably provoke an epileptic fit, and this teaching is supposed to be based on a statement by Valnet (1980 p. 11) but what he actually wrote is 'Even in weak doses the essences of sage, rosemary and hyssop can produce *a tendency to epilepsy under certain conditions and in persons whose resistance is low*' (author's italics). Cases of poisoning by sage and hyssop oils in the south of France have been investigated and the sage culprit has been identified as *Salvia lavandulaefolia*, rich in camphor. The epileptogenic effects of these two oils were extrapolated from animal tests and for humans the subclinical doses for *Hyssopus officinalis* and sage were found to be up to 0.1 ml/kg and 0.4 ml/kg, while lethal doses were more than 1.6 ml/kg and 4.0 ml/kg respectively; the greatest toxicity was due to a combination of pinocamphone and isopinocamphone (Steinmetz et al 1980). According to Renzini et al (1999) *Hyssopus officinalis* begins to exhibit cytotoxicity at a concentration of 100 μg/ml and is due mainly to the component linalool. Millet et al (1979) investigated – in animals – the convulsant activity of *Hyssopus officinalis* and *Salvia lavandulaefolia* and found the subclinical dose for hyssop to be less than 0.08 g/kg, while above 0.13 g/kg convulsions appeared and were lethal at 1.25 g/kg; this effect they also found to be due to the presence of pinocamphone and isopinocamphone.

SUMMARY

While some essential oils do present hazards, which frighten off the inadequately trained, the properly trained therapist will recognize the hazard and deal with it appropriately so as to reduce or obviate any risk whatsoever to the client. He or she will do this by applying the training received to the best advantage, assessing the situation and also using common sense. These powerful oils should not be available to the general public who may know nothing about their chemistry and effects.

Chapter 3 (Part II)

Power and hazards

Len Price

SPECIFIC HAZARDS

DERMAL TOXICITY

This term includes irritation, phototoxicity and sensitization. When considering this topic it must be borne in mind that the essential oils used for aromatherapeutic purposes must be of the highest quality, that is to say botanically identified, well stored and not adulterated (many cases of dermal toxicity can be traced back to substances which have been added for commercial reasons); it is imperative to procure the oils from an ethical source (from the standpoint of aromatherapy). For safe aromatherapy use, steam distilled essential oils are superior to other extracts such as absolutes, concretes, carbon dioxide extracted, etc: lavender absolute was involved in two cases, one a therapist with a 3-year history of dermatitis extending to face and neck (Bleasel, Tate & Rademaker 2002). Often the quantity of essential oils used in reported cases of dermal toxicity is excessive; in normal aromatherapy use essential oils are always used in quite high dilution.

Skin irritation, sensitization

This is a reaction to an irritant which produces inflammation and itchiness. Some essential oils are irritating to the skin and, usually but not exclusively, these are found to contain high proportions of either aldehydes or phenols. Oils in common use which have been found to be irritant are listed in Appendix B.6. Because there appears to be a wide variation in tolerance between people, a given oil might not cause a reaction in the majority of people yet be irritant to one or two more sensitive individuals. However, dermal irritation produced by essential oils is usually localized and short lived. Assuming that one oil has a 50% presence of an offending component, this is present in the total mix at only 0.5% when the oil is used in a normal massage mix along with two or three other oils at the standard dilution of 3% essential oils in a carrier.

When spread over a large area of skin the possibility of irritation is remote; the degree of irritation is proportional to the strength of the mixture applied. The essential oils which are potentially irritant to the skin include:

Cinnamomum verum (fol) [cinnamon leaf]
Origanum vulgare [oregano]
Satureia hortensis [summer savory]
Satureia montana [winter savory]
Syzygium aromaticum (flos) [clove bud]
Syzygium aromaticum (fol) [clove leaf]
Syzygium aromaticum (lig) [clove stem]
Thymus vulgaris ct. phenol [red thyme]
Thymus capitatus [Spanish oregano]
Thymus serpyllum [wild thyme] (depending on chemotype).

Tagetes

An aromatherapist presented with acute bilateral hand eczema 24 hours after spraying roses with an insecticide and patch testing gave a strong reaction to *Tagetes patula* [French marigold]: the acute eczema was attributed to a cross reaction with pyrethroid in the insecticide (Bilsland & Strong 1990). Dermatitis caused by the leaves and flowers of *Tagetes minuta, T. patula, T. erecta* and *T. glandulifera* is common in South Africa and the essential oil of *Tagetes glandulifera* is sometimes cited as being a skin irritant, but we have not found this to be the case in practice, although it is a photosensitizer.

Brassica nigra and Armoracia rusticana

Two oils from the Cruciferae family – *Brassica nigra* [mustard] and *Armoracia rusticana* [horseradish] – are not normally recommended for aromatherapy use, because both consist almost entirely of allylisothiocyanate. These oils applied neat to the skin will provoke severe burning and blistering

but it has been known for them to be recommended at the extremely low concentration of one drop of essential oil in 500 ml of carrier oil for rheumatism.

Melaleuca alternifolia

There are many cases reported of skin irritancy and dermatitis involving tea tree oil (Bhushan & Beck 1997, Southwell, Freeman & Rubel 1997). It should be borne in mind that tea tree oil is cultivated, grown from seed, and therefore the composition of the oil when distilled is variable. This oil is then adjusted at source to conform to laid down parameters (especially the 1,8-cineole content) and so may not have the natural synergy that may be expected. Tea tree oil has a relatively simple composition (about 30 compounds) and therefore is easily synthesized in the laboratory; and this is indeed carried out: such oils are known as reconstructed oils (RCO) and are not natural products and may have unwanted side-effects.

Seven people had been applying commercial tea tree oil **undiluted** on the skin for conditions such as fungal infections, pimples and skin rashes, and all developed eczematous dermatitis, some with vesiculation: a common allergen was (−)-limonene: application of **diluted** oil to the skin caused no reaction (Knight & Hausen 1994). Use of the commercial oil undiluted was ill advised.

Treatment of chronic atopic dermatitis by application of undiluted *Melaleuca alternifolia* was unsuccessful and then oral ingestion of the oil mixed with honey was advised, which led to exacerbation of the dermatitis: 1,8-cineole was the allergen (De Groot & Weyland 1992). The reasoning behind this treatment is hard to understand.

Santalum album

Overdose due to long-term use, namely daily application for 8 years, of a sandalwood paste to the forehead lead to a hyperpigmented, erythematous plaque and lesions and fissures on thumb and forefinger; sandalwood paste patch test proved positive (Sharma, Bajaj & Singh 1987). The offending compound was not identified.

Sensitivity

A Japanese study showed that the skin of men tends to be more than twice as sensitive as that of women, and when in situations of severe stress, lack of sleep, etc., then all skins are rendered more sensitive (Hosokawa & Ogwana 1979).

Other oils potentially irritant to the skin are *Origanum vulgare* [oregano], *Satureia hortensis* and *S. montana* [summer and winter savory respectively] and *Thymus vulgaris*, carvacrol or thymol chemotypes [red thyme]. The following oils are known to cause sensitivity in some people.

Pimpinella anisum [aniseed], *Syzygium aromaticum* [clove – bud, leaf and stem] can irritate the skin if used in high concentration because of their phenolic ether and phenol content respectively, as can the aldehydic oil, *Cinnamomum verum* [cinnamon – bark and leaf]. Cinnamon bark oil contains cinnamic aldehyde which is a known skin sensitizer, but the whole oil proves to be less so. Nonetheless, a patch test should always be carried out prior to using this oil.

Of 1500 dermatitis patients who were patch tested 21 had a reaction to essential oils (which were not botanically specified) of pine needle, dwarf pine, clove and eucalyptus and it was found that some components of the essential oils – carene, phellandrene and eugenol – were sensitizers (Woeber & Krombach 1969). Regional provenance of the essential oils had no great influence on sensitization potency; good quality and lack of ageing were more important. A therapist with a 3-year history of forearm dermatitis was sensitive to a range of oils containing geraniol but was also sensitive to yarrow, laurel and peppermint oils which do not contain geraniol (Bleasel, Tate & Rademaker 2002).

Mucous membrane irritation

Generally speaking, essential oils with a substantial content of phenols (chiefly thymol, carvacrol and eugenol) can be responsible for irritating a mucous membrane. Oils containing aldehydes may also be implicated. In the past it was believed that the hydrocarbon terpenes caused mucous membrane irritation (Gattefossé 1937 p. 40) but this is now thought not to be the case. Any of the oils listed in Appendix B.6 may cause irritation of the mucous membranes of the alimentary, respiratory and genitourinary tracts. A possible exception is lemon oil, which contains less than 5% aldehyde and consists mainly of hydrocarbon terpenes.

Contact sensitization

There are some oils which do not produce any reaction on first contact with the skin, but may do so on a subsequent application; there seems to be no common denominator to the essential oils which are sensitizing. The body's reaction involves the immune system, via the cells in the basal layer of the epidermis. Poor storage of oils containing a significant amount of monoterpenes can lead to the formation of sensitizing hydroperoxides: an infamous example is turpentine, which is responsible for skin allergies in workers in the paint industry. Oils to be wary of in this respect are shown in Appendix B.8.

Cross-sensitization

Once a person is sensitized to one substance, then that person is more likely to be susceptible to other similar substances, although the risk is low. This need not cause concern, but any aromatherapist who is sensitive to substances should be aware of the possibility. This is a complex topic, not well understood, but one example is when people become sensitive to benzoin after sensitization to Peru balsam or turpentine. There is a similar relationship between turpentine and peppermint and a case of turpentine induced sensitivity to peppermint oil involved a laboratory technician who suffered swelling of tongue, lips and gums after a dental operation. Tests revealed sensitivity to peppermint oil, an ingredient in dental spray and mouthwash and this was due to α-pinene, limonene and phellandrene which are also present in turpentine from which he had previously developed severe eczema of the hands (Dooms-Goossens et al 1977).

An aromatherapist had a 12-month history of hand and forearm dermatitis which improved when away from work. Patch testing revealed positive reactions not only to oils of lavender, geranium and lemongrass but also to oils to which she had not been previously exposed (palmarosa, frankincense, rose, neroli, myrrh) which implied cross reactivity (Bleasel, Tate & Rademaker 2002). Dermatitis recurred after eating lemongrass flavoured food – systemic contact dermatitis (see Appendix B.8).

A man allergic to turpentine breathed in the vapour of tea tree oil in hot water to help his bronchitis and developed acute exudative dermatitis of face, trunk and arms (De Groot 1996). Origin of the essential oil was not stated. A woman who had been treating her acne for a long period of time with undiluted *Melaleuca alternifolia* essential oil without reaction presented with dermatitis on forehead and mouth: patch testing was positive to tea tree and colophony (an oleo resin from which turpentine is distilled): cross reaction between turpentine and colophony was already established (Selvaag, Erikson & Thune 1994).

Phototoxicity, photosensitivity

Photosensitization is a process in which reactions to normally ineffective radiation are induced in a system by the introduction of a radiation-absorbing substance: the photosensitizer (Blum 1964, Johnson 1984, Kochevar 1987, Lamola 1974, Spikes 1977). Photosensitivity may occur when certain essential oil components, particularly the expressed oils, react with the skin under the influence of ultraviolet rays, yet does not occur on skin protected from natural or artificial sunlight. It may result in erythema, hyperpigmentation and perhaps vesicles, depending on the severity of the reaction. Furanocoumarins (psoralens) appear to be primarily responsible for phytophototoxic reactions in humans (Lovell 1993) so care needs to be taken with the citrus essences, which are expressed from the peel and contain large furanocoumarin molecules: this is particularly so with bergamot (see below). Other oils exhibiting this characteristic at aromatherapeutic doses are *Angelica archangelica* rad. [angelica root], *Juniperus virginiana* [Virginian cedarwood], *Ruta graveolens* [rue], *Lippia citriodora* [lemon verbena] and *Cuminum cyminum* [cumin] (Opdyke 1974) (see Appendix B.7).

Factors which influence the phototoxic response to psoralens are the presence of a suntan, natural pigmentation (dark skin), site of application, skin hydration and the interval between application of the psoralen and irradiation (it is worth mentioning that aromatherapy oils are applied mainly to areas not normally exposed to sunlight). A particularly notable culprit is the expressed oil of *Citrus bergamia* [bergamot] (Opdyke 1973), which has been studied by Zaynoun, Johnson & Frain-Bell (1977) and its use in aromatherapy needs consideration; tests by Pathak & Fitzpatrick (1959)

have shown the time interval between applying psoralens and the maximal phototoxic effect to be 30–45 minutes (tested on guinea pig and human skin), and a later test (Arora & Willis 1976) indicated a time interval of up to 75 minutes.

Tests probably carried out for the benefit of the perfumery trade on bergamot oil in ethyl alcohol showed no phototoxic responses at a concentration of 0.5%, and at 1.0% no phototoxic response after 8 hours; the tests were carried out on five subjects (Zaynoun, Johnson & Frain-Bell 1977 p. 231) and also showed that intervals of 1 to 2 hours between application and irradiation yielded a maximal phototoxic response. Applying this directly to aromatherapy is questionable as aromatherapists do not use ethyl alcohol as a medium for application, and the flow of psoralen through the horny layer of the skin is dependent on the carrier used (Kaidbey & Kligman 1974, Kammerau et al 1976). It is known that the horny layer is a major barrier to the penetration of psoralens; in tests, 70–90% of topically applied 8-methoxypsoralen (8-MOP, xanthotoxin, which is not present in bergamot oil) did not enter the horny layer and was finally lost through sloughing (Kammerau et al 1976). Bergamot oil itself is resorbed through the skin in 40–60 minutes (Römelt et al 1974, Valette 1945).

The tests by Zaynoun, Johnson & Frain-Bell (1977 p. 232) also showed that using paraffin molle flavum (PMF) as the carrier resulted in increased speed of penetration through the horny layer and produced a shorter period in which phototoxicity persists than when using ethanol, and it is possible that the effects using a vegetable oil as a carrier more closely resemble those results using PMF than those using alcohol.

The IFRA Committee recommends a level of 5-MOP (bergapten, a naturally occurring analogue of psoralen) of 75 ppm in a (fragrance) compound, and assuming a 5-MOP content of 0.35% this equates to a level of expressed bergamot oil in the compound of 2% (Jouhar 1991) and this translates to 0.4% (about eight drops in 100 ml) in the aromatherapy preparation applied to the skin. The use of 5-MOP is forbidden in the EU except as a normal component of essential oils.

In our practical experience over two decades, there has been no reported problem for thousands of therapists who have followed our training and numerous clients who have followed our advice. On this basis, it is suggested that following application of bergamot oil using the normal aromatherapy dilution (usually less than 1%, as essential oils are usually used in synergistic blends, and not individually) it is reasonably safe to expose the skin of normal people to sunlight provided that more than 2 hours have elapsed since the application. This advice may be tempered by the holistic approach and any unusual sensitivity of the individual client.

On the other hand, it is interesting to note that some other simple coumarin derivatives, such as umbelliferon, herniarin and aesculetin have a sunlight filter effect because they absorb ultraviolet light of 280–315 nm (Schilcher 1985 p. 228).

It is today necessary to be especially wary of reported cases now that the fragrance industry relies so heavily on synthetic materials. An example is a middle-aged man who used a sandalwood aftershave lotion for 3 weeks which brought about weeping, lichenified dermatitis of the face which worsened in sunlight, even after discontinuing the aftershave lotion. On analysis the commercial sandalwood was found to be composed of synthetic and natural geranium, synthetic and natural sandalwood, cedarwood oil and patchouli oil: he tested positive to the synthetic and natural geranium. For aromatherapeutic use it is essential to use authentic essential oils of known provenance; with such oils and proper advice such an incident would not occur.

OTHER SENSITIVITIES AND TOXICITIES

Prolonged use

If any one oil is used for a very long period of time then there may be a risk of sensitization even though none exists for normal usage. It is relevant to note here that when eau de Cologne (which contains bergamot and other citrus essences) was much in vogue many people wore it daily over a period of years and developed raised erythematous rough skin where the eau de Cologne had been applied – usually on the neck (berloque dermatitis). This reaction can be semi-permanent, lasting for years after cessation of use of the fragrance before disappearing (Shirley Price's personal experience). Many perfumes have ingredients in common with

eau de Cologne and may produce similar reactions. A 47-year-old woman who had sold food which was smoked and spiced with juniper berry oil for 25 years developed a rash which became generalized, followed by a dry cough and asthma. Skin tests with juniper and pine oils proved positive (Rothe, Heine & Rebohle 1973).

Melaleuca alternifolia [tea tree] oil was identified as a possible cause of relapsing eczema in a 53-year-old woman who had prolonged exposure to the oil (Schaller & Korting 1995). She was also allergic to other essential oils including lavender, jasmine and rosewood, which may have resulted from prolonged exposure to the oils, but was in addition allergic to laurel and eucalyptus, to which she had not been previously exposed. This report emphasizes the importance of treating essential oils with respect, especially when using them for prolonged periods of time. To obviate toxicity as a result of overuse of any one oil, it is good aromatherapy practice to change the oils used during a treatment of long duration.

A survey of effects on therapists

A survey of 120 aromatherapists carried out by Wong (1995), in conjunction with Aromatherapy Quarterly, of the personal effects of essential oils on therapists using essential oils in treatments, revealed that they took place on many levels. A few suffered adverse effects but it was felt that these were due to reactions to clients rather than to the oils themselves. It is emphasized that this was a survey, not a properly constituted trial. Of the 120 therapists surveyed:

- most felt the effects were beneficial
- only two were men
- most had been in practice for less than 4 years
- most gave fewer than 10 treatments per week
- 40 different oils were mentioned.

Effects on particular systems included the following:

1. **The skin**
   - 105 therapists experienced insignificant or no effect.
   - Several therapists experienced skin irritation, often between the fingers, and sweet almond oil and geranium were mentioned by two therapists as the offenders.

- Two therapists appeared to have developed eczema, and one previous dermatitis had disappeared.

2. **Emotional and mental state**
   - Only seven therapists surveyed felt that the oils had had no effect, with a majority feeling a moderate to great effect, usually beneficial, helping to calm, relieve headache and help sleep.
   - Sleeplessness was mentioned in connection with geranium, bergamot, lemongrass, peppermint and rosemary.

3. **Female reproductive system**
   - About 28% of the women surveyed felt some effect on their reproductive system, but most did not know whether this was due to the essential oils or to other factors.
   - Some said they felt no effects when using oils on clients, but experienced considerable effects when using oils on themselves.
   - Most experienced positive effects such as an improvement in PMS, period pains, and menopausal symptoms, and a more regular menstrual cycle.
   - Clary sage was mentioned many times in this context.
   - Six aromatherapists had been pregnant while practising; some found their sense of smell became more acute and they could not tolerate strong aromas.
   - A few therapists felt adverse effects such as tender breasts, irregular or heavy menstruation, a change in menstrual cycle and fluctuating hormone levels, but these are common and may not be linked to essential oil use.

4. **Digestive system**
   - 109 found a slight or no effect.
   - Some found that the calming effect of the essential oils helped digestive problems; a few reported flatulence; others had disturbed bowel movements.

5. **Urinary system**
   - 106 reported a slight or no effect, with 11 reporting moderate to great effect.

6. **Lymphatic system**
   - 96 felt no effects.
   - Of the 22 who reported effects, about half were positive and half negative regarding fluid retention, congestion and swollen glands (some felt their symptoms were due to standing).

7. **Immune system**
   - 96 felt a positive effect on their immune system and three felt negative symptoms.

8. **Respiratory system**
   - Approximately half of those surveyed felt improved symptoms in catarrh, coughs, hay fever, asthma, breathing or chest infections.
   - A few thought that their symptoms were made worse.

9. **Circulation, muscles and joints**
   - Any adverse effects were felt to be due to performing massage rather than to essential oils.
   - Some felt their joint and muscle problems had improved.

(Note: the quality and purity of the oils used by those surveyed is unknown and it is well known that synthetics added to essential oils can have effects of their own. In a general survey such as this other circumstances may well have had an effect, e.g. diet, medication, general state of health, allergies, etc.; the performance of the massage itself may be responsible for some of the joint and circulation problems reported.)

It is undeniable that, along with the undoubted positive powers of essential oils, there will be some unwanted effects. However, it is safe to say that these are rare, mostly only following an overdose or overuse. The general safety of essential oils normally used in aromatherapy may be judged by the health of workers who handle and inhale significant quantities of essential oils in the course of their daily work. Some members of our own staff handled, bottled and breathed a wide range of oils during the whole of their working day for over a decade, with no reported bad effects. There are many therapists (including ourselves) who have been working full-time with the oils over an even longer period of time (three decades) who have experienced nothing but good effects, and it may therefore be inferred that aromatherapy is basically a safe therapy. There are one or two therapists who have developed sensitivity to a few oils; unfortunately if the sensitivity is due to a specific chemical in the oil then wherever that chemical occurs the person may have a reaction. It should be noted that in some cases a reaction may be due to an adulterant rather than a natural essential oil component. Therapists who do not use perfumes run less risk of developing sensitivities to essential oils, as the overall quantity of synthetics employed in perfumes in day-to-day situations plays a large part in the growing number of people developing allergies and substance sensitivities (Bennett 1990) – quite an alarming fact.

Mutagenicity and teratogenicity

There is no available evidence that any natural essential oil has ever provoked mutagenicity or teratogenicity in an embryo or developing foetus. No tests have been carried out because the possibility of fragrant materials causing either genetic mutation or malformation is regarded as unlikely.

Carcinogenicity

A few oils have been tested for carcinogenicity on animals and the essential oil components safrole and dihydrosafrole have been implicated in the formation of hepatic tumours in rats; calamus oil containing β-asarone produced duodenal tumours (Taylor et al 1967). For this reason sassafras, which contains safrole as an important constituent, is not used in aromatherapy. Safrole is also significantly present in Brazilian sassafras oil, and in trace amounts in white camphor oil. Wiseman et al (1987) found that β-asarone produced malignant liver tumours in rodents but another study failed to confirm the carcinogenicity of β-asarone and calamus oil in rats (Ramos-Ocampo 1988). β-asarone (found in calamus oil) is restricted in foods and drinks to 0.1–1 mg/kg.

Despite the evidence from animal testing (where the doses used were large), it is thought that there is minimal risk in humans undergoing aromatherapy treatment; Tisserand & Balacs (1995 p. 101) suggest that a safe level for external use in aromatherapy is 0.1% maximum of β-asarone (also estragole, methyl eugenol and safrole).

Neurotoxicity

Special care must be taken with a few essential oils containing significant amounts of a ketone, which can be aggressive to nerve tissue. Not all ketones are neurotoxic (Tisserand 1985 p. 61, Winter 1984

pp. 62–63), but as a class they must be regarded as hazardous in this respect. Particular care must be exercised when using oils containing apiole (e.g. *Petroselinum sativum* (fruct.) [parsley seed]) and ascaridole (e.g. *Peumus boldus*). (For risks of using neurotoxic oils in pregnancy see Ch. 12.) The molecules in essential oils are lipid soluble and as such can pass the blood–brain barrier and access the central nervous system. The degree of lipid solubility varies from one class of molecule to another; e.g. esters are more fat soluble than are alcohols. Once past this barrier there is a potential for toxicity; accidental overdose of *Syzygium aromaticum* [clove] (5–10 ml) produced convulsions in a child (Hartnoll et al 1993). It is thought that the ketone thujone (found in *Thuja occidentalis*, *Salvia officinalis*, *Tanacetum vulgare*, *Artemisia vulgaris* and *A. absinthium*) is toxic to the central nervous system, as is the ketone asarone (found in *Acorus calamus*) (Wenzel & Ross 1957).

Hepatotoxicity

When using essential oils having appreciable quantities of aldehydes there is a risk of toxicity due to build-up in the liver. People taking fennel essential oil over a long period of time show a colour change in the liver tissue (Franchomme & Pénoël 2001 p. 105). Thujone, thymol and turpentine oil may damage the liver following oral ingestion in high doses (Schilcher 1985 p. 229). Liver toxicity seems to arise when innocuous essential oil components are metabolized to toxic chemicals, as with pulegone, found in many of the mint oils. Also to be treated with caution (based largely on animal testing using very high doses) are methyl chavicol (found in *Artemisia dracunculus* [tarragon]), safrole (in *Sassafras albidum*), myristicin and elemicin (in *Myristica fragrans* [nutmeg]) and apiole (in *Petroselinum sativum* (fruct.) [parsley seed]).

Nephrotoxicity

Some essential oils have an effect on the kidneys which is regarded as stimulating and beneficial in low doses, but could be classed as toxic if the quantity of oil used is excessive or it is used for too long a time. *Juniperus sabina* [savin] is mentioned by Schilcher (1985 p. 229) as causing damage to the kidneys, even when applied externally.

Large quantities of the ester methyl salicylate, found in the oils of *Gaultheria procumbens* [wintergreen] and *Betula lenta* [sweet birch], and of safrole (found in *S. albidum* [sassafras]) are nephrotoxic. Sandalwood and turpentine taken orally in excessive doses can also cause kidney damage (Tukioka 1927).

Respiratory sensitivity

See Chapter 5, section on inhalation.

POWERFUL OILS IN PREGNANCY

There are several essential oils which may have unwanted therapeutic effects during the first trimester of pregnancy, e.g. they may be emmenagogic and are therefore best avoided at this time, especially as, once in the body fluids, they may pass through the placenta. It is known that, although the placenta acts as a barrier against both neutral and positively charged molecules, those which are negatively charged can cross it fairly easily (Maickel & Snodgrass 1973); it is also known that small molecules with a molecular weight of less than 1000 are able to pass through the placenta (Baker 1960). Therefore, as many essential oil molecules are negatively charged and all have molecular weights of less than 250, it can be assumed that essential oils do pass through the placenta. Their effects on a newly formed foetus have not yet been studied. However, essential oils may be used correctly and safely later in the pregnancy, and it is our wish to try and clarify this potentially confusing situation. 'Crossing the placenta does not necessarily mean that there is a risk of toxicity to the foetus; this will depend on the toxicity and the plasma concentration of the compound' (Tisserand & Balacs 1995).

Many books on aromatherapy are derivative and consequently few authors are able to explain their recommendations of particular oils. This lack of firm information has led many aromatherapists to avoid using any allegedly unsafe oils during the whole gestation period, even though some of the proscribed oils are not necessarily unsafe in relation to pregnancy.

For example, essential oils which appear on a general 'never to be used' list are sometimes conflated with those oils which may need to be used during pregnancy, but with care. Also, many lists of oils to be avoided during pregnancy include those containing aldehydes and phenols (such as *Cymbopogon citratus* [lemongrass] and *Syzygium aromaticum* [clove bud], whose toxicity is mainly a potential irritant effect on the skin), and contraindications do not specifically relate to pregnancy (see Appendix B.6). Some oils listed contain coumarins and are therefore photo-sensitizers (Appendix B.7), but again this does not affect their use with particular regard to pregnancy. The essential oils listed in Appendices B.6 and B.7 should be treated with caution by everyone, not just those who are pregnant. Balacs (1992) began the clarification of this area by giving reasons for his list of oils to be avoided in pregnancy. His article and 'The Aromatherapy Workbook' (Price 2000 p. 131) are intended to be more informative and to put back into perspective the use of powerful and extremely useful essential oils during pregnancy. Another interesting point to consider is that a woman is often unaware of being pregnant at first – sometimes for up to 4 weeks (or more, in certain cases) and could be using several essential oils regularly during that time! Where this is known to have happened, no ill effects have been reported.

To save confusion and misuse, members of the general public (and inadequately qualified aromatherapists) are best advised not to use an essential oil appearing on any restrictive list during pregnancy without having been given advice by a competent aromatherapist; there are a number of essential oils which can be used by them with safety during this 9-month period.

EFFECTS OF GROSS MISUSE OF ESSENTIAL OILS

Because of the complexity of essential oil chemistry, a number of essential oils are labelled as toxic without any evidence of their causing harm to human beings, except by gross misuse. Toxicity of the main component of an essential oil does not always constitute proof that the whole essential oil is toxic to humans, whatever the results of research on rats and mice (which are injected with or made to ingest essential oils – see Ch. 3 Part I). Other research has shown that the results of animal testing cannot be directly extrapolated to humans and that because of the small amounts used in aromatherapy massage the effects of the essential oils would be 100 000 times less hazardous than the amounts used in animal testing (Tisserand & Balacs 1991).

Empirical evidence accumulated over many years would seem to be a truer test than animal research. Such evidence illustrates that when used in small doses (and for a restricted length of time), even the so-called toxic oils on the lists referred to do not normally present a hazard. However, the dangers of gross misuse of essential oils – whether generally considered to be safe or toxic – are also amply documented. Take *Mentha pulegium* [pennyroyal], which is reputed to be a strong abortifacient and a much impugned oil so far as pregnancy is concerned. The following cases of women who took large doses of pennyroyal deliberately are all recorded in medical journals.

■ To induce menstruation, one woman took about 15 ml of pennyroyal and suffered acute gastritis, recovering fully (Allen 1897).
■ Another made herself an infusion with about 15 ml of pennyroyal and 'threepennyworth of rum'. She felt sick after 10 minutes and later became unconscious; she vomited when roused shortly afterwards and recovered by the next day (Braithwaite 1906).
■ To induce abortion, a 22-year-old American took approximately 10 ml of pennyroyal and felt dizzy within an hour, recovering the same day. Tests showed her liver and renal functions to be normal and she was discharged 2 days after admission (Sullivan & Peterson 1979).
■ A 24-year-old mother of two, taking an unknown amount of pennyroyal in two separate doses (evening and the following morning) succeeded in aborting on the second day but was admitted to hospital seriously ill. Towards the end of 10 days her general condition was recorded as being satisfactory – all damaged tissues seemed to have recovered fully, except the kidneys. However, she developed pneumonia and died 3 days later (Vallance 1955).
■ An 18-year-old American girl took about 30 ml of pennyroyal, thinking she was pregnant. After severe vomiting and vaginal bleeding, she suffered a cardiopulmonary arrest 4 days

after ingestion. She died 2 days later following a second cardiopulmonary arrest (Sullivan & Peterson 1979).

Mentha pulegium can contain anything from 26.8–92.6% of the powerful ketone pulegone (see Potential toxicity below) depending on the country of origin and whether it is cultivated or wild. Lawrence (1989) quotes the pulegone content found in *M. pulegium* from the following countries:

Uruguay (1985): 26.8%
Angola (1976): 42%
Greece (1972): 61.9%
Chile (1986): 92.6%.

The average content is normally around 65%, but it is not known what percentage of pulegone was in the oils used by the women quoted above. It is difficult therefore to be certain about what dosage level is safe and when the amount begins to pose a danger. What is clear is that swallowing large quantities (15–25 ml) of any essential oil, even one considered to be safe, constitutes gross misuse, and may cause significant side-effects (see Ch. 3 Part I).

EMMENAGOGIC ESSENTIAL OILS

Emmenagogic essential oils are recommended to promote menstrual flow in non-pregnant women suffering from amenorrhoea, or irregular or scanty menstruation. The oils listed below are considered by the majority of writers to be emmenagogic. Such oils should not be used in the first trimester of pregnancy, unless needed in an emergency or for a short period of time. In such instances they should be used exclusively under the direction of an aromatherapist or aromatologist. Where there is a history of miscarriage, they should not be used at all.

■ *Achillea millefolium* [yarrow] contains little or no thujone as opposed to sage oil, which may contain 50% (Leung & Foster 1996 p. 458), but the plant has been used as an abortive in the past (Chandler, Hooper & Harvey 1982) and so the essential oil must be regarded as emmenagogic until proven otherwise. There is also a taxonomic problem with yarrow; Lawrence (1984) speaks of yarrow being a complex of hardly separable species, which is another reason for caution.

- *Foeniculum vulgare* var. *dulce* – also hormone-like, diuretic and galactagogic, facilitates delivery (average phenolic ether content 60%).
- *Myristica fragrans* [nutmeg] – also facilitates delivery; is hallucinogenic in overdose (average phenolic ether content 6%).
- *Pimpinella anisum* [aniseed] – also hormone-like; facilitates delivery (average phenolic ether content 83%).
- *Salvia officinalis* – also hormonelike; prepares uterus for labour (average ketone content 35%).

The following essential oils are those which some books, but not all, suggest are emmenagogic and should be used with caution during pregnancy. No evidence has yet been produced to support or refute these suggestions and, under the guidance of adequately trained aromatherapists, it would appear from the facts below that their use may not be detrimental to the well-being of a pregnant woman. However, this does not necessarily mean that all of them should automatically be regarded as safe oils, because even safe oils can be used wrongly, and far from safely.

- *Chamaemelum nobile* syn. *Anthemis nobilis* [Roman chamomile] (contains around 13% of a ketone). The link to amenorrhoea is due to nervous problems (Valnet 1980 pp. 104–105).
- *Matricaria recutita* [German chamomile] – hormonelike (Franchomme & Pénoël 2001 p. 396) (contains around 30% oxides).

These two essential oils are recommended for amenorrhoea, but their emmenagogic properties are generally considered to be very mild.

- *Commiphora myrrha, C. molmol* [myrrh]. Myrrh is thought to be an emmenagogue perhaps because it is hormonal; in Grieve (1991 p. 572) it is not made clear whether the plant or the essential oil is responsible for the therapeutic action (see *Levisticum officinale* below). As a result it appears in many British aromatherapy books as a proven emmenagogue. None of the French books cite it as such and Balacs (1992) considers it to have 'doubtful toxicity'.
- *Juniperus communis* (fruct. ram. fol.) [juniper berry, twig, leaf] – diuretic. Formacek & Kubeczka (1982) found *J. communis* to contain approximately 87% terpenes, with a small percentage of alcohols and no ketones, yet a

J. communis cited in Franchomme & Pénoël (2001 p. 389) is given as containing ketones (percentages not given). It is cited occasionally as an essential oil to be avoided in pregnancy, yet Franchomme cites no contraindications for this oil. Valnet (1980) gives it as an emmenagogue, though he does not cite amenorrhoea as an indication for its use – only painful menstruation, and it is not clear whether he means the essential oil or a decoction of the berries; this is crucial, as larger plant molecules can have different effects from the smaller volatile molecules. Franchomme makes no reference to the reproductive system whatsoever, nor do four other French aromatherapy books. The property of *J. communis* upon which all are agreed is its diuretic effect. This is sometimes suggested as the reason to avoid its use during early pregnancy, though it is an accepted fact that the baby draws all its needs from the mother, sometimes at her expense.

- *Levisticum officinale* [lovage] – diuretic (contains around 50% phthalides, about which not much is known). The essential oil is distilled from the roots. The leaves were once used as an emmenagogue (Grieve 1991 p. 500), which may be the reason why the essential oil has been assumed to be emmenagogic also.
- *Melaleuca cajuputi* [cajuput] – hormonelike (contains around 30-40% oxides). Franchomme (Franchomme & Pénoël 2001 p. 397) is the only person to advocate prudent use of this essential oil during pregnancy. He does not give it as emmenagogic.
- *Mentha* x *piperita* [peppermint] – hormonelike (contains 20-50% alcohols, 15–40% ketones). Like several essential oils, the main constituents in peppermint essential oil are variable, making decisions regarding its emmenagogic properties difficult. The pulegone content is usually 0.3–0.6%, though American peppermint may be just under 3% (Gilly, Garnero & Racine 1986). Peppermint is sometimes distilled after drying the plant, when the ratio of menthone (16–36.1%) to menthol (46.2–30.8%) is radically different (Fehr & Stenzhorn 1979). Valnet (1980 p. 173) and Tisserand (1977 p. 269) list it as an emmenagogue, though Franchomme & Pénoël (2001 p. 401–402) list it as a hormonelike oil which regulates the ovaries; they do not

contraindicate it for pregnant women. Bardeau (1976 p. 216) states that it calms painful periods.

■ *Ocimum basilicum* [European basil]. Because of its phenolic ether content (methyl chavicol), which varies within wide limits, depending on the species, the origin and the time of harvesting, basil is often cited as an emmenagogue. Valnet (1980) cites it as such, though Franchomme & Pénoël (2001 p. 408) give no mention of its use for any gynaecological condition and state that regardless of the percentage of methyl chavicol there are no known contraindications. Most of the basil oils available to aromatherapists contain a high percentage of methyl chavicol, the lowest being around 50% (and often as high as 75–80%). The plants from which the authors obtain their European basil oil have a very low methyl chavicol content, usually around 12%.

■ *Origanum majorana* [sweet marjoram] (contains around 40% terpenes and 50% alcohols). When this essential oil is contraindicated for pregnancy it is no doubt being confused, by the use of the common name, with *Thymus mastichina* [Spanish marjoram]. The latter essential oil is a species of thyme and has totally different constituents, with an oxide content of 55–75%. There is no mention of any emmenagogic effect or of having to treat *O. majorana* with caution in any of the French aromatherapy literature (including Franchomme & Pénoël 2001, Valnet 1980) and no evidence has yet been produced to support the contraindication of *T. mastichina*, despite its high oxide content. Until there is, it may be prudent to use this latter oil with care. 'Marjoram' essential oil should not be purchased without knowing its botanical name.

■ *Rosa damascena, R. centifolia* [rose otto] – hormonelike (contains over 60% alcohols). Rose otto is cited several times as being antihaemorrhagic (Bardeau 1976 p. 268, Franchomme & Pénoël 2001 p. 421, Roulier 1990 p. 298), but no sources mention its having any emmenagogic properties. Wabner (1992 personal communication) states that it regulates menstruation because of its hormonal influence, but that it is not emmenagogic.

■ *Rosmarinus officinalis* [rosemary] – different chemotypes (ketone content 14–35%, oxide content 18–40%). The chemotype labelled by Franchomme (Franchomme & Pénoël 2001 p. 421) as an emmenagogue is the camphoraceous rosemary. He cites the verbenone chemotype as neurotoxic and abortive (which would indicate care when used with pregnant women), but gives no contraindications regarding the reproductive system for the cineole chemotype. Roulier (1990 p. 298), on the other hand, gives no contraindications regarding the verbenone chemotype, yet warns against use of both the cineole and the camphoraceous type on pregnant women. He gives neither of them as an emmenagogue. The rosemary quoted in Valnet (1980 p. 177), which is not given as a specific chemotype and does not appear to contain verbenone, is given as an emmenagogue.

■ *Salvia sclarea* [clary] – hormonelike (contains 60–70% esters). The French authors mentioned above cite clary, referring only to its hormonal properties (Roulier 1990 p. 302) specifically in regard to amenorrhoea, but with no mention of its being emmenagogic. It is considered emmenagogic by Holmes (1993), although no authority is given. According to Culpeper (1983), the juice of the herb (not the essential oil), drunk in beer, accelerates menstruation. This could be due to its hormonal properties, as sclareol (the diterpenol responsible for the hormonelike property of clary) is present in the juice in a much higher quantity than in the essential oil, due to its molecular weight (see Ch. 1).

■ *Vetiveria zizanioides* [vetiver] (average ketone content 22%). Only one source has been found to cite *V. zizanioides* as an emmenagogue, i.e. Franchomme & Pénoël (2001 p. 433).

TRAINING AND EDUCATION

The purpose of training is to ensure minimum risk and maximum benefit to clients, but some training programmes instil fear and insecurity by insufficient, inadequate and often incorrect teaching. It is important that aromatherapy schools and colleges adopt a sensible approach to the subject of toxicity and do not – as many appear to do – sensationalize and exaggerate possible harmful effects of essential oils. It may be that it is lack of adequate education of teachers that brings about this situation. While this is true, it is up to aromatherapists to have an inquiring mind and make sure that the toxicity information they have been taught is constructive to their work, not destructive to it. This is not to say that essential oils, even if carefully chosen, can be used carelessly; it goes without saying that relevant knowledge and care in use are required.

To address the subject of safe use of essential oils, one must first remember that their use in aromatherapy in this country first developed from a beauty therapy aspect, where low dosage was combined with a gentle approach – unlikely to be in sufficient concentration to have any risks in use. Teaching avoided (and usually still does) any mention of the possibility of intensive or internal use, where possible risks would be more likely to occur. In aromatherapy today essential oils are not used in their concentrated form, but in such high dilution (usually 1–4%) that the only precaution necessary is to be aware of contraindications to their use in specific circumstances – i.e. epilepsy, pregnancy, skin sensitivity, etc. Nevertheless, at the 'risk' end of the 'safety' scale, it is possible to use certain essential oils intensively and/or internally, but only when extra training in the chemical constituents and their possible effects has been undertaken, as not all essential oils can be used in these two ways! However, with comprehensive knowledge, applied intelligently and with prudence, these advanced uses are as safe as any other method. Users of essential oils are most likely to do harm through ignorance of possible hazards (Battaglia 2003 p.121)

CLIENT TREATMENT

The therapist must make an informed oil choice and note, not only any possible contraindication against a particular oil, but also possible contraindications pertinent to the client which would affect the method of treatment, the concentration of oil used and the overall length of time an oil is expected to be used. The age and physical and mental state of the individual client at the time of treatment are factors which are all of paramount importance before selecting the essential oils.

The concentration of the oils to be used depends on the correct assessment of the client's state of health. The length of time an oil is used depends on the reason for its use in the first place. To attack an infection, a strong dose of a powerful – and possibly so-called 'toxic' oil – is required for a short length of time; for a chronic problem such as asthma, a much smaller dose of 'safe' oils is effective and can be used for a longer time. These choices can be made only if the therapist has sufficient knowledge of the essential oil properties and chemistry, applied with common sense, to know whether or not a 'toxic' oil could be used successfully on a particular client, giving speedier beneficial results.

Many therapists will not recommend the application or use of a dilute blend of essential oils on one patient for longer than 3 weeks, because of possible build up of toxins in the liver, which is always to be considered. On the other hand, clients have been using the author's arthritis and asthma blends twice daily for much longer periods (even up to a year or more) without problem, where daily use makes movement easier and reduces pain in arthritis and rheumatism, and makes breathing much easier for someone with chronic asthma.

GENERAL PRECAUTIONS REGARDING THE USE OF ESSENTIAL OILS

- Keep out of the reach of children.
- Essential oils are not to be ingested without specific professional advice.
- Never remove a dropper insert from a bottle of essential oils to prevent accidental ingestion; if this should happen then medical assistance must be sought immediately.
- Do not apply neat to the skin unless under the direction of a suitably qualified therapist.
- Idiosyncratic reactions to essential oils are possible; immediate medical assistance must be sought.
- Neat essential oils can be removed from the hands by washing thoroughly with a mild detergent to prevent transference to other parts of the body (e.g. the eyes).
- If essential oil does get into the eye then the eye should be flushed with a good quality carrier oil which will dissolve the oil (water does not).

SUMMARY

The need for a dispassionate and scientific attitude towards media charges of the dangers of essential oils has been demonstrated, as has the need for skill in their selection and prescription. Various types of potentially toxic situations have been identified. These should not occur if the guidelines for safe administration are followed. Despite this, essential oils must be treated as hazardous substances. In order to comply with the requirements of COSHH, a thorough assessment of the potential risks associated with their use must be carried out in order to prevent anyone who may come into contact with them from being harmed.

References

Allen W T 1897 Note on a case of supposed poisoning by pennyroyal. The Lancet i: 1022–1023

Arctander S 1960 Perfume and flavor materials of natural origin. Published by the author, Elizabeth New Jersey, p. 4

Arora S K, Willis I 1976 Factors influencing methoxsalen phototoxicity in vitiliginous skin. Archives of Dermatology 112: 327

Baker J B E 1960 The effects of drugs on the fetus. Pharmacological Reviews 12: 37–90

Balacs M A 1992 Safety in pregnancy. International Journal of Aromatherapy 4(1): 12–15

Bardeau F 1976 La médecine aromatique. Laffont, Paris

Battaglia S 2003 The complete guide to aromatherapy. International Centre of Holistic Aromatherapy, Brisbane

Baudoux D 2000 L'aromathérapie: se soigner par les huiles essentielles. Atlantica, Biarritz

Bennett G 1990 Allergy and substance sensitivity. Course notes. Shirley Price Aromatherapy College, Hinckley

Bhushan M, Beck M H 1997 Allergic contact dermatitis from tea tree oil in a wart paint. Contact Dermatitis 36(2): 117

Bilsland D, Strong A 1990 Allergic contact dermatitis from the essential oil of French marigold (*Tagetes patula*) in an aromatherapist. Contact Dermatitis 23: 55–56

Bischof C, Holthuijzen J, Löwenstein C, Stengele M, Stahl-Biskup E, Wilhelm E 1992 Essential oil analysis in the European pharmacopoeia. 23rd International Symposium on Essential Oils, West of Scotland College, Ayr, Scotland. Copies available from Lehrstuhl für Pharmakognosie der Universität Hamburg, Bundesstrabe 43, D-2000 Hamburg 13

Bleasel N, Tate B, Rademaker M 2002 Allergic contact dermatitis following exposure to essential oils. Australasian Journal of Dermatology 43: 211–213

Blum H F 1964 Photodynamic action and diseases caused by light. Hafner, New York

Braithwaite P F 1906 A case of poisoning by pennyroyal: recovery. British Medical Journal 2: 865

British Pharmacopoeia 1993 HMSO, London, p. 273

Chandler R F, Hooper S N, Harvey M J 1982 Ethnobotany and phytochemistry of yarrow, *Achillea millefolium*, Compositae. Economic Botany 36(2): 203

Culpeper N 1983 Culpeper's colour herbal. Foulsham, London, p. 47

De Groot A C 1996 Airborne allergic contact dermatitis from tea tree oil. Contact Dermatitis 35(5): 304–305

De Groot A, Weyland W 1992 Contact allergy to tea tree oil. Contact Dermatitis 26: 309

Deans S G, Noble R C, Penzes L, Imre S G 1993 Promotional effects of plant volatile oils on the polyunsaturated fatty acid status during aging. Age 16: 71–74

Dooms-Goossens A, Degreef H, Holvoet C, Maertens M 1977 Turpentine induced hypersensitivity to peppermint oil. Contact Dermatitis 3(6): 304–308

Duraffourd P 1982 En forme tous les jours. La Vie Claire, Périgny: p. 16

Dürbeck K 2003 The procurement of genuine authentic essential oils: professional aromatherapy's challenge. IFPA Conference, Bristol 12 October

Fehr D, Stenzhorn G 1979 Untersuchungen zur Lagerstabilität von Pfefferminzblättern, Rosmarinblättern und Thymian. Pharmazeutische Zeitung 124: 2342–2349

Formacek K, Kubeczka K H 1982 Essential oils analysis by capillary chromatography and carbon-13 NMR spectroscopy. John Wiley, New York

Franchomme P, Pénoël D 2001 L'aromathérapie exactement. Jollois, Limoges

Gattefossé R-M 1937 Aromatherapy (trans 1993). Daniel, Saffron Walden, p. 34

Gilly G, Garnero J, Racine P 1986 Menthes poivrées-composition chimique analyse chromatographie. Parfumerie Cosmétiques Aromates 71: 79–86

Grieve M 1991 A modern herbal. Penguin, London

Griggs B 1977 New green pharmacy. Vermilion, London, p. 305

Gurr F W, Scroggie J G 1965 Eucalyptus oil poisoning treated by dialysis and mannitol infusion, with an appendix on the analysis of biological fluids for alcohol and eucalyptol. Australasian Annals of Medicine 14(3): 238–249

Hall C 1904 cited in Valnet J 1980 The practice of aromatherapy. Daniel, Saffron Walden, p. 34

Hartnoll G et al 1993 Near fatal ingestion of oil of cloves. Archives of Disease in Childhood 69: 392–393

Hay R K M, Waterman P G 1993 Volatile oil crops. Longman, Harlow, pp. 175–176

Holmes P 1993 Clary sage. International Journal of Aromatherapy 5(1): 15–17

Hosokawa H, Ogwana T 1979 Study of skin irritations caused by perfumery materials. Perfumer and Flavorist 4(4): 7–8

Hotchkiss S 1994 How thin is your skin? New Scientist (29 January) 141(1910): 24–27

Howes A, Chan U, Caldwell J 1990 Structure specificity of the genotoxicity of some naturally occurring alkenylbenzenes determined by the unscheduled DNA synthesis assay in rat hepatocytes. Food and Chemical Toxicology 28(8): 537–542

IFRA (International Fragrance Association) 1992 Code of practice. IFRA, Geneva

Jenner P M, Hagan E C, Taylor J M, Cook E L, Fitzhugh O G 1964 Food flavourings and compounds of related structure. I. Acute oral toxicity. Food and Cosmetics Toxicology 2: 327

Johnson B E 1984 Light sensitivity associated with drugs and chemicals. In: Jarrett A (ed) The physiology and pathophysiology of the skin. Academic Press, New York, pp. 541–606

Jouhar A J (ed) 1991 Poucher's perfumes, cosmetics and soaps, vol. 1, 9th edn. Blackie, Glasgow, p. 40

Jürgens U R, Stober M, Schmidt-Schilling L, Kleuver T, Vetter H 1998 Antiinflammatory effects of eucalyptol (1,8-cineole) in bronchial asthma: inhibition of arachidonic acid metabolism in human blood monocytes *ex vivo*. European Journal of Medical Research 3: 407–412

Kaidbey K H, Kligman A M 1974 Photopigmentation with trioxsalen. Archives of Dermatology 109: 674

Kammerau B, Klebe U, Zesche A, Schaefer H 1976 Penetration, permeation and resorption of 80-methoxypsoralen. Comparative *in vitro* and *in vivo* studies after topical application of four standard preparations. Archives of Dermatological Research 255: 31

Kligman A M 1966 The identification of contact allergens by human assay. III. The maximization test, a procedure for screening and rating contact sensitisers. Journal of Investigative Dermatology 47: 393

Kligman A M, Epstein W 1975 Updating the maximization test for identifying contact allergens. Contact Dermatitis 1: 231

Knight T E, Hausen B M 1994 Melaleuca oil (tea tree oil) dermatitis. Journal American Academy of Dermatology 30(3): 423–427

Kochevar I E 1987 Mechanisms of drug photosensitization. Photochemistry and Photobiology 45: 891–895

Lamola A A 1974 Fundamental aspects of spectroscopy and photochemistry of organic compounds; electronic energy transfer in biologic systems; and photosensitization. In: Fitzpatrick T B (ed) Sunlight and man. University of Tokyo Press, Tokyo, pp. 17–55

Lautié R, Passebecq A 1984 Aromatherapy. Thorsons, Wellingborough, p. 15

Lawrence B M 1984 Progress in essential oils: yarrow oil. Perfumer and Flavorist 9(4): 37

Lawrence B M 1989 Progress in essential oils: pennyroyal. Perfumer & Flavorist 14(3): 71

Leung A Y, Foster S 1996 Encyclopedia of common natural ingredients used in food, drugs and cosmetics. John Wiley, New York, p. 458

Levenstein I 1976 Report to RIFM 18 August. Cited in Food and Cosmetics Toxicology 16: 673

Lovell R C 1993 Plants and the skin. Blackwell Scientific, London, p. 65

Low D, Rawal B D, Griffin W J 1974 Antibacterial action of the essential oils of some Australian Myrtaceae with special references to the activity of chromatographic fractions of oil of Eucalyptus citriodora. Planta Medica 26: 184–189

Mabey R 1988 The complete new herbal. Elm Tree, London

Maickel R P, Snodgrass W R 1973 Physiochemical factors in maternal-fetal distribution of drugs. Toxicology and Applied Pharmacology 26: 218–230

Millet Y, Tognetti P, Lavaire-Pierlovisi M, Steinmetz M D, Arditti J, Jouglard J 1979 Experimental study of the toxic convulsant properties of commercial preparations of essences of sage and hyssop. Rev E. E. G. Neurophysiology 9(1): 12–18

Mills S 1991 The essential book of herbal medicine. Penguin Books Ltd., London, p. 282

Müller J, Brèuer H, Mensing J, Beck C 1984 The H&R book of perfumes, vol. 1. Johnson, London, p. 111

Opdyke D L J 1973 Bergamot oil expressed. Food and Cosmetics Toxicology 11: 1031–1033

Opdyke D L J 1974 Monographs on fragrance raw materials: cumin oil. Pergamon, Oxford p. 274

Opdyke D L J 1976a Lemon grass oil West Indian. Food and Cosmetics Toxicology 14: 457

Opdyke D L J 1976b Inhibition of sensitisation reactions induced by certain aldehydes. Food and Cosmetics Toxicology 14(3): 197–198

Opdyke D L J 1979 Fragrance raw materials monographs. Food and Chemical Toxicology 17(3): 253–258

Opdyke D L J 1992 Monographs on fragrance raw materials. Food and Chemical Toxicology vol 30 special issue viii: 137s

Patel S, Wiggins J 1980 Eucalyptus oil poisoning. Archives of Disease in Childhood 55(5): 405–406

Pathak M A, Fitzpatrick T B 1959 Relationship of molecular configuration to the activity of furocoumarins which increase the cutaneous responses following long wave ultraviolet radiation. Journal of Investigative Dermatology 32: 255

Pénoël D 1992/93 Winter shield. International Journal of Aromatherapy 4(4): 11

Price L 1990a Clinical practitioners aromatherapy course notes. Shirley Price International College of Aromatherapy, Hinckley

Price L 1990b Lecture notes: theory and philosophy of aromatherapy. Shirley Price International College of Aromatherapy, Hinckley

Price S 2000 The aromatherapy workbook. Thorsons, London, p. 131

Ramos-Ocampo V E 1988 Mutagenicity and DNA damaging activity of calamus oil, asarone isomers and dimethoxypropenylbenzene analogues. Philippine Entomologist 7(3): 275–291

Raynor L 1999 The genus Echinacea. Herbs 24(2): 5

Renzini G, Scazzocchio F, Lu M, Mazzanti G, Salvatore G 1999 Antibacterial and cytotoxic activity of *Hyssopus officinalis* L. oils. Journal of Essential Oil Research 11: 649–654

Römelt H, Zuber A, Dirnagl K, Drexel H 1974 Münchner Medizinische Wochenschrift 116: 537 cited in Schilcher H 1985 Effects and side effects of essential oils. In: Baerheim Svendsen A, Scheffer J J C (eds) Essential oils and aromatic plants. Martinus Nijhof/Junk, Dordrecht, p. 228

Rothe A, Heine A, Rebohle E 1973 Oil from juniper berries as an occupational allergen for the skin and respiratory tract. Berufsdermatosen 21(1): 11–16

Roulier G 1990 Les huiles essentielles pour votre santé. Dangles, St-Jean-de-Braye

Schaller M S, Korting H C 1995 Allergic airborne contact dermatitis from essential oils used in aromatherapy. Clinical and Experimental Dermatology 20(2): 143–145

Schilcher H 1985 Effects and side-effects of essential oils. In: Baerheim Svendsen A, Scheffer J J C (eds) Essential oils and aromatic plants. Martinus Nijhof/Junk, Dordrecht, p. 229

Schnaubelt K 1998 Advanced aromatherapy. Healing Arts Press, Vermont

Schroeder J 1689 Pharmacopoeia medico-chymica, thesaurus pharmacologus. (Ulm 1641, 1649, 1655, 1662, 1705) (Frankfurt 1640, 1669, 1677) (Lyons 1649, 1656, 1665, 1681) (Leyden 1672) (Geneva 1689) (Nürnberg 1746)

Selvaag E, Erikson B, Thune P 1994 Contact allergy due to tea tree oil and cross sensitisation to colophony. Contact Dermatitis 31: 124–125

Sharma R, Bajaj A K, Singh K G 1987 Sandalwood dermatitis. International Journal Dermatology 26(9): 597

Simpson E 1994 Essential oils and the ageing process. Aroma 93: harmony from within. Conference Proceedings. Aromatherapy Publications, Brighton, pp. 107–110

Southwell I A, Freeman S, Rubel D 1997 Skin irritancy of tea tree oil. Journal of Essential Oil Research 9: 47–52

Spikes J D 1977 Photosensitization. In: Smith K C (ed) The science of photobiology. Plenum, New York, pp. 87–110

Spoerke D G, Vandenburg S A, Smolinske S C, Kulig K, Rumack B H 1989 Eucalyptus oil: 14 cases of exposure. Veterinary and Human Toxicology 31(2): 166–168

Steinmetz M D, Tognetti P, Mourgue M, Jouglard J, Millet Y 1980 Concerning the toxicity of certain commercial essential oils – essences of hyssop and sage. Plantes Med Phytother 14(1): 34–45

Stewart D 2004 The chemistry of essential oils made simple. Care Publications, Missouri

Sullivan J B, Peterson R G 1979 Pennyroyal poisoning and hepatoxicity. Journal of the American Medical Association 242(26): 2873–2874

Taylor J M et al 1967 Toxicity of oil of calamus (Jammu variety). Toxicology and Applied Pharmacology 10: 405

Temple W A, Smith N A, Beasley M 1991 Management of oil of citronella poisoning. Journal of Toxicology: Clinical Toxicology 29(2): 257–262, Discussion 263

Tibbals J 1995 Clinical effects and management of eucalyptus oil ingestion in infants and young children. Medical Journal of Australia 163(4): 177–180

Tisserand R 1977 The art of aromatherapy. Daniel, Saffron Walden

Tisserand R 1985 The essential oil safety data manual. Association of Tisserand Aromatherapists, Brighton

Tisserand R, Balacs M A 1991 Research reports. International Journal of Aromatherapy 3(1): 6

Tisserand R, Balacs M A 1995 Essential oil safety. Churchill Livingstone, New York, p. 105

Trease G E, Evans W C 1983 Pharmacognosy, 12th edn. Baillière Tindall, London

Tukioka M 1927 Proceedings. Imperial Academy Tokyo 3: 624

Tyman J H P 1990 Essential Oils Trade Association Symposium, Brunel University, June

Valette C 1945 Société de Biologie Comptes Rendus 13 October cited in: Katz A E 1947 Pénétration transcutanée des essences. Parfumerie Modern 39: 64–66

Vallance W B 1955 Pennyroyal poisoning: a fatal case. The Lancet ii: 850–851

Valnet J 1980 The practice of aromatherapy. Daniel, Saffron Walden

Vilaplana , Romaguera C, Grimalt F 1991 Contact dermatitis from geraniol in Bulgarian rose oil. Contact Dermatitis 24: 301

Webb N J A, Pitt W R 1993 Eucalyptus oil poisoning in childhood: 41 cases in south east Queensland. Journal of Paediatric Child Health 29: 368–371

Wenzel D G, Ross C R 1957 Journal of the American Pharmaceutical Association 46: 77

Winter R 1984 A consumer's dictionary of cosmetic ingredients. Crown, New York

Wiseman R W et al 1987 Structure-activity studies of hepatocarcinogenicities of alkenylbenzenes derivatives related to estragole and safrole on administration to preweanling male C57BL/6J x C3H/HeJF1 mice. Cancer Research 47: 2275–2283

Woeber K, Krombach M 1969 Sensitisation from volatile oils. Berufsdermatosen 17(6): 320–326

Wong M 1995 The healing touch: survey results. Aromatherapy Quarterly 46: 26–29

Zaynoun S T, Johnson B E, Frain-Bell W 1977 A study of bergamot and its importance as a phototoxic agent. II. Factors which affect the phototoxic reaction induced by bergamot oil and psoralen derivatives. Contact Dermatitis 3: 225–239

Zhiri A 2002 Huiles essentielles chémotypées et leurs synergies. Amyris, Bruxelles

Sources

AOC 1997 Report from research and scientific sub-committee for Executive and Council meetings, 27 November

Guba R 2000 Toxicity myths – the actual risks of essential oil use. International Journal of Aromatherapy 10(1–2): 37–49

Lamy J 1985 De la culture à la distillerie: quelques facteurs influant sur la composition des huiles essentielles. Chambre d'Agriculture de la Drôme, Valence, p. 5

Chapter **4**

Traditional use, modern research

Len Price

INTRODUCTION

The use of essential oils as part of traditional plant-based medicine has led to the accumulation of a large body of empirical knowledge about their effectiveness in different conditions. This chapter looks systematically at their therapeutic properties, and shows where possible how modern science confirms traditional usage.

ORTHODOX MEDICINE AND PHYTOTHERAPY

There have always existed many different approaches to the healing of people. Today these approaches are generally viewed as being complementary and supplementary to each other rather than competitive and antagonistic. Two of the different medical approaches are contrasted here: orthodox medicine and phytotherapy.

THE ORTHODOX APPROACH

The predominant contemporary approach is that adopted by orthodox allopathic medicine, where illness is regarded as being due to an outside agent. Throughout the ages this outside agent concept has been looked upon in various ways and illness attributed to 'evil spirits', 'ill will' or 'microbes' and, in more modern times, 'bacteria' and 'viruses'. In classical medicine the aim is to target and exterminate this outside agent, so freeing the body from further attack; the body is left to repair itself (Verdet 1989). It has, however, been estimated that 85% of all illness is self-limiting (see Ch. 8).

This selective focusing on the causative agent has brought about an enormous increase in the knowledge of the separate body systems and organs. However, the sheer volume of knowledge acquired has resulted in specialization and compartmentalization becoming the norm, and it is left to the general practitioner to preserve an overview of the whole person.

For many decades now medicine, and consequently pharmacy, has lived under the reign of analysis, of simplification. This philosophy shows itself in the production of medicines which are for the most part composed of a single well-defined molecule, well-known regarding its structure and properties, particularly the pharmacodynamics or therapeutic action on the organism. This style of analysis and simplification is the heritage of Descartes, who said quite rightly that to know the body better it was necessary to divide it into its constituent parts (Duraffourd 1982 p. 14).

This excellent principle has, however, been pursued to such a degree that there now exists a detrimental imbalance in medical care as the large number of iatrogenic illnesses shows.

DIFFERENT APPROACHES

- **Phytotherapy** (herbal medicine, but without the old-fashioned connotation of 'herbalism') deals exclusively in whole plants or isolated plant principles, and aromatherapy may be considered to be one of its branches (unlike homoeopathy, which uses plant, animal and mineral materials). Phytotherapy is essentially an empirical medicine, which recognizes the importance of the individual, and that each person lives his/her own ill health. This means that each person must receive individual treatment and care in his/her own environment, which may take longer than orthodox medicine but has a long-lasting effect. As well as treating illness, phytotherapy and aromatherapy are valuable for everyday prophylactic use, reinforcing weak points in the person to maintain good health. The following theoretical comparison illustrates the different approaches taken by orthodox and complementary practitioners in treating a person.

- **Allopathy.** Should an apparently healthy person suddenly develop a gastroenteric problem, a gastroenterologist will investigate only the digestive system and not pay too much attention to neighbouring organs and systems. The offending bacteria will be identified in the laboratory and an antidote will be prescribed, most probably an antibiotic. After treatment the symptoms will disappear and the client is said to have regained health.

- **Aromatherapy.** The aromatherapist will look at the patient and will say that the defence system has broken down, allowing the bacteria to enter and thrive, and that this is the cause of the illness. The weakness will then be considered in relation to other systems – kidneys, liver, lungs, skin – and all this is then studied in the context of the living environment. The illness may be a problem relating to food, a stressful experience or climate, and a balance must be sought; the aromatherapist using the properties of essential oils has the necessary weapons to effect this.

I had seen the miracles of modern medicine in Intensive Care; in daily practice it was not the same. Sick people fell ill again; sick people suffered side effects; new sicknesses appeared when I treated them with chemical medicines. But what struck me most of all was the complete absence of the human dimension.

Dr Jean-Claude Lapraz, quoted in Griggs (1997)

RECENT HISTORY OF PLANT–BASED MEDICINE

At the beginning of this century many medicines were based on plants and plant extracts. One reason for the former popular use of plants in healing was their easy availability in a still largely rural environment – people could gather plants and process their own medicines. Another reason for their use was the prevailing poverty at the time. In many areas of Europe money was scarce, there was little state assistance and private health insurance was practically unknown. Bonnelle (1993) quotes some older people's memories:

Before the social security, when people had to pay, they didn't call the doctor out … That's why people used to treat themselves with plants then.

My mother had 50 plants which she used to dry ... The doctor never came to our house. 20 franc pieces came in but never went out, except to buy a field.

However, after the Second World War, orthodox medicine took advantage of recent developments in science and technology. This resulted in an accelerating shift in emphasis from natural medicines to rapidly acting drugs. Dr Jean-Claude Lapraz made this observation:

When I was a boy my grandfather had a farm in the country, and I noticed that everybody used plants: they drank them in infusions, they made an oil to treat burns – Oh yes, plants worked, I saw that clearly. But later, in all the years I spent in medical school, nobody ever mentioned plants. Not a single one.

Quoted in Griggs (1997)

Decline and fall of popular plant medicine

As part of the fresh start after the Second World War, state medicine was introduced in some Western European countries, including France and the UK. This was one of the greatest advances in civilization the world has seen, and we should all be very much the worse off, both as individuals and as a society, if it did not exist. Unwittingly though, this wonderful step forward struck a near-mortal blow at folk plant medication because, with the availability of free treatment and advice from doctors, the knowledge of centuries was discarded, or at best put to one side and little used. People were no longer content with the gentle use of plants which took rather a long time both to prepare and to bring about healing. They had great expectations of the new synthetic drugs, which genuinely appeared then to produce immediate and startling results without any real effort on the part of the sufferer.

Nowadays, speaking for myself, plants are not strong enough. I used nothing else before but now you have to get the doctors' medicines. When they discovered the new drugs, everyone forgot about the plants.

Bonnelle (1993)

Both doctors and vets have used antibiotics extensively and liberally since 1945, and people's expectations of medical practice have changed, in that instant cures are asked for, without any effort, responsibility or participation on the part of the sufferer. In a broad sense the relationship of people to their own health has changed and, as plant remedies have fallen into disuse and lost ground to high tech instant medicine, popular knowledge has disappeared inexorably. The older generation who used to practise self-healing with plants still talk about plants but no longer use them and do not pass on their knowledge to their successors.

In the flower-power and Beatles age of the 1960s and 1970s there was a resurgence of many ideas, including caring for the ecological balance of nature, the use of natural as opposed to synthetic products, and the idea of eating organically grown foods. This new vision also encompassed the field of medicine and as a result many alternative (as they were viewed then) approaches to healing took root and flourished. These are now known as energetic, parallel or complementary approaches and, in contradistinction to the idea of conquering the illness by destroying the disease, there is much attention paid to a holistic style of treatment, of strengthening the body's own natural defences to cope with attacks by pathogens, of helping a person to live in harmony with their own body, with other people and with the environment. When a person is successful in this, then good health is enjoyed: illness strikes when the balance of the person within the environment is disturbed.

Today plant remedies are beginning to become more popular again, chiefly for small problems (such as headaches and twinges) which are too insignificant to warrant troubling the busy doctor and for chronic complaints (which by definition are not easily susceptible to orthodox treatment). Here, people are prepared to try, at their own expense, alternative procedures for the 'you must learn to live with it' conditions. It is significant that the most popular aromatherapy treatment and therefore one which might be regarded as successful is, in the author's experience, for chronic arthritis and rheumatism.

ACCEPTANCE OF AROMATHERAPY

Litigation in all fields of medicine has increased dramatically over the last decade and it has now reached a significant level of cost. Where midwifery is concerned, the Congenital Disabilities (Civil Liabilities) Act 1976 provides for a child to be entitled to recover damages where he/she has suffered as a result of a breach in duty of care, and litigation can be instigated up to 25 years after the event. With this in mind it is understandable to a degree that 'unproven' complementary treatments and medicaments are viewed with a certain amount of caution. Nevertheless, the attitude of doctors to alternative and complementary therapies is changing, as is shown by the following surveys carried out in the UK, Canada, Israel and USA.

- **UK:** A survey of doctors revealed that 93% of all general practitioners (GPs) and 70% of hospital doctors had suggested a referral to alternative treatment at least once; 20% of GPs and 12% of house doctors practised an alternative therapy (Perkin, Pearcy & Fraser 1994). Researchers at the University of Exeter reviewed 12 surveys of doctors and found that, on average, 46% considered complementary therapies to be effective, but noted that young doctors were significantly more favourable to complementary therapies than were older doctors (Ernst, Resch & White 1995).
- **Canada:** 73% of doctors surveyed wanted to know more about the major alternative/complementary therapies; they believed that alternative therapies were most needed for chronic pain or illness and musculoskeletal disorders (Verhoef & Sutherland 1995).
- **Israel:** There were similar findings in a survey of Israeli doctors, where 60% of all physicians had made referrals to complementary health practitioners at least once (Borkan et al 1994).
- **USA:** Doctors are showing growing interest in alternative/complementary remedies, with over 70% in one survey indicating that they would like to learn more about the available therapies (Berman et al 1995).

The intrinsically safe practice of aromatherapy is finding acceptance in many hospital departments today. The following comparison may help to explain why.

Orthodox drugs

These are predominantly synthetic but may include isolated natural components, and are mostly used in a symptomatic way. Side-effects (iatrogenic disease) are always present to some degree which may necessitate further medication. The newer antidepressants (e.g. fluoxetine) can cause side-effects including nausea, vomiting and diarrhoea, and this may be the reason for the continued use of tricyclic drugs (e.g. dothiepin hydrochloride) despite the risks shown by research. The drugs themselves are usually available only on prescription, but less powerful drugs and tablets are sometimes available over the counter.

The clinical testing of drugs is rigorous but carried out over a comparatively short timescale compared with traditional plant usage.

The United States Patent Office is ready to grant patents for medicines, although it is an open question in professional ethics whether a physician should patent a remedy. Synthetic medicines, prepared by chemical processes, often coal tar products, are now invading the field of Nature's simples, and it is possible that there may yet be a number of patentable compounds invented, to replace quinine and other vegetable alkaloids and extracts (Scientific American 1886).

Side-effects not only come from the drug itself but also are due to additives, such as colouring. Pollock et al (1989) carried out a survey of 2204 orthodox drugs and found 419 different additives present in 930 formulations; these additives may cause a variety of reactions in some people, e.g. nettle rash, watery eyes and nose, blurred vision, oedema, bronchoconstriction (Bowker undated) and hypersensitivity reactions and photo allergy (Lawrence 1987). Artificial colourings and preservatives are not added to essential oils.

Essential oils

These are natural products extracted by steam distillation, those used in aromatherapy being obtained from a single, specified botanical source. Only whole, non-standardized, unadulterated oils should be used in aromatherapy.

Aromatherapy seeks to instil respect for the therapeutic powers inherent in natural aromas that have not been tampered with by humans. It also tries to show how the wider ecosystem which produces natural essential oils is of ultimate importance, for this wider ecosystem will have a profound effect on the intimate ecosystem of human health. The way we treat nature – either by polluting it or by maintaining its integrity – will ultimately have a bearing on the natural products (such as the essential oils) that we use for our own well-being. And therein lies the importance of holism (Eccles 1997).

For aromatherapists to be able to carry out this aspect of holism, they have to depend on honest suppliers with a similar philosophy to their own suppliers who can guarantee not only the exact source of their oils, but also that they are not the 'commercial' products used by the perfume and food industries. Pharmacists look for cost effectiveness; they do not always realize that any essential oil conforming to a BP formula will have been modified to fit a specification.

Side-effects – fringe benefits

As a general rule the quantity of essential oils used is extremely small and unwanted side-effects are rare in practice; most side-effects are positive and wanted. It is usual for ample time to be devoted by the aromatherapy practitioner both for discussion with the client and for the treatment. Individual treatment is necessary because clients are regarded as individuals: germs do not necessarily produce the same reaction in different hosts, and it may be necessary to specify different oils to tackle the same infection in different people (Valnet 1980 p. 42). With one mix of essential oils it is possible to care for more than one health problem (the shotgun effect – see Ch. 3 Part I p. 58).

THE THERAPEUTIC PROPERTIES OF ESSENTIAL OILS

There are many reasons why essential oils need to be included in the armoury of weapons in the fight against disease. They have many positive properties and effects which are desirable – and few drawbacks. They are capable of being antiinflammatory, antiseptic, appetite stimulating, carminative, choleretic, circulation stimulating, deodorizing, expectorant, granulation stimulating, hyperaemic, insecticidal, insect repelling and sedative (Schilcher 1985 p. 217). They are natural antimicrobial agents able to act on bacteria, viruses and fungi, and many trials have been

performed in this field (see below). Tropical countries have traditionally used lots of spices in their cuisines, not only for the flavour, but also to kill the microbes which flourish in hot climates. It is thought that the antiseptic powers of essential oils are due to their lipid solubility (Malowan 1931) and their surface activity (Rideal, Rideal & Scriver 1928).

Essential oils are applied to the skin by various methods, ingested or inhaled (see Ch. 5), and all of these are harmless unless used incorrectly. A significant point in their favour is their pleasant aroma. They are much used in products for the home (examples are lemon and lavender) and are well accepted – they are much more pleasant and safer in use than bleach or carbolic acid. The aroma itself has effects on the person using them (see Ch. 8).

The aromatherapist should have precise control over, and full knowledge of, the substances being employed in the treatment. If this is the case, and the aromatherapist determines the therapeutic materials to be used, not some faraway laboratory, the medicine may be tailored precisely to the individual patient. Generally speaking there is an absence of unwanted side-effects arising from the use of essential oils in a healing situation (see Synergism in Ch. 3 Part I), and plant extracts are ecologically sound, causing no pollution, unlike antibiotics, which are flushed down the drain and pollute the land (Verdet 1989).

ANTISEPTIC, ANTIBACTERIAL

Essential oils have multiple actions and effects, e.g. when used for a respiratory infection an oil may be not only antiseptic, but also mucolytic, antiinflammatory and so on (Duraffourd 1987 p. 17). Another example is the use of oils on the digestive system, where the oils are antiseptic but do not act unfavourably on the flora and on the digestive secretions, in contrast to the unwelcome effects of antibiotics. The molecules of essential oils occur naturally and are not inimical to the human body. They support the immune system and can be considered as pro- and eubiotic as opposed to the synthetic antibiotics.

There is a natural variation in the chemical composition and physical characteristics of essential oils from year to year but this variation does

Case study 4.1a Antiseptic and antibacterial – Dr D Pénoël – *Aromatologist, France*

Chronic bacterial infection

Patient assessment

One month after a premature birth, A began to suffer from recurrent ENT infections that were repeatedly treated by antibiotics. Neither did homeopathic treatment prevent the recurrence of the infections and A's health became worse by the time she reached 10 months. Tetracyclines had rotted her teeth and her knees hurt whenever the weather was wet. After repeated infections having been artificially suppressed, her immune system was beginning to be affected.

When A was 7 years old, the ENT children's specialist asked for an X-ray of the sinuses. The radiography showed a complete blockage of the left maxillary sinus, a thickening of the wall of the right maxillary sinus and an infectious condition of the enlarged adenoids. The chronic inflammatory state of the mucous membrane was the result of the infection and excess production of mucus – and the specialist decided to operate, to flush the pus out of the sinuses. A's parents decided they would prefer to try aromatherapy first.

When she first went to the aromatherapy clinic, A had tubes in her ears and impaired hearing, frequent pains in her knees and her breathing was affected by her permanent chronic infection. She was skinny, pale, permanently tired and sad, and she was backward at school due to absence due to illness.

Intervention

A complete programme of treatment was established, involving both visits to the clinic each day and treatments at home. Her parents were given nutritional advice, which they followed scrupulously.

The essential oils to be used were considered from an analytical perspective, regarding the individual molecules and their percentages, linking this data with pathological aspects of the case. Several methods of treatment were used:

- High-tech aerosol equipment, with sonic vibrations, was used to penetrate deeply into the sinuses, using the synergy within *Inula graveolens* [inula] – which is strongly mucolytic as well as being antiinfectious, antiinflammatory and an immune system regulator.
- 10 ml of the following essential oils were applied neat daily – mainly on the back and thoracic area: *Rosmarinus officinalis* ct. cineole/camphor [rosemary] – mucolytic and antiinflammatory, *Melaleuca alternifolia* [tea tree] – antiseptic and *Thymus satureioides* [Moroccan thyme] – anti-infectious, antiinflammatory, immunostimulant.
- Orally, 5–6 drops of the following essential oils were blended in honey and taken 4 times a day with warm water, like a herbal tea: *M. alternifolia, Mentha. x piperita* [peppermint], *T. satureioides* and *Satureia montana* [mountain savory].
- Swiss reflex massage was carried out on the relevant foot reflexes.
- Drainage of the face area was done using suction cups and magnetic field therapy on the face, liver, spleen and kidney areas.

Outcome

After 2 weeks, and 11 clinical sessions it was clear that an overall and local improvement had taken place. When the new X-ray was taken it showed that the sinus and adenoid infections had totally cleared. The ENT specialist, on seeing the X-ray, simply said 'cases of spontaneous healing are known among children'. Nevertheless, aromatic medicine had succeeded where everything else had failed.

---

not seem materially to affect their antiseptic properties, although it is necessary to know the analysis of the actual sample of oil being tested. It is possible to have two antibacterial powers for one essential oil, depending on the method of use, e.g. the antiseptic use of liquid or vaporized oil.

Essential oils are especially valuable as antiseptics because their aggression towards microbial germs is matched by their total harmlessness to tissue – one of the chief defects of chemical antiseptics is that they are likely to be as harmful to the cells of the organism as to the cause of the disease. It is very important to remember that (chemical) antiseptics will destroy not only the micro-organisms but also the surrounding cells (Valnet 1980 p. 44).

Case study 4.1a Antiseptic and antibacterial – Dr D Pénoël – *aromatologist, France (cont'd)*

Treatments at home were continued, but shortly afterwards, A had acute tonsillitis, a quantity of thick brown mucus being found on A's pillow every morning for 4 days. It was assumed that her whole organism had gained enough strength from the aromatherapeutic treatments to expel the accumulated toxins and waste matters from all the previous medication and accumulated infections which had been locked inside until then.

Essential oils were therefore applied intensively as before, and after 4 more days, her throat was completely cleansed, the fever stopped, and A was once more feeling like a new child!

Conclusion

When acute stages of a disease are dealt with successfully by implementing natural medicine treatments, it marks a turning point in the underlying illness. A is now 15 years old and has taken no antibiotics since she was 7. She is strong, healthy, excels at school in art and in sport and believes that the intervention of aromatic medicine definitely changed her life.

Case study 4.1b   Antiseptic and antibacterial – U Rädlein –
nurse aromatherapist, Germany

Wound infection

Patient assessment

A 45-year-old woman had a motor vehicle accident, resulting in a comminuted fracture of the ankle. It was operated on but the operation site became infected and was open for 4 months. At this stage the orthopaedic surgeon gave his permission to try and treat the wound with essential oils. First, a wound swab was taken and *Staphylococcus aureus*, *Streptococcus pseudomonas* and *Escherichia coli* were isolated, from which the programme was formulated.

Intervention

The treatment consisted of a daily footbath with 3 drops each of:

- *Thymus vulgaris* ct. alcohol
- *Citrus limon*
- *Melaleuca alternifolia*

(The essential oils were put on a small spoon of salt to emulsify them and then put into the footbath water.)

The wound was then cleaned – and a dry gauze compress (on which was put 3 drops of tea tree) put on. This was covered with a mull bandage, the whole treatment being carried out once daily. During this time the patient was given no antibiotics – only 20 drops of Tramal when needed for her pain.

Outcome

After 3 days she no longer needed any analgesics. 2 weeks later, when a wound swab was tested none of the original bacteria were present.

The wound closed after 3 weeks of using aromatherapy.

The use of essential oils is a sure way of avoiding the phenomenon of developed resistance in microbes as experienced with antibiotics, because the aromatic essences are able to destroy even the resistant strains selectively (Pellecuer, Allegrini & De Buochberg 1974). Germs resistant to synthetic antibiotics are susceptible in certain cases to some essences in dilutions as low as 1 in 16 000, e.g. *Satureia montana* (Belaiche 1979 p. 31) (see Table 4.1).

It is wise to avoid any possible resistance on the part of a germ by always prescribing the use of three or four essential oils in combination. This multimix approach will tend to minimize any risk of acquired resistance to any one oil, and it is unlikely that bacteria will be resistant at the same time to the other oils in the mix. This is one of the reasons why the Authors strongly advise using a powerful synergistic mix of oils in any treatment.

Table 4.1 Antibacterial spectrum of *Satureia montana* on some species and strains resistant to antibiotics (after Pellecuer et al 1976)

Bacteria tested	Origin of bacteria	Type of resistance	Active dose in mg/ml
Staphylococcus aureus	IP 6454	penicillin	0.250
Staphylococcus aureus	IP 6455	penicillin streptomycin tetracycline	0.250
Staphylococcus aureus	IP 52149	penicillin streptomycin tetracycline	0.250
Staphylococcus aureus	IP 52150	streptomycin	0.250
Sarcina lutea	natural	100γ of tetracycline	0.062
Bacillus subtilis	natural	streptomycin	0.250
Escherichia coli	natural	ampicillin colomycin	0.250
Staphylococcus pathogen	natural no. 1		0.062
Staphylococcus pathogen	natural no. 2	Resistant to 500γ of	0.062
Staphylococcus pathogen	natural no. 3	virginiamycin	0.062
Staphylococcus pathogen	natural no. 5		0.125
Staphylococcus pathogen	natural no. 8		0.250
Staphylococcus pathogen	natural no. 10		0.125

Moreover this risk is further reduced, even though the metabolism of the microbe changes continually, because essential oils are natural products and their composition varies with each fresh batch.

Testing for antiseptic and antibacterial activity

Tests have been carried out on the antiseptic and antibacterial properties of essential oils for more than a century. Two of the first were Chamberland's in 1887, concerning the activity of cinnamon oils, angelica and geranium (Valnet 1980 p. 33), and Koch's 1881 investigation of turpentine with respect to the anthrax bacillus. Since then the antiseptic and bactericidal powers of well known natural essential oils have been tested many times in laboratories across the world using the aromatogram technique (see below). This is a recognized standard test and the results obtained are repeatable (provided the essential oils themselves are repeatable) and are universally acceptable: it is virtually the same as the antibiogram test.

Tests proving the antiseptic effects of essential oils are numerous, and the following are cited as examples: Belaiche (1985a,b), Beylier (1979), Bonnaure (1919), Carson & Riley (1993), Carson et al (1995), Cavel (1918), Chamberland (1887), Courment, Morel & Bay (1938), Deans & Svoboda (1988), Deans & Svoboda (1990a,b), Gattefossé (1919, 1932), Gildemeister & Hoffmann (1956), Hinou, Harvala & Hinou (1989), Holland (1941), Jalsenjak, Pelinjak & Kustrak (1987), Jasper, Maruzella & Laurence Liguori (1958), Jasper et al (1958), Juven et al (1994), Kienholz (1959), Knobloch et al (1989), Low, Rowal & Griffin (1974), Martindale (1910), Moleyar & Narasimham (1992), Onawunmi (1988, 1989), Onawunmi & Ogunlana (1986), Onawunmi, Yisak & Ogunlana (1984), Pellecuer, Allegrini & De Buochberg (1974), Pellecuer et al (1975, 1976), Raharivelomanana et al (1989), Ramanoelina et al (1987), Ritzerfeld (1959), Shemesh & Mayo (1991), Tukioka (1927) and Yousef & Tawil (1980).

There is a wide variation in the antiseptic and bactericidal effects between different individual essential oils as shown by their phenol coefficients (Martindale 1910, Poucher 1936, Rideal, Sciver & Richardson 1930). This is illustrated in Table 4.2.

Table 4.2 The phenol coefficients of some essential oils and their isolated compounds

Whole essential oil	Compound	Phenol coefficient
Aniseed		0.4
Peppermint		0.7
	menthol	0.9
Lavender		1.6
Lemon (Java)		2.2
	cinnamaldehyde	3.0
	citral	5.2
	camphor	6.2
Clove		8.0
	eugenol	8.6
Fennel		13.0
Thyme		13.2
	thymol	20.0
	synthetic chlorothymol	75.0

From Schilcher 1985, p. 221, reprinted by permission of Kluwer Academic Publishers. The phenol coefficient gives an indication of the antiseptic strength or weakness of a substance compared with that of phenol (which has a coefficient of 1.0).

It is well known that essential oils provide a very pleasant and effective means of disinfecting the air in an enclosed area (Kellner & Kober 1954, 1955, 1956) and are therefore ideal for use in sick rooms, burns units, reception areas, waiting rooms, etc. A test describing the use of a blend of pine, thyme, peppermint, lavender, rosemary, clove and cinnamon essential oils for the bacteriological purification of the air concluded that 'the atmospheric dispersion of the prepared liquid brought about a very marked disinfection of the air, as demonstrated by the considerable reduction in the number of pre-existing micro-organisms, some types being destroyed completely' (Valnet 1980 pp. 36–38).

Poucher (1936) quotes the results of an early investigation of the effect of 33 essential oils and phenol on beef tea which had been infected with water taken from a sewage tank. The trial referred to was originally carried out by Cavel (1918) and a selection from the results is shown in Table 4.3. The figures denote the dilution per 1000 at which the oils no longer showed effective antiseptic action, hence the lower the figure the greater the antiseptic power. It is interesting to note that

Table 4.3 Antiseptic effect of essential oils in sewage water

Essential oil	Dilution
Thyme	0.70
Origanum	1.00
Orange (sweet)	1.20
Verbena	1.60
Cassia	1.70
Rose	1.80
Clove	2.00
Eucalyptus	2.50
Peppermint	2.70
Vetiver	2.25
Gaultheria	3.00
Palmarosa	3.10
Spikenard	3.50
Star anise	3.70
Cinnamon (Ceylon)	4.00
Anise	4.20
Rosemary	4.30
Cumin	4.50
Neroli	4.75
Lavender	5.00
Melissa	5.20
Ylang ylang	5.60
Phenol	5.60
Fennel (sweet)	6.40
Lemon	7.00
Angelica	10.00
Patchouli	15.00

From Poucher 1936, vol.2, p. 361 with permission.

phenol (the standard for comparison) appears fairly low in the table.

Methicillin resistant *Staphylococcus aureus* (MRSA)

Recent experience has indicated that essential oils have an important part to play in dealing with this resistant bacterium. At a presentation to the Royal Society of Medicine it was stated by Michael Smith, pathologist, that several essential oils (including *Ormenis mixta, Origanum vulgare, Thymus vulgaris* ct. thymol, *Lavandula* x *intermedia* 'Super', *Cupressus sempervirens, Mentha* x *piperita, Ravensara aromatica, Juniperus communis* (unspecified), *Citrus limon, Cymbopogon martinii, Eucalyptus globulus, Eucalyptus smithii*) were effective against MRSA (cited in Buckle 1997 p. 125). Later, Sherry et al (2001) used a blend of phytochemicals (*Eucalyptus globulus, Melaleuca alternifolia, Thymus* species, *Syzygium aromaticum*, citrus extracts and bioethanol) successfully in two cases to treat methicillin resistant *Staphylococcus aureus*; it was reported that there was no subsequent recurrence of infection.

Antibiogram and aromatogram

An antibiogram can test the validity of an antibiotic agent for the treatment of, say, a chest infection. A sample of sputum is taken and a culture grown in a dish. The antibiotic is introduced into the centre of the culture and its activity against the offending micro-organism may be measured by the appearance of a clear 'killing zone'. The diameter of this clear area indicates the power of the antibiotic: the greater the diameter, the greater the effectiveness of the antibiotic agent. The aromatogram is carried out in exactly the same way as the antibiogram, except essential oil is used instead of an antibiotic. Both methods are subject to the proviso that *in vitro* activity is not always echoed *in vivo*, which is modified by absorption, metabolism, bioavailability, etc. Finding the most effective and appropriate essential oil to counteract any particular germ can be a lengthy undertaking: if there were no previous experience to go on it would be necessary to test all the oils in the therapist's repertory, perhaps 60 or more. It goes without saying that the essential oils used in the treatment should be from the same batch as the sample tested, because essential oils from different sources can vary in chemical composition. This testing procedure has confirmed the antiseptic powers of many oils but at the same time has revealed in some other oils antiseptic powers which were hitherto unsuspected, or at least underrated. At one time in aromatherapy, fennel (*Foeniculum vulgare* var. *dulce*) was known only for being an appetite stimulant, nutmeg (*Myristica fragrans*) as a stomachic and tarragon (*Artemisia dracunculus*) as an antispasmodic, but now the antiseptic qualities of these oils are also recognized. These tests allow essential oils to be used precisely and effectively, without the consequences which sometimes follow the use of antibiotics (such as tiredness, lowered immune system activity and destruction of intestinal flora). Because of the huge number of aromatogram results which have now been published, it is possible to list the major essential oils by their antimicrobial properties (Roulier 1990 p. 55), see Table 4.4.

OTHER PROPERTIES

Analgesic

Many essential oils have analgesic properties to some degree and there seems to be no single reason why they do, just as pain itself is complicated. It is thought that the effect is partly due to the antiinflammatory, circulatory and detoxifying effects of some oils and to the anaesthetic effect of others. The phenol eugenol found in the oil of clove is well known for its use in calming dental pain, wintergreen oil (containing methyl salicylate, an ester) has traditionally been used in rubs for muscle pain, and menthol has been used specifically for headaches. On the skin, oils rich in terpenes have an analgesic effect, especially those containing *p*-cymene (Franchomme & Pénoël 2001 p. 99). Many aromatherapists report that the oil of *Melaleuca alternifolia* has this effect. Azulene and chamazulene (found in the chamomiles) also can be used on the skin. Some essential oils have a universal sedative or soporific action leading to an easing of pain, e.g. *Chamaemelum nobile, Cananga odorata, Citrus reticulata* (fol.) (Rossi et al 1988), *Citrus bergamia* (per. and fol.) (Franchomme & Pénoël 2001 p. 99). According to Roulier (1990), the analgesic and

Case study 4.2a   Analgesic – Jill Baxter – *nurse aromatherapist, UK*

Pain relief

Patient assessment

Four years ago, when J's wart first needed surgery, it was found to be benign. Following that, a severe injury against the angle of a piece of furniture was thought to trigger malignant growths. His main problem area was on the sciatic nerve, left hand side. He had had several operations and the deep creases, puckering and scar tissue on the site meant that surgeons were against further incisions – they said there is little that can be done, apart from giving him morphia for the pain.

When he was first seen by the aromatherapist he moved very stiffly indeed, lying on the couch most awkwardly.

Intervention

J's back, shoulders, legs and feet were massaged with *Lavandula angustifolia* [lavender] and *Rosmarinus officinalis* [rosemary] in a blend of wheatgerm and grapeseed oil, neat lavender being applied freely afterwards to the site of the wound.

Outcome

J said he would never have believed the measure of relief he has found since having aromatherapy treatments – immediate relief from constant aching, a greater range of movement and a good night's sleep. He has also noticed that his skin is more supple.

---

antalgic essential oils are: white birch, chamomile, frankincense, wintergreen, clove, lavender, mint (common names only given).

A study into the use of complementary therapies to help treat patients suffering chronic pain was carried out at Monklands Hospital in Scotland. More than 75% of patients referred by local GPs suffering from a range of complaints (e.g. back or shoulder pain, long-term problems, premenstrual tension, depression, anxiety or mood swings) found that such therapies helped to provide short-term relief of their symptoms. The patients were treated with essential oils, reflexology or acupuncture during an 8-week trial (Anderson 1998). (See Appendix B.9 for a list of effective oils.)

Antifungal

Many essential oils have been reported as having an antifungal effect (Table 4.5) and many investigations have taken place, some more than half a century ago (Schmidt 1936) showing the fungicidal and fungistatic effects of cinnamon, clove, fennel and thyme; these were active against *Candida albicans*, *Sporotrichon* and *Trichophyton* species (Gildemeister & Hoffmann 1956 p. 140). The fungicidal activity of the oil of *Chamomilla recutita* and its components, including chamazulene and (–)-α-bisabolol, has been well investigated and shown to be effective against *Trichophyton rubrum*,

T. mentagrophytes, T. tonsurans, T. quinckeanum and *Microsporum canis* in concentrations of 200 mg/ml (Janssen et al 1984, 1986, Szalontai, Verzar-Petri & Florian 1976, 1977, Szalontai et al 1975a,b). *Satureia montana* also has been found to be active against *Candida* (Pellecuer et al 1975). A general review of some essential oils with antifungal properties has been carried out (Pellecuer et al 1976) and in other trials a number of compounds found in essential oils, especially the aldehydes and esters, are effective against various fungi, including *Candida* infection (Larrondo & Calvo 1991, Maruzella 1961, Thompson & Cannon 1986). The oil of *Melaleuca alternifolia* has been investigated in vaginal infection with *Candida* and has been found to be effective (Belaiche 1985c, Pena 1962, Shemesh & Mayo 1991). Rosemary, savory and thyme also have antifungal properties (Pellecuer, Roussel & Andary 1973) and *Ocimum basilicum* has both antifungal and insect-repelling properties (Dube, Upadhyay & Tripath 1989).

Antiinflammatory

The oils of *Lavandula angustifolia* and *Chamomilla recutita* are widely used to soothe minor inflammations such as sunburn, small burns and insect bites, and plenty of people can testify to their effectiveness in this respect. Jakovlev, Isaac & Flaskamp (1983) showed the antiinflammatory

Table 4.4   Antibacterial effects of essential oils

Latin name	Common name	Bacillus megaterium	Bacillus mycoides	Bacillus pumilis	Bacillus subtilis	Bacterioides fragilis	Clostridium perfringens	Clostridium sporogenes	Corynebacterium diphtheriae	Diplococcus pneumoniae	Enterobacter aerogenes	Enterobacter cloaceae	Enterococci	Escherichia coli	Helicobacter pylori	Klebsiella species	Klebsiella ozonae	Klebsiella pneumoniae	Lactobacillus plantarum	Mycobacterium phlei	Mycobacterium tuberculosis
Abies balsamea	balsam fir needle													x							
Artemisia dracunculus	tarragon									x			x	x		x					
Boswellia carteri	frankincense				xx									x						x	
Carum carvi	caraway										xx			x		x					
Chamaemelum nobile	Roman chamomile																				
Cinnamomum verum (cort.)	cinnamon bark									xxx			xxx	xxx		xxx					
Cistus ladaniferus	labdanum													x							
Citrus aurantium var. amara (flos)	neroli												x	x		x					
Citrus aurantium var. amara (fol.)	petitgrain									x			x	x		x					
Citrus bergamia (per.)	bergamot											x				x					
Citrus limon (per.)	lemon									x			x	x							x
Coriandrum sativum (fruct.)	coriander									x	x			x		xx					
Cupressus sempervirens	cypress													x							x
Cymbopogon citratus	lemongrass																				
Cymbopogon martinii	palmarosa																				
Eucalyptus citriodora	lemon scented gum	x												xx							
Eucalyptus dives	broad leaved peppermint													xx							
Eucalyptus globulus	Tasmanian blue gum									xxx			x	xx		xx					
Eucalyptus radiata	narrow leaved peppermint													xx							
Eucalyptus smithii	gully gum																				
Eucarya spicata	Australian sandalwood																				
Foeniculum vulgare var. dulce (fruct.)	fennel									x				x							
Helichrysum angustifolium	everlasting											x		x				x			
Hyssopus officinalis	hyssop							xx													xxx

Moraxella species	MRSA	Neisseria catarrhalis	Neisseria gonorrhoeae	Neisseria meningitidis	Proteus species	Propionibacterium acnes	Pseudomonas aeruginosa	Salmonella species	Salmonella pullorum	Salmonella typhi	Salmonella typhimurium	Sarcina species	Shigella sonnet	Staphylococcus species	Staphylococcus albus	Staphylococcus aureus	Staphylococcus epidermidis	Staphylococcus faecalis	Streptococcus species	Streptococcus faecalis	Streptococcus beta-haemolytic	Vibrio cholerae	Vibrio parahaemolyticus	Yersinia enterocolitica
														x										
							X		X						x	x					x			x
												x				x	x							
					xx				x							xx								
																x								
					xxx		xx		xxx						xxx	xxx			xx	xxx				xx
																x								
					x																x			
															x	xx					x			
									x							x			xx					
x				x												x								
					x				x							x								xx
x																x					x			
																						x		
x																xx								
																xx								
x					xx				x						xx	xx		x			?			
							x									x								
x																								
																xxx								
					x				x							x								
							x									x	x							
															x	x			x		x			

Table 4.4 Antibacterial effects of essential oils (*cont'd*)

Latin name	Common name	Bacillus megaterium	Bacillus mycoides	Bacillus pumilis	Bacillus subtilis	Bacterioides fragilis	Clostridium perfringens	Clostridium sporogenes	Corynebacterium diphtheriae	Diplococcus pneumoniae	Enterobacter aerogenes	Enterobacter cloaceae	Enterococci	Escherichia coli	Helicobacter pylori	Klebsiella species	Klebsiella ozonae	Klebsiella pneumoniae	Lactobacillus plantarum	Mycobacterium phlei	Mycobacterium tuberculosis
Laurus nobilis	bay																				
Lavandula angustifolia	lavender								x	xx	xx		xx	xx		xx					
Leptospermum scoparium	manuka																				
Matricaria recutita	German chamomile																				
Melaleuca alternifolia	tea tree					x	xx	xx	xx	xx	x			xx		x					
Melaleuca leucadendron	cajuput									xxx			xx	xx		xxx					
Melaleuca viridiflora	niaouli												x	x							x
Mentha x piperita	peppermint				xx					x				xx		xx					xx
Myristica fragrans (sem.)	nutmeg										x			xx		xx					
Ocimum basilicum var. *album*	basil									x	x			x							
Origanum majorana	marjoram							xx		x	xx			xx		xx					
Origanum vulgare, O. heracleoticum	oregano				xx									xx							
Ormenis mixta	Moroccan chamomile													xx							
Pelargonium graveolens P. x asperum	geranium									xx	xx		x			x					
Pimpinella anisum	aniseed																				
Pinus sylvestris	pine									xx			xx	xx		xx					
Piper nigrum	black pepper													x						x	
Ravensara aromatica	ravensara																				
Rosa damascena	rose otto														x						
Rosmarinus officinalis	rosemary							xx	x	x	xx			x		xx					
Rosmarinus officinalis ct. verbenone	rosemary verbenone																				
Salvia officinalis	sage				x					x				xx			x				
Satureia hortensis	summer savory									xxx			xx	xx		xx					x
Satureia montana	winter savory									xxx			xx	xx		xx					x
Syzygium aromaticum (flos)	clove bud						xx			xxx	xx		xxx	xx		xx					xx

Moraxella species	MRSA	Neisseira catarrhalis	Neisseira gonorrhoeae	Neisseria meningitidis	Proteus species	Propionibacterium acnes	Pseudomonas aeruginosa	Salmonella species	Salmonella pullorum	Salmonella typhi	Salmonella typhimurium	Sarcina species	Shigella sonnet	Staphylococcus species	Staphylococcus albus	Staphylococcus aureus	Staphylococcus epidermidis	Staphylococcus faecalis	Streptococcus species	Streptococcus faecalis	Streptococcus beta-haemolytic	Vibrio cholerae	Vibrio parahaemolyticus	Yersinia enterocolitica
											x					x							x	
x	x				x				x						x	xx				xx	xxx		x	
																x								
																x								
	x		x		x	x	xx			xxx				x		xx	x							
					xx									xx		xx				x				
					x											xx				x		x		
	x				xx		xx		xx							xx		x		x				xx
			x						x															x
							x		x							x				x				x
					xx		x		xx							xx								xx
	x						xx				xx					xx								
	x																							
					x		x		xx					xx		x					xx			xx
								x						x		x				xx		x	x	
					xx									xx		xx					xx			
									x										x	x				x
	xx																							x
					x				x					x		x				xx	x	x		
													x				x							
					x		x	x	x				x			xx			x	x	x			
					x		xx		xx						xxx	xxx				x	xxx			xx
					x		xx		xx						xxx	xxx				xxx	xxx			xx
	x				xx		xx		xx						xxx	xx				x	xx			xx

Table 4.4   Antibacterial effects of essential oils (*cont'd*)

Latin name	Common name	Bacillus megaterium	Bacillus mycoides	Bacillus pumilis	Bacillus subtilis	Bacterioides fragilis	Clostridium perfringens	Clostridium sporogenes	Corynebacterium diphtheriae	Diplococcus pneumoniae	Enterobacter aerogenes	Enterobacter cloaceae	Enterococci	Escherichia coli	Helicobacter pylori	Klebsiella species	Klebsiella ozonae	Klebsiella pneumoniae	Lactobacillus plantarum	Mycobacterium phlei	Mycobacterium tuberculosis
Tagetes patula, Tagetes minuta	taget, French marigold		x	x	x									x							
Thymus capitatus	Spanish oregano									xxx			xxx	xxx		xxx					
Thymus serpyllum	wild thyme									x			x	x		x					
Thymus mastichina	Spanish marjoram																				xx
Thymus vulgaris ct. thymol	thyme									xxx	xxx		xxx	xxx		xxx					

Not all the oils in this table have been tested for all the bacteria shown. References used include:

Belaiche P 1979 Traite de Phytotherapie et d'Aromatherapie. 3 vols. Maloine, Paris

Deans S G, Ritchie G A 1987 Antibacterial properties of plant essential oils. International Journal of Food Microbiology 5: 165–180

Deans S G, Svoboda K P 1988 Antibacterial activity of French tarragon [*Artemisia dracunculus* L] essential oil and its constituents during ontogeny. Journal of Horticultural Science 63: 503–508

Deans S G, Svoboda K P 1989 Antibacterial activity of summer savory [*Satureia hortensis* L] essential oil and its constituents. Journal of Horticultural Science 64: 205–211

Franchomme P, Pénoël D 2001 L'aromatherapie exactement. Jollois, Limoges

Mentioned as antibacterial but unspecified:

Illicium verum	star anise
Inula helenium	elecampane
Melissa officinalis	lemon balm
Mentha arvensis	cornmint
Terebinth	turpentine
Pogostemon patchouli	patchouli

Moraxella species	MRSA	Neisseria catarrhalis	Neisseria gonorrhoeae	Neisseria meningitidis	Proteus species	Propionibacterium acnes	Pseudomonas aeruginosa	Salmonella species	Salmonella pullorum	Salmonella typhi	Salmonella typhimurium	Sarcina species	Shigella sonnet	Staphylococcus species	Staphylococcus albus	Staphylococcus aureus	Staphylococcus epidermidis	Staphylococcus faecalis	Streptococcus species	Streptococcus faecalis	Streptococcus beta–haemolytic	Vibrio cholerae	Vibrio parahaemolyticus	Yersinia enterocolitica
										x					x	x								
			xxx												xxx	xxx				xx				
			x													x				xx				
x			xxx		x		xxx		xx	xxx					xxx	xxx			xxx	xxx				

Case study 4.2b   Analgesic – R.A.H. *aromatherapist, UK*

Back pain

Patient assessment

Mr H had acute back pain in July after lifting heavy weights at work. He was treated with conventional drugs by his GP and returned to work fairly quickly after using the analgesics prescribed. However, the pain recurred and he was off sick from work in September, again not benefiting from the conventional treatment, which this time consisted of analgesics, antiinflammatory drugs and physiotherapy. He developed an allergy to the anti-inflammatory drug Ibuprofen, but this was detected before any harm was done. Several of the doctors in the practice had been called out to administer analgesia, by tablet, injection or suppository. Obviously, this could not go on and Mr H was admitted to hospital over Christmas with chronic back pain.

It was decided to see whether aromatherapy could bring him some relief.

Intervention

The essential oils selected were:

- 3 drops *Chamaemelum nobile* [Roman chamomile]
- 2 drops *Lavandula angustifolia* [lavender]
- 1 drop *Origanum majorana* [sweet marjoram] in 10 ml grapeseed oil

20–23 December: Having given him a full back massage, special attention was given to his lower legs and feet, as it had been observed how rigid his feet were, with virtually no flexibility in his ankles. He was taught some foot exercises, his lower extremities were massaged and counselling was given to him. That night he slept very well without sedation.

26–29 December: Massaged as before. Mr H was walking better during day and had less pain.

As the aromatherapist was to be off duty for several nights, a lotion containing the same essential oils was prepared for him so that the other night nurses could stroke this on his back every night. He promised to continue his foot exercises.

7–11 January: Mr H's back and feet were massaged as before by the aromatherapist, with excellent effect. He was confident and talking about the possibility of going on holiday. He had been to physiotherapy and had used the exercise bike, but disliked it (legs aching); however, he had continued with his leg and foot exercises.

Outcome

On the 29th January Mr H said he was completely pain free.

Case study 4.3   Antifungal – A Barker – *aromatologist, UK*

Candida albicans

Patient assessment

In July 1990 Mrs F (aged 40) was referred to a consultant, suffering from a continuous urinary tract infection (with inflammation, incontinence and pain) which antibiotics failed to control. She was given intermittent self-catheterization (ISC) and by April 1992 major surgery (removal of the bladder) was considered.

Mrs F also developed a vaginal inflammation – thrush – and by September 1992, she was unable to perform the ISC due to this, and a cystectomy was again discussed.

The sister suggested to the consultant that aromatherapy be tried and the agreed consultation took place in March 1993 with the continence advisor and Mrs F's husband also present.

Mrs F complained of constant pain and swelling of the abdomen (caused by having to have residual catheterization using microcatheters). It was apparent that her vagina was the consistency of 'raw liver' and she suffered frequent discharges, thus intercourse had been impossible. The husband was asked to attend with her so that he could be checked over, as this side of the partnership, although important, is often overlooked – Mrs F had had this recurrent form of *Candida* for several years and the relationship was beginning to suffer; credit was due to the couple for the level of understanding shared.

Intervention

The couple's normal diet plan for an average week was looked at and gradual changes – over a period of time, so as not to add to the stress of the situation – were arranged to help the body balance itself.

A colonic massage with essential oils was decided upon, to benefit the swelling, pain and infection:

- *Citrus bergamia* (per.) [bergamot]
- *Eucalyptus globulus* [blue gum]
- *Melaleuca alternifolia* [tea tree]
- *Melaleuca viridiflora* [niaouli]

These were mixed together in equal quantities and a 15-minute massage given. At the first treatment a high concentration of 2.5 ml of the essential oils was put into 5 ml grapeseed oil – a 50% dilution.

Mr F was taught how to perform a very simple abdominal massage in a clockwise direction, to be carried out once daily to aid Mrs F's constipation. This was a good morale booster for him, as he had previously felt helpless – and he now became part of her recovery process. For his contribution, he was given a 3% mix of:

Zingiber officinale (antispasmodic and laxative)
Foeniculum vulgare var. *dulce* (appetite stimulant, laxative and circulation stimulant)
Mentha x *piperita* (analgesic, antiinflammatory and stomachic)

Treatment with live yogurt and essential oils was discussed and as the client's vagina was too swollen to use a tampon soaked in this mix, it was decided to pour the yogurt mixture into the vagina, the client being propped up, legs raised, to allow the mix to penetrate. Although messy and difficult, the swelling had reduced enough after several days to insert a tampon, changing it morning and night.

Colonic massage treatment at the hospital involved using different strengths of essential oil; for 3 days a dilution of 5 drops in 5 ml was used. Several weekly treatments followed, using only 1 drop of the synergistic blend in 5 ml grapeseed oil.

Treatment at home involved:

- Tea made with marigold flowers plus 1 drop bergamot 3 times a day for 3 weeks
- 6 acidopholus tablets daily
- Essential oils for the bath
- Abdomen massage oil – 3% mix for Mr F to use as above
- 10 ml yogurt with 5 drops tea tree – used as above

Outcome

By the end of the month Mrs F was already feeling benefits from the treatment and the yogurt treatment was changed to oral yogurt tablets.

By June, the abdominal swelling was going down.

By the end of July the urinary tract was almost clear. Mrs F was on 3 acidopholus tablets daily, marigold tea and occasional yogurt with tea tree internally.

Abdomen massage was still carried out by her husband once or twice a week with a reduced concentration of oils to 1.5%.

The couple's relationship is now close once more, partially due to Mr F's eagerness to help.

effect of yarrow, chamomile containing chamazulene, arnica flower and turpentine. Azulenes are sesquiterpene derivatives and have the empirical formula $C_{15}H_{18}$. While chamazulene and (–)-α-bisabolol found in chamomile oils are antiinflammatory agents (Weiss 1988 p. 24), other azulenes which may be added to anti-inflammatory preparations are not so effective, e.g. guaiazulene (manufactured from guaiol) and elemazulene (from elemol). Also (+)-α-bisabolol and synthetic (–)-α-bisabolol are not as effective as the natural form. [There do appear to be differences in effect between natural occurring and synthesized molecules: synthetic myristicin does not produce hallucinations (D'Arcy 1993), unlike natural myristicin extracted from nutmeg oil (in which it is present at 4%)].

Otitis media is an infectious and inflammatory disease which may lead to impairment of hearing; over a 2 year period Kang Mok Yoo, an otolaryngologist in S. Korea, used aromatherapy to treat 200 patients suffering from chronic mucoid otitis media with effusion and found that the success rate was 90% achieved in just 13 days on average (personal communication). See Table 4.6 and Appendix B.9.

Antipruritic

Lavender and tea tree (both unspecified) were diluted in Jojoba and sweet almond oils employed

---

Case study 4.4 Antiinflammatory – L Cooke – *aromatherapist, UK*

Gangrene

Client assessment
Mr A developed gangrene on the toes of his left foot – and the whole area was inflamed. There was also a large patch on his shin and a smaller area below his knee. As the gangrene was in its acute stage, Mr A wanted to see an aromatherapist that he knew, to try anything she may suggest, before it reached the stage of needing amputation. The consultant was in agreement, as there was nothing the hospital could do except amputation.

Intervention
To reduce the inflammation, the following oils were applied in a cold compress to each area and left for 60 minutes:

- 8 drops *Eucalyptus globulus* [blue gum] – antiinflammatory, bactericidal, rubifacient
- 8 drops *Lavandula angustifolia* [lavender] – analgesic, antibacterial, antiinflammatory, cicatrizant
- 150 ml cold water

The three pieces of cotton – the sizes of the areas to be treated – were first wetted (and squeezed well) in cold water, before immersing in this well stirred blend – making sure all the liquid was absorbed. Each was squeezed lightly to remove excess liquid before applying to the areas concerned.

The foot and leg were then massaged using the following blend:

- 16 drops *Juniperus communis* fruct. [juniper berry] – analgesic, depurative
- 16 drops *Pelargonium graveolens* [geranium] – analgesic, antibacterial, antiinfectious, antiinflammatory, cicatrizant, haemostatic
- 16 drops *Eucalyptus globulus* – as above
- 75 ml carrier lotion
- 25 ml hypericum

Mr A was given the rest of the blend to apply at home twice a day.

Outcome
The inflammation died down quickly and after several days the dark patches on his leg formed a hard scaly skin, which subsequently flaked off.

The recovery was put down to the fact that the gangrene was treated in its acute stage.

Two and a half years later Mr A had an accident and the patches had reappeared on the same three areas as before. He had refused to go into hospital, sending instead for the aromatherapist, who repeated the treatment above. In between visits, the district nurse was given permission to apply the lotion on every visit.

The leg made a complete recovery once again.

Table 4.5 Antifungal effects of essential oils

Latin name	Common name	General antifungal properties*	Acinetobacter calcoacetica	Aspergillus species	Aspergillus flavus	Aspergillus fumigatus	Aspergillus nidulans	Aspergillus niger	Aspergillus ochraceous	Aspergillus parasiticus	Candida species	Candida albicans	Candida glabrata	Chaetomium species	Clamidia sporogenes	Clostridium perfringens	Colletotrichum gloeosporioides	Cryptococcus neoformans	Epidermophyton species	Fusarium species	Fusarium oxysporum	Fusarium moniliforme	Listeria monocytogenes	Malassezia furfur
Artemisia dracunculus	tarragon											X												
Cinnamomum verum (cort)	cinnamon bark				X			X		X		XX	X					X						
Cinnamomum verum (fol.)	cinnamon leaf				X			X				X	X											
Cistus ladaniferus	labdanum											X												
Citrus aurantifolia (per.)	lime			X																X				
Citrus aurantium var. amara (fol.)	petitgrain bigarade	X										XXX												
Citrus aurantium var. amara (flos)	neroli	X																						
Citrus aurantium var. amara (per.)	bitter orange			X																X				
Citrus aurantium var. sinensis (per.)	sweet orange			X	X			X		X														
Coriandrum sativum	coriander									X														
Cuminum cyminum (fruct.)	cumin				X			X		X														
Cymbopogon martinii	palmarosa			X							X													
Cymbopogon citratus	lemongrass			X							X													
Ellettaria cardamomum	cardamom				X				X	X														
Eucalyptus citriodora	lemon scented gum	X						X				X												
Eucalyptus dives	broad leaved peppermint							X				X												
Eucalyptus globulus	Tasmanian blue gum											X												
Eucalyptus radiata	narrow leaved peppermint							X				X												
Eucaria spicata	Australian sandalwood											XXX												
Foeniculum vulgare var. dulce	fennel											X												
Hyssopus officinalis	hyssop					X																		

Moraxella species	Mycobacterium fortuitum	Mycobacterium smegmatis	Microsporum audounii	Microsporum canis	Microsporum cookei	Microsporum gypseum	Mucor species	Nigrospora oryzae	Penicillium species	Penicillium chrysogenum	Pitysporum ovale	Rhizopus species	Saccharomyces cereviciae	Sclerotium rolfsii	Sporotrichium species	Tinea capitis	Tinea pedis	Trichoderma viride	Trichophyton species	Trichophyton beigelii	Trichophyton mentagrophytes	Trichophyton quinckeanum	Trichophyton rubrum	Trichophyton souclanense	Trychophyton tonsurans	Trichophyton violaceum	Trichothecium roseum	Zygorrhynchus species
				X											X				X		X		X					
				X																	X		X					
												X																
												X																
							X																X			X		
							X																X			X		
									X																			
	X												X								X							X
															X					X								

Table 4.5   Antifungal effects of essential oils (*cont'd*)

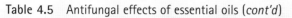

Latin name	Common name	General antifungal properties*	Acinetobacter calcoacetica	Aspergillus species	Aspergillus flavus	Aspergillus fumigatus	Aspergillus nidulans	Aspergillus niger	Aspergillus ochraceous	Aspergillus parasiticus	Candida species	Candida albicans	Candida glabrata	Chaetomium species	Clamidia sporogenes	Clostridium perfringens	Colletotrichum gloeosporioides	Cryptococcus neoformans	Epidermophyton species	Fusarium species	Fusarium oxysporum	Fusarium moniliforme	Listeria monocytogenes	Malassezia furfur
Illicium verum	star anise	X																						
Inula helenium	elecampane	X																	X					
Kunzea ericoides	kanuka																							
Lavandula angustifolia	lavender											XX			XX									
Lavandula x intermedia 'Super'	lavandin																							
Leptospermum scoparium	manuka											X												
Matricaria recutita	German chamomile																							
Melaleuca alternifolia	tea tree	X						XX				XX					X						X	
Melaleuca leucadendron	cajuput	X										XX												
Melaleuca viridiflora	niaouli							X																
Melissa officinalis	lemon balm	X																						
Mentha arvensis	cornmint	X																						
Mentha x piperita	peppermint											X												
Mentha spicata	spearmint																							X
Myrtus communis	myrtle	X						X				X												
Nardostachys jatamansi	spikenard	X		X		X	X														X	X		
Nepeta cataria	catnep							XX				XX												
Ocimum basilicum	basil	X		X		X	X		X					X							X	X		
Origanum heracleoticum	Greek oregano	X						XX				XX												XX
Origanum majorana	sweet marjoram	X																						
Pelargonium graveolens	geranium											?					X							
Pelargonium asperum	geranium											X												
Pinus sylvestris	pine											XX												
Pogostemon patchouli	patchouli	X																	X					
Rosmarinus officinalis	rosemary									X		X											X	

Moraxella species	Mycobacterium fortuitum	Mycobacterium smegmatis	Microsporum audounii	Microsporum canis	Microsporum cookei	Microsporum gypseum	Mucor species	Nigrospora oryzae	,Penicillium species	Penicillium chrysogenum	Pitysporum ovale	Rhizopus species	Saccharomyces cereviciae	Sclerotium rolfsii	Sporotrichium species	Tinea capitis	Tinea pedis	Trichoderma viride	Trichophyton species	Trichophyton beigelii	Trichophyton mentagrophytes	Trichophyton quinckeanum	Trichophyton rubrum	Trichophyton souclanense	Trychophyton tonsurans	Trichophyton violaceum	Trichothecium roseum	Zygorrhynchus species
					X													X		X						X		
																						X						
																X												
																X												
															X	X												
				X																X	X	X		X				
		X									X					X		X										
																											X	
																			X			X						
																	X											
								X		X																		
										X				X														
																			XX			XX						
				X		X												X		X		X	X		X			
																						X						

Table 4.5 Antifungal effects of essential oils (*cont'd*)

Latin name	Common name	General antifungal properties*	Acinetobacter calcoacetica	Aspergillus species	Aspergillus flavus	Aspergillus fumigatus	Aspergillus nidulans	Aspergillus niger	Aspergillus ochraceous	Aspergillus parasiticus	Candida species	Candida albicans	Candida glabrata	Chaetomium species	Clamidia sporogenes	Clostridium perfringens	Colletotrichum gloeosporioides	Cryptococcus neoformans	Epidermophyton species	Fusarium species	Fusarium oxysporum	Fusarium moniliforme	Listeria monocytogenes	Malassezia furfur
Rosmarinus officinalis ct. verbenone	rosemary verbenone											X												
Salvia officinalis	sage		X									X			X			X						
Satureia montana S. hortensis	winter savory	X										X												
Syzygium aromaticum (flos)	clove bud							XX	XX	XX		XX												
Tagetes glandulifera, T. patula	marigold							X																
Thymus capitatus	Spanish oregano											XXX												
Thymus mastichina	Spanish marjoram											X												
Thymus serpyllum	wild thyme											X												
Thymus vulgaris (population)	thyme	X										X												
Thymus vulgaris ct. linalool, geraniol	sweet thyme											X												
Thymus vulgaris ct. thymol, carvacrol	thyme	X								X		XXX						X						XX
Santalum spicatum	Australian sandalwood							X																

* Oils mentioned as having antifungal properties but without mention of a specific fungus

Moraxella species	Mycobacterium fortuitum	Mycobacterium smegmatis	Microsporum audouinii	Microsporum canis	Microsporum cookei	Microsporum gypseum	Mucor species	Nigrospora oryzae	Penicillium species	Penicillium chrysogenum	Pitysporum ovale	Rhizopus species	Saccharomyces cerevisiae	Sclerotium rolfsii	Sporotrichium species	Tinea capitis	Tinea pedis	Trichoderma viride	Trichophyton species	Trichophyton beigelii	Trichophyton mentagrophytes	Trichophyton quinckeanum	Trichophyton rubrum	Trichophyton souclanense	Trychophyton tonsurans	Trichophyton violaceum	Trichothecium roseum	Zygorrhynchus species
	X																											
X																												
															X				X									
																	X	X										
															X				X									
															X				X									

Table 4.6   Antiinflammatory effects of essential oils

Latin name	Common name	Unspecified	Acne	Boils	Arteritis	Arthritis	Blepharitis	Bronchitis	Bursitis	Cellulitis	Colitis	Coronaritis	Cystitis	Dermatitis	Eczema	Emphysema	Enterocolitis	Gall bladder inflammation	Gastritis
Achillea millefolium	yarrow																		
Acorus calamus	sweet flag							x					x						x
Aloysia triphylla	verbena												x						
Boswellia carteri	frankincense																		
Cinnamomum verum (fol.)	cinnamon leaf																		
Cistus ladaniferus	labdanum				x									x					
Citrus aurantium var. amara (fol.)	petitgrain		x																
Citrus aurantium var. amara (per.)	orange bitter	x																	
Citrus limon (per.)	lemon			x															
"*Commiphora myrrha C. molmol*"	myrrh	x																	
Coriandrum sativum	coriander																		x
Cuminum cyminum	cumin					x											x		
"*Cymbopogon citratus C. flexuosus*"	lemongrass				x						x								
Elettaria cardamomum	cardamum	x																	
Eucalyptus citriodora	lemon scented gum					x							x	x					
Eucalyptus globulus	Tasmanian blue gum							x					x						
Eucalyptus radiata	narrow leaved peppermint		x					x											
Eucalyptus staigeriana	lemon scented ironbark	x																	
Foeniculum vulgare var. dulce	fennel												x						
Helichrysum angustifolium	everlasting					x					x			x					x
Hyssopus officinalis	hyssop							x					x			x			
"*Inula helenium I. graveolens*"	elecampane							x					x	x					
Juniperus communis (ram)	juniper twig	x																	
Lavandula angustifolia	lavender		x										x		x				
Litsea cubeba	may chang													x					
Matricaria recutita	German chamomile													x	x				x
Melaleuca alternifolia	tea tree																		
Melaleuca viridiflora	niaouli						x	x			x								
Melissa officinalis	melissa	x																	
Mentha x piperita	peppermint							x			x		x		xx		x		x
Mentha spicata	spearmint												x						
Myrtus communis	myrtle																		
Nepeta cataria	catnep					x													

Gingivitis	Gout	Hepatitis	Insect bites, stings	Laryngitis	Neuritis	Orchitis	Otitis	Pericarditis	Phlebitis	Pleurisy	Prostatitis	Rheumatism	Rheumatoid arthritis	Rhinitis rhinopharyngitis	Salpingitis	Sinusitis	Stomatitis	Tendonitis	Tonsillitis	Tracheitis	Urethritis	Vaginitis
					x						x	x										
x																						
												x										
												x										
															x		x					
													x									
x			x									x										
		x				x						x										
								x														x
				x						x							x					
							x							x								x
x																						
													x				x					
												x	x				x					
				x																x		x
			x				x		x								x					
												x										
							x										x					x
											x			x			x				x	x
		x		x													x					
											x											
												x										
x			x																			

Table 4.6 Antiinflammatory effects of essential oils (*cont'd*)

Latin name	Common name	Unspecified	Acne	Boils	Arteritis	Arthritis	Blepharitis	Bronchitis	Bursitis	Cellulitis	Colitis	Coronaritis	Cystitis	Dermatitis	Eczema	Emphysema	Enterocolitis	Gall bladder inflammation	Gastritis
Ormenis mixta (flos)	Moroccan chamomile										x		x	x	x				
Pelargonium graveolens	geranium					x					x								
Picea mariana	black spruce																		
Pinus mugo var. *pumilio*	dwarf pine	x																	
Pinus sylvestris	pine					x												x	
"*Pogostemon cablin P. patchouli*"	patchouli		x											x	x				
Ravensara aromatica	ravensara																		
"*Rosa centifolia R. damascena*"	rose														x				
Rosmarinus officinalis	rosemary												x					x	
Syzygium aromaticum (flos)	clove bud					x		x	x										
Thymus satureioides	Moroccan thyme					xx							x						
Thymus vulgaris ct. geraniol	sweet thyme					x								x					
Thymus vulgaris ct. linalool	sweet thyme							x					x		x				
Thymus vulgaris ct. thujanol-4	thujanol thyme				x									x					
"*Valeriana officinalis V. walachii*"	valerian	x																	
Zingiber cassumunar	plai, phrai					x			x		x								
	fol(ium) = leaf																		
	flos = flower																		
	caul(is) = stem																		
	cort(ex) = bark																		
	sem(en) = seed																		
	rad(ix) = root																		
	ram(unculus) = twig																		
	per(icarpium)																		
	lig(num) = wood																		
	rhiz(oma) = rhizome																		

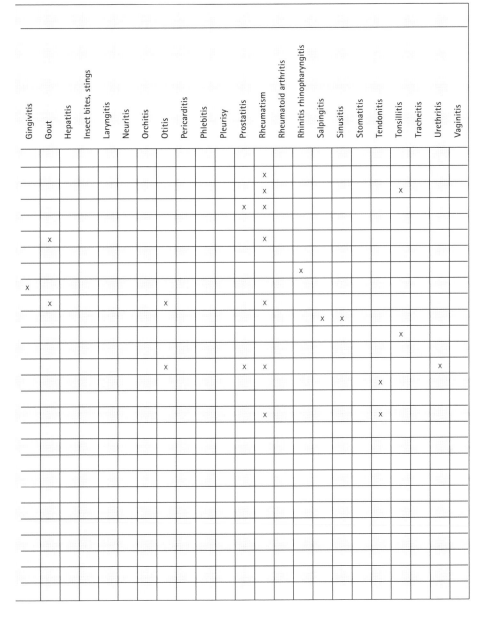

Gingivitis	Gout	Hepatitis	Insect bites, stings	Laryngitis	Neuritis	Orchitis	Otitis	Pericarditis	Phlebitis	Pleurisy	Prostatitis	Rheumatism	Rheumatoid arthritis	Rhinitis rhinopharyngitis	Salpingitis	Sinusitis	Stomatitis	Tendonitis	Tonsillitis	Tracheitis	Urethritis	Vaginitis
												X										
												X							X			
											X	X										
	X											X										
													X									
X																						
	X								X			X										
															X	X						
																			X			
									X		X	X									X	
																		X				
												X						X				

in massage in a study to determine the effects of aromatherapy on pruritus and stratum corneum hydration pruritus in patients undergoing haemodialysis. Results showed pruritus to be significantly decreased and skin hydration greatly enhanced (You-Ja Ro et al 2002).

Antitoxic

Chamomile oil has been found to be capable of inactivating toxins produced by bacteria. The amount of oil obtained by distilling 0.1 g of chamomile is sufficient to destroy, within 2 hours, three times that amount of staphylococcal toxins – the highest concentration of toxin so far found in the human organism. Streptococcal toxins proved even more sensitive (Weiss 1988 p. 26).

Antiviral

Most people practising aromatherapy have reported success in the control of Herpes viruses causing *Herpes simplex* type I, but there is no consistency in the choice of oils used (as can be seen from Table 4.7). Speaking from personal experience, we have always found the oils of *Melissa officinalis* and *Eucalyptus smithii* to be helpful for *Herpes simplex* type I. The use of melissa agrees with tests showing this plant to be antiviral (Cohen, Kucera & Herrman 1964, Herrman & Kucera 1967, Kucera & Herrman 1967). For herpes zoster (shingles) the oil of *Pelargonium graveolens* [geranium] is specifically recommended, but it is best applied at the first sign of an attack to prevent the viruses from replicating. Used early it prevents blisters from forming and damps down the pain. Although attempts have been made to treat *Herpes simplex* type II – the many oils suggested include *Melaleuca alternifolia* [tea tree] and *M. viridiflora* (Franchomme & Pénoël 2001 pp. 397, 398) – little success has been reported. Despite the lack of scientific support, many aromatherapists still feel that *Herpes simplex* type II and other viral infections such as glandular fever and influenza do respond to essential oil treatment. There is also some research to support the use in this area of black pepper oil (*Piper nigrum*) (Lembke & Deininger 1988). The oils of *Cymbopogon flexuosus* [lemongrass], *Mentha arvensis* and *Vetiveria zizanioides* [vetiver] (Pandey et al 1988) and *Eucalyptus viminalis*, *E. macarthurii* [woolly-butt] and *E. dalrympleana* appear to be effective *in vitro* and *in ovo* on two strains of influenza virus (Vichkanova, Dzhanashiya & Goryunova 1973). There have been other papers published on this topic in India, Russia and China and a Swiss patent was filed in 1979 for an antiviral preparation using essential oils.

Table 4.7 shows the essential oils which have been recommended for antiviral use. The information has been culled from many sources, which often used only the common name for the plant volatile oil.

The following oils are also mentioned as having antiviral properties, but without specific indications (Franchomme & Pénoël 2001): *Aniba rosaeodora*, *Cinnamomum camphora* var. *glavescens* Hayata, *C. cassia*, *C. zeylanicum* and *C. zeylanicum* ct. eugenol, *Cistus ladaniferus* ct. pinene and *C. ladaniferus*, *Citrus limon* (per.), *Corydothymus capitatus*, *Cymbopogon martinii* var. *motia* and *C. martinii* var. *sofia*, *Eucalyptus polybractea* ct. cryptone and *E. radiata*, *Hyssopus officinalis* var. *decumbens* and *H. officinalis*, *Lantana camara* ct. davanone, *Lavandula* x *intermedia* 'Reydovan', *Ocimum gratissimum* ct.

eugenol and *O. gratissimum* ct. thymol, *Origanum compactum* and *O. heracleoticum*, *Ravensara aromatica*, *Satureia hortensis*, *Thymus vulgaris* ct. geraniol, *T. vulgaris* ct. linalool and *T. vulgaris* ct. thujanol-4, *Trachyspermum ammi*.

Several constituents which are found naturally in a wide range of essential oils (anethole, β-caryophyllene, carvone, cinnamic aldehyde, citral, citronellol, eugenol, limonene, linalool, linalyl acetate, α-sabinene, γ-terpinene) were found to be active against *Herpes simplex* (Lembke & Deininger 1985, 1988). Thus it can be seen that there is no one molecule or even one class of molecule involved. If the oils are effective it could well be because of some property common to all of them – perhaps lipid solubility.

Balancing

Aromatherapists are well aware of the remarkable balancing powers of essential oils. At times this can cause puzzlement because of the apparently contradictory effects of the oils, but essential oils are complex mixtures of many natural constituents, some of which are stimulating and others sedative, so a single oil may demonstrate an arousing effect on one occasion and a sedative effect on another. This is known as the adaptogenic effect.

Hyssop essential oil contains the ketone pinocamphone and is said to be toxic in high doses, causing epileptic attacks in those so predisposed (Valnet 1980). Yet this oil is used in Case study 4.6 (and has been used by the authors in an epilepsy case) with beneficial effects. *Lavandula angustifolia* is well known for its sedative effect but rather less known for its ability to prevent sleep at high doses (observed and experienced by many aromatherapists). Similarly hawthorn berries (used in herbal medicine) can lower blood pressure in some but raise it in others (Mabey 1988 p. 179). In aromatherapy this balancing of blood pressure is often ascribed to *Cananga odorata* but is not proven. The skill of the aromatherapist lies in using such effects in skilful blends to the best advantage of the client.

Deodorant

Bad smells sometimes arise from the disease process, and the sweet-smelling oils act to prevent

Table 4.7 Antiviral effects of essential oils

Latin name	Common name	Unspecified	Adenovirus	Childhood infections	Herpes genitalis	Glandular fever	Herpes simplex	Herpes varicella	Influenza	Viral enteritis	Viral enterocolitis	Viral hepatitis	Viral infections	Viral meningitis	Viral neuritis	Warts	Verrucae	Zoster	Multiple sclerosis	Poliomyelitis
Aniba rosaeodora	rosewood								×											
Cinnamomum verum (fol.)	cinnamon leaf	×																		
Cinnamomum verum (cort.)	cinnamon bark												×			×	×			
Cistus ladaniferus	labdanum			×																
Citrus aurantifolia (per.)	lime								×							×	×			
Citrus aurantium var bergamia (per.)	bergamot						×													
Citrus limon (per.)	lemon						×		×							×	×			
Commiphora molmol	myrrh											×								
Cuminum cyminum	cumin	×																		
Cupressus sempervirens	cypress								×											
Eucalyptus dives	broad leaved peppermint	×																		
Eucalyptus globulus	Tasmanian blue gum						×		×											
Eucalyptus radiata	narrow leaved peppermint								×											
Eucalyptus smithii	gully gum								×		×									
Helichrysum angustifolium (flos)	everlasting								×		×									
Hyssopus officinalis	hyssop						×													
Inula helenium	elecampane									×										
Laurus nobilis (fol.)	bay leaf														×					
Lavandula x intermedia 'Super'	lavandin Super									×										
Lavandula latifolia L. spica	spike lavender										×									
Litsea cubeba	may chang														×					
Melaleuca alternifolia	tea tree						×		×	×										
Melaleuca leucadendron	cajuput														×					
Melaleuca viridiflora	niaouli				××		×			×		××								
Melissa officinalis	melissa						×											×		
Mentha x piperita	peppermint									×		×			×			×		
Nepeta cataria	catnep						××													
Ocimum basilicum	basil											×			×					
Origanum majorana	sweet marjoram						×													

Table 4.7 Antiviral effects of essential oils (*cont'd*)

Latin name	Common name	Unspecified	Adenovirus	Childhood infections	Herpes genitalis	Glandular fever	Herpes simplex	Herpes varicella	Influenza	Viral enteritis	Viral enterocolitis	Viral hepatitis	Viral infections	Viral meningitis	Viral neuritis	Warts	Verrucae	Zoster	Multiple sclerosis	Poliomyelitis
Pelargonium graveolens P. x asperum	geranium						X											X		
Pimenta dioica (fol.)	pimento																	X	x	x
Pimenta racemosa (fruct.)	West Indian bay								x		x	x	x		x					
Piper nigrum	pepper		X																	
Ravensara aromatica	ravensara							x	X	X		X						xx		
Rosmarinus officinalis	rosemary						X					X								
Rosmarinus officinalis ct. verbenone	rosemary verbenone									xx	X	X								
Satureia montana	winter savory																			
Salvia officinalis	sage				x	X			X	X				x	X			X		
Satureia hortensis	summer savory												x							
Satureia montana	winter savory												x							
Syzygium aromaticum (flos)	clove bud						xx		x	xx	x	X								
Thymus serpyllum	wild thyme								X											
Thymus vulgaris ct. phenol	thyme					X			X											
Thymus vulgaris ct. geraniol	sweet thyme									xx			x				x			
Thymus vulgaris ct. linalool	sweet thyme									xx			x				x	X		
Thymus vulgaris ct. thujanol–4	sweet thyme	x																		

Case study 4.5 Antiviral – Dr. D. Pénoël – *Aromatologist, France*

Viral infection

Client assessment

Clément was suffering from *Molluscum contagiosum*, a serious viral infection, which had developed while the family were on holiday in Corsica. His whole body (including his genitals) was covered with boils; he was feverish and screaming with pain day and night.

The parents firmly believed in natural medicine and did not wish to send Clément to the hospital, knowing that no allopathic cure existed for viral diseases. The boy was also prone to eczema and allergic reactions. Not only was the medical condition of the child assessed, but the family were asked to undertake the therapeutic program prescribed.

Intervention

A toxic free diet was established for Clément to help the detoxification process which accompanies any infectious disease.

Because of the extreme cutaneous condition, the hydrolat of *Melissa officinalis* [melissa] (undiluted) - antiviral, antiinflammatory, calming - was selected first and sprayed around the little boy, who felt relief for the first time in many days of intense suffering.

The following essential oils were then chosen and blended:

Chamaemelum nobile [Roman chamomile] – antiinflammatory, calming, vulnerary

Matricaria recutita [German chamomile] – cicatrizant, antiallergic, antiinflammatory

Melaleuca alternifolia [tea tree] - analgesic, antiinfectious, antiinflammatory, antiviral, immunostimulant

Thymus vulgaris ct linalol [sweet thyme] – antiinfectious, antiinflammatory, antiseptic, antiviral, immunostimulant

Juniperus communis fruct. [juniper berry] - analgesic, antiseptic, antiviral, depurative

These were made up in three ways:

– A 5% concentration with a 95% blend of vegetable carrier oils, also active in the healing process: macerated oils of calendula (60%) and St John's Wort (25%) and oil of *Calophyllum inophyllum* (5%). The parents were asked to apply this blend on each boil, using a fine paint brush.
– A blend of the essential oils above was given to the parents to be used internally - 1 drop blended in honey six times per day.
– 3 drops, diluted in vegetable oil, were put into capsules, to use as suppositories.

A second blend of essential oil was made with equal quantities of:

Melaleuca cajuputi (cajuput)
Melaleuca alternifolia
Myrtus communis (red myrtle)

This was to be applied without dilution on the sole of the each foot six times a day.

After the first treatment at the clinic, the blends and suppositories were given to the parents to continue treatment at home; the spraying equipment was lent to them for the period of intensive care.

The parents were asked to telephone every day to report Clément's progress and to return to the clinic after nine days.

Outcome

After three days the problem had enormously improved. The treatment was continued, but reducing the number of applications per day.

Nine days later the family returned to see me. Clément's skin was almost perfect and he had regained his vitality. This remarkable and speedy result was helped not only by the determination of the parents, but also by the high quality aromatic and vegetable oils.

Case study 4.6   Balancing – A Barker – *aromatologist, UK*

Epilepsy

Patient assessment

7-year-old M was hyperactive and epileptic: going in a few seconds from daydreaming to petit mal convulsions.

He was on a high dose of Epanutin, which his mother was not very happy about.

The following essential oils were used in high concentration as recommended in Valnet (1980):

- 15 drops *Hyssopus officinalis* [hyssop]
- 20 drops *Salvia officinalis* [sage]
- 25 drops *Ocimum basilicum* [sweet basil]

These were used in 30 ml of carrier oil (10% dilution) – only on the kidney area of M's back, thus the quantity of essential oils being applied was in reality quite small.

Outcome

The convulsions ceased within a week. M now being on a minimum dose of Epanutin. The massage oil concentration was reduced to 1.5% and treatments to one a month. M's mother is now looking at withdrawing conventional drug therapy.

---

degradation, replace the odours and tackle the bacteria causing these effects. The use of sweet-smelling and familiar essential oils is more accept-able to the client (who may be in a weakened state) than is the imposition of harsh synthetics. This attribute is also helpful in a healing situation where bad smells are generated, for example in some severe burn injuries. Essential oils do not merely disguise these unpleasant odours which clients and nurses have to suffer, but actually cancel them out.

> *The odour of essential oils does not cover up the bad smells of infected gangrenous or cancerous wounds; it suppresses them by physicochemical action.*
>
> Valnet (1980 p. 44)

The authors have supplied a mixture of essential oils designed for this purpose for a number of years to a burns unit at the request of the consultant surgeon. The nurses find it particularly useful when bathing patients with burns. Essential oils find a similar use in incontinence cases, making life a great deal more pleasant for all concerned. Bad-smelling wounds can be deodorized by the use of *Hypericum* oil (see p. 106), thyme and citrus oils (Schilcher 1985 p. 222). Chamomile preparations, *Myristica fragrans* and lavandin are also known for their deodorizing effect.

Because of the deodorizing effect of some fragrant materials they are useful in underarm and foot deodorants. Compounds and oils recommended as effective against body odour are eugenol, linalool and the essential oil *Pogostemon patchouli* (Decazes 1993). Elsewhere *Salvia sclarea, Cymbopogon flexuosus, Zingiber officinale* and *Myristica fragrans* are also mentioned in this respect.

Digestive

Essential oils have strong effects on the digestive system (Table 4.8) and are used in appetite-stimulating and digestive drinks as carminatives and stimulants for the stomach, liver and gall bladder. The carminative effect of many essential oils is strong, and there are other benefits, such as increased secretory activity of the stomach and gall bladder, antiseptic and spasmolytic effects. The essential oils concerned are mainly from the Apiaceae botanical family – *Carum carvi, Coriandrum sativum, Foeniculum vulgare* var. *dulce, Pimpinella anisum* and also *Mentha* x *piperita, Ocimum basilicum* and the chamomiles (Schilcher 1985 p. 224). Wild thyme (*Thymus serpyllum*) has been shown to stimulate bile production (Chabrol et al 1932), and essential oils containing the alcohols menthol and thujanol-4 seem to be beneficial to liver function (Gershbein 1977, Zara 1966).

The citrus oils generally have a favourable effect on the digestive system, being mildly appetite stimulating and digestive. *Citrus aurantium* var. *amara* (per.) is given as a treatment for constipation as it encourages intestinal peristalsis and also acts as a cholagogue (Duraffourd 1982 p. 95); this oil is also mentioned for dyspepsia, flatulence and

Case study 4.7a   Balancing – R Toon – *aromatherapist, UK*

Constipation

Patient assessment

Mr A was an epileptic, deaf blind man in his twenties with profound learning disabilities. Prior to coming into the residential home his diet was very poor and he had almost no exercise. As a result, he had to take three types of medication three times a day for his constipation. He was immediately introduced to a balanced high fibre diet incorporating wholemeal bread and fresh fruit and vegetables. He also began an exercise programme involving swimming (once a week) and walking (3–4 times a week).

Intervention

It was decided to make massage a part of Mr A's new lifestyle. The oils selected were:

- 3 drops *Citrus reticulata* [mandarin]
- 3 drops *Rosmarinus officinalis* [rosemary]
- 3 drops *Zingiber officinale* [ginger]
- 50 ml grapeseed oil

Mr A received massage of his abdomen and lower back daily, after his evening bath. At first he would not tolerate the texture of the oil-based blend, so the same essential oils were blended into a white lotion and used for a week.

Once he had become accustomed to receiving massage, the grapeseed oil was reintroduced as the carrier without further difficulty.

Outcome

Within 6–8 weeks a definite improvement could be observed. Mr A was opening his bowels regularly and there had also been a reduction in the number of epileptic seizures. As a result his GP reviewed his medication as part of a programme to reduce his drug intake.

It was felt that the holistic approach of using essential oils together with diet, exercise and massage was particularly effective in helping Mr A to deal with his constipation.

Case study 4.7b   Digestive – L Cantele – *nurse aromatherapist, USA*

Flatulence – twin babies

Client assessment

The clients, 5-week-old twin babies, were suffering from severe flatulence problems, with constipation. They were in pain and constantly crying. Neither of the children was sleeping well due to the stomach pain and inconsolable crying fits.

Intervention

The following massage oil was prepared for the mother to use at home every evening:

- 5 drops *Rosmarinus officinalis* [rosemary] – analgesic, digestive (sluggish and painful digestion)
- 3 drops *Chamaemelum nobilis* [Roman chamomile] – calming, digestive
- 4 drops *Origanum majorana* [sweet marjoram] – analgesic, digestive (flatulence)
- 50 ml sweet almond oil

After a treatment by the therapist, the babies' mother was shown how to give her babies a simple abdomen massage herself. She was also asked to apply a little of the blend to the soles of the babies' feet.

Outcome

After 2 days, the mother called to say that the results were so encouraging after the initial treatment and her massage the following night that she was going to continue over the next few days.

After a week, the babies were sleeping better – they were no longer waking up during the night from flatulence and pain.

The babies are now 7 months old. From time to time they become constipated, but the mother simply applies the essential oil mix twice during the day – abdomen and feet – and before they go to bed, which solves the problem straightaway.

Table 4.8 Essential oils and the digestive system. Sources same as for Appendix A

Latin name	Common name	Antispasmodic	Aperitive	Astringent	Carminative	Choleretic	Hepatic stimulant	Litholytic U=urinary K=kidney G=gall	Pancreatic stimulant	Colic	Colitis, gastroenteritis	Constipation	Diarrhoea	Digestion painful	Digestive stimulant	Diverticulitis	Enteritis, gastritis	Indigestion	Nausea	Ulcers (gastric and duodenal)
Achillea millefolium	yarrow	×				×		K							×					
Carum carvi	caraway				×	×				×								×		
Chamaemelum nobile (flos)	Roman chamomile		×		×	×					×		×					×		
Citrus aurantium var. amara (flos)	neroli						×		×											
Citrus aurantium var. amara (fol.)	petitgrain																	×		
Citrus aurantium var. amara (per.)	orange bitter	×					×			×		×				×		×		
Citrus bergamia (per.)	bergamot	×	×		×					×					×			×		
Citrus limon (per.)	lemon	×	×	×	×			G,U	×	×			×	×	×			×	×	
Citrus reticulata (per.)	mandarin				×	×	×					×			×			×		
Commiphora myrrha	myrrh															×				
Coriandrum sativum	coriander	×			×						×				×					
Cupressus sempervirens	cypress	×		×									×							
Eucalyptus smithii	gully gum														×					
Foeniculum vulgare var. dulce (fruct.)	fennel				×	×		U			×				×			×		
Hyssopus officinalis	hyssop						×	U		×					×			×		
Juniperus communis (fruct.)	juniper berry		×	×	×		×	U,K	×	×	×				×	×				
Matricaria recutita (flos)	German chamomile	?													×	×			×	×
Melaleuca alternifolia	tea tree												×							
Melaleuca leucadendron	cajuput	×																		
Melaleuca viridiflora	niaouli				×		×	G			×		×				×			
Melissa officinalis	melissa	×		×		×	×			×	×		×		×	×		×	×	
Mentha x piperita	peppermint	×		×	×	×	×			×	×		×		×	×		×	×	
Myristica fragrans (sem.)	nutmeg	×			×										×			×	×	×

Table 4.8 Essential oils and the digestive system. Sources same as for Appendix A (cont'd)

Latin name	Common name	Properties								Indications										
		Antispasmodic	Aperitive	Astringent	Carminative	Choleretic	Hepatic stimulant	Litholytic U=urinary K=kidney G=gall	Pancreatic stimulant	Colic	Colitis, gastroenteritis	Constipation	Diarrhoea	Digestion painful	Digestive stimulant	Diverticulitis	Enteritis, gastritis	Indigestion	Nausea	Ulcers (gastric and duodenal)
Nepeta cataria	catnep							G												
Ocimum basilicum var. album	basil	×			×		×			×		×	×		×			×		
Origanum majorana	marjoram	×			×					×	×	?	×		×		×	×		×
Pelargonium graveolens	geranium			×			×		×		×		×			×				
Pimpinella anisum	aniseed	×	×		×					×					×		×	×		
Pinus sylvestris	Scots pine							G												
Piper nigrum	pepper						×					×			×					
Rosmarinus officinalis	rosemary				×	×	×	G		×		×	×	×	×		×	×		
Salvia officinalis	sage		×	?		×				×					×			×		
Santalum album	sandalwood			×							×									
Satureia montana, S. hortensis	winter and summer savory	×			×	×				×		×	×	×	×					
Syzygium aromaticum (flos)	clove bud	×																		
Thymus serpyllum	wild thyme									×										
Thymus vulgaris 'Population'	thyme				×							×	×	×	×					
Zinziber officinale	ginger				×					?		×	×	×	×				×	

gastric spasm (Franchomme & Pénoël 2001 p. 365). *Rosmarinus officinalis* has always been associated with improving the liver function. In animals an intravenous infusion of rosemary doubled the volume of bile secreted (Valnet 1980 p. 177); it is given as a carminative and cholagogue (Lautié & Passebecq 1984 p. 74) and to stimulate hepatobiliary secretions (Duraffourd 1982 p. 107).

Diuretic

Just as rosemary oil is traditionally associated with the liver, so juniper berry oil – *Juniperus communis* (fruct.) – is associated with the kidneys. At normal dosage it is a beneficial stimulant, although it has a toxic effect on inflamed kidneys. There is a diuretic effect (Duraffourd 1982, p. 67, Franchomme & Pénoël 2001 p. 389, Lautié & Passebecq 1984 p. 51, Viaud 1983) although this is denied by Schilcher (1985 p. 226) and omitted by Roulier (1990). However, one authority (Gattefossé 1937 p. 71) states that nearly all essences (essential oils) are diuretic and endorses juniper oil. It is also claimed that terpene-free oil containing mainly terpinen-4-ol has marked diuretic effects (Schneider 1975), although juniper oils consist of more than 90% hydrocarbon monoterpenes and the level of this alcohol may be only 2–5%.

Energizing

Plants capture electromagnetic energy from the sun and some of this is stored in the essential oil. The biosynthesis of the terpenes has as a starting point acetyl coenzyme A (Hay & Waterman 1993 p. 52) and in certain plants this process of synthesis goes beyond terpenes to the production of steroids with hormonal properties. Plant metabolic mechanisms have much in common with those of humans, and this starting point of acetyl coenzyme A is analogous to the process in the human body by which steroids are synthesized – cortisone, vitamin D and cholesterol. The phenylpropanoids, another building block of essential oils, provide a further example. They are in effect the precursors of some of the amino acids, the basic elements for the synthesis of proteins. Proteins are the building blocks of the human body, the agents for transformation and energy transfer which maintain the fabric of the body and all the physiological activity (Duraffourd 1987 p. 26). This may help us in understanding the special nature of essential oils; because of their

---

Case study 4.8a   Diuretic – S Price – *aromatologist, UK*

Water retention

Client assessment
Mrs L was suffering from oedema in her legs and ankles, which had been under control with diuretic tablets from her doctor. She had come off these of her own accord, as she was unable to support the frequency of toilet visits which they caused – at most awkward moments.

She had heard of aromatherapy and asked if anything could help her swollen legs. As she said she had stopped taking her diuretic tablets, it was ethically possible to treat her with essential oils.

Intervention
The essential oils chosen for Mrs L were those with diuretic properties: *Citrus limon* [lemon], *Cupressus sempervirens* [cypress], *Foeniculum vulgare* [fennel] and *Juniperus communis* [juniper].

10 drops of each were put into 50 ml grapeseed oil and Mrs L was shown how to apply it firmly in an upward direction only. This she had to do every night – and report back in 2–3 weeks.

Outcome
When Mrs L returned, she was delighted with the reduction of swelling in her legs – with no over frequent visits to the toilet. A few days before, she had paid her regular visit to the doctor, who had looked at her legs and said 'Ah, Mrs L, I see you have gone back onto your tablets!', whereupon she explained that that was not the case – and that she had visited an aromatherapist. 'H'm!' was the reply!

Case study 4.8b   Diuretic – A James – *aromatherapist, UK*

Lymphoedema

Client assessment

Pam has suffered swollen legs and ankles for many years; it affected her whole body in that wounds took a long time to heal and she is allergic to stitches. Around 5 years ago she was referred to a circulatory specialist who diagnosed primary lymphoedema, which is quite a rare condition, usually occurring in its secondary form after lymph glands have been removed, i.e. cancer surgery. There seems to be a lack of information surrounding the condition and little treatment available. Her GP has been very sympathetic and understanding and has tried his best to keep up to date with new information or clinical trials that may be taking place concerning the condition.

Intervention

The treatment consisted of a leg massage carried out on a weekly basis for 8 weeks. Pam was given a blend of oils to use twice daily before using her leg massage machine, given to her by her GP to increase the circulation and assist drainage of the lymphatic system.

It was decided to use the following oils for both clinical and home treatments (the quantities below are for the home blend):

- 8 drops *Rosmarinus officinalis* [rosemary] – cicatrizant, decongestant (also increases arterial and peripheral circulation), detoxifying, diuretic and generally fortifying the system. It is said also to promote the circulation of Chi energy in the body

- 8 drops *Cupressus sempervirens* [cypress] – decongestant, diuretic, phlebotonic
- 6 drops *Cymbopogon citratus* [lemongrass] – antiinflammatory, increases blood and lymphatic circulation, detoxifying and activates T-lymphocytes
- 8 drops *Chamaemelum nobile* [Roman chamomile] – antiinflammatory, vulnerary

The essential oils above were added to the following carrier oils:

- 70 ml Sweet almond (*Prunus amygdalis* var. dulcis) – nourishes dry skin, soothes inflammation
- 15 ml Passion flower (*Passiflora incarnata*) – improves the skin's elasticity
- 15 ml Evening primrose oil (*Oenethera biennis*) – contains gamma-linoleic acid to enhance skin care

Outcome

Over the 8 weeks of treatment Pam reported that after each one her legs felt much lighter and calmer. They did not ache as much and there was a great improvement in the quality and texture of her skin, which became less dry and flaky, with more elasticity. The blemishes she had had at the start of the study cleared up quite quickly, without many new ones appearing. There was also a reduction in the lumpiness of her skin – these were thought by her GP to be lumps of coagulated lymph.

She continues to be seen on a regular basis and her legs remain in good health.

---

molecular energy and because they have elements in common with human physiology, they can help to correct either deficits or blockages (Duraffourd 1987 p. 27).

Granulation promoting, cicatrizant

This effect helps in healing where there has been damage or removal of tissue. Probably the best-known use is that of lavender oil for minor burns,

which yields positive and rapid results (Gattefossé 1937). Hypericum oil and chamomile oils have been used traditionally for wound healing, and the validity of this has been borne out in the case of chamomile by studies (Glowania, Raulin & Swoboda 1987, Thiemer, Stadler & Isaac 1973). Red oil of hypericum is available: it is a fixed oil – usually with a base of olive oil or sunflower oil – in which the flowers of St John's wort (*Hypericum perforatum*) have been macerated. This oil contains as active constituents not only the essential oil but also hypericin and was much used in the past for the external treatment of wounds and burns (Weiss 1988 p. 296); the authors have found *Pelargonium graveolens* [geranium] to be most effective in this respect.

Hormonelike activity

Some essential oils have a tendency to normalize hormonal secretions, and it is thought that this action may be direct or effected via the hypophysis (Franchomme & Pénoël 2001). No work

---

Case study 4.9   Cicatrizant – J Hinchliffe – *aromatherapist, UK*

Wound healing

Client assessment
DH was 61 years old, having retired at 50 on medical grounds due to rheumatoid arthritis (since the age of 24), for which he had had gold injections to ease the pain and increase movement. The side-effects from long-term injections resulted in an outbreak of sores on his lower legs.

The gold injections were stopped when the sores first appeared (age 45); there were two or three around each ankle and were red and itchy. Having remained unchanged for 16 years, suddenly, at the age of 61, they began to increase in size and became extremely itchy, very sore and very red. Eventually they began to join together in one great mass of extremely red and angry looking skin that bled easily. D scratched them in his sleep, which of course made the condition worse. D was very anxious about the state of his legs and wearing trousers was very uncomfortable.

The doctor prescribed a steroid cream, which at first seemed to help, but after a couple of weeks, they actually looked worse. D was referred to a dermatologist and whilst waiting for an appointment, he turned to aromatherapy.

Intervention
D was advised to wear either shorts or loose-fitting trousers, preferably cotton, to avoid irritating the skin and to let air circulate around his legs.

The method of treatment chosen was by self-application, as it was more convenient than applying a compress and D was just about to go on holiday.

The selected oils were:

- *Lavandula angustifolia* [lavender] – anti-infectious, cicatrizant, antiinflammatory, regenerative

- *Melaleuca leucadendron* [cajuput] – analgesic, antiinfectious and indicated for sores and skin diseases (Valnet 1980)
- *Syzygium aromaticum* [clove bud] – analgesic, antiinfectious, cicatrizant and immunostimulant

These were placed in a carrier lotion with 25% of calendula oil – antiinflammatory and vulnerary, therefore excellent for wounds.

Outcome
When D returned from holiday a week later, his lower legs appeared to be 50% better. The redness had reduced to a pale pink and some of the sores had disappeared. The area had not itched enough to need scratching, so had not bled. D was very pleased indeed.

After 2 weeks, the sores had decreased further, had stopped itching and were looking and feeling better each day.

After 6 weeks, all the sores had disappeared apart from two pale and no longer itchy ones on his right leg.

Although these two sores did not disappear altogether, they do not often itch and are not very noticeable. The healing was excellent, with very little scarring and D is glad to be out of pain.

He now uses the mix once a week, or if the two remaining patches feel at all itchy. No more sores have appeared since and the dermatologist appointment was cancelled. The doctor was amazed at the result and said he would be happy to refer similar cases to the aromatherapist.

(From The Aromatherapist 5(4).)

has so far been done to establish precisely how the oil molecules could do this. For the present, treatment is easy and pleasant for the client and, so far as is known, without any unwanted side-effects. The hormonelike action of some plant extracts has been widely noted. Extracts of fennel seed have a slight oestrogenic effect in animal experimental models (Foster 1993) and fennel has been used for thousands of years as a menstrual cycle regulator and for premenstrual syndrome (Stewart 2005 p. 411); Bernadet (1983) and others advise the use of essential oils for such disorders as dysmenorrhoea and amenorrhoea.

There are compounds in some volatile oils that have a structural similarity to natural human hormones, and these promote efficient endocrine gland activity by natural means. Sclareol (Fig. 2.7), viridiflorol (Fig. 2.6a) and *trans*-anethole (Fig. 4.1a) are examples of compounds that have struc-

tures similar to folliculin or analogous to oestrogen. Other compounds, found in *Pinus sylvestris*, are similar to cortisone (Franchomme & Penoël 2001 p. 417).

The essential oil of *Vitex agnus-castus* balances progesterone levels and moderates excess oestrogen by direct action on the pituitary (Lucks 2003 p. 15) and cypress contains a chemical structure which is a homologue of the ovarian hormone (Valnet 1980 p. 71).

The essential oils of pine (needles), borneol, geranium, basil, sage, savory and rosemary are said to stimulate the cortex of the suprarenal gland, while anise excites the anterior pituitary body, as does mint (Valnet 1980 p. 70). Monoterpenes, in particular α-pinene and β-pinene and δ-3-carene, which are found in many essential oils, mimic the action of cortisone in so far as they have a modulating effect on the activity

---

Case study 4.10   Hormonal – C. O'Malley – *aromatherapist, UK*

Hormonal (PMS)

Kay worked in an office with several other girls – and the therapist. She was a chatty, happy person, well liked. However, when her period was due, she became a different person – snapping people's heads off and generally reacting with bad temper at the slightest challenge. She realised after a while that her behaviour was affecting the others in the office. The therapist suggested she try aromatherapy and Kay accepted.

Intervention
The essential oils chosen were those which are hormonelike, alleviating PMS:

- 2 drops *Chamomilla recutita* [German chamomile]
- 5 drops *Pimpinella anisum* [aniseed]
- 8 drops *Salvia sclarea* [clary]
- A few drops of *Lavandula angustifolia* were added – to her liking, as she was not too keen on the aroma without it
- 30 ml grapeseed carrier oil

Kay was asked to apply this blend to her abdomen every night and morning immediately after she finished menstruating each month until the next period commenced.

She was also given a pure blend of the oils (in the same proportions) to use in the bath which she took twice a week.

Outcome
After the first month, the girls felt that Kay was marginally easier to live with.

By the second month there was a noticeable difference and by the third month, Kay herself felt much more relaxed and able to cope. She continued the two treatments for 6 months, then decided she was so much better – and happier – that she would stop the night and morning applications.

The therapist suggested she stop only the morning application first, continuing to apply it at night for 2 months, before stopping altogether. This she did, but never gave up the bath blend, as she loved the aroma while bathing. Kay was with the firm for a further 3 years before getting married and moving away and in all that time Kay was her original happy and efficient self – her PMS was non-existent.

of the adrenal cortex. They cause release of the adrenocortical hormone cortisol, which additionally alleviates pain, inflammation and, to some extent, allergic reactions (von Braunschweig 1999 p. 17).

The following plant volatile molecules are said to be hormonelike: anethole (*para*-anol methyl ether), citral, eugenol, carvacrol, thymol, gingerol, lachnophyllum methyl ester, matricaria methyl ester, viridiflorol, sclareol.

Anethole, p-anol methyl ether

This molecule (Fig. 4.1a) is generally believed to have oestrogen-like properties, being emmenagogic, lactogenic. This phenol methyl ether is found in *Foeniculum vulgare* var. *dulce* [fennel] oil 52–86% (Tisserand & Balacs 1995 p. 74) and anethole, fennel oil and aniseed oil have all been shown to have oestrogenic activity (in rats) (Zondec et al 1938). The structure of the molecule has a similarity to a derivative of stilben, viz diethyl stilbestrol (Fig. 4.1c), to which its mode of action may be compared. Essential oils containing this molecule e.g. *Pimpinella anisum* [aniseed] should be used in the menstrual cycle before ovulation (Franchomme & Pénoël 2001 p. 189, 193). *trans*-Anethole has weak oestrogen-like properties (Zondec et al 1938). Albert-Puleo (1980 2:337) suggests that polymers of anethole such as dianethole and photoanethole are active oestrogenic compounds. N.B. Essential oils rich in anethole are to be used with caution orally in people with oestrogen dependent cancers, in endometriosis, pregnancy, breast feeding (Tisserand & Balacs 1995 p. 75). Mills (1991 p. 425) states:

> anethole has structural similarity to the catecholamines adrenaline, noradrenaline and dopamine: this may account for some of the sympathomimetic effects of fennel and anise (which also contain large quantities of anethole) such as ephedrine like bronchodilator action and amphetamine like facilitation of weight loss. The traditional lactogenic effect may be due to competitive inhibition of dopamine inhibition of prolactin secretion as much as to any direct hormonal activity. The relationship of anethole to psychoactive chemicals like mescaline, asarone and myristicin from nutmeg has been noted and may account for a psychoactive and aphrodisiac tradition for fennel and anise.

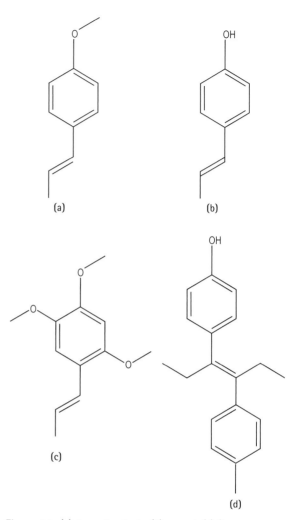

Figure 4.1 (a) *trans*-Anethole; (b) *p*-anol; (c) β-asarone; (d) diethyl stilbestrol.

Some plant materials have long been regarded as psychotropic agents and this property may arise from the myristicin and elemicin compounds: these have a structural similarity to amphetamines which exert hallucinogenic effects (see Fig. 4.2). Apiole found in parsley and dillapiole also bear a relationship to these compounds (Trease & Evans 1983 p. 691).

Citral (Figs 2.11a, 2.11c)

This molecule was shown to have an oestrogenic effect causing prostatic hyperplasia (in rats) (Abramovici et al 1985, Geldof et al 1992). Balacs & Tisserand (1995 p. 146) referring to *Cymbopogon flexuosus* [lemongrass] say that a mild hormone-

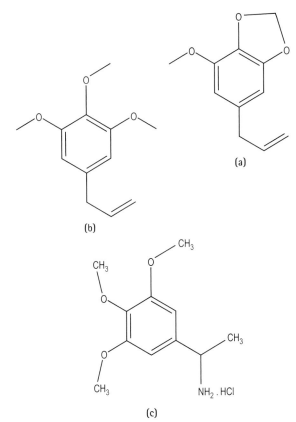

Figure 4.2 (a) Myristicin; (b) elemicin; (c) amphetamine corresponding to elemicin.

like (oestrogenic) action may be assumed from the citral content but that as used in aromatherapy it is not known whether there will be an oestrogenic or androgenic effect.

Eugenol, carvacrol (Fig. 2.9c), thymol (Fig. 2.8b), gingerol

Hormones play a part in the mechanisms of prostaglandins and these molecules, found in the essential oils of *Syzygium aromaticum*, *Thymus vulgaris* and *Zingiber officinale* have an influence on prostaglandin E (Bennett & Stamford 1988, Wagner et al 1986).

Lachnophyllum methyl ester, matricaria methyl ester

Esters as a rule are not hormonelike but these two esters are exceptions, the only ones known at the present time. They are used in the treatment of delayed puberty (Franchomme & Pénoël 2001 p. 207). *Cis-* and *trans-* forms of Lachnophyllum

methyl ester occur at 40–60% in the essential oil of *Coniza bonariensis* (Asteraceae); this essential oil has no known contraindications

Viridiflorol (Fig. 2.6a)

This is a sesquiterpenol that occurs up to 15% in the essential oil of *Melaleuca quinquenervia* [niaouli] (Myrtaceae) and has an oestrogen like influence in ovaries and testicles (Franchomme & Pénoël 2001 p. 398).

Sclareol (Fig. 2.7)

This is a diol (diterpenic alcohol) occurring up to 7% in the essential oil of *Salvia sclarea* [clary] (Lamiaceae) that has a similarity to the oestrogens; allegedly aphrodisiac according to Franchomme & Pénoël (2001 p. 424).

Essential oils affecting the thyroid gland

Allium sativum [garlic] thyroid stimulant (Franchomme & Pénoël 2001 p. 349).

Onion (*N*-propyl disulphide) and garlic (methyl disulphide, allyl disulphide) inhibit iodine metabolism (rats) (Cowan et al 1967, Salji et al 1971).

Daucus carota [carrot seed] helps the pituitary gland to regulate the production of thyroxin.

Commiphora myrrha [myrrh] balances the production of thyroxin. Rose (1992 p. 118) advises myrrh be used in inhalation in the early morning to stimulate and regulate the thyroid.

Pinus sylvestris [pine] is a thyroid stimulant.

Cymbopogon martinii [palmarosa] considered having a normalizing effect on the thyroid gland (Rose 1992 p. 122).

Picea mariana [black spruce] is said to be cortisone like and useful in cases of hyperthyroidism.

Sassafras: In rats, oral administration of safrole or sassafras oil gives rise to cellular changes in the adrenal, pituitary and thyroid glands; also to the testes or ovaries (Abbot et al 1961).

Not referenced: many essential oils are said to have a tendency to normalize hormonal secretions by encouraging the endocrine glands naturally to work more efficiently. In my searches I have found these mentioned – artemisia, basil, cinnamon, clary sage, cumin, cypress, lavender, melissa, myrtle, pepper, mint, pine, thyme, valerian. Both *Pimenta dioica* [allspice] and eugenol are said to enhance trypsin activity and have larvicidal properties (Harkiss personal communication). See Table 4.9.

Hormones and herbal extracts

It is interesting to note that many herbal preparations are reputed to have hormonelike activity.

- **Plants having oestrogenic activity:** according to Bartram (1995 p. 316) more than 300 plants are known to possess oestrogenic activity including wholewheat and soya products; he gives important oestrogenics as aniseed, beth root, black cohosh, elder don quai, evening primrose, fennel, helonias, hop, liquorice, sage, sarsaparilla, aletris.
- **Plants affecting the thyroid:** *Fucus vesiculosus* [bladder wrack, kelp] contains up to 0.1% iodine; raises hormone production by the thyroid gland in poorly functioning thyroids (Bartram 1995 p. 60, Chevallier 1996 p. 211). Kelp is nourishing for the thyroid and is thought an ideal diet for this gland (Mills 1991b p. 515). *Lycopus virginicus* [bugleweed] has sedative properties and is used for overactive thyroid (Bartram 1995 p. 76, Chevallier 1996 p. 229). *Sargassum pallidum* [hai zao] used to treat thyroid problems due to low level of iodine in the body; do not take without professional supervision (Chevallier 1996 p. 264).

Hyperaemic

Essential oils promote local peripheral circulation owing to a primary irritation of the skin, and the effects of this are twofold:

- The freeing of mediators (e.g. bradykinin) which cause vasodilatation.
- Humoral reactions resulting in the anti-inflammatory effect.

On the skin there is a sensation of warmth, comfort and pain relief following the use of rubefacients such as *Eucalyptus globulus, Rosmarinus officinalis* and *Juniperus communis*, which cause increased local blood circulation. Local skin irritation may also have some effect on internal organs (e.g. cardiac ointment used in angina). Some essential oils are vesicants, e.g. *Brassica nigra* [mustard] and *Armoracia lapathifolia* [horseradish]

due to the principal constituent allylisothiocyanate. Croton oil also is a vesicant, and its use is proscribed by the Medicines Act 1968.

Immunostimulant

Melaleuca viridiflora has been reported to have an immunostimulant effect by increasing the level of immunoglobulins (Pénoël 1981), and many other oils have been mentioned by various writers as strengthening the immune system. There is a wide variety and no common agreement, and this may be so because many oils possess a range of properties (antifungal, antiseptic, antiviral, etc.) that are beneficial to the immune system (see Ch. 15). (See Appendix B.9 for a list of effective oils.)

Insecticidal and repellent

Plant volatile oils may be used over a long period of time without promoting resistance – some plants use essential oils to repel attacking insects, and they are still effective after millions of years. In the south of France, citronella is universally used as an insect repellent, and tests show other oils to have this property too, e.g. *Ocimum basilicum* (Dube, Upadhyay & Tripath 1989). Of a number of essential oils and some of their components investigated for insecticidal activity, only a few demonstrated this attribute – *Cinnamomum camphora, C. verum, Cymbopogon nardus, Syzygium aromaticum* and Eucalyptus oils, plus two aldehydes and a ketone (cinnamic aldehyde, citral and carvone) (Gildemeister & Hoffmann 1956). Our past experience indicates that *Thymus vulgaris* ct. thymol and *Melaleuca alternifolia* are effective parasiticides (head and pubic lice), and tests in which the authors were involved tend to confirm this. See Table 4.10 and Appendix A for more information.

Mucolytic and expectorant

Accumulated secretions in the mucous linings can hold germs and it is necessary to break down the mucus in order to kill them. Many oils are mucolytic thanks to their content of powerful ketones (carvone, menthone, thujone, pinocamphone, etc.) and in some cases lactones. The expectorant effect is due to the breaking down of secretions and to cilial activity, and several oils have in the past

Table 4.9   The influence of essential oils on the hormonal system

Latin name	Common name	Adrenal (cortex)	Adrenal (medulla)	Amenorrhoea	Antidiabetic	Choleretic cholagogic	Cortisone-like	Dysmenorrhoea	Emmenagogic	Hypophysis/gonads	Hypophysis	Hypothalamus	Impotence/frigidity
Achillea millefolium	yarrow			x		x		x					
Aloysia triphylla	verbena				x								
Anethum graveolens	dill seed					x							
Angelica archangelica (rad.)	angelica root								x				
Cananga odorata	ylang ylang				x								
Carum carvi	caraway								x				
Chamaemelum nobile	Roman chamomile			x				x	x				
Cinnamomum verum (cort.)	cinnamon bark								x				
Citrus aurantium var. *amara* (per.)	orange bitter					x					x	x	
Citrus limon (per.)	lemon										x	x	
Commiphora myrrha	myrrh								?				
Cupressus sempervirens (fol. strob.)	cypress												
Cymbopogon citratus C. flexuosus	lemongrass												
Foeniculum vulgare var. *dulce* (fruct.)	fennel			x				x	x				
Hyssopus officinalis	hyssop							x	x				
Illicium verum	star anise												
Laurus nobilis	bay leaf								x				
Lavandula angustifolia	lavender								x				
Matricaria recutita	German chamomile			x									
Melaleuca leucadendron	cajuput								?				
Melaleuca viridiflora	niaouli			x				x	x	x			
Melissa officinalis	lemon balm					xx							
Mentha x *piperita*	peppermint							x					
Mentha spicata	spearmint					x							
Myristica fragrans	nutmeg								x				x
Myrtus communis	myrtle			x				x					
Nardostachys jatamansi	spikenard												
Origanum majorana	sweet marjoram												
Pelargonium graveolens P. x *asperum*	geranium				x								
Picea mariana	black spruce						x						
Pimenta racemosa	West Indian bay							x	x				
Pimpinella anisum	aniseed			x					x				
Pinus sylvestris	pine	x						x			x		x
Piper nigrum	black pepper												x

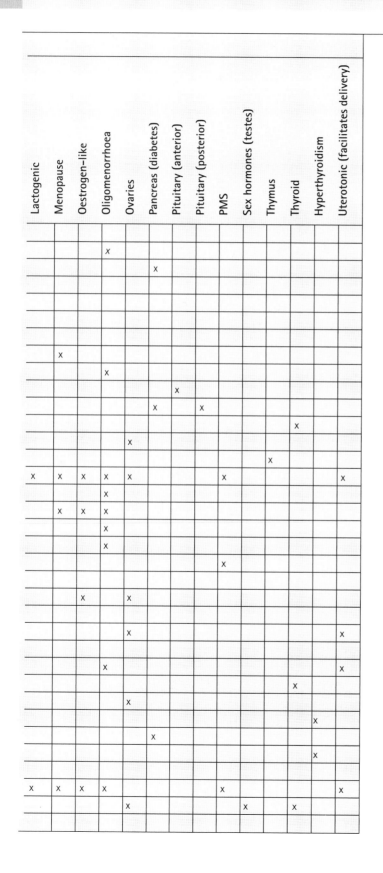

Table 4.9   The influence of essential oils on the hormonal system (*cont'd*)

Latin name	Common name	Adrenal (cortex)	Adrenal (medulla)	Amenorrhoea	Antidiabetic	Choleretic cholagogic	Cortisone-like	Dysmenorrhoea	Emmenagogic	Hypophys/gonads	Hypophysis	Hypothalamus	Impotence frigidity
Rosa centifolia R. damascena	rose otto								?				x
Rosmarinus officinalis	rosemary	x		x	x				x				x
Rosmarinus officinalis ct. verbenone	rosemary verbenone												x
Salvia officinalis	sage		x	x	x			x	x				
Salvia sclarea	clary			xx				x	?				
Santalum album	sandalwood												x
Syzygium aromaticum (flos)	clove bud												x
Tagetes patula, T. glandulifera	French marigold			x					x				
Thymus vulgaris ct. linalool	sweet thyme												
Thymus vulgaris ct. thujanol	thujanol thyme					x							
Thymus vulgaris ct. thymol	thyme	x											
Vetiveria zizanioides	vetiver			x					x				
Zingiber officinale	ginger												x

Lactogenic	Menopause	Oestrogen-like	Oligomenorrhoea	Ovaries	Pancreas (diabetes)	Pituitary (anterior)	Pituitary (posterior)	PMS	Sex hormones (testes)	Thymus	Thyroid	Hyperthyroidism	Uterotonic (facilitates delivery)	
			x											
		x		x					x					
x	x	x										x		
x	x	x												
									x					
											x		x	
													x	
			x	x										

Case study 4.11   Immunostimulant – R Holder – *aromatologist, UK*

Immunostimulant

Client assessment

Mrs X, a middle-aged teacher, had chronic bronchitis every winter, exacerbating her usually well controlled asthma. We discussed aromatic medicine and she was keen to try a prophylactic aromatic mixture in the period before the approaching winter. Meanwhile, she attended every 2 months for an aromatherapy massage, mainly for stress-related muscular aches.

Intervention

For her 2-monthly massage, the following oils were selected – for muscular aches and bronchitis:

- 1 drop *Abies balsamea* – antispasmodic (muscle relaxant), antiseptic (pulmonary)

- 1 drop *Eucalyptus smithii* [gully gum] – analgesic, anticatarrhal, antiinfectious, decongestant, expectorant
- 2 drops *Melaleuca alternifolia* [tea tree] – analgesic, antiinfectious, immunostimulant
- 2 drops *Rosmarinus officinalis* ct. camphor [rosemary] – analgesic, mucolytic, muscle relaxant
- 10 ml carrier oil

For home use she was given:

- 1 ml *Abies balsamea* – as above
- 4 drops *Eucalyptus dives* ct. pipiterone [broad leaved peppermint] – anticatarrhal, anti-infectious, mucolytic
- 3 ml *Eucalyptus smithii* [gully gum] – analgesic, anticatarrhal, antinfectious, decongestant, expectorant

---

Case study 4.11   Immunostimulant – R Holder – *aromatologist, UK (cont'd)*

- 12 drops *Melaleuca alternifolia* [tea tree] – as above
- 3 ml *Melaleuca leucadendron* – analgesic, anti-infectious, expectorant
- 4 drops *Myrtus communis* – anticatarrhal, anti-inflammatory, expectorant
- 2 drops *Cinnamomum verum* (fol.) – immunostimulant, neurotonic
- 4 drops *Rosmarinus officinalis* ct. camphor – analgesic, muscle relaxant
- 22 ml *Echinacea purpurea* (macerated in sunflower oil) – helps raise tissue permeability and stimulates phagocytosis

Six drops of this mixture were to be applied to the pre-warmed soles of both her feet night and morning – and once in between, if possible.

Several months later, just before the end of the Christmas term, she reported that it was the first time she had ever managed to work through that particular term without being off sick with bronchitis and subsequent further problems. She was so pleased with these results, that she decided to use the same mixture every year, starting at the end of the summer holidays.

---

been tested to determine expectorant properties (Boyd & Pearson 1946, Gordonoff 1938, Schilcher 1985 p. 223). Besides *Eucalyptus globulus* and other essential oils containing the oxide 1,8-cineole, *Pimpinella anisum*, *Foeniculum vulgare* var. *dulce*, *Pinus sylvestris* and *P. mugo* var. *pumilio*, *Thymus vulgaris* ct. phenol and *T. serpyllum* are also expectorants. These oils, whether used by external application or by inhalation, reach the bronchi and are eliminated from the lungs in the exhaled air. Russian research endorsed this property of some essential oils when inhaled (Eremenko et al 1987); all 96 patients suffering from chronic bronchitis showed a significant increase in the permeability of the respiratory tracts and clearing of the airway as well as a decrease in immunoglobulin E, indicating reduced infection levels. The study shows that the vapour of some essential oils (camphor, eucalyptus, peppermint and menthol) can improve the function of the lungs and bronchials, and so relieve mucous congestion, chest infections, colds and influenza.

Sedative

In the past there has been little apart from anecdotal evidence for the sedative properties of essential oils, but now several oils have been investigated and found to be effective. They include *Melissa officinalis*, which is calming to the central nervous system because of its citronellal and other monoterpene content (Becker & Förster 1984, Mills 1991), and the valerian oils, which contain small amounts of valepotriates (Becker 1983, Becker & Reichling 1981, Boeters 1969, Schmiedeberg 1913). *Valeriana officinalis* contains only about 1.5% of these but this figure can rise to 12% in other species. Recently other tests have been carried out which prove for the first time the sedative, calming effects of other oils, such as *Citrus aurantium* var. *amara* (flos) [neroli] and *Passiflora incarnata* [passion flower] (Buchbauer 1993, Buchbauer, Jirovetz & Jäger 1992, Buchbauer et al 1993) (Table 4.11). The aromatic water collected during the distillation of orange flowers (orange flower water) also has sedative properties, and more effective still is the essential oil of petitgrain *C. aurantium* var. *amara* (fol.) (Duraffourd 1982 p. 97). Lavender is recognized as a calming oil (Guillemain, Rousseau & Delaveau 1989) (Table 4.11) and is now used in many hospital wards to aid sleep (see Ch. 14). It is thought that the sedative effect of *Lavandula angustifolia* is due in part to the presence of coumarins in the oil, even though the content is low at 0.25% (Franchomme & Pénoël 2001 p. 391). *Cymbopogon citratus* essential oil was shown in rats to have a marked depressive effect on the central nervous system producing an effect comparable to chlorpromazine hydrochloride (Seth, Kokate & Varma 1976).

Case study 4.12 Mucolytic and expectorant – Anonymous – *aromatherapist*

Bronchial inflammation

Client assessment

Tim had suffered with bronchial inflammation and accumulation of mucus in his lungs for 5 years, since undergoing treatment for cancer in the throat/pharynx area – with radiotherapy to the thorax. The resultant scarring reduced his lung capacity, causing fibrosis to the lung. His dependency on antibiotics increased as chest infections increased also. He was experiencing difficulty in expectoration of accumulated mucus, usually dark brown, thick and tenacious. In addition, he was often very tired.

An intensive application of the following essential oils was used:

- 25 ml *Eucalyptus smithii*
- 10 ml *Abies balsama* [Canadian balsam]
- 5 ml *Eucalyptus radiata*
- 5 ml *Lavandula spica* [spike lavender]
- 5 ml *Melaleuca alternifolia* [tea tree]
- 5 ml *Cymbopogon citratus* [lemongrass]
- 5 ml *Thymus vulgaris* ct. geraniol [sweet thyme]
- 4 ml of the blend was applied twice a day to the soles of his feet, having first warmed them with a heater

Outcome

Within 10 minutes of applying the blend, some sputum was expectorated, with very little effort or coughing, continuing to be produced for about an hour. Almost at the same time, his nose began to run, accompanied by short bursts of sneezing. Within 1 week, the mucus was coming up more easily, was a lighter colour and less thick.

After 3 weeks the sputum was whitish-clear and Tim was not coughing at all during the night. He felt brighter, more alert and relaxed.

Case study 4.13 Sedative – H Charlesworth – *aromatherapist, UK*

Menopausal headaches

Assessment

Mary, 53, had suffered from severe headaches and muscular fatigue for more than 2 years. Her doctor had prescribed hormone replacement therapy to help her through the menopause, but this had not helped her headaches or fatigue. Her life was stressful due to the responsibility of her disabled mother, which kept her confined to her home except for shopping, as she worried should she be absent for long periods.

Mary wanted to be helped, but was very tense and apprehensive.

Intervention

Mary did not want a full body massage, so was given a neck and shoulder massage with a blend of:

Eucalyptus globulus [blue gum] – antimigraine, decongestant
Lavandula angustifolia [lavender] – sedative
Mentha x *piperita* [peppermint] – analgesic, antimigraine, hormonelike (hot flushes)
Origanum majorana [sweet marjoram] analgesic, calming

She was given the same blend in a lotion base for home treatment to massage onto her forehead and neck whenever she felt a headache approaching. She was also given essential oils to put in her bath:

Lavandula angustifolia – as above
Chamaemelum nobile [Roman chamomile] – antispasmodic, calming, menstrual
Pelargonium graveolens [geranium] – analgesic, decongestant

Outcome

On her return to the clinic 2 weeks later, she reported having had only one headache – after a particularly stressful time with her mother. I suggested that when she felt particularly stressed to practise deep breathing and inhale the oils prescribed for her bath.

After two more visits she reported being completely free from headaches and her energy had returned.

She now visits occasionally when she requires a relaxing shoulder massage or needs to replace her oils.

Table 4.10   Insecticidal, larvicidal and repellent properties of essential oils

Latin name	Common name	Clothes moths	Fleas	Cockroaches	Gnats	Houseflies	Insects (unspecified)	Lice	Mosquitoes (unspecified)	Mosquito larvae	Aedes aegypti	Allocophora foveicollis	Anopheles funestus	Anopheles gambiae	Anopheles stephensi	Culex quinquefasciatus	Culicoides variipennis	Dermatophagoides pteronyssinus (house dust mites)	Pediculosus capitis	Pediculosus pubis
Acorus calamus (rad.)	calamus					RS	S													
Cymbopogon nardus	citronella								R											
Eucalyptus globulus	Tasmanian blue gum				R				R									I		
Laurus nobilis	bay leaf			R																
Melaleuca alternifolia	tea tree																			I
Melaleuca leucadendron	cajuput		R					R	R											
Myrtus communis	myrtle																		IL	
Mentha x piperita	peppermint		R		R				RI	L				R						
Ocimum basilicum	sweet basil					RI	RI		RI					R		I				
Pelargonium graveolens	geranium				R				RI											
Syzygium aromaticum (flos)	clove bud	R							R											
Thymus vulgaris (population)	thyme								I	L										

R = repellent
I = insecticidal
L = larvicidal
S = makes sterile

Compiled from information in Appendix A q.v.

Table 4.10 Insecticidal, larvicidal and repellent properties of essential oils (cont'd)

Compound	Common name	Clothes moths	Fleas	Cockroaches	Gnats	Houseflies	Insects (unspecified)	Lice	Mosquitoes (unspecified)	Mosquito larvae	Aedes aegypti	Allocophora foveicollis	Anopheles funestus	Anopheles gambiae	Anopheles stephensi	Culex quinquefasciatus	Culicoides variipennis	Dermatophagoides pteronyssinus (house dust mites)	Pediculosus capitis	Pediculosus pubis
Carvone (unspecified)							I													
Cinnamal							I													
Citral							I													
p-Menthane-3, 8-diol	found in Eucalyptus oil													R			R			
p-Menthane-3, 8-diol + Isopulegol + Citronellol													R	R						
(Z, E)-Ocimenone	found in Tagetes patula									L										

R = repellent
L = larvicidal

I = insecticidal
S = makes sterile

Compiled from information in Appendix A q.v.

Table 4.11 Effects of fragrance compounds and essentials oils on the motility of mice after a 1-hour inhalation period (from Buchbauer et al 1993 p. 661)

Compound	Effect on motility %[a]	Effect on motility after caffeine %[b]
Anethole	−10.81	−1.26
Anthranilic acid methyl ester	+17.70	+38.22
Balm leaves oil (Austria)	−5.21	+16.29
Benzaldehyde	−43.69	−34.28
Benzyl alcohol	−11.21	−23.68
Borneol	−3.05	−1.88
Bornyl acetate	−7.79	+2.27
Bornyl salicylate	−17.29	−2.99
Carvone	−2.46	−47.51
Citral	−1.43	+17.24
Citronellal	−49.82	−37.40
Citronellol	−3.56	−13.71
Coumarin	−15.00	−13.75
Dimethyl vinyl carbinol	+5.36	−2.11
Ethylmaltol	+9.73	+2.09
Eugenol	+2.10	−38.73
Farnesol	+5.76	+36.34
Farnesyl acetate	+4.62	−30.71
Furfural	+3.04	−4.51
Geraniol	+20.56	+1.20
Geranyl acetate	−29.18	−7.46
Isoborneol	+46.90	−11.23
Isobornyl acetate	+3.16	−22.35
Isoeugenol	+30.05	−74.34
β-Ionone	+14.20	−27.97
Lavender oil (Mont Blanc)	−78.40	−91.67
Lime blossom oil (France)	−34.34	+30.41
Linalool	−73.00	−56.67
Linalyl acetate	−69.10	−46.67
Maltol	+13.74	−50.04
Methyl salicylate	+16.64	−49.88
Nerol	+12.93	+29.31
Nerol oil	−65.27	+1.87
Orange flower oil (Spain)	−4.64	−14.62
Orange terpenes	+35.25	−33.19
Passion flower oil (USA)	+8.15	−27.93
2-phenyl ethanol	+2.67	−30.61
2-phenyllethyl acetate	−45.04	+12.42
α-pinene	+13.77	+4.73
Rose oil (Bulgaria)	−9.50	+4.31
Sandalwood oil (East India)	−40.00	−20.70
α-Terpineol	−45.00	−12.50
Thymol	+33.02	+19.05
Valerian root oil (China)	−2.70	−12.01

[a]motility of untreated control animals = 100%
[b]motility of control animals after pretreatment with 0.1% caffeine solution (0.5 mL, ip) = 100%

Spasmolytic

Essential oils have been found to relieve smooth muscle spasm (Debelmas & Rochat 1964, 1967a,b, Taddei et al 1988), hence their usefulness for some problems of the digestive tract. The oils with this property are chamomile oils containing (−)-α-bisabolol (Achterrath-Tuckerman et al 1980, Melegari et al 1988), *Carum carvi*, *Cinnamomum zeylanicum* (cort.), *Citrus aurantium* var. *amara* (per.), *Foeniculum vulgare* var. *dulce*, *Melissa officinalis* and *Mentha* x *piperita* (Schilcher 1985 p. 225).

There is value in successful practical experience, and essential oils have been used to ease spasm in skeletal muscle also, despite the lack of clinical trials. The authors have used *Ocimum basilicum* and *Origanum majorana* successfully over the years, and a fuller list has been published (Price 2000 pp. 266–287). *Cupressus sempervirens* is also credited with this property (Franchomme & Pénoël 2001 p. 373).

OTHER CONSIDERATIONS

ESSENTIAL OIL INTERACTION WITH DRUGS

Essential oils are composed of chemicals which are known to be active, gain access to cells by virtue of being fat soluble, and are metabolized by the body. It has been found by experience that some oils are relaxing, some are sedative, some sharpen the memory, some promote the circulation and so on. Therefore it may be assumed that as active agents they may react with other drugs present in the body, although there has been no evidence so far which would imply any adverse significant reaction between essential oils and allopathic drugs, and they have been used together successfully in hospitals (Barker 1994 personal communication). In a study on rats, eucalyptol administered subcutaneously or by aerosol was found to increase the *in vitro* liver metabolism of aminopyrine, *p*-nitro-anisol and aniline, and *in vivo* the metabolism of pentobarbital (Jori, Bianchetti & Prestini 1969). Animal studies have shown enhanced skin penetration for some drugs with eucalyptus oil, camphor and limonene, and,

---

Case study 4.14   Spasmolytic – S Price – *aromatologist, UK*

Chronic leg cramp

Client assessment

Mrs P had suffered with cramp in her calves and feet for several years, occurring most of the time during the night. Her doctor had not taken much interest, telling her to rub them when it occurred – and this would ease it. Having heard of aromatherapy, she decided to see if it could help her.

Intervention

Mrs P was asked first if she would be prepared to apply an oil blend to her legs every night before retiring. Having been assured that she would do anything to help, the following prescription was made up for her:

- 16 drops *Ocimum basilicum* [European basil] – analgesic, antispasmodic
- 16 drops *Origanum majorana* [sweet marjoram] – analgesic, antispasmodic
- 100 ml grapeseed carrier oil

She was asked to telephone if there was no improvement after a week – and to make another appointment for a month's time.

Outcome

There was no phone call and Mrs P arrived after a month to say that she had had no cramp at all for a week. Because of this, the frequency of use of her essential oil mix was reduced to once every 2 nights – and an appointment made for another 4 weeks' time.

At her next appointment, Mrs P reported that she had still had no cramp at night, so her frequency of use was reduced to twice a week.

At the next visit, Mrs P reported having cramp during the last week, but she had forgotten to apply her oil the night before. This showed that twice a week was the minimum number of applications to achieve good results.

When Mrs P went to Australia to live with her daughter, she took with her a 5 litre can of the blended oils – she didn't want to risk being without them!

---

in laboratory tests on excised human skin, penetration of 5-fluorouracil was increased with aniseed oil (2.8 times), ylang oil (7.8 times) and eucalyptus oil (34 times) (Williams & Barry 1989). Drug interaction with essential oils is discussed in Tisserand & Balacs (1995).

Nevertheless this is a cloudy area and, until laboratory investigations into possible reactions between essential oils and other drugs have been carried out and results made known, it is possible only to surmise what may happen. If sedative pills to help sleep are being prescribed then it may be unwise with our present level of knowledge to use an essential oil such as rosemary, which keeps the mind alert. It would be better to choose oils like lavender, vetiver and valerian, which are known to aid relaxation and sleep. It has been suggested that when a person is on medication the drugs involved could possibly affect metabolization of essential oil molecules. In some cases metabolism may be increased, e.g. with clofibrate (a blood lipid level reducer), steroids and phenobarbitones (antiepileptic). In other cases the drugs involved may reduce the metabolism of essential oil molecules, e.g. imidazole (antifungal), plant drugs, caffeic acid, myristicin or tannic acid. The study by Buchbauer et al (1993) indicates an area of possible future study in that some essential oils or their components may interact with caffeine, e.g. neroli, methyl salicylate, isoeugenol.

Some essences have been found to complement the action of antibiotics. Laboratory tests have shown that the essence of niaouli will increase the activity of streptomycin, cocaine and, more especially, of penicillin (Quevauviller & Parousse-Perrin 1952a,b). Reporting the results obtained when using turpentine derivatives in conjunction with antibiotics, Mignon has shown, from tests *in vitro* and on mice, the action of the antibiotics to be considerably augmented by being administered in a solution of oxygenated turpentine derivatives. There are, however, some constituents of some essential oils (aldehydes, ketones and some alcohols) which inactivate antibiotics and so limit their use in ointment form (Valnet 1980 p. 39).

The aroma of jasmine has been shown to shorten pentobarbital-induced sleeping time (in mice); *cis-* and *trans-*phytol were considered the stimulant-like compounds in solvent extracted oil (Kikuchi et al 1989) and *Cymbopogon citratus* injected peritoneally (in rats) was found to be analgesic, to prolong phenobarbitone induced sleeping time and to potentiate the effects of morphine (Seth, Kokate & Varma 1976).

Molecular structure

A relationship between the molecular structure of the essential oil components and their therapeutic effect has been studied and published (Franchomme & Pénoël 2001). This is an interesting piece of work and although not proven rigorously is nevertheless very useful to therapists when studying and selecting oils; the principles involved are to be found in Price (2000 pp. 52–54). Balacs (1991) comments that it is based on the presence of key chemical groups in the oil molecules. If this approach is valid, then it may well be that essential oil molecules are interacting with the same receptors on nerve cells and in other tissues which respond to drugs. See also Hormonelike above.

Homoeopathy

For many years now we have been questioning practitioners of homoeopathy as to whether homoeopathic treatment is affected in any way by the concurrent use of essential oils, and the answers have varied from the total prohibition of all essential oils to the unrestricted use of any. However, the chief common ground is that peppermint should be avoided and probably eucalyptus and camphor as well, perhaps due to their strong aroma, and this is what is advised in the absence of a definitive answer.

SUMMARY

The numerous therapeutic properties of essential oils have been examined in some detail, and scientific confirmation of traditional wisdom given where possible. It is to be hoped that more controlled trials will take place, and the importance of the totality of effects of any essential oil will be given precedence over the activity of its components.

References

Abbot D D et al 1961 Chronic oral toxicity of oil of sassafras and safrole. Pharmacologist 3(73): 62

Abramovici A et al 1985 Benign hyperplasia of ventral prostate in rats induced by a monoterpene (preliminary report). The Prostate 7: 389–394

Achterrath-Tuckerman U, Kunde R, Flaskamp O, Theimer I, Theimer K 1980 Pharmacological investigations with compounds of chamomile. V. Investigations on the spasmolytic effect of compounds of chamomile. Planta Medica, Stuttgart 39: 38–50

Albert-Puleo M 1980 Fennel and anise as oestrogenic agents. Journal of Ethnopharmacology 2: 337–344

Anderson M 1998 Sweet smell of success for Monklands hospital. Scottish Nurse 1998 2(8): 7

Balacs T 1991 Essential issues. International Journal of Aromatherapy 3(4): 24

Bartram T 1995 Encyclopedia of herbal medicine. Grace, Christchurch

Becker H 1983 Deutsche Apotheker Zeitung 123: 2470

Becker H, Förster W 1984 Biologie, Chemie und Pharmakologie pflanzlicher Sedativa. Zeitschrift Phytotherapie Stuttgart 5: 817–823

Becker H, Reichling J 1981 Deutsche Apotheker

Zeitung 121: 1185

Belaiche P 1979 Traité de phytothérapie et d'aromathérapie, 3 vols. Maloine, Paris

Belaiche P 1985a L'huile essentielle de *Melaleuca alternifolia* (Cheel) dans les infections cutanées. Phytothérapie 15 September: 15–18

Belaiche P 1985b L'huile essentielle de *Melaleuca alternifolia* (Cheel) dans les infections urinaires colibacillaires chroniques idiopathiques. Phytothérapie 15 September: 9–12

Belaiche P 1985c L'huile essentielle de *Melaleuca alternifolia* (Cheel) dans les infections vaginales à *Candida albicans*. Phytothérapie 15 September: 13–14

Bennett A, Stamford F 1988 The biological activity of eugenol, a major constituent of nutmeg, on prostaglandins, the intestine and other tissues. Phytotherapy Research 2: 124–129

Berman B M, Singh B K, Lao L, Singh B B, Ferentz K S, Hartnol S M 1995 Physicians' attitudes towards complementary or alternative medicine: a regional survey. Journal of the American Board of Family Practitioners 8(5): 361–366

Bernadet M 1983 La phyto-aromathérapie pratique. Dangles, St-Jean-de-Braye

Beylier M F 1979 Bacteriostatic activity of some Australian essential oils. Perfumer & Flavorist 4(23) (April/May): 23–25

Boeters M 1969 Behandlung vegetativer Regulationsstörungen mit Valepotriaten (Valmane). Münchner Medizin Wochenschrift 11: 1873–1876

Bonnaure F 1919 Essais sur les propriétés bactericides de quelques huiles essentielles. Parfumerie Moderne 12: 151

Bonnelle C 1993 Des hommes et des plantes. Editions du Parc Naturel Régional du Vercors, Lans-en-Vercors, p. 32

Borkan J, Neher J O, Anson O, Smoker B 1994 Referrals for alternative therapies. Journal of Family Practitioners 39(6): 545–550

Bowker (undated) Food additives and the patients they affect. CBA and Associates Ltd, London (leaflet)

Boyd E M, Pearson G L 1946 The expectorant action of volatile oils. American Journal of Medical Science 211: 602–610

Buchbauer G 1993 Biological effects of fragrances and essential oils. Perfumer & Flavorist 18 (January/February): 19–24

Buchbauer G, Jirovetz L, Jäger W 1992 Passiflora and lime blossoms: motility effects after inhalation of the essential oil and of some of the main constituents in animal experiment. Archiva Pharmaceutica (Weinheim) 325: 247–248

Buchbauer G, Jirovetz L, Jäger W, Plank C, Dietrich H 1993 Fragrance compounds and essential oils with sedative effects upon inhalation. Journal of Pharmaceutical Sciences 82(6) (June): 660–664

Buckle J 1997 Clinical aromatherapy in nursing. Arnold, London, p. 125

Carson C F, Riley T V 1993 Antimicrobial activity of the essential oil of *Melaleuca alternifolia*. Applied Microbiology 16(2): 49–55

Carson C F, Cookson B D, Farrelly H D, Riley T V 1995 Susceptibility of methicillin-resistant *Staphylococcus aureus* to the essential oil of *Melaleuca alternifolia*. Journal of Antimicrobial Chemotherapy 35: 421–424

Cavel L 1918 Sur la valeur antiseptique de quelques huiles essentielles. Comptes Rendus Académie des Sciences, p. 827

Chabrol E, Charonnat R, Maximum M, Busson A 1932 Le serpolet: cholagogue. Comptes Rendus Société Biologie 109: 275–276

Chamberland M 1887 Les essences au point de vue de leurs propriétés antiseptiques. Annales Institut Pasteur 1: 153–154

Chevallier A 1996 Encyclopedia of medicinal plants. Dorling Kindersley, London

Cohen R A, Kucera L S, Herrman E C 1964 Antiviral activity of *Melissa officinalis* extract. Proceedings of the Society of Experimental Biology and Medicine 117: 431–434

Courmont P, Morel P, Bay I 1938 The antiseptic action of essential oils. Parfumerie Moderne 21: 161

Cowan J W et al 1967 Antithyroid activity of onion volatiles. Australian Journal of Biological Sciences 20: 683–685

D'Arcy P F 1993 Drug reactions and interactions. International Pharmacy Journal 7(4) (July/August): 140–142

Deans S G, Ritchie G A 1987 Antibacterial properties of plant essential oils. International Journal of Food Microbiology 5: 165–180

Deans S G, Svoboda K P 1988 Antibacterial activity of French tarragon (*Artemisia dracunculus* L.) essential oil and its constituents during ontogeny. Journal of Horticultural Science 63: 135–140

Deans S G, Svoboda K P 1989 Antibacterial activity of summer savory [*Satureia hortensis* L.] essential oil and its constituents. Journal of Horticultural Science 64: 205–211

Deans S G, Svoboda K P 1990a Essential oil profiles of several temperate and tropical aromatic plants: their antimicrobial and antioxidative properties. Proceedings 75th International Symposium of Research Institute for Medicinal Plants, Budakalasz, Hungary, pp. 25-27. (Copies obtainable from authors at Scottish Agricultural College, Ayr)

Deans S G, Svoboda K P 1990b The antimicrobial properties of marjoram (*Origanum majorana* L.) volatile oil. Flavor & Fragrance Journal 5(3): 187–190

Debelmas A M, Rochat J 1964 Etude comparée sur la fibre lisse des solutions aqueuses saturées d'essence de thym, de thymol et de carvacrol. Bulletin des Travaux. Société de Pharmacie de Lyon 4: 163–172

Debelmas A M, Rochat J 1967a Action des eaux saturées d'huiles essentielles sur la musculature lisse. 25th International Congress of Pharmaceutical Science. Butterworth, London, pp. 601–607

Debelmas A M, Rochat J 1967b Activité antispasmodique étudiée sur une cinquantaine d'échantillons différents. Plantes Médicinales et Phytothérapie 1: 23–27

Decazes J-M 1993 The masking effect of perfume ingredients. Symposium at Stoke-on-Trent: Fragrance – more than just a pleasant smell? Society of Cosmetic Chemists

Dube S, Upadhyay P D, Tripath S C 1989 Antifungal, physiochemical, and insect-repelling activity of the essential oil of *Ocimum basilicum*. Canadian Journal of Botany 67(7): 2085–2087

Duraffourd P 1982 En forme tous les jours. La Vie Claire, Périgny, p. 107

Duraffourd P 1987 Les huiles essentielles et la santé. La Maison du Bien-Etre, Montreuil-sous-Bois

Eccles S 1997 Editorial. Aromatherapy Quarterly 55: 5

Entertainer 21–27 April 94 The Entertainer Costa del Sol edition

Eremenko A E, Nikolaevskii V V, Kostin N F, Meshkov V V 1987 Letuchie fraktsii fitontsidov na osnove efirnykh masel v sostav lechebno-reabilitatsionnykh kompleksov pri khronicheskikh bronkhitakh. Volatile fractions of essential oil based phytoncides as a component of therapeutic-rehabilitative complexes in chronic bronchitis (in Russian). Tikhomirov AA Ter. Arkh. 59(3): 126–130

Ernst E, Resch K L, White A R 1995 Complementary medicine. What physicians think of it: a meta analysis. Archives of Internal Medicine 155(22): 2405–2408

Foster S 1993 Herbal renaissance. Gibbs Smith, Layton, Utah, p. 93

Franchomme P, Pénoël D 2001 L'aromathérapie exactement. Jollois, Limoges

Gattefossé R M 1919 Propriétés bactéricides de quelques huiles essentielles. Parfumerie Moderne 13: 152

Gattefossé R M 1932 Rôle antiseptique de la lavande. Parfumerie Moderne 26: 543–553

Gattefossé R M 1937 Aromatherapy (transl 1993). Daniel, Saffron Walden, p. 87

Geldof A A et al 1992 Oestrogenic action of commonly used fragrance agent citral induces prostatic hyperplasia. Urological Research 20: 139–144

Gershbein L E 1977 Regeneration of rat liver in the presence of essential oils and their components. Food and Cosmetics Toxicology 15: 173–181

Gildemeister E, Hoffmann F 1956 Die ätherischen Öle, vol 1. Akadamie Verlag, Berlin, p 119

Glowania H J, Raulin C, Swoboda M 1987 Effect of chamomile on wound healing – a clinical double-blind study. Zeitschrift für Hautkrankheiten (Berlin) 62(17): 1262, 1267–1271

Gordonoff T 1938 Ergebnisse der Physiologie, biologischen Chemie und experimentallen. Pharmakologie 40: 53

Griggs B 1997 New green pharmacy. Vermilion, London, p. 293

Guillemain J, Rousseau A, Delaveau P 1989 Neurodepressive effects of the essential oil of Lavandula angustifolia Mill. Annales Pharmaceutiques Franìaises 47(6): 337–343

Hay R K M, Waterman P G 1993 Volatile oil crops. Longman, Harlow, p. 52

Herrman E C Jr, Kucera L S 1967 Antiviral substances in plants of the mint family (Labiatae). II. Nontannin polyphenol of Melissa officinalis. Proceedings of the Society for Experimental and Biological Medicine 117: 369–374

Hinou J B, Harvala C E, Hinou E B 1989 Antimicrobial activity screening of 32 common constituents of essential oils. Pharmazie 44(4) (April): 302–303

Holland E H 1941 Results of a series of investigations carried out on the germicidal, disinfectant and bacteriostatic action of Melasol (Melaleuca alternifolia). Unpublished paper, Sydney University

Jakovlev V, Isaac O, Flaskamp E 1983 Pharmacological investigations with compounds of chamomile. VI. Investigations on the antiphlogistic effects of chamazulene and matricin. Planta Medica 49: 67–73

Jalsenjak V, Peljnjak S, Kustrak D 1987 Microcapsules of sage oil: essential oils content and antimicrobial activity. Pharmazie 42(6) (June): 419–420

Janssen A M, Scheffer J J C, Baerheim Svendsen A, Aynehchi Y 1984 Pharmazeutisch Weekblad (scientific edn) 6: 157

Janssen A M, Chin N L J, Scheffer J J C, Baerheim Svendsen A 1986 Screening for antimicrobial activity of some essential oils by the agar overlay techniques. Pharmazeutisch Weekblad (scientific edn) 8: 289–292

Jasper C, Maruzella J C, Laurence Liguori L 1958a The in vitro antifungal activity of essential oils. Journal of the American Pharmaceutical Association 47(4): 294–296

Jasper C, Maruzella J C, Percival A, Henry P AsThe antimicrobial activity of perfume oils. Journal of the American Pharmaceutical Association 47(7): 471

Jori A, Bianchetti A, Prestini P E 1969 Effect of essential oils on drug metabolism. Biochemical Pharmacology 18: 2081–2085

Juven B J, Kanner J, Schved F, Weisslowicz H 1994 Factors that interact with the antibacterial action of thyme essential oil and its active constituents. Journal of Applied Bacteriology 76: 626–631

Kellner W, Kober W 1954 Möglichkeiten der Wewendung ätherischer Öle zur Raumdesinfektion. I. Mitteilung: Die Wirkung gebrèuchlicher ätherischer Öle auf Testkeime. Arzneimittel-Forschung [Drug Research] 4(5): 319

Kellner W, Kober W 1955 Möglichkeiten der Werwendung ätherischer Öle zur Raumdesinfektion. II. Arzneimittel-Forschung [Drug Research] 5(4): 224

Kellner W, Kober W 1956 Möglichkeiten der Werwendung ètherischer Öle zur Raumdesinfektion. III. Arzneimittel-Forschung [Drug Research] 6(12): 768

Kienholz M 1959 Action antibactérienne des huiles essentielles. Arzneimittel-Forschung [Drug Research] 9(8): 518–519

Kikuchi A, Tsuchiya T, Tanida M, Uenoyama S, Nakayama Y 1989 Stimulant like ingredients in absolute jasmine. Chemical Senses 14(2): 304

Knobloch K, Pauli A, Iberl B, Weigand H, Weis N 1989 Antibacterial and antifungal properties of essential oil components. Journal of Essential Oil Research 1: 119–128

Kucera L S, Herrman J C Jr 1967 Antiviral substances in plants in the mint family (Labiatae). 1. Tannin of *Melissa officinalis*. Proceedings of the Society for Experimental and Biological Medicine 124: 865

Larrondo J V, Calvo M A 1991 Effect of essential oils on *Candida albicans*: a scanning electron microscope study. Biomedical Letters 46(184): 269–272

Lautié R, Passebecq A 1984 Aromatherapy. Thorsons, Wellingborough, p. 74

Lawrence F (ed) 1987 Additives – your complete survival guide. Century, London

Lembke A, Deininger R 1985 Preparation and method for stimulating the immune system. German Patent 3508875 A 1 21 November 1985

Lembke A, Deininger R 1988 Virus inactivating pharmaceutical containing formates and black pepper oil. European Patent (EP) 259617 A 2 16 March 1988

Low D, Rowal B D, Griffin W J 1974 Antibacterial action of the essential oils of some Australian Myrtaceae. Planta Medica 26: 184

Lucks B C 2003 Essential oils in holistic menopause management. In Essence Winter (2) (3)

Mabey R 1988 The complete new herbal. Elm Tree, London

Malowan S L 1931 Zeitschrift für Hygiene 1(1): 93

Martindale W H 1910 Antiseptic powers of essential oils. Perfumery & Essential Oil Record 1: 266, 274

Maruzella J C 1961 Antifungal properties of perfume oils. Journal of the American Pharmaceutical Association 50: 655

Medicines Act 1968 HMSO, London

Melegari M, Albasini A, Pecorari P, Vampa G, Rinaldi M, Rossi T, Bianchi A 1988 Chemical characteristics and pharmacological properties of the essential oil of *Anthemis nobilis*. Fitoterapia 59(6): 449–455

Mills S Y 1991a Essential book of herbal medicine. Penguin, London, p. 452

Mills S Y 1991b The essential book of herbal medicine. Arkana, London

Moleyar V, Narasimham P 1992 Antibacterial activity of essential oil components. International Journal of Food Microbiology 16: 337–342

Onawunmi G O 1988 In vitro studies on the antibacterial activity of phenoxyethanol in combination with lemongrass oil. Pharmazie 43(1) (January): 42–43

Onawunmi G O 1989 Antifungal activity of lemongrass oil. International Journal of Crude Drug Research 27(2): 121–126

Onawunmi G O, Ogunlana E O 1986 A study of the antibacterial activity of the essential oil of lemongrass *Cymbopogon citratus* (DC) Stapf. International Journal of Crude Drug Research 24(2): 64–68

Onawunmi G O, Yisak W A, Ogunlana E O 1984 Antibacterial constituents in the essential oil of *Cymbopogon citratus* (DC) Stapf. Journal of Ethnopharmacology 12(3): 279–286

Pandey M P, Prasad J, Awasthi L P, Kaushik P 1988 Antiviral effect of the essential oils from lemongrass (*Cymbopogon flexuosus*), mint (*Mentha arvensis*) and vetiver (*Vetiveria zizanioides*). Indigenous medicinal plants including microbes and fungi. National seminar on conservation and ethnobotanical aspects. Today and Tomorrows Printers and Publishers, New Delhi, pp. 47–49

Pellecuer J, Allegrini J, De Buochberg S 1974 Etude in vitro de l'activité anti-bactérienne et antifongique de l'essence de *Satureia montana* L. Labiées. Journal de Pharmacie de Belgique 29(2): 137–144

Pellecuer J, Allegrini J, De Buochberg S, Passat J 1975 Place de l'essence de *Satureia montana* L. Labiées dans l'arsenal thérapeutique. Plantes Médicinales et Phytothérapie 9(2): 99–106

Pellecuer J, Allegrini J, Seimeon M, De Buochberg S 1976 Huiles essentielles bactéricides et fongicides. Revue de l'Institut de Lyon 1(2): 135–159

Pellecuer J, Roussel J L, Andary C 1973 Propriétés antifongiques comparatives des essences des trois Labiées méditerranéennes: romarin, sariette et thym. Travaux de la Société de Pharmacie de Montpelier 33(4): 587

Pena E F 1962 Melaleuca alternifolia oil – its use for trichomonal vaginitis and other vaginal infections. Obstetrics and Gynaecology June: 793–795

Pénoël D 1981 Phytomédecine. CIMP, La Courtête 1/2: 63

Perkin M R, Pearcy R M, Fraser J S 1994 A comparison of the attitudes shown by general practitioners, hospital doctors and medical students towards alternative medicine. Journal of the Royal Society of Medicine 87(9): 523–525

Pollock I, Young E, Stoneham M, Slater N, Wilkinson J, Warner J 1989 Surveys of colourings and preservatives in drugs. British Medical Journal 299: 649–651

Poucher W A 1936 Perfumes, cosmetics and soaps, 3 vols. Chapman & Hall, London

Price S 2000 The aromatherapy workbook. Thorsons, London

Quevauviller A, Panousse-Perrin J 1952a Exaltation du pouvoir anesthétique local de la cocaïne par l'essence de Niaouli purifiée. Anesthésie 9: 421

Quevauviller A, Panousse-Perrin J 1952b Influence du Gomenol sur l'activité in vitro de certains antibiotiques. Revue de Pathologie Comparée et Hygiène Générale 637: 296

Raharivelomanana P J, Terrom G P, Bianchini J P, Coulanges P 1989 Study of the antimicrobial action of various essential oils extracted from Malagasy plants. II: Lauraceae. Archives Institut Pasteur de l'Afrique (Madagascar) 56(1): 261–271

Ramanoelina A R, Terrom G P, Bianchini J P, Coulanges P 1987 Antibacterial action of essential oils extracted from Madagascar plants. Archives Institut Pasteur de l'Afrique (Madagascar) 53(1): 217–226

Rideal S, Rideal E K, Sciver A 1928 An investigation into the germicidal powers and capillary activities of certain essential oils. Perfumery & Essential Oil Record 19: 285

Rideal E K, Sciver A, Richardson N E G 1930 Perfumery & Essential Oil Record 21: 341

Ritzerfeld W 1959 Arzneimittel-Forschung 9: 521

Rose J 1992 The aromatherapy book. North Atlantic Books, Berkeley

Rossi T, Melegari M, Bianchi A, Albasini A, Vampa G 1988 Sedative, antiinflammatory and antidiuretic effects induced in rats by essential oils of varieties of Anthemis nobilis: a comparative study. Pharmacology Research Communications 5 (December 20): 71–74

Roulier G 1990 Les huiles essentielles pour votre santé. Dangles, St-Jean-de-Braye

Salji J P et al 1971 The antithyroid activity of Allium volatiles in the rat – in vitro studies. European Journal of Pharmacology 16: 251–253

Schilcher H 1985 Effects and side effects of essential oils. In: Baerheim Svendsen A, Scheffer J J C (eds) Essential oils and aromatic plants. Martinus Nijhof/Junk, Dordrecht

Schmidt P W 1936 Zentralblad für Bakteriologie, Parasitenkunde und Infektionskrankenheiten 138: 104

Schmiedeberg O 1913 Grundriss der Pharmakologie, 7th edn. Pharmakologie, Leipzig

Schnaubelt K 1994 Aromatherapy and chronic viral infections. In: Aroma 93 Conference Proceedings. Aromatherapy Publications, Brighton, pp. 34-41

Schneider G 1975 Pharmazeutische Biologie. Wissenschaftsverlag, Mannheim, p 128

Scientific American 1886 [quoted in Scientific American 1996 50, 100 and 150 years ago.] September: 14

Seth G, Kokate C K, Varma K C 1976 Effect of essential oil of Cymbopogon citratus Stapf. On the central nervous system. Indian Journal of Experimental Biology 14(3): 370–371

Shemesh A U, Mayo W L 1991 Tea tree oil – natural antiseptic and fungicide. Journal of Alternative and Complementary Medicine 9 (12 December): 11–12

Sherry E, Boeck H, Warnke P H 2001 American Journal of Infection Control 29: 346

Stewart D 2005 The chemistry of essential oils made simple. Care, Marble Hill, Missouri

Szalontai M, Verzar-Petri G, Florian E 1976 Acta Pharmaceutica [Hungary] 46: 232

Szalontai M, Verzar-Petri G, Florian E 1977 Contribution to the study of antimycotic effect of biologically active components of Matricaria chamomilla L. Parfümerie und Kosmetik [Hungary] 58: 121

Szalontai M, Verzar-Petri G, Florian E, Gimpel F 1975a Pharmazeutische Zeitung 120: 982

Szalontai M, Verzar-Petri G, Florian E, Gimpel F 1975b Deutsche Apotheker Zeitung 115: 912

Taddei I, Giachetti D, Taddei E, Mantovani P, Bianchi E 1988 Spasmolytic activity of peppermint, sage and rosemary essences and their major constituents. Fitoterapia 59: 463–468

Thiemer K, Stadler R, Isaac O 1973 Arzneimittel-Forschung 23: 756

Thompson D P, Cannon C 1986 Toxicity of essential oils on toxigenic and nontoxigenic fungi. Bulletin of Environmental Contamination and Toxicology 36(4) April: 527–532

Tisserand R, Balacs T 1995 Essential oil safety. Churchill Livingstone, New York, pp. 41–43

Trease G E, Evans W C 1983 Pharmacognosy, 12th edn. Baillière Tindall, London

Tukioka M 1927 Proceedings, vol 3. Imperial Academy, Tokyo, p. 624

Valnet J 1980 The practice of aromatherapy. Daniel, Saffron Walden

Verdet 1989 Why phytotherapy? Aromatherapy Study Trip Lecture notes. Price Publishing, Hinckley, p. 10

Verhoef M J, Sutherland L R 1995 General practitioners assessment of and interest in alternative medicine in Canada. Society Scientific Medicine 41(4): 511–515

Viaud H 1983 Huiles essentielles. Présence, Sisteron

Vichkanova S A, Dzhanashiya N M, Goryunova L V 1973 Antiviral activity displayed by the essential oil of Eucalyptus viminalis and of some frost-hardy eucalypti. Farmakologiia Toksikologiia 36(3): 339–341

von Braunschweig R 1999 Powerful contents of the angelica root: the monoterpenes. Forum E1

Wagner H, Wierer M, et al 1986 In vitro Hemmung der Prostaglandin Biosynthese durch étherische Öle und phenolische Verbindungen. Planta Medica 184–187

Weiss R F 1988 Herbal medicine. Arcanum, Göteborg, p. 296

Williams A C, Barry B W 1989 Essential oils as novel human skin penetration enhancers. International Journal of Pharmaceutics 57: R7–R9

You-Ja Ro, Hyae-Chung Ha, Chun-Gill Kim, Hye-A Yeom 2002 The effects of aromatherapy on pruritus in patients undergoing hemodialysis. Dermatology Nursing August 14(4): 231–238

Yousef R T, Tawil G G 1980 Antimicrobial activity of volatile oils. Pharmazie 35(11): 698–701

Zara M 1966 Association atoxique de dérivées terpéniques d'huiles essentielles possédant une triple action en hépatologie (cholérétique, antispasmodique, lipotrope). Vie Médicinale 47(10): 1549–1553

Zondec B et al 1938 Phenol methyl ethers as oestrogenic agents. Biochemical Journal 32: 641–645

SECTION 2

The foundations of practice

Chapter 5

How essential oils enter the body

Len Price

INTRODUCTION

Essential oils follow three main pathways to gain entry to the body: ingestion, inhalation and absorption through the skin (Fig. 5.1). Ingestion is little used in the UK. Of the two remaining pathways, inhalation is a very effective method and indeed is regarded by some (e.g. Buchbauer 1988) as the only method truly deserving the name aromatherapy. However, topical application via the skin has also been found to be effective – the route selected depends on the problem being helped.

INHALATION

Access via the nasal passages is indisputably the quickest effective route in the treatment of emotional problems such as stress and depression (and also some types of headache). This is because the nose has direct contact with the brain, which is responsible for triggering the effects of essential oils regardless of the route they use to gain access to it. The nose itself is not the organ of smell, but simply modifies the temperature and humidity of the inhaled air and collects any foreign matter which may be breathed in. The first cranial (olfactory) nerve is responsible for the sense of smell and serves the receptor cells, of which there are two groups of about 25 million, each occupying a small area (of about 4 cm^2) at the top of the nostrils (Van Toller 1993).

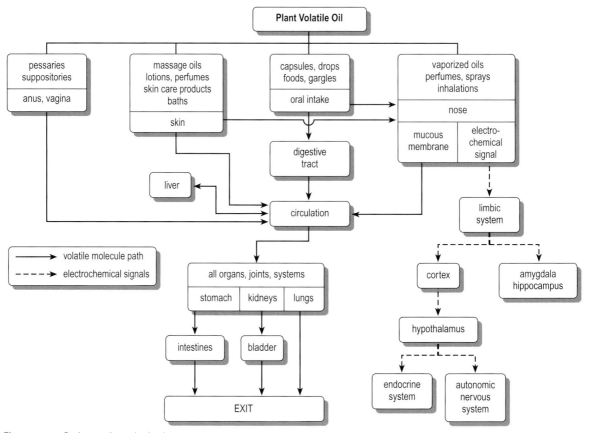

Figure 5.1 Pathways into the body.

INHALATION AND THE MUCOUS MEMBRANES

When inhaling any vapour, some molecules from it inevitably travel down the pathway to the lungs where, if they are appropriate essential oils, they can have an immediate and beneficial impact on many breathing difficulties. In the nose the endothelium is thin and the site is close to the brain, therefore it must be assumed that essential oil molecules reach the local circulation and the brain fairly easily and quickly. On their journey to the lungs some molecules are undoubtedly absorbed by the mucous linings of the respiratory pathways, the bronchi and multitudinous bronchioles, where access is very easy. Arriving at the point of gaseous exchange in the alveoli, the tiny molecules are transferred to the blood circulating the lungs. It can be seen that deep breathing will increase the quantity of any essence or essential oil taken into the body by this route. Ill effects from inhalation

of essential oils normally used in aromatherapy are rare.

METHODS OF INHALATION

Inhalation is an unobtrusive way of using essential oils in a health-care setting. They may be given via a tissue, the hands (in an emergency), a vaporizer, etc., and all are effective in the appropriate situation. To select oils for particular conditions, see the tables in Chapter 4 and Appendix B.9.

Tissues

Inhalation from a tissue with five to six drops of essential oil (three drops for children, the elderly and pregnant women) is most effective for immediate results, requiring two or three deep breaths to ensure good contact with the cilia. To give further benefit, and easier with children and the elderly, the tissue can be placed inside the shirt, blouse or nightwear so that the effects may continue as the heat of the body causes the oil molecules to evaporate and float upwards to the nose. Firm tissues such as kitchen towels hold the aroma longer than do paper handkerchiefs.

Q-tips

This method uses less essential oil than does a tissue, because it is concentrated in a small area. The Q-tip is held against the dropper and one drop allowed to wet it. Unlike a crumpled tissue, it cannot be placed next to the skin, but has the advantage of slower evaporation, so it can be used for longer.

Hands

This is an excellent method, but should be confined to emergencies only and is not suitable for children. A solitary drop of essential oil (single, or from a mix) can be put into one of the patient's palms, which is then rubbed briefly against the other palm to disperse and warm the oil. With eyes closed, the patient places the cupped hands over the nose, avoiding the eye area, taking a deep nasal breath. It is usually respiratory or stress conditions which require this sort of help.

Steamers

Allowing a patient to hold a basin of hot water is not acceptable in many hospital situations, on account of the Health and Safety Act (1994). Even if the nurse holds it there is always the possibility that some people, especially those with learning difficulties, may strike out (involuntarily or other-wise) and knock the scalding water over themselves or the nurse. Home-visiting health professionals may find in certain circumstances, and with people whose movements are stable, that the method can be used safely, but it is our opinion that dry inhalation is safer for those not enjoying full health and living alone, unless a proprietary brand electric diffuser is used – which can be expensive.

Nebulizers are safer but unfortunately essential oils, especially if undiluted, can attack some kinds of plastic, so care must be taken not to damage the equipment. A precautionary test is advisable for any plastic which may come into contact with essential oils. This applies also to facial steamers. These methods are normally used for respiratory problems and the common cold, though any problem which can benefit from inhalation may obtain speedier relief when steam is used. The heat of the water evaporates the oil molecules more quickly, increasing the strength of the vapour and for this reason only half the number of drops (i.e. three) are needed compared with inhalation from a tissue (or one to two drops for a child, elderly person or pregnant woman). The following cautions may be helpful:

- Ensure the patient's eyes are kept closed and watch carefully for any adverse reaction such as choking or coughing, which can happen if too many drops have been used or too deep a breath is taken.
- One drop only – with water of not too high a temperature – is adequate for asthmatics because the overpowering effect of the vapour (stronger because of the speedy evaporation referred to above) may have an adverse effect.

Baths

Treatment by putting oils into the bath is effective because not only do they come into gentle contact with the skin, but also they are inhaled at the same time; thus a double benefit is derived. For details, see Methods of percutaneous absorption below.

Spray bottle

A quick way of freshening the air when dressings are being changed for patients with bed sores, gangrene, etc. is using 10–12 drops of essential oil in 250 ml of water, shaking the bottle well before spraying the room. The essential oils to use in this case are *Pinus sylvestris* [Scots pine], *Thymus vulgaris* [thyme] (all chemotypes, though phenolic thymes are the most powerful antiseptics), *Syzygium aromaticum* [clove], *Eucalyptus smithii* [gully ash], *Mentha* x *piperita* [peppermint].

Vaporizers and diffusers

Possibly the most favoured way of using inhalation in a health-care setting at the moment is from a vaporizer. This liberates the lightest molecules from the oil first, releasing the heavier ones progressively. Although there are many different types of vaporizers available, only electric ones are considered safe where patients are concerned (the British Safety Standard mark should be looked for on the model to be used). Electric vaporizers should be thermostatically controlled at a low temperature, preventing the essential oils from becoming too hot. If this occurs, not only are they used up too quickly to be economical but the heaviest molecules burning off last may produce an unpleasant acrid smell.

Diffusers (units with a small blown-glass container for the essential oils) are more efficient in that they push out all the differently sized molecules at the same time. Unlike vaporizers using heat, there is no burning of residue when the essential oil is used up. Their only disadvantage is cost: the oils are used up fairly rapidly and the equipment cost which can be up to three times greater than that of an electric vaporizer. A recent development on the market uses a new technique to deliver evenly and economically all sizes of molecules contained in the essential oils into the atmosphere. The essential oils are released in a regulated manner so that the air does not become overloaded; there are time switches for selecting both operating and rest times, making this method suitable for clinical use.

Ethical considerations

A few hospitals use vaporizers and diffusers in single-occupancy rooms only – not in general ward areas, as it is felt by some therapists to be unethical to impose aromas (which may be disliked or unwanted by some) on other occupants. Nevertheless, when the effects required for a whole ward are the same for each occupant, e.g. when conducting a trial or keeping a ward free from infection, the method is viable and effective; it can also be useful in the reduction of stress and insomnia as well as in the destruction of germs. It seems strange that there is not equal ethical consideration regarding piped music, the wearing of perfume, the use of perfumed spray cleaners or

---

Box 5.1   Use of fragranced cleaning materials

When lecturing abroad, the authors' room in the hotel was on the 24th floor.

They stepped into the lift and began to ascend. After one or two breaths, Len's breathing began to be laboured. I could smell immediately that the lift had just been cleaned with a synthetic lavender product and it was this which was affecting Len's lungs.

At the 10th floor, his breathing was noticeably worse, so I placed his handkerchief over his mouth and nose, telling him to hold his breath as long as he could. I also pressed the 12th floor button, but the lift was already programmed for its first stop at the 24th.

When we reached the 24th floor, Len stumbled out of the lift – and tried to take a breath. However, he was now in the throes of an asthma attack and breathing was very difficult.

Fortunately, our room was near the lift and as soon as we entered, I took out the bottle of Len's 'Rescue' blend of undiluted essential oils – which I carry everywhere with me.

Putting a few drops on his handkerchief for his nose and mouth, I quickly removed his shirt and applied about 20 drops down his spine, rubbing them well into his spinal column and across each side of his back in the area of his lungs, adding more drops to ensure full coverage.

With my first and second fingers, I then 'drew' firm lines several times in the spinal channel, repeating these together with the rubbing of the lung area for several minutes.

Almost immediately, Len's breathing began to improve, his shoulders more relaxed – and without heaving.

The essential oils in this blend are equal quantities of:

- *Abies balsamica* [Canadian balsam]
- *Aloysia triphylla* [verbena]
- *Boswellia carteri* [frankincense]
- *Eucalyptus smithii* [gully gum]
- *Hyssopus officinalis* [hyssop]
- *Pinus mugo* var. *pumilio* [dwarf pine]

the pollution of air through cigarette fumes, the last three of which can adversely affect the health of those in the vicinity. Unfortunately, large vaporizer units used in hotels and offices are often run on commercial-grade essential oils and aromas to keep costs down, without taking into account what effect long-term exposure may have on people's health. It is already known that artificial perfumes and adulterated essential oils cause sensitivities in asthmatics and skin reactions in those susceptible to such effects (see Box 5.1). 'Environmental fragrancing', as this practice is termed, is most advanced in the USA, where there is growing concern at the use of synthetic aromas (see Ch. 8). The liberty of the individual is an important consideration and, unlike shoppers irritated by 'muzak' or 'fragrancing' designed to alter their mood, hospital patients are not free to walk away from an environmental influence which they may not like.

ABSORPTION VIA THE SKIN

Until the second half of the 20th century the skin was thought to be almost impermeable (Maibach & Marzulli 1977, Stoughton 1959). This old idea still persists, even though the skin is now known to be a poor barrier to lipophilic substances (Brun 1952) and essential oils in a base oil applied to the skin are absorbed into the bloodstream (Jäger et al 1992). Most chemicals are absorbed to some degree and this is made use of in patch therapy, e.g. glyceryl trinitrate must penetrate the skin to reach the blood vessels and heart to treat angina, and many other substances – including oestradiol, scopolamine and nicotine – are administered in this way, while others are being tested – e.g. beta blockers, testosterone and antihistamines (Cleary 1993).

TRANSDERMAL DELIVERY

Many drugs are unsuitable for use in therapeutic transdermal delivery systems due to their low permeability through the skin, so the use of penetration enhancing agents is advantageous and various studies suggest that essential oils offer a useful selection of safe penetration enhancers to aid topical drug delivery. In tests by Williams & Barry (1989) eucalyptus and chenopodium essential oils caused a 30-fold increase in the drug 5-fluorouracil (5-FU) permeability coefficient using excised human skin. The skin permeation of the neuroleptic drug haloperidol was increased in the presence of cineole and (+)-limonene but that of chlorpromazine was not; in fact (+)-limonene reduced it (Almiral et al 1996): terpenes have been shown to have an enhancing effect on the transdermal permeation of hydrophilic drugs and chlorpromazine is more lipophilic than haloperidol.

The principal component of eucalyptus oil was investigated to determine whether 1,8-cineole could be detected in effective amounts in skeletal muscles after dermal application; the bioavailability of 1,8-cineole was 320% greater when using an applicator compared to using an occlusive dressing (Weyers & Brodbeck 1989). Takayama & Nagai (1994) studied the promoting effects of terpenes present in essential oils on the percutaneous absorption of indomethacin from hydrogels was investigated in rats *in vivo* and found that absorption was remarkably enhanced by cyclic monoterpenes such as limonene, terpinene and terpinolene. It was noted that the terpenes had a strong fluidizing effect on the lipid bilayer structure and (+)-limonene in the presence of ethanol changed the barrier structure of the skin, accelerating the transfer of ethanol and thus permeation of indomethacin was promoted due to its affinity with alcohol.

Sesquiterpenes also have been shown to increase 5-FU absorption across human (cadaver) skin; the increase was thought to be brought about by disrupting intercellular lipid bilayers and by forming complexes with 5-FU: sesquiterpenes with polar functional groups produced the best absorption improvements (Cornwall & Barry 1994). The mechanisms by which penetration enhancers increase the permeability of the stratum corneum are discussed by Cornwall et al (1996).

THE SKIN AS A WATER BARRIER

Water comprises 90% of any cell and therefore the skin has developed as a barrier specifically to resist water; nevertheless it is slightly permeable to water soluble substances, to water itself and to lipids (Riviere 1993). The absorption of drugs and poisons through the skin was studied by Macht

(1938) and there has been a considerable amount of research on pesticides and the skin. Pesticides, which dissolve in essential oils, are lipid-like and can therefore get through the skin – every farmer is aware of this health hazard, and thousands of people are killed each year by pesticides, mostly in developing countries. The amount absorbed through human skin varies enormously; for example less than 1% of cypermethrin pesticide is absorbed whereas up to 65% of the antifungal agent benzoic acid may penetrate the skin (Hotchkiss 1994).

The skin's success as a barrier is due in the main to the stratum corneum, the tough and durable, self-repairing keratinized layer, which is 20 layers of dead cells thick. Once a chemical gets past the epidermis – the only great obstacle – the rest of the journey into the body is easy, because the presence of lipids in all cell membranes negates the dermis's effectiveness as a barrier. For example, the antibacterial substance hexachlorophene is absorbed through the skin and was shown in 1969 to cause microscopically visible brain damage in rats (Winter 1984 p. 138) and chloasma in humans; in the 1970s hexachlorophene was used as an antiseptic in baby soaps and talcum powders, causing brain damage and even death in some babies after it had penetrated the skin (Jackson 1993). The lipid solubility of essential oil components allows these compounds to cross the blood–brain barrier (where certain substances are held back by the endothelium of cerebral capillaries) and make contact with the fluids around the brain (Anthony & Thibodeau 1983).

There are many factors which dictate the rate and quantity at which any given substance penetrates the skin, but it is now generally recognized that the skin is a semi-permeable membrane susceptible of penetration by substances to a greater or lesser degree (Lexicon Vevy 1993a). The physicochemical properties of the molecules, such as the molecular weight, spatial arrangement, polarity, optical activity, liposolubility, coefficients of diffusion and dissociation, are fundamental to skin penetration. Mills (1993) states that an advantage of the percutaneous route for remedies is the avoidance of the 'first-pass liver' effect, i.e. they are not subject to immediate metabolization by the liver as they are in oral administration.

THE SKIN AS A GATEWAY

On account of their solubility in the lipids found in the stratum corneum, lipophilic substances (such as essential oils) are considered to be easily absorbed. The absorption of organic compounds with anionic or cationic groups (weak acids and alkalis) takes place when they are found in undissociated form – then they are more lipophilic than when dissociated; it also depends on their dissociation constant and on the pH of the substance and of the skin. The majority of essential oils and their components pass through the skin and the organism and can be detected in exhaled air within 20–60 minutes (Katz 1947). Some examples of the times recorded are 1,8-cineole and α-pinene take 20 minutes; eucalyptus, eugenol, linalyl acetate, geranyl acetate, anethole and thyme oil take between 20 and 40 minutes; bergamot, aniseed and lemon oils, take between 40 and 60 minutes; true lavender, pine, geranium and citronella oils and cinnamaldehyde take between 60 and 80 minutes; coriander, rue and peppermint oils, geraniol and citrals take up to 2 hours.

Once the essential oil constituents have passed the epidermis and entered the complex of lymph and blood vessels, nerves, sweat and oil glands, follicles, collagen, fibroblasts, mast cells, elastin and so on (known as the dermis), they are then carried away in the circulation to pervade every cell in the body. There is no research at the moment comparing percutaneous absorption with the gastrointestinal route (Torii et al 1991).

The main factors affecting the penetration of the skin by essential oils are detailed below.

Intrinsic factors

- **Area of skin.** The very large area of the skin – in the region of 2 m^2 – makes it possible for a significant quantity of essential oils to be applied to the skin and so taken into the body. If a set quantity of essential oil in a carrier is applied to a small area of skin, then less will enter than if the same quantity were to be applied to a greater area.
- **Thickness and permeability of the epidermis.** On palmar and plantar skin sites where the epidermis is quite thick and there are no oil glands, the time taken to cross the skin is longer,

especially for any lipid soluble components. There is less resistance to water soluble components, however, e.g. garlic placed on the feet is soon detected on the exhaled breath. Easy penetration may occur on parts of the body where the skin is thinner, e.g. behind the ears, eyelids and inside wrist. The skin regions of the legs, buttocks, trunk and the abdomen area are less permeable than are those of the soles, palms, forehead, scalp and armpits (Balacs 1993).

■ **Gland openings and follicles.** Hydrophilic molecules can find a path through the skin using the sweat glands; lipophilic molecules may use the sebaceous glands as a pathway, also travelling between the cells through the fatty cement and through the cells themselves, all of which contain lipids (Lexicon Vevy 1993b). The skin of the forehead and scalp contains numerous oil glands, and here the epidermis is thinner. This again makes for easy penetration of lipophilic substances, although the water layer on the skin must present a partial barrier for the lipophilic molecules. The number of follicles and sweat glands is another factor; generally speaking, the more openings the speedier the access. When sweating, because of a fever or after a sauna for example, the body is exuding and ingress of essential oils is hindered.

■ **Reservoirs.** Essential oils, being lipid soluble, gain access to lipid rich areas of the body (Buchbauer 1993), therefore it is possible that essential oils may be sequestered (stored apart) in the body, as happens in the plants that produce them. If so, there would be reservoirs of essential oils (or at least of some of their constituent molecules) in the outer layers of the epidermis and subcutaneous fat, and these may persist for some time. It might be considered that lipophilic components can, at least temporarily, be retained in this layer and consequently will not be available for rapid diffusion to other adjacent levels (Lexicon Vevy 1993b). Subcutaneous fat has a poor blood supply and although essential oils are slow to enter they probably tend to stay there for a long time. A Dutch Government Commission report in 1983 showed that many MAC (maximum acceptable concentrations) for toxic chemicals failed to take into account the significant physiological differences between the sexes. Women's skin is more permeable to toxic chemicals than that of men and because they carry more fat, their body levels of fat soluble chemicals are generally higher and take longer to disperse (Eisberg 1983).

■ **Enzymes.** Enzymes in the skin can activate and inactivate many drugs and foreign compounds. They can also activate and inactivate the body's own natural chemicals such as hormones, steroids and inflammatory mediators. The activities of these skin enzymes may vary greatly between individuals and with age (Hotchkiss 1994). The skin contains many enzymes and therefore provides a 'laboratory' where metabolism can take place. Certainly some enzymes will effect a change in some essential oil molecules and even a slight change of shape in an essential oil molecule will mean a change in the effect on the body. In the case of some phthalic esters, enzymatic action effects complete metabolization during skin absorption; enzymes in the skin can either activate or inactivate drugs and other alien compounds and there is great variation between individuals and with age. Bacterial action breaks down the triacylglycerides in sebum to organic free fatty acids and incompletely esterified glycerol derivatives, and it is reasonable to suppose that similar sorts of processes may happen with the essential oils.

■ **Damaged skin.** Broken, inflamed and diseased skin is not a great barrier and ingress is rapid through cuts, abrasions, ulcers, psoriasis, burns, etc. Aged skin and skin dehydrated through exposure to sunlight does not accept substances easily: some dermatological problems (e.g. ichthyosis) may also have this same effect.

Other physiological factors

■ **Rate of circulation.** Where there is an increase in the rate of blood flow, perhaps due to rubbing (massage) or inflammation, there is an increased rate of absorption. Massage not only increases the speed of blood flow (causing hyperaemia) but also raises the local skin temperature slightly, hence we can expect an increased rate and degree of absorption of essential oils owing to the lowering of the viscosity and dilation of the blood vessels (Pratt & Mason 1981). Proof that essential oils in a base oil applied to the skin are absorbed into the bloodstream has been provided by Jäger et al (1992) by the detection of linalyl acetate and linalool in a blood sample taken 5 minutes after the oil was applied.

■ **Rate of distribution.** As far as distribution is concerned, the speed of the lymph and blood circulation is a limiting factor because the circulation is slower in the capillary loops than in the veins. The speed may be increased, for example, by massage or by warmth (e.g. infrared). Both these methods may be used to increase the rate of distribution of essential oils. It has been proved that the blood vessels constantly resorb and expel terpenes so that a balance of flow results (Römmelt et al 1974, Schilcher 1985).

External factors

■ **Hydration.** Hydrated skin is very permeable, hence the effectiveness of what the authors term aromabalneotherapy (the use of essential oils in a bath). It has been shown that in a bath the essential oils penetrate the skin 100 times faster than does water and 10 000 times more quickly than do the ions of sodium and chloride (Römmelt et al 1974). Conversely, if the stratum corneum is dehydrated its permeability is decreased.

■ **Degreased skin.** Although detergents, degreasants, soaps, etc. increase the permeability of the skin to essential oils, they are not necessarily recommended.

■ **Warmth.** A warm room, warm oils, warm hands and body all help to speed up absorption. Care must be taken that the body is not made too warm (e.g. after exercise) as it is then exuding and eliminating, making ingress of oils difficult.

■ **Occlusion.** Occlusion due to a covering, e.g. a compress, has a sealing-in effect and decreases the ability of the essential oils to volatilize and aids warming. Oils applied under occlusion, as with all other substances, have an enhanced effect because of the increase in the quantity absorbed, due probably to local warming, and reduced loss of molecules from the site of appli-

cation through evaporation: as evaporation is reduced, absorption may be increased (Bronaugh et al 1990). Clothing may be regarded as being partially occlusive.

Oil-related factors

■ **Viscosity.** All essential oils have a low viscosity, but some oils with a relatively high viscosity, e.g. sandalwood, which comprises 90% sesquiterpenols, will still cross the skin at a rate similar to other oils. Viscosity plays a more important part with regard to the carrier oils because some, such as hazelnut, are quite viscous and others, such as grapeseed and sunflower, are less so.

■ **Molecular size.** If the molecular weight exceeds 500 then it is unlikely to pass the skin. Essential oils, being products of distillation, are limited to a maximum molecular weight of 225 (rarely reaching 250). In some cases it may be worth considering the use of a carrier that is partially hydrophilic (e.g. wheatgerm oil, walnut oil) even if to a small extent. The size and shape of the individual essential oil molecules also has a bearing on the speed at which they penetrate the skin. Small molecules pass easily down the follicular and sebaceous ducts, and the smaller the molecule the faster it penetrates. Dissociation may also be relevant. When dissolved in a carrier the essential oil molecules may split into ions, thus becoming even more tiny. The bigger molecules, being less volatile, are less likely to be lost to the atmosphere, stay on the skin longer and therefore have a greater opportunity for penetration. Even though essential oils are quite volatile and evaporate from the warm surface of the skin, absorption may be 20–40% of the oil applied, and up to double that, depending on the extent of occlusion.

■ **Frequency of use.** There is some evidence that repeated use of the same oil makes the skin more permeable.

■ **Carriers.** The carrier medium can have a significant effect on absorption of essential oils (see discussion on phototoxicity in Ch. 3 Part II, p. 64). In a laboratory test using rat skin, absorption of phenol was enhanced when a barrier cream was used; in humans, penetration of fragrance chemicals was increased when mixed with ethanol (Hotchkiss 1994). Saturated oil carriers such as lard, wool-fat and mineral oil (e.g. baby oil) all prevent or seriously delay absorption: the higher the degree of unsaturation of a fat the easier the absorption process becomes. Zatz (1993) found that when phenol was applied to the skin in a saturated fat the antiseptic effect was inhibited.

METHODS OF PERCUTANEOUS ABSORPTION

Many of the techniques used on the skin entail the use of water, vegetable oil or a bland lotion to dilute and spread the essential oils over an area of skin.

Compresses

Compresses are sometimes required on open wounds such as leg ulcers, bedsores, boils, etc., and on bruising or areas of severe localized pain such as arthritis, stomach pain, fractures, etc. A non-adherent silicon dressing such as Mepitel should be used on ulcers, and a low adherent absorbent dressing such as Melolin on open wounds. The size of compress, number of drops of essential oils and amount of water used are dependent upon the size of the area to be treated. A septic finger requires only a minuscule square of the dressing material chosen, and an eggcupful of water to which two drops of essential oil have been added, whereas a swollen rheumatic knee

---

Case study 5.1 Back and menstruation pain – A Windsor– *aromatherapist, UK*

Client assessment

Edna had suffered lower back pain during the last 3 months of her first pregnancy – and following the birth, this had recurred, though less intense and not so frequent. When her periods recommenced, they were usually preceded by a headache and accompanied by menstrual pain for the first 2 days. She didn't want medication, but approached her GP, whom she knew accepted aromatherapy for certain disorders and after showing her the proposed treatment plan, she was happy for Edna to go ahead, so long as she reported back after a month – whether or not the results were beneficial.

Intervention

Back massage, abdomen massage and compress were the treatments decided upon, the abdomen being massaged first, after which a compress was applied under Edna's abdomen, on a warm towel, whilst her back was massaged – her weight keeping the compress in place.

Equal quantities of the following oils were chosen for both massage and compress treatments:

- *Angelica archangelica* rad. [angelica] – antispasmodic, sedative
- *Chamaemelum nobile* [Roman chamomile] – anti-inflammatory, antispasmodic, calming, menstrual (dysmenorrhoea), sedative

- *Pelargonium graveolens* [geranium] – analgesic, antiinflammatory, antispasmodic, decongestant
- *Salvia sclarea* [clary] – decongestant, hormone regulator

For the massage, 2 drops of each were used in 10 ml sweet almond oil and 3 drops of each in 200 ml warm water for the compress.

Edna was given 4 drops of each of the above oils in 50 ml carrier oil for her husband to apply to her back and herself to her abdomen each night. Edna herself was shown how to prepare a compress to use the 3–4 nights before her period was expected, being given a 10 ml bottle of the blended essential oils she needed for this.

Treatment 2: one month later, Edna said she had felt more relaxed and the headache she had had at the start of her period had been less intense, as had her period pain.

Treatment 3: one month later, there had been no headaches or back pain, so the compress was omitted from the treatment and the next appointment was made for 2 months' time.

Outcome

After 4 months, there was still no pain during menstruation and the backache had not recurred.

would require a piece of cloth large enough to cover the swelling, and a small basinful of water (about 200 ml) containing five to six drops of essential oils. As always, the quantities of essential oil should be halved for children and the elderly.

The chosen material should be immersed in the mixture (well stirred) of water and essential oil, squeezed gently and placed over the required area. It should be covered in the normal manner, and a piece of Clingfilm can be ideal as a first layer to prevent evaporation of the essential oils. The compress should be left on for about 2 hours, or overnight if practicable. Some therapists apply essential oils diluted in a vegetable oil to the site, if the skin is unbroken, then cover it. During the 1914–1918 war, other media used for wet dressings for large wounds with considerable tissue loss were ether and ointment bases, into which the essential oils were mixed (Valnet 1980 p. 67). For open wounds a cream or lotion base can be applied directly on to the dressing.

Case study 5.2 Leg ulcers – P Price– *aromatologist, UK*

Client assessment
Joe, a widower of 91 years, was retired and lived alone. He had few hobbies except cleaning his house and working in his garden, taking little exercise outside of these activities. His diet was simple yet sufficient.

Joe had a leg ulcer which was being treated with compression bandages by a community nurse once a week. She was reluctant to give information on the dressing used.

Presenting symptoms
The ulcer was 3 inches in diameter, situated on the outside calf of the left leg. Joe had been told that he could not expect any improvement because everything possible was being done for him and the condition had remained static for some considerable time.

Intervention
For the first week of treatment essential oils were to be used in distilled water in a spray. The four oils selected were:

- 15 drops *Citrus bergamia* [bergamot] – anti-infectious, cicatrizant
- 20 drops *Commiphora myrrha.* [myrrh] – anti-inflammatory, antiseptic, cictrizant
- 25 drops *Lavandula angustifolia* [lavender] – analgesic, antiinflammatory, antiseptic, cicatrizant
- 10 drops *Melaleuca alternifolia* [tea tree] – analgesic, antiinflammatory
- 100 ml warm water

The oils were selected very carefully for their constituent properties, which collectively addressed the pain, the infection and the healing.

After consultation with the doctor it was agreed that for the aromatherapy intervention the bandage could remain off for 3 days during the daytime, being replaced at night.

First visit (morning): Joe's wound was sprayed when the nurse removed his bandage (shaking the bottle well before use), Joe himself spraying the leg himself at intervals six times during the day (thereby involved in his own care) until the nurse replaced the bandage at night. This was repeated each day.

Second visit (evening 3 days later): after these 3 days the commencement of healing was evident. Wearing protective gloves, the same synergy of essential oils was applied directly to the wound (in a 3% dilution using *Calendula* as a carrier) before the nurse applied the compression bandage. This was to be left for a week until the next bandage. During this week Joe's feet were massaged every day with the same blend, resulting in a noticed improvement in the circulation.

Third evening visit: The above procedure was repeated.

Outcome
After 3 months the ulcer was closed – the only evidence of it having been there being a small area of discoloured skin, which later improved.

Joe was consistent in the use of his oil blend once a day for the rest of his life and the ulcer did not recur. The quality of Joe's life was greatly improved as a result of the treatment – not least because his improved mobility meant he could work again in his beloved garden.

Gargles and mouthwashes

After the removal of tonsils or complicated dental surgery, gargling with essential oils helps to relieve any pain or inflammation, stem blood flow and aid healing; at the same time the oils are antiseptic to the mucous surfaces. Two to three drops in quarter of a tumbler of water is all that is needed – the most important rule to follow being that the water should be well stirred before each mouthful to disperse the essential oils each time. For children, blend one drop only of essential oil in a teaspoonful of honey before adding the water. *Syzygium aromaticum* (flos) [clove bud] is the most used for pain in this context (but see Appendices also).

Sprays

The spray method mentioned above (see Methods of inhalation, p. 141) can also be used as a method of application when the client is unable to be touched, e.g. in the case of severe burns, zoster or wounds. A higher concentration is needed when treating burns this way, e.g. 15–20 drops in 50 ml of distilled or sterilized water. Appropriate essential oils in this case are *Citrus limon* [lemon], *Lavandula angustifolia* [lavender], *L.* x *intermedia* 'Super' [lavandin], *Matricaria recutita* [German chamomile], *Melaleuca viridiflora* [niaouli] and *Pelargonium graveolens* [geranium].

Baths

A valuable method of use involving water and inhalation is the addition of six to eight drops of essential oils to the bath water after running it to the correct temperature. This amount of essential oil in a bathful of water can appear to be too little, but it must be borne in mind, as mentioned above, that skin penetration is increased 100 times in this method and that inhalation also plays a significant part. There are those who advise adding the essential oils to another medium first, such as vegetable oil, dried milk, high proof vodka, bubble bath mix, etc. While useful for certain skin conditions, vegetable oil is not necessary in most circumstances (and it can leave an oily ring on the bath which is difficult to remove). Although the essential oils are not completely soluble in water, it is a simple matter to disperse them by vigorously agitating the water (efficiently, so no globules can get into the eyes). For water births the essential oils are best dissolved first in a small amount of powdered milk (adding enough water to make a thin paste). Blend three to four drops in honey or dried milk for children and the elderly. For maximum benefit, the patient should remain in the bath for 10 minutes if possible.

Foot, hand and sitz baths

It is sometimes easier to use a washing-up bowl for bathing individual areas – the sitz bath, for example, is ideal for haemorrhoids and stitches after childbirth. Three to four drops of essential oils are needed, and a kettle should be available to keep the bath warm during the 10 minutes. Arthritic hands and ankles can be successfully treated in this way. This method may not be found to be necessary for children but, should the occasion arise, remember to halve the number of drops of essential oil.

Topical application

Application means the 'putting on' of oils – either for self-use or via a third party. Treatment by massage employs an organized routine using specific movements to achieve specific aims, e.g. lymph drainage, relaxation, etc. Professional aromatherapists mostly employ essential oils with massage, and this subject is covered in detail in Chapter 7 together with massage techniques suitable for nurses to administer without having qualified in whole-body massage.

Unless aromatherapists are paid by the health authority or the patient concerned, or they are offering their services voluntarily, there is not usually time in a busy nursing schedule for a nurse to spend an hour or more with a patient requiring an aromatherapy treatment. However, nurses do have time to apply a ready-diluted oil or lotion on the relevant area daily as an embrocation. It takes no longer than giving more usual forms of medication and adds the magic of touch and care to the prescription.

The normal dilution is 15–20 drops in 50 ml of suitable carrier oil or lotion, but for the very young, elderly, heavily medicated or those with learning difficulties half this amount is advised. When essential oils are to be applied daily, it is less messy to dilute them in a non-greasy lotion base of emulsified oil and water (garments and bed linen can become permanently soiled by vegetable oil). A number of rheumatology wards apply an aromatherapy lotion as part of the daily treatment, resulting in a reduction in the use of painkillers (see Ch. 14). For effectiveness in certain conditions, e.g. lowered immune system activity or toxic build-up, an essential oil lotion should be applied liberally to the lymph node areas such as the armpits and groin (see also Ch. 9).

THE SIGNIFICANCE OF MACERATED CARRIER OILS

It is well worth taking care to select a carrier which is of holistic and/or symptomatic use, e.g. one of the macerated oils such as calendula. Lime blossom carrier oil can help to induce sleep or soothe rheumatic pain, carrot or hypericum carrier oils will help to reduce skin inflammation or accelerate the healing of burns, calendula or hypericum carrier oils will help to soothe and heal bruising, and calendula, hypericum or rosehip carrier oils will relieve skin rashes, etc. (Price 2000, Price et al 1999). The quantity of essential oil added should be the same as when using a basic carrier oil.

FIXED OILS AND SKIN PENETRATION

It has generally been considered that triacylglycerol molecules are too large to penetrate the skin but this observation has perhaps been brought into question. Tests on rat skin suggested that the oils of linseed, safflower and avocado were of interest in carrying active substances into the skin (Valette & Sobrin 1963).

Essential fatty acid deficiency is recognized as a complication of long term fat-free parenteral nutrition, and consideration has been given to the use of cutaneously applied vegetable oils as a way of avoiding this problem. Sunflower seed oil was used on three patients who had developed essential fatty acid deficiency after major intestinal resections (Press, Hartop & Prottey 1974, Prottey, Hartop & Press 1975). The deficiency was corrected by the application of 2–3 mg of the oil per kg of body weight per day for 12 weeks. Friedman et al (1976) reported the correction of essential fatty acid deficiency in two infants given 1400 mg/kg per day of topically applied sun-

flower oil. In order for the essential fatty acid to be made available the molecules of triacylglycerol have to undergo hydrolysis. This implies that the topically applied oil has been metabolized and so skin penetration has taken place. In a report assessing the safety of sweet almond oil it is stated that pharmacological studies reveal that sweet almond oil is slowly absorbed through intact skin (Expert Panel 1983). Sweet almond oil has been used as a solvent for parenterally administered drugs (Hizon & Huyck 1956).

Miller et al (1987) examined the use of safflower oil on five patients, and deduced that topical application may improve plasma fatty acid profiles but adequacy of tissue stores remained unanswered. However, other investigators have reported that essential fatty acid deficiency cannot be influenced by cutaneously applied vegetable oils (Hunt et al 1978, McCarthy et al 1983, O'Neill, Caldwell & Meng 1976).

Clearly, uncertainty remains. However, there is evidence that oils rich in bonded essential fatty acids do benefit the skin. A deficiency in essential fatty acids increases transepidermal water loss resulting in dryness; this may be corrected by the topical application of borage and evening primrose oils for 14 days with a resulting 2% increase in the level of γ-linolenic acid in the stratum corneum (Hoffmann-La Roche 1989). (See fixed oils in Ch. 7).

INGESTION

Ingestion is the main route employed by aromatologists and doctors in France, but is not widely used by aromatherapists in other countries. In the UK and elsewhere there are wide variations in training standards, ranging from those designed for simple beauty therapy to that enabling a therapist to practise clinical aromatherapy/aromatology. Therapists who have successfully completed an advanced training in aromatic medicine accredited by the IAM (see Useful addresses) are in a position to advise the use of essential oils per os.

Most of the research carried out by medical aromatologists in France has involved internal use of essential oils. In this case every drop of oil used reaches the body systems, unlike inhalation, when only a tiny amount of essential oil vapour enters the body, and external application, where some of the essential oils are lost by evaporation.

METHODS OF INGESTION

Per os (see also Ch. 3 Part I)

When essential oils are taken by mouth, knowledge of the constituents of the essential oils is of paramount importance. This is not to say that an oil containing a potentially hazardous component cannot be ingested – these components are sometimes effective for certain disorders. It simply means that it is essential to know the strength of concentration, the nature of any diluent used and the length of time for which it is to be taken.

Alcohol and honey water are the most usual diluents (Valnet 1980) though vegetable oils (such as hazelnut and olive oils) are excellent for this purpose and are preferred by many doctors and naturopaths practising in France (Collin 1994 personal communication), who have studied phytotherapy and are experienced in prescribing essential oils for internal use. Special dispersants are available for use to ensure essential oils dissolve thoroughly in an excipient, including water. Although higher doses can be found in aromatherapy books (particularly those written by French authors) a rough guide to the maximum safe dose is three drops, three times a day, for 3 weeks (see Ch. 3 Part I), although the individual and the particular oils used must be taken into consideration. As mentioned above, all the oil is

---

Case study 5.3 Spondolytis – S Gelzer – *aromatologist, Switzerland*

Client assessment (self)
I was hospitalized with complete bed rest for 8 weeks, with inflammation of the spinal vertebrae and discs, caused by infection of the vertebrae through *Staphylococcus*, which literally ate away pieces of my lumbar vertebrae. I was fed intravenously with 6 g antibiotics every day.

Intervention
Being an aromatologist, I made an essential oil mix to compensate for – and support – the effects of the antibiotics. I mixed equal quantities of the following essential oils and after blending 3 drops into honey, I diluted this in a cup of herbal tea, drinking one cup three times a day for 8 weeks:

- *Melaleuca alternifolia* [tea tree] – analgesic, antibacterial, antiinfectious, antiinflammatory, immunostimulant
- *Origanum vulgare* [origanum] – antiinfectious, immunostimulant
- *Satureia montana* [savory] – analgesic, antibacterial, antiinfectious, immunostimulant
- *Syzygium aromaticum* [clove bud] – analgesic, antibacterial, antiinfectious, antiinflammatory, immunostimulant
- *Thymus vulgaris* ct. phenol ['red' thyme] – antibacterial, antiinfectious

I also gave myself two other forms of treatment:

1. Application – to the part of my back I could easily reach, I applied a lotion daily, containing:
   - *Melaleuca alternifolia*, properties as above
   - *Thymus vulgaris* ct geraniol – antiinfectious, antiinflammatory, neurotonic
   - *Ravensara aromatica* [ravensara] – antibacterial, antiinfectious, anti-inflammatory, neurotonic
   - *Eucalyptus smithii* [gully gum] – analgesic, antiinfectious, balancing
2. Swiss reflex treatment – I made up a Swiss reflex cream using the same oils as for the lotion above with which to massage my spinal reflexes every day.

Outcome
As a result, I was taken off the oral antibiotics 2 months earlier than normal and off the intravenous antibiotics 3 weeks earlier than most spondylodiscitis cases.

Not only that, but my general vitality level was better throughout than previous cases the hospital had treated.

In addition I had no side-effects – except that I was in very good spirits, which amazed the medical team. I was the first person who did not need Valium – and I had virtually no pain.

taken into the body via ingestion, so extra training is essential. Although not harmful when used correctly, continual ingestion for too long a period of time can eventually lead to toxic build-up in the liver. This is particularly true of the powerful oils. It is for this reason that, after 3 weeks, several days' rest from the oils is indicated, to allow the liver the opportunity to eliminate any accumulated toxic matter.

Because they are usually tasteless and do not cause irritation, many conventional drugs are given by mouth. Essential oils often taste quite bitter and may irritate the mucous lining; for this reason essential oils to be taken by mouth are frequently put into capsules. Most aromatherapists are cautious about using ingestion, because of greater danger of an excessive dose reaching the liver than by external application. Further, there is the possibility of change in the essential oil molecules by digestive enzymes, strong acids and metabolization. Nevertheless, the authors have used essential oils in this way for nearly two decades for sore throats, stomach upsets, etc., with no reported adverse effects. After specialized training in this field (i.e. aromatology), therapists should be confident in using this method. Aromatherapists often advocate tisanes (herbal teas) and while these can be helpful they are not the same as essential oils in composition and do not have exactly the same action.

Per rectum or vagina

Another method of internal use is by means of suppositories and pessaries, which can be useful in cases of irritable bowel syndrome, haemorrhoids, vaginal infections and *Candida*. Suppositories, though not much favoured in the UK, allow the essential oils direct access to the bloodstream with little chance of metabolization. The maximum dose for suppositories and pessaries is six drops (Collin 1994 personal communication). Toxic or irritant essential oils should not be used (see Ch. 3).

SUMMARY

This chapter has identified the principal routes by which essential oils can enter the body – and the principal hindrances. Detailed information has been given so that the aromatherapist can select the optimum pathway to achieve the desired therapeutic effect.

References

Almiral M, Montana J, Escribano E, Obach R, Berrozpe J D 1996 Effect of *d*-limonene, α-pinene and cineole on the *in vitro* transdermal human skin penetration of chlorpromazine and haloperidol. Arzneimittelforschung 46(7): 676–680

Anthony C P, Thibodeau G A 1983 Nervous system cells in anatomy and physiology. Mosby, St Louis

Balacs T 1993 Essential oils in the body. In: Aroma '93 Conference Proceedings. Aromatherapy Publications, Brighton, pp. 12–13

Bronaugh R L, Webster R C, Bucks D, Maibach H I, Sarason R 1990 In vivo percutaneous absorption of fragrance ingredients in rhesus monkeys and humans. Food and Chemical Toxicology 28(5): 369–373

Brun K 1952 Les essences végétales en tant qu'agent de pénétration tissulaire. Thèse Pharmacie, Strasbourg

Buchbauer G 1988 Aromatherapy: do essential oils have therapeutic properties? In: International Conference on Essential Oils, Flavours, Fragrances and Cosmetics, Beijing. International Federation of Essential Oils and Aroma Trades, London, pp. 351–352

Buchbauer G 1993 Molecular interaction. International Journal of Aromatherapy 5(1): 11–14

Cleary G 1993 Transdermal drug delivery. In: Zatz J L (ed) Skin permeation: fundamentals and applications. Allured, Wheaton, pp. 207–237

Cornwall P A, Barry B W 1994 456 Sesquiterpene components of volatile oils as skin penetration enhancers for the hydrophilic permeant 5 fluorouracil. Journal of Pharmacy and Pharmacology 46(4): 261–269

Cornwall P A, Barry B W, Bouwstra J A, Gooris G S 1996 Modes of action of terpene penetration enhancers in human skin: differential scanning calorimetry, small angle X-ray diffraction and enhancer uptake studies. International Journal of Pharmaceutics 127: 9–26

Eisberg N 1983 Male chauvinism in toxicity testing? Manufacturing Chemist 3 (July): 3

Friedman Z, Shochat S, Maisels M, Marks K, Lamberth E 1976 Correction of essential fatty acid deficiency in newborn infants by cutaneous application of sunflower seed oil. Pediatrics 58: 650–654

Health and Safety Commission 1994 The health and safety at work act. HMSO, London

Hizon R P, Huyck C L 1956 The stability of almond and corn oils for use in parenteral solutions. Journal of the American Pharmaceutical Association 45: 145–150

Hoffmann-La Roche 1989 Information leaflet HHN-5379A/589

Hotchkiss S 1994 How thin is your skin? New Scientist 141(1910): 24–27

Hunt C E, Engel R R, Modler S, Hamilton W, Bissen S, Holman R T 1978 Essential fatty acid deficiency in neonates: inability to reverse deficiency by topical application of EFA-rich oil. Journal of Pediatrics 92(4): 603–607

Jackson E 1993 Toxicological aspects of percutaneous absorption. In: Zatz J L (ed) Skin permeation: fundamentals and applications. Allured, Wheaton, pp. 177–193

Jäger W, Buchbauer G, Jirovetz L, Fritzer M 1992 Percutaneous absorption of lavender oil from a massage oil. Journal of the Society of Cosmetic Chemists 43(1) (January–February): 49–54

Katz A E 1947 Parfümerie Modern 39: 64

Leung A Y, Foster S 1996 Encyclopedia of common natural ingredients used in food, drugs and cosmetics. John Wiley, New York

Lexicon Vevy 1993a La peau: siège d'absorption et organ cible. In: Skin Care Instant Reports (Vevy Europe, Genova) 10(4): 35–41

Lexicon Vevy 1993b La peau: siège d'absorption et organ cible. In: Skin Care Instant Reports (Vevy Europe, Genova) 10(6): 68

McCarthy M C, Turner W, Whatley K, Cottam G 1983 Topical corn oil in the management of essential fatty acid deficiency. Critical Care in Medicine 5: 373–375

Macht D 1938 The absorption of drugs and poisons through the skin and mucous membranes. Journal of the American Medical Association 110: 409–414

Maibach H I, Marzulli F N 1977 Toxicologic perspectives of chemicals commonly applied to skin. In: Drill V A, Lazar P (eds) Cutaneous toxicity. Academic Press, New York

Miller D G, Williams S K, Palombo J D, Griffin R E, Bistrian B R, Blackburn G L 1987 Cutaneous application of safflower oil in preventing essential fatty acid deficiency in patients on home parenteral nutrition. American Journal of Clinical Nutrition 46: 419–423

Mills S 1993 The essential book of herbal medicine. Penguin, London, pp. 333, 334

O'Neill J A, Caldwell M D, Meng H C 1976 Essential fatty acid deficiency in surgical patients. Annals of Surgery 185(5): 535–541

Pratt J, Mason A 1981 The caring touch. Heyden, London

Press M, Hartop P J, Prottey C 1974 Correction of essential fatty acid deficiency in man by the cutaneous application of sunflower-seed oil. The Lancet 6 April: 597–599

Price L, Smith I, Price S 1999 Carrier oils for aromatherapy and massage. Riverhead, Stratford upon Avon

Price S 2000 The aromatherapy workbook. Thorsons, London, pp. 162–172

Prottey C, Hartop P J, Press M 1975 Correction of the cutaneous manifestations of fatty acid deficiency in man by application of sunflower seed oil to the skin. Journal of Investigative Dermatology 64(4): 228–234

Riviere J E 1993 Biological factors in absorption and permeation. In: Zatz J L (ed) Skin permeation: fundamentals and applications. Allured, Wheaton, pp. 113–125

Römmelt H, Drexel H, Dirnagl K 1978 Heilkunst 91(5): 21

Römmelt H, Zuber A, Dirnagl K, Drexel H 1974 Münchner Medezin Wochenschrift 116: 537

Schilcher H 1985 Effects and side effects of essential oils. In: Baerheim Svendsen A, Scheffer J J C (eds) Essential oils and aromatic plants. Kluwer Academic, Dordrecht, p. 218

Stoughton R B 1959 Relation of the anatomy of normal and abnormal skin to its protective function. In: Rothman S (ed) The human integument, normal and abnormal. American Association for the Advancement of Science: 3–24

Takayama K, Nagai T 1994 Limonene and related compounds as potential skin penetration promoters. Drug Development and Industrial Pharmacy 20(4): 677–684

Torii S, Fukada H, Kanemoto H, Miyanchi R, Hamauzu Y, Kawasaki M 1991 Contingent negative variation (CNV) and the psychological effects of odour. In: Van Toller S, Dodd G (eds) Perfumery: the psychology and biology of fragrance. Chapman & Hall, London, pp. 107–118

Valette G, Sobrin E 1963 Percutaneous absorption of various animal and vegetable oils. Pharmica Acta Helvetica 38(10): 710–716

Valnet J 1980 The practice of aromatherapy. Daniel, Saffron Walden

Van Toller S 1993 The sensory evaluation of odours. Paper on clinical practitioner's course, Shirley Price International College of Aromatherapy, Hinckley

Weyers W, Brodbeck R 1989 Skin absorption of volatile oils. Pharmacokinetics. Pharmazie in Unserer Zeit 18(3): 82–86

Williams A C, Barry B W 1989 Essential oils as novel human skin penetration enhancers. International Journal of Pharmaceutics 57: R7–R9

Winter R 1984 A consumer's dictionary of cosmetic ingredients. Crown, New York

Zatz J L 1993 Modification of skin permeation by solvents. In: Zatz J L (ed) Skin permeation: fundamentals and applications. Allured, Wheaton, pp. 127–148

Chapter 6

Hydrolats – the essential waters

Len Price

CHAPTER CONTENTS

INTRODUCTION

The subject of aromatic waters is intriguing, yet not one on which very much has been written. It has been necessary to search many books on herbalism and aromatherapy to glean snippets of information. Even then the quality of information is not always very good, and very little would stand up to rigorous examination (save for the information on kekik water (Aydin, Baser & Öztürk 1996)). Most has been found in French literature, the country that most uses hydrolats, although even there not to a great extent today.

Water has the remarkable capability of picking up information relating to the vibrational energy found in a living plant, of storing this information and, under certain circumstances, of transferring this to the human body. This means that distilled hydrolats pick up and store not only physical plant particles (Roulier 1990) but possibly also subtle energetic information; consequently such products have an almost homoeopathic aspect.

There are several kinds of water-based aromatic products used in therapies, including infusions, teas (it has been estimated that over 1 000 000 cups of chamomile tea are taken every day worldwide (Foster 1996)), tisanes, wines, vinegars, as well as aromatic waters, which may be distilled or prepared. Distilled aromatic waters – hydrolats – contain the water soluble compounds of the plant, but not the tannic acid and bitter substances, and make an excellent complement to that other product of distillation, the powerful essential oils. They are, however, very different in nature from the volatile essential oils, even though obtained from the same plant, in as much as they are without aggression and are active on a different level; these 'gentle giants' are subtle, safe and effective, although any treatment must be carried out over a longer period of time than when using essential oils.

Some plants, whether containing essential oils or not, are distilled specifically for the hydrolat and not for the essential oil; when plants are distilled specifically for the hydrolat the quality of the water used is of great importance. Although there may be no volatile or aromatic molecules in these plants, and hence no aromatic oil, all water soluble molecules within the plant are taken up by the steam; thus the hydrolats stand intermediate between, and represent to some extent a fusion of, aromatherapy and herbalism, containing as they do some of the useful plant molecules from both worlds. Hydrolats are used in conjunction with both essential oil treatments and herbalism, as well as on their own.

As these valuable products of the distillation process are so safe in use, they deserve to be much better known and far more widely used, especially by aromatherapists already familiar with that other product of the distillation process, the essential oils. Hydrolats last featured in the French Codex in 1965.

TERMINOLOGY

In France the term hydrolat is used to describe the condensed steam which has passed through the plant material; the translation of hydrolat is given as 'aromatic, medicated water' (Mansion 1971) and this is the nomenclature adopted by Price & Price (2004 p. 31–34) to describe distilled plant waters, but many names are in use, some more accurate than others.

Terms used for these products are:

■ Aromatic water – this term does not imply distillation and so is inaccurate.
■ Floral waters – this is inaccurate and incomplete as by no means all distilled waters are from flowers.
■ Hydrosol – this is inappropriate, as it is a generic term applied to a wide range of products (including hydrolats) and is not specific: a

hydrosol may be defined as a colloidal solution (i.e. a dispersion of material in a liquid, characterized by particles of very small size, of between 0.2 and 0.002 micrometres) where water is the dispersant medium.
■ Essential water – this is an ancient name and aptly describes the aromatic distilled water from the still.
■ Prepared water – this is an assembly of products to simulate a natural product.

PREPARED AROMATIC WATERS

These are not produced by the distillation process but are put together in a laboratory. They consist of distilled water with the addition of one or more essential oils; these oils may be genuine plant extracts (volatile oil, absolute or concrete) or they may be partly or wholly artificial or synthetic. Essential oils are not generally soluble in water – probably on average only about 20% of any given oil is water soluble – but many of the oils can be 'knocked' into solution by shaking to produce a saturated solution. For each litre of distilled water 2–3 grams (40–60 drops) of essential oil can be added; this must be shaken frequently and vigorously for 2 or 3 days and then stored in a cool place; it can be stored successfully at 10–15°C for several months. Essential oils suitable for use by this method are anise, basil, Borneo camphor, caraway, chamomile, cinnamon, citron, coriander, cypress, eucalyptus, fennel, garlic, geranium, hyssop, juniper, lavender, lemon, marjoram, melissa, niaouli, nutmeg, orange, origanum, peppermint, rosemary, sage, savory, tangerine, tarragon, verbena and ylang ylang (Lautié & Passebecq 1979 p. 91).

They may be used for gargles, mouthwashes, bathing wounds and for ingestion, where 20 ml of the made water contains one drop of essential oil and therefore one teaspoonful contains about a quarter of a drop (about 0.25% concentration). Many essential oils exhibit significant bactericidal power at a concentration of 0.25%, as found in prepared waters, e.g. in a concentration of 0.18% clove essential oil kills the tubercular bacillus in a few minutes without causing any tissue damage or risk of toxicity, in contrast to some other preparations and antibiotics (Lautié & Passebecq 1979 p. 92).

Prepared waters do not have the same make-up as essential (distilled) waters, and therefore cannot have the same therapeutic properties. Some prepared waters are made with the use of alcohol, and these are not recommended for use alongside aromatherapy. The main volume of sales of prepared waters is to skincare manufacturers for use in 'natural' skin toners, refreshers and washes. Water which has had essential oil(s), synthetics or alcohol added to it is not a hydrolat and the two should not be confused. To achieve a genuine plant water, distillation alone is the true method.

WHAT ARE HYDROLATS?

Hydrolats are a product of distillation and can be considered as true partial extracts of the plant material from which they are derived. They may be byproducts of the distillation of volatile oils, e.g. chamomile water and lavender water, or of the distillation of plant material which has no volatile oil, e.g. elderflower, cornflower, plantain. Their method of preparation, by definition, necessitates that they be totally natural products with no added synthetic fragrance components. Hydrolats are obtained from aromatic and other plants by steam distillation, and during this process a proportion of the water soluble compounds of the essential oil contained in the plant matter is absorbed and retained by the water. As some essential oils have a relatively high proportion of water soluble compounds, much of the essential oil can be lost to the water during the distillation process, e.g. *Melissa officinalis* [lemon balm]; in such cases it is imperative to use cohobation. This is a system whereby the water/steam in contact with the biomass during distillation is continuously recirculated, giving maximal opportunity for the water soluble elements of the essential oil and the plant to pass into the water. Eventually this water reaches saturation point, when no more of the essential oil components can pass into solution (it is at this stage that the complete essential oil is gained); thus a water is produced that is rich not only in some essential oil molecules but also in other hydrophilic molecules found in the plant which are not usually part of the essential oil. When distilling for hydrolats, it is important that the

water used in the distillation process should be of good quality, preferably from a non-polluted spring, and free of any chemical cleansers that may have been used to clean the still.

Aromatic waters contain about 0.02% to 0.05% (or perhaps more, according to the plant) of the water soluble parts of the essential oil freely dispersed in an ionized form: this is equivalent to up to 10 drops approximately per litre of hydrolat (Price & Price 2004 p. 47). They may have similar properties to the parent oils but not to the same degree, and often their properties are different.

WHICH PLANTS YIELD A HYDROLAT?

Many aromatherapists think that only plants containing an essential oil are distilled but this is not so. Many plants containing very little or no essential oil at all are processed primarily to gain the hydrolat. The hydrolat from each plant, like the essential oil, is unique and reacts according to its constituents. *Hypericum perforatum*, often macerated in olive oil to gain its therapeutic properties (see Carrier oils in Ch. 7) is an example of a plant that contains an essential oil but which is rarely distilled for this on account of the minute yield, which would cause the price to be prohibitive; it is therefore distilled for its hydrolat. *Plantago lanceolata* [plantain] is an example of a non-aromatic plant which is distilled only for its hydrolat. This illustrates that water soluble molecules other than volatile essential oil molecules can be taken into the steam, yielding a therapeutic water at the end of the process.

YIELD

It is not possible to gain an almost unlimited or even a large quantity of water from a small amount of plant material. The quantity of hydrolat is proportionately limited to the plant weight and therefore hydrolats of excellent quality are obtained when cohobation is an integral part of the distilling process. This method is used to produce a number of hydrolats, e.g. rose, and yields a saturated hydrolat; *Melissa* is another case where a whole essential oil cannot be achieved until the steam water is saturated with the water soluble molecules of the essential oil, thus preventing the loss of these from the essential oil.

Yields of distilled waters usually lie between the limits of 1 to 1.5 and 2 to 5 litres per kilogram of plant matter, and vary according to the particular plant. The waters of thyme, savory and rosemary require a less quantity of plant than do lettuce, hawthorn, yarrow or hemp agrimony. Some waters are known as 'weight for weight' products since the quantities of plant matter and water product are equal, e.g. 100 lb of roses are distilled with sufficient water to yield 100 lb of fragrant rose water (Poucher 1936).

APPEARANCE AND AROMA

Distilled waters are not strongly coloured and are clear, with the exception of cinnamon water, which is always opalescent; for the most part they have only slight, delicate colouration (Viaud 1983 p. 23). Their smell may be generally reminiscent of the original plant material, but this is not always the case; an example is distilled lavender water, which often disappoints (Price & Price 2004 p. 58–59)

KEEPING QUALITIES AND STORAGE

Waters need to be stored at a temperature of less than 14°C, and in the shade. At higher temperatures certain waters tend to show flocculation. The maximum storage period under the conditions given must not, in general, exceed 1 year as some hydrolats are fragile and break down after a relatively short time. They are best purchased in small quantities, although Rouvière & Meyer (1989) say that the plant waters resulting from the distillation process of essential oils have a life of 2 to 3 years, owing to the presence of soluble compounds from the essential oils, which inhibit bacterial growth: this has been confirmed by the authors (Price & Price 2004 p. 56–57). Those hydrolats which have a good content of antiseptic phenols keep well; the distilled waters of *Satureia hortensis* and *Origanum vulgare* can be kept for more than 2 years with no discernible change.

COMPOSITION

It is known that, besides certain volatile compounds (isovalerianic, cyanhydric, benzoic and cinnamic acids), distilled plant waters can contain many other volatile principles, although these are rarely properly identified. Analysis of three hydrolats

(*Lavandula angustifolia, Salvia officinalis, Matricaria recutita*) showed that they contain substances present in the plant (Montesinos 1991 p. 24, Price & Price 2004). The pH of a hydrolat is closely linked to the concentration of alcohols and phenols present and to the degree of dissociation; they are sometimes neutral but usually have a weak acid reaction (Price & Price 2004 p. 58).

QUALITY

The basic criteria for obtaining a good quality hydrolat are the same as those for the procurement of a genuine essential oil, i.e. using a known botanical species, grown organically or wild, with a known chemical make-up; a distillation of sufficient duration and at low pressure; and a hydrolat that itself has had nothing added and nothing extracted. It is imperative that only products obtained during steam distillation and without colouring matter, stabilizers and preservatives be used. Products procured from a high-street chemist shop do not usually conform to this high standard, often containing synthetic materials; alternatively, they may be entirely artificial.

As with an essential oil, it is difficult to judge the quality of a distilled water from the smell; a true distilled water does not necessarily smell the same as the oil from the same plant because it has a different chemical make-up; when freshly distilled it may have an odour and taste of the still, although this is not long lasting.

Unfortunately, most hydrolats from plants distilled for their essential oils are discarded and are saved only if ordered beforehand. It is generally thought that because hydrolats are often thrown away, they should be inexpensive; unhappily this is not the case, as the cost of transporting the bulk (volume and weight) of the product is reflected in the final cost.

USES OF HYDROLATS

A nice attention, however, is certainly necessary in the use of them.

John Farley (1783), principal cook at the London Tavern, Dublin, referring to the water and infusions of bay.

Waters are ultra mild in action compared with essential oils and are useful for the treatment of the young, the elderly and those in a state of delicate health. The less volatile odorous molecules are integrally dispersed in the water in ionized form, therefore irritation of the skin and mucous surfaces is avoided. Hydrolats have a higher concentration of volatile elements than do teas and so are more efficacious and quicker acting, with a very easy method of use, i.e. drinking small quantities.

Hydrolats work synergistically with essential oils and so they can be prescribed as a complement to either phytotherapy (Streicher 1996) or aromatherapy. Herbalists in France do not use these waters on their own to any great extent, but they are used as a complement to other phytotherapeutic treatments both internally and externally; they are used both singly and as ready-prepared mixes.

GENERAL

Being non-aggressive, waters can be used safely for disinfection of open wounds and on mucous surfaces; they have been mentioned for use in cases of eczema, ulcers, bronchitis, tracheitis, colitis, burns and pain, whether local or generalized (e.g. *Chamaemelum nobile* [Roman chamomile] is said to ease post-zoster pain). They are used in gargles, nasal sprays, skin sprays, compresses and vaginal douches.

Case study 6.1 Severe burns – A Hanson – *aromatherapist, Sweden*

Client assessment
One day, when Harry, 36, lit a ring in his gas stove, the whole space exploded into flames, burning his face and neck. Although he managed to put some cold water on his face, he had to extinguish the fire and comfort his four children. The aromatherapist arrived half an hour after the burning occurred and Harry was in great pain. The hospital was over 25 kilometres away, the burn needed immediate treatment and Harry was reluctant to go to the hospital anyway.

Intervention
Day 1 – afternoon: Burnt hair was sticking to Harry's face and neck and he was in shock. First, he was asked to stand in the shower with cold water pouring over his face and neck, for 10 minutes. Meanwhile, 3 basins were prepared as follows:

1. Ice cubes, 200 ml of lavender hydrolat (*Lavendula officinalis* – all the therapist had with her) and 50 ml of peppermint hydrolat (*Mentha x piperita*) to help cool the skin.
2. $\frac{1}{2}$ litre of cold water, 5 ml lavender essential oil and 50 ml of peppermint hydrolat.
3. Ice cubes and cold water.

- A clean tea towel was torn in half, and wrung into basin 1 (keeping it fairly wet) and applied to Harry's face and neck.

- The second piece was dipped into basin 2 and applied – then the last two applications repeated many times, as they immediately turned warm on his burn. Ice cubes were continually added to the 1st and 2nd basins – plus another 50 ml peppermint hydrolat to basin 1 and another 5 ml lavender essential oil to basin 2.

This went on for 2 hours, during which time he was given a strong painkiller.

As the skin had cooled down somewhat, the following gel was prepared – and thickly (but very gently) applied on the whole area:

- 25 ml fresh aloe vera (direct from the plant)
- 10 drops *Lavandula officinalis* – analgesic, anti-inflammatory, antiseptic, cicatrizant
- 20 drops *Melaleuca alternifolia* [tea tree] – analgesic, antiinfectious, antiinflammatory

Harry felt immediate relief and after 5–10 minutes the pain lessened. After 1 hour the gel had formed a strong film (stronger than that on healthy skin) and the pain was gone.

His eyes and lips were very swollen, his face red and on his upper lip blisters were forming where he had licked off the gel. More was applied there, after which Harry went to bed and slept soundly.

Case study 6.1 Severe burns – A Hanson – *aromatherapist, Sweden* (cont'd)

Day 2 – morning: The whole face was sore, the nose having an open wound where the skin was burned off. It was not bleeding though it was weeping and swollen. There were brown dry patches under his eyes, his eyelids were swollen and red, his lips swollen and cracked and his cheeks streaked in red and white.

The whole area was sprayed with rose hydrolat (*Rosa damascena*), a very wet compress was made with the hydrolat, to try and help remove the burned hair still stuck on his skin. When it was removed – and the skin was dry the gel blend was applied again to the whole face, upper lip and neck. Photographs were taken.

Day 2 – evening: During the day the brown patches had paled somewhat. His chin and neck were still painful. The nose had dried up and a scab was forming around the edges of the wound. Harry had slept during the day.

The spraying and compress treatments were repeated with the rose hydrolat, and more burned hair came away. As the emergency was over, a weaker gel blend was then made, using 25 ml aloe vera gel with only 5 drops each of *Lavandula officinalis* and *Melaleuca alternifolia*.

Day 3 – morning: The skin was cleansed again with rose hydrolat to remove the last of the burned hair; the nose and lip had started to dry up, the area was less swollen and the patches under the eyes were almost gone. The whole area was still sensitive.

Day 3 – evening: The nose and lip had started bleeding slightly, but as the face and neck showed only a faint redness by then, the gel blend was applied only to the nose and lip and carrot oil, which is antiinflammatory and helpful to burns, to the rest of the area.

Day 4 – morning: This was the turning point! No pain, only itching. Harry's nose and lip had small scabs and looked clean, without any suggestion of impending infection. A doctor representing the insurance company arrived – and said that the nose and lip had second degree burns, the face and neck, first degree. He did not believe the burn had been as bad as reported, until he was shown the photographs.

Harry took a lukewarm shower, the gel dissolving in the water. Carrot oil was then applied to the whole area except nose and lip, which was given the gel blend again. The procedure was repeated in the evening.

Table 6.1   Properties and indications: essential waters

Essential water	General	Skin	Emotion
Achillea millefolium [yarrow]	Circulatory problems (women)		
Calendula officinalis [marigold]	Emmenagogue, hypertension, staphylococcus	Eczema, skin drainer, pyodermatitis	
Centaurea cyanus [cornflower]	Skin problems of intestinal origin		
Chamaemelum nobile [Roman chamomile]	Cardiac calmative? Healing, ophthalmic	Antiinflammatory, infections	Calming
Citrus sinensis [orange flower]	Cardiac calmative, anticollibacillus		Seasonal nervous depression, uplifting
Cupressus sempervirens [cypress]	Haemorrhoids, broken veins		
Eucalyptus globulus [Tasmanian blue gum]	Bronchi, kidneys, pancreas, antidiabetic	Acne	
Foeniculum vulgare [fennel]	Galactogen, antiseptic		

Table 6.1   Properties and indications: essential waters (*cont'd*)

Essential water	General	Skin	Emotion
Helichrysum angustifolium [everlasting]	Diabetes, aerophagy, pulmonary depurative	Bruises, abscesses, couperose skin, cicatrizant	Nervous depression, sedative
Hypericum perforatum [St John's wort]		Soothing	
Hyssopus officinalis [hyssop]	Low dose – clears the lungs; high dose – antiepileptic		
Juniperus communis [juniper]	Diuretic, kidney deflocculant, rheumatoid arthritis	Skin astringent, oily skin, refreshing	
Lavandula angustifolia [lavender]	Intestinal antibiotic, rheumatism	Soothing, pimples, burns, insect bites	
Lavandula x intermedia [lavandin]		Acneic skin, herpes	
Melissa officinalis [lemon balm]	Blepharitis, conjunctivitis, digestive, headaches	Irritated skin, insect bites, herpes	Sedative, relaxing, uplifting, depression
Mentha x piperita [peppermint]	Eupeptic, antiseptic	Itching, inflammation, cooling	Refreshing
Myrtus communis [myrtle]	Soothing antiseptic		
Ocimum basilicum [basil]	Carminative, digestive		
Origanum majorana [marjoram]	Clears the liver, gall bladder		
Origanum onites [kekik]	Cardiovascular stimulant		
Pinus syvestris [Scots pine]	Balsamic, diuretic		
Rosa damascena [rose]	Mouth ulcers	Toning all skin types, dermatitis, wrinkles, couperose	Mental strain, calming, sedative
Rosmarinus officinalis [rosemary]	Emmenagogue, rheumatism, circulation stimulant	Toning oily and mixed skins	Stimulating, alertness
Salvia officinalis [sage]	Emmenagogue, pelvic congestion, diuretic, rheumatism, ulcers	Astringent, oily skin, acne, eczema	
Salvia sclarea [clary]	Sore throat, period pain	Astringent, oily skin, acne, inflamed, mature skin	Depression, anxiety
Satureia montana [savory]	Revitalizing		
Thymus serpyllum [wild thyme]	Intestinal antiseptic, Gram −ve		
Thymus vulgaris (population) [thyme]	Intestinal antiseptic, Gram +ve	Acne, dermatitis, insect bites, eczema	Stimulating, revitalizing
Thymus vulgaris ct. alcohol [sweet thyme]	Eye problems		

SKIN CARE

Hydrolats are nearly free of irritating components, and their mild action and lack of toxicity make them ideal for use as skin care products; they have long been used in this way in the form of cleansers, toners (all skin types especially sensitive skin), conditioning creams and lotions. They are also used in baby care, bath preparations, hair rinses, aftershave preparations and facial sprays.

CHILDREN

Hydrolats produced for therapeutic use should not contain added alcohol as a preservative (care must be taken when procuring the hydrolat; concentrated waters do contain alcohol (Price & Price 2004 p. 38)), and so are suitable for children, especially as they may be sweetened with sugar if necessary. They are recommended for young children for external and internal use because they do not irritate the skin or mucous surfaces.

EYE CARE

Some hydrolats are used in preparations for eye-washes; e.g. *Myrtus communis* [myrtle] and *Chamaemelum nobile* [Roman chamomile] soothe pains resulting from inflammatory states of the eyes.

TRADITIONAL MEDICINE

Hydrolats are often prescribed by some complementary practitioners to adjust the 'energy balance' and the 'environment' (both internal and external) of the person, for instance according to Chinese medicine. The conditions treated include disorders of the digestive system such as constipation, rheumatism, migraine (from liver irritation), parasites, and ear, nose and throat problems.

ROUTES OF ABSORPTION

First there is the oral route through the walls of the digestive tract. The culinary aspect is attractive here as hydrolats are easily added to foods and are palatable (Price & Price 2004 pp. 173–177).

The rectal route using an enema is also used, and the active substance is here absorbed across the mucous surfaces of the large intestine.

Finally there is the skin; here the substance is absorbed from the whole surface of the body.

METHODS OF USE AND DOSAGE

- Put 50 ml of hydrolat into a bath to aid relaxation and promote a soothing effect.
- Use it on a cotton wool pad as a skin tonic after cleansing.
- Use it as a mouthwash or gargle.
- Put a teaspoonful (5 ml) into tea (without milk), fruit juice or fruit salads, coffee (petitgrain or orange flower water is delicious in coffee and fruit salads) or in a morning glass of water.
- Oral (internal) use may safely be recommended where appropriate; up to three teaspoonfuls (15 ml) per day may be ingested.

Duration of treatment is dependent on the particular organ and person being treated:

- For treatment of the liver, two teaspoonfuls should be taken before supper or before going to bed.
- For treatment of the kidneys and bladder, three teaspoonfuls should be taken between 3 p.m. and 7 p.m.
- For treatment of the lungs, six teaspoonfuls should be spread throughout the day in acute cases or three teaspoonfuls for chronic cases.
- For gargles hydrolats may be used neat, but in general use they should be diluted, up to 1 in 10 depending on the water.

Table 6.1 lists the properties and indications for use of hydrolats for general conditions, skin conditions and emotional states: it is based, almost wholly, on anecdotal evidence in the absence of any other kind of proof. There is a general table giving the properties of these waters in Price & Price (2004). Waters have certainly been in continual use for three and a half centuries, and perhaps longer, in cooking, for medicine and for personal cleanliness (Genders 1977).

CAUTIONS

It should be noted that preservative is often added to shop bought natural hydrolats to improve the shelf-life and these should be avoided for culinary or therapeutic purposes. When purchasing waters it may also be necessary to obtain a certificate

---

Case study 6.2 Menopausal problems – P Price – *aromatologist, UK*

Client assessment

Norma, aged 52, suffered from menopausal symptoms, such as sleepless nights, hot flushes and restless legs. Occasionally she had migraines or severe headaches. She felt tired all the time and was forgetful. The worst symptom was the flushing, which Norma had been suffering from for over 4 years, the problem being so severe that during that time she had not been able to have a cover on her, otherwise she wakened up drenched with sweat, needing to change the bed.

Intervention

After a thorough consultation, the following was advised:

- Cut down on processed foods and alcohol.
- Walk rather than drive whenever possible.
- Go to her GP for a thyroxin level check – this can fall during menopause, thus being a contributory factor to tiredness, memory loss and headaches.

The following hydrolats were blended together 50/50:

- *Rosa damascena* [rose]
- *Ribes nigrum* [blackcurrant]

Both are beneficial for menopausal symptoms, in particular hot flushes, and help to balance the natural hormone levels in the body. Norma was asked to drink 25 ml of this three times a day, in 25 ml warm water and to contact the therapist in 7 days to let her know how she was coping. She was also reminded about starting her lifestyle changes.

Outcome

After 5 days an excited Norma phoned to say that she had just had her first good night's sleep for years, and that she had slept with a sheet over her. She was delighted and amazed that the hydrolats had worked so quickly – as was the therapist! She had not had time to make any serious lifestyle changes – just increase her walking time and practise deep breathing.

Within the month, the intake of hydrolats was reduced to twice a day and the next month to once a day, by which time Norma was sleeping with a duvet and the headaches had notably improved.

Norma enjoyed the taste and was happy to continue the treatment, which she is still on at the time of writing.

Her thyroid test showed that she needed slight supplementation and within 3 months her tiredness had improved.

---

from the supplier to ensure that the proper conditions of harvesting, processing and stocking have been observed.

Hydrolats, as with other partial plant extracts, will possess the claimed activity of the plant only if its constituents giving this activity are contained within that fraction of the plant forming the partial plant extract. Many partial plant extracts, particularly distillates, have the advantage of being virtually colourless, making them easy to incorporate into a range of products. Unfortunately, this has led over the years to the production of distillates from a wide range of plant materials which are not suitable for this form of processing, and therefore little credence can be given to any claimed activity of the plant material or to its extract (Helliwell 1989).

SUMMARY

Continued use of hydrolats over centuries indicates that these substances have a potential for therapeutic use and are worthy of investigation. Physically they contain some water soluble molecules known to be therapeutic, in common with essential oils and some compounds found in other types of herbal preparations, and it may be that they also carry information and energy in a manner somewhat analogous to homoeopathic remedies. They are gentle in use and may safely be used in some cases where the use of the more powerful essential oils would be inadvisable, and may also be used to complement other forms of treatment; they have the advantage of being relatively inexpensive.

References

Aydin, Baser & Öztürk 1996 The chemistry and pharmacology of origanum (kekik) water. 27th International Symposium on Essential Oils, September, Vienna

Farley J 1783 Handbook on the art of cookery and housekeepers complete assistant, p. 307

Foster S 1996 Chamomile: *Matricaria recutita & Chamaemelum nobile*. Botanical series 307. American Botanical Council, Austin, p. 6

Genders R 1977 A book of aromatics. Darton, Longman and Todd, London, p. 13

Helliwell K 1989 Manufacture and use of plant extracts. In: Grievson M, Barber J, Hunting A L L (eds) Natural ingredients in cosmetics. Micelle, Weymouth, pp. 26–27

Lautié R, Passebecq A 1979 Aromatherapy; the use of plant essences in healing. Thorsons, Wellingborough

Mansion J E 1971 Harrap's new standard French and English dictionary.

Montesinos C 1991 Eléments de reflexion sur quelques hydrolats. Study written for Ecole Lyonnaise de Plantes Médicinales, Lyons

Poucher W A 1936 Perfumes, cosmetics and soaps, vol II. Chapman & Hall, London, pp. 34–35

Price L, Price S 2004 Understanding hydrolats: the specific hydrosols for aromatherapy. Churchill Livingstone, Edinburgh

Roulier G 1990 Les huiles essentielles pour votre santé. Dangles, St-Jean-de-Braye, p. 115

Rouvière A, Meyer M-C 1989 La santé par les huiles essentielles. M A Editions, Paris, pp. 82–83

Streicher C 1996 Hydrosols – the subtle complement to essential oils. Plexus 1: 22

Viaud H 1983 Huiles essentielles – hydrolats. Présence, Sisteron

Sources

Claeys G 1992 Précis d'aromathérapie familiale. Equilibres, Flers, p. 74

de Bonneval P 1992 Votre santé par les plantes. Equilibres, Flers

Grace U-M 1996 Aromatherapy for practitioners. Daniel, Saffron Walden, pp. 84–85

Price S 1997 Aromatic water. The Aromatherapist 3(2): 44–47

Price L, Price S 1999 Essential waters. Riverhead, Stratford upon Avon

Rose J 1994 Hydrosols: the other product of distillation. Aromatherapy correspondence course notes, California

Chapter 7

Touch and massage

Shirley Price

INTRODUCTION

Because the word 'massage' cannot be used in certain countries by aromatherapists, unless one holds a massage certificate recognized by that country, for example, in France and America, another name is often used for the same thing – 'therapeutic touch'; this enables those not sanctioned by the government, yet with a massage qualification, to carry out massage, but under a different name. However, the intention of the therapist is the same – to relieve tension and enable a beneficial result to take place.

Most aromatherapy schools teach their own specialized massage (or therapeutic touch); however, patients and clients can still benefit greatly from touch from an inexperienced or non-qualified person. Some massage movements are illustrated in this chapter for the benefit of those already qualified in aromatherapy and/or massage, but also to encourage other nurses with an inborn feeling for massage to use the simpler methods described. For the lay person or the busy nurse, knowledge of a few of the simpler techniques is an extremely valuable asset which can only bring benefit to those needing care.

TOUCH AND MASSAGE

Life takes it out of you, but massage puts it back.

Maxwell-Hudson (1999)

Massage begins with touch, which all of us need; it conveys a feeling of warmth, relaxation and security – all beneficial to good health. There are many empirical examples of massage therapy effects, including reduction of pain during childbirth and lower back pain (Field 2000 p. 45), even without essential oils. The addition of essential oils with analgesic properties will enhance the relief obtained by massage alone.

Massaging babies and infants can reduce pain associated with teething, constipation and colic, as well as inducing sleep (Auckett 1981). Studies carried out on preterm infants nearly 20 years ago showed without doubt that massage was beneficial to their growth and development (Field et al 1987). The babies were massaged for 15 minutes three times a day for 10 days – in an incubator. Compared with the control group, 47% of the treated infants gained more weight and were hospitalized for 6 days less.

PATIENT BENEFITS

Whether the causes of ill-health are bio-mechanical, psychosocial, biochemical – or a combination of these elements, massage seems to be able to exert a beneficial influence (Chaitow 2000). Touch itself is a basic human behavioural need (Sanderson, Harrison & Price 1991) and 'may be the only therapy which is instinctive; we hold and caress those we wish to comfort; when we hurt ourselves, our first reaction is to touch and rub the painful part' (Vickers 1996).

As research and scientific developments in the efficacy of drugs forged ahead, close patient contact diminished and massage had more or less lost its therapeutic status in medical care by the 1960s. However, there was a great deal of evidence in the late 1980s and 1990s of a renewed interest by nurses in the value of touch where patients are concerned and at the time of writing (2005) many hospitals and hospices are using massage to benefit their patients. During this same period of time, massage has been enhanced in many hospitals by the addition of essential oils, transforming the treatment into one of aromatherapy (Buckle 1997), when the benefits can be enhanced by the choice of essential oils used (Wilkinson 1995); increased energy levels, reduced side-effects from drugs, symptoms not treated by the hospital relieved and emotional problems eased. The effects can last longer than those of massage alone owing to the therapeutic action of the essential oil components (see Chs 10–15).

Patients can benefit greatly from a massage (simple or involved) given by any of the following people:

- a physical therapist – without essential oils
- a physical therapist using essential oils ready blended by an aromatherapist or aromatologist
- a nurse with no professional massage, but with a sound theoretical knowledge of essential oils
- a nurse using essential oils under the direction of an aromatherapist or aromatologist
- a nurse using touch and gentle non-manipulative massage movements, without essential oils (see Introducing massage, p. 173).

The most important thing to remember is that nothing can replace hands-on, when the giver (whether or not a qualified masseur/se) is caring and works within his/her capabilities, combining gentle touch with a loving attitude. With the right approach, once a small non-intrusive movement is made, both the giver and the receiver can come to enjoy the care they are sharing – making it easier for the receiver to open up and to become not only more relaxed in body, but also happier in mind (Worrell 1997). Authors agree that it is not necessary to spend an hour on a massage in order for it to be effective, as people can benefit from a short period of dedicated time.

PHYSIOLOGICAL BENEFITS

Massage increases the circulation of both the blood and the lymph (helping in the elimination of toxins from the body); it slows down the pulse rate, lowers blood pressure, releases muscle tension, tones under-worked or weak muscles and relieves cramp.

PSYCHOLOGICAL BENEFITS

Although these are perhaps not so easy to evaluate, they are significant and play their part in the holistic healing effect: relaxing an apprehensive mind, uplifting depression and despair, relieving panic or anger and, importantly, giving a person the feeling that someone cares enough to spend time giving the specialized contact brought by touch and massage.

Case study 7.1 Anxiety – N Darrell – *aromatologist, Eire*

Client assessment

Kay, a 42-year-old woman working in a family business, was referred for treatment by her GP, with severe anxiety and stress. Over the past 3 weeks, due to business problems, she had become increasingly withdrawn and anxious. She was experiencing panic attacks (which left her clammy and freezing) in crowded places and also at night, which was disturbing her sleep pattern, thus she found it hard to wake up in the morning. She had extreme tension in her neck and shoulders, suffering headaches as a consequence. Her breathing tended to be shallow and rapid and she had lost more than a stone in weight over the 3 weeks, partly due to lack of appetite.

Intervention

Due to the amount of anxiety she was experiencing she was taken through some breathing exercises before a full body massage, which was carried out using:

- 3 drops *Chamamaelum nobile* [Roman chamomile] – antispasmodic, calming, sedative
- 1 drop *Rosa damascena* [rose otto] – neurotonic
- 3 drops *Origanum majorana* [sweet marjoram] – analgesic, calming, neurotonic, respiratory tonic
- 10 ml grapeseed carrier oil

Kay opted for treatment twice a week and after the first treatment said she felt much calmer and more relaxed. She was standing upright rather than being bent over with the shoulder tension and said that her head felt much clearer.

She was given a blend of the following neat essential oils to use at home in the bath and as an inhalant if required:

- 1 ml *Valeriana officinalis* [valerian] – sedative, tranquillizing
- 1 ml *Chamaemelum nobile* – properties as above
- 2 ml *Lavandula angustifolia* [lavender] – analgesic, balancing, calming and sedative, tonic
- 2 ml *Origanum majorana* – properties as above
- 3 ml *Cananga odorata* [ylang ylang] – balancing, calming, sedative

On her next visit Kay reported that she found inhaling the oils when particularly anxious had relieved the hyperventilation and helped her to relax; she had also started to incorporate breathing exercises into her routine.

After 6 treatments over 3 weeks, Kay felt sufficiently confident to go shopping without anxiety. She had also been able to resolve some of the problems at work. She was beginning to put weight back on and her appetite had returned to normal.

She therefore decided to reduce her treatments to once a week and after 3 more weeks, she felt able to resume some of her work duties, when she reduced her treatments to once a month. She had not ceased taking her medication during her aromatherapy treatment time, but 6 months after first commencing aromatherapy, her doctor felt he could reduce her medication over the next 3 months.

At this time, she found she was able to carry out her normal work schedule and once again enjoy social activities. . . . She now goes for aromatherapy treatments when she feels the need.

MASSAGE AND AROMATHERAPY – THERAPIES IN THEIR OWN RIGHT

PROFESSIONAL MASSAGE

Numerous books on massage have been written for the general public and several colleges run short courses which are not sufficiently comprehensive to confer a recognized massage qualification. To meet professional standards, and be able to give a full, professional massage, the therapist must know anatomy and physiology, understand the relationship between the structure and function of the tissues being treated, be knowledgeable in pathology – as well as being skilled in the proper manipulation of tissues (Beard & Wood 1964 p.1).

Massage and aromatherapy

It would prevent misunderstanding of the word aromatherapy if the qualification in massage were totally separate from that of essential oil knowledge. As Vickers (1996 p. 15) so rightly says, 'massage and aromatherapy should be judged on their own merits'. This 'combined' situation arose because aromatherapy was originally intended to be studied only by beauty therapists, whose massage training is comprehensive.

Aromatherapy schools in the 1970s taught only their own specialized massage – not presenting a problem when students were already qualified in the therapy, as they were when the field was extended to physical therapists. However, when the general public wanted to learn aromatherapy, the situation was more difficult and although many schools then held basic massage courses for them, the situation evolved where many schools placed too much emphasis on the massage (though generally not enough to attain an independent qualification) and barely any emphasis on the essential oils. This situation has been regulated to a certain degree by the aromatherapy associations, who stipulate the number of hours to be spent on massage and the number of hours to be spent on essential oil knowledge for an aromatherapy course wishing to be accredited by them.

Because the two subjects are linked, neither is taken to its full potential; the massage training of aromatherapists is not usually as thorough as that of a physical therapist and the essential oil training is not as deep as that of an aromatologist (therapist qualified in complete aromatic medicine) and member of the Institute of Aromatic Medicine – see Ch. 9.

BENEFICIAL EFFECTS OF MASSAGE

Massage is widely recognized as providing the following benefits; it:

- induces deep relaxation, relieving both mental and physical fatigue
- releases chronic neck and shoulder tension and backache
- improves circulation to the muscles, reducing inflammation and pain
- relieves neuralgic, arthritic and rheumatic conditions
- helps sprains, fractures; breaks and dislocations heal more readily
- promotes correct posture and helps improve mobility
- improves, directly or indirectly, the function of every internal organ
- improves digestion, assimilation and elimination
- increases the ability of the kidneys to function efficiently
- flushes the lymphatic system by the mechanical elimination of harmful substances (especially toxins due to bacteria) and waste matter
- helps to disperse many types of headache (or migraine) originating from the gall bladder, liver, stomach and large intestine, and also those of emotional origin (including premenstrual syndrome or PMS)
- stimulates both body and mind without negative side-effects
- helps to release suppressed feelings, which can be shared in a safe, confidential setting
- is a form of passive exercise, partially compensating for lack of active exercise.

These combined benefits not only result in increased body awareness, but also produce better overall health. Furthermore, studies carried out in hospitals and private practice have shown that massage with essential oils greatly enhances and prolongs the health-giving effects.

Case study 7.2 Depression – L Bischoff – *aromatherapist, South Africa*

Client assessment

After suffering a major depressive episode where she had brief reactive psychosis, Miss L was hospitalized for 1 week.

Shortly after her return from hospital she stopped taking her medication. She was advised against this, as it is possible for a relapse to occur – but she was adamant as she said it was making her feel worse. She also suffered from lower back pain through sitting for long periods at her knitting machine – an improved posture for knitting was suggested, although Miss L had not felt able to do any since leaving hospital. She used to do aerobics, but again, not since leaving hospital. She was not sleeping well and had PMS before her periods.

Intervention

It was felt important to tackle her emotional problems as well as the physical and six weekly massage treatments were undertaken, using the following essential oils:

Boswellia carteri [frankincense] – analgesic, antidepressive, antiinflammatory, immunostimulant
Chamaemelum nobile [Roman chamomile] – antispasmodic, calming, stimulant
Citrus aurantium var. *amara* flos [neroli] – antidepressive, neurotonic
Coriandrum sativum [coriander] – analgesic, euphoric, neurotonic

Foeniculum vulgare [fennel] – analgesic, antiinflammatory, oestrogen-like

Miss L was given a full body massage on each treatment.

Outcome

She experienced great relief after the first massage and that night had a good night's sleep, feeling relaxed for several days afterwards.

After the second one, her back felt much better – she was able to move more freely, although her sleeping pattern was not back to normal. It was therefore decided to give Miss L the same essential oils to use at home, in two blends:

- $1\frac{1}{2}$ ml of each oil in a 10 ml bottle, 6–8 drops of which was to be put into a bath – at least 2–3 times a week
- 3 drops of each oil in 50 ml in oil of *Vitis vinifera* [grapeseed], to massage into her shoulders and neck every night before retiring

By the fourth treatment, Miss L had recommenced her aerobic classes, as her back felt so much better all the time. She was also sleeping as well as before her illness.

Because of this, a month was left before each of the remaining two treatments, the improvements remaining stable.

SIMPLE MASSAGE SKILLS

The most easily acquired skills of massage are:

- **Stroking**, which comes under the heading of *effleurage* movements (perhaps the most important for hospital use), for which the whole of both hands from fingertips to wrist are usually used. Stroking is simply an extension of touch and, as well as being one of the simplest, is one of the most important movements in massage.
- **Frictions**, which come under the heading of *petrissage* (a deeper and more energetic series of movements than effleurage), and in which either the thumb or one or more fingers are employed. 'Rubbing it better' is nothing other than a simple friction movement. The Hippocratic writings (from the Hippocratic collection 460–357 BC, quoted in Beard & Wood 1964 p. 3) contain the remark that 'the physician must be experienced in many things, but assuredly also in rubbing, for rubbing can bind a joint that is too loose and loosen a joint that is too hard'.

All of us have an innate ability to perform these two movements correctly and safely without the necessity of long training; both are taught thoroughly on aromatherapy and aromatology/ aromatic medicine courses.

Three further techniques, requiring greater skill and best learned on an accredited massage course, may be mentioned:

- **Kneading** (a form of petrissage), involving use of the palm, palmar surface of the fingers, the thumb, or thumb and fingers working together, is a squeezing and 'pulling' movement, often used on the shoulders and the thighs.
- **Percussion**, where hands and fingers continually make and break contact with the body in a definite rhythm is not normally used in aromatherapy.
- **Lymph drainage**, which is only briefly covered in an aromatherapy training programme, is fully covered on a Vodder technique course.

EFFLEURAGE

Effleurage is the basis of all good massage. It can be used on its own, at the beginning and ending of a massage involving other movements on a given area, and also in between other types of movements. It consists of two types of stroking movement, normally using the whole hand or hands, which should mould themselves to the shape of the part of the body being massaged. The strokes are either deep (i.e. with pressure) or superficial (without pressure). Sometimes only part of the hand is used – perhaps only two fingers on a small area or on a baby.

Deep stroking with both hands is accomplished by moving up the part of the body being massaged with pressure, usually towards the heart (see below); its purpose is to assist the venous and lymphatic circulation by its mechanical effects on the tissues.

Superficial stroking is effected without pressure of any kind, and in any direction (the pressure is so light that the circulation is not directly affected). The perfection of this technique can require skill and long practice. However, in simple massage, superficial effleurage is mostly used as the return movement of deep effleurage, moving away from the heart back to the starting position.

Effleurage is used mainly to relax the recipient both mentally and physically and to improve the vascular and lymphatic circulation. Many different types of strokes come under this heading, but all should follow the basic principles above.

FRICTIONS

Frictions are another form of compression massage, or kneading. They may be performed with the whole or proximal part of the palm of the hand, or with the palmar surface of the distal phalanx of the thumb or of the fingers, which carry out circular movements over a restricted area. There are two types of frictions:

1. **Fixed frictions** move the superficial tissues over the underlying structures, i.e. the part of the hand used is 'stuck' firmly to the client's skin, which is moved over the tissues beneath by the act of making circles.
2. **Gliding frictions** move part of the hand over a small area of the skin surface and may also progress along a specific path.

Frictions are primarily used to break down fibrous knots, loosen adherent skin, loosen scar tissue, relieve tension nodules in the muscles and increase the circulation in a specific area.

OTHER SKILLS REQUIRED

Learning the different types of movements is only part of massage training. Equally important is the way in which these movements are performed. Essential factors to consider are the direction of movement, the amount of pressure, the rate and rhythm of the movements, the medium used, the position of both patient and therapist and the duration and frequency of the treatment (Beard & Wood 1964 pp. 37–40). Further factors include the need for full contact with the patient and complete relaxation of the masseur's own hands and arms because hard, tense hands transfer tension (and possibly pain) to the recipient. The mind should also be cleared of any intruding, disruptive thoughts.

The following principles need to be absorbed at the same time as the actual movements are learned.

Contact

No part of the human body is flat; nevertheless, when using effleurage (stroking movements) there should be full hand contact with every part of any large area to be massaged (Price 1999). Hands and fingers when fully relaxed can maintain this contact by following the body's contours closely, draping themselves over the body like silk. The hands should remain in contact with the body for both outward and return journeys of all movements made in sequence. Neither should the hands be lifted off between changes in movements, because this disrupts the flow of the massage as a whole (Price 2000 p. 203).

Pressure

In effleurage, when using the whole hand on a large area, pressure should always be concentrated on the palm of the hand (Price 2000 p. 201). The fingers should be kept completely relaxed because pressure from them at this time does not provide the relaxation required from effleurage – finger pressure should be kept for friction movements only. Normally, palm pressure should be applied only when moving towards the heart, with none on the return journey. One of the aims of massage is to stimulate the circulation, and the return of the venous blood is not as easily accomplished by the pumping action of the heart as is the movement of the arterial blood – therefore pressure towards the heart increases the rate of circulation. The lymphatic flow is also increased, ridding the body more quickly of any harmful substances.

Pressure in frictions, using the thumb or finger pads needs to be firm, but care must be taken to use the whole finger pad and not to dig in with the tip.

In Japanese shiatsu massage, pressure usually follows the acupuncture meridian lines and can therefore sometimes be applied moving away from the heart. This kind of massage works on body energy – not necessarily the circulation of blood and lymph – and this technique should be learned independently from Western techniques.

Speed

This depends to a certain extent on the effects to be achieved. Generally speaking, massage is given to relax the recipient, and a rate of approximately 15 strokes a minute for a long stroke (e.g. hand to shoulder) is considered correct (Mennell 1945) or 18 cm (7 inches) per second (Beard & Wood 1964 p. 38). Anything faster than this can induce a state of agitation, and is used only if the massage is intended to be stimulating.

Rhythm

Uneven or jerky movements are not conducive to relaxation and care should be taken to maintain a smooth, unbroken rhythm (Price 2000 p. 203). While practising, relaxing music with a regular gentle beat can be of great help in sustaining continuous, fluent and flowing effleurage movements. Frictions should also be performed rhythmically (Beard & Wood 1964 pp. 10–11).

Continuity

Nothing breaks the relaxing effect of massage more than the repeated lifting off and replacing of the hand or hands. Because most massage is carried out to relax both mind and body, the movements themselves (and the changeover from one movement to another) should be smooth and unnoticeable to the recipient. The whole area receiving massage should be covered without a break in continuity, contact or rhythm. Nevertheless, should a stimulating effect be required then staccato-type massage (percussion) can be effective.

Duration

The duration of a massage session depends on how much of the body is to be massaged, the age of the individual, the size of the body and by no means least, the enjoyment level of the recipient. The massage sequences suggested in this book each last between 5 and 15 minutes, taking into consideration only the size of the area to be massaged. Ten minutes of massage normally provides sufficient relaxation to induce a good night's sleep.

Frequency

The frequency of massage treatment depends to a great extent on the pathological condition of the patient, as does the type of massage given. 'It is generally believed that massage is most effective daily, although some investigators have suggested that it is more beneficial when administered more frequently and for a shorter duration' (Beard & Wood 1964 p. 39).

CONTRAINDICATIONS FOR MASSAGE

Contraindications for massage depend very much on the type of condition suffered. The lists below should be consulted to determine whether massage of any kind is appropriate or not.

ILLNESS

Whole-body massage is not taught in this book and is contraindicated in the situations described below. Although whole-body massage should not be given, specific area massage (e.g. shoulders, hands and arms, feet and lower legs, face and scalp) is acceptable in most instances.

■ **Infection.** The advice of the microbiologist or the infection control nurse should be sought if considering any type of massage for the infectious or contagious patient.
■ **Pyrexia.** If the client feels well enough an appropriate specific area could be massaged gently, using oils to give a cooling effect (e.g. include 0.5–1% peppermint in the blend).
■ **Severe heart conditions.** Permission from the doctor or specialist must be obtained for whole-body massage.
■ **Medication.** If on strong (and/or many types of) medication, specific-area massage only should be used.
■ **Cancer.** There is some controversy over massage where this condition is present, and reports from aromatherapists show that consultants can give conflicting advice. Some consultants say that it is not advisable to encourage movement of the lymph, because this may promote migration of the cancer to another area of the body; others say that to move the lymph and therefore encourage the elimination of toxins, and possibly some of the cancer cells also, could be beneficial (see Ch. 15). Horrigan (1991) offers the opinion that, although surface massage will not cure cancer by natural means, equally it will:

  ■ not make the cancer grow owing to an increased blood supply
  ■ not make the cancer spread
  ■ not interfere with chemotherapy and radiotherapy.

LOCALIZED DAMAGE

In the following situations, the site of any trauma should be avoided, although other areas can be massaged:

■ **Inoculations.** The site of an inoculation given within the previous 24 hours should not be massaged.
■ **Recent fractures and recent scar tissue.** The healing of scar tissue can be hastened by the gentle application of essential oils in a carrier oil or lotion, or spraying them in a water carrier on to the site if touch cannot be tolerated.
■ **Bruises, broken skin, boils and cuts.** If small, they can be covered with thin transparent tape, proceeding then with the massage.

NORMAL PHYSIOLOGY

In the following situations, whole-body massage is contraindicated, although specific-area massage is allowed:

■ **Hunger.** If 6 hours or more have passed since any food intake, or if the patient feels hungry, fainting may occur with whole-body massage.
■ **Digestion.** Immediately following a heavy meal, the digestive system is working full time and whole-body massage could cause either nausea or fainting.
■ **Alcohol.** After recent alcohol intake, massage and certain essential oils can intensify the effects of alcohol, possibly causing dizziness, or a floating feeling. Specific-area massage does not have this effect, and the amount of any essential oil used (in the recommended dilution) would be too small to make their use contraindicated.
■ **Perspiring.** Immediately after exertion, sport, a long hot bath or sauna, the body absorbs essential oils with difficulty. It is advisable to wait 20–30 minutes before whole-body massage, although a wait of 10–15 minutes is adequate for specific-area massage.
■ **Menstruation.** During the first 2 days of menstruation, bleeding could be increased by whole-body massage. However, specific-area massage can help to relieve congestion and soothe any pain or discomfort.

VARICOSE VEINS AND OEDEMA

These two conditions are often believed to be unsuitable for massage. In fact, they can both be alleviated by essential oils used in light massage. Special care is needed in the execution of the massage, and only gentle, almost superficial, *upward* effleurage strokes should be used.

- **Varices.** The area above the damaged valve should be cleared first with deep, firm, upward effleurage strokes, before commencing the light upward strokes on the affected area itself.
- **Oedema.** This condition must be treated by a precise technique. When it is present in an extremity, then the massage should begin with the proximal portion, because it is important to clear and improve the circulation in this area first before attempting to relieve the oedema. Treatment of the distal part should then be carried out, returning to the proximal part at intervals during the massage and to finish with. The affected part must be elevated while giving the massage (Beard & Wood 1964 pp. 38, 60, 104).

MASSAGE SEQUENCES

First is a technique for introducing massage and essential oils to a client or patient, followed by some simple massage techniques, easily carried out after attending an introductory course on the subject.

INTRODUCING MASSAGE

For some, close contact with patients can be 'a daunting commitment. Staff may need training to deal with the emotions massage may bring up in the patient' (quoted in Tattam 1992). In order not to take the patients' anxieties on board, the therapist (or nurse) should endeavour to be empathetic, rather than sympathetic.

Also, not everyone enjoys the thought of touching others (or being touched) – perhaps a lack of love in childhood or a bad experience may be responsible. However, if a strong desire to help the patient in any way possible is there, this can be overcome and the pleasure of seeing a positive reaction is more than worth the effort.

The easiest part of the body to start with is the hand, as few people have a hang-up about shaking hands – we all do it as a matter of course. The 'handshake technique' is also an excellent way of introducing the aroma of essential oils. Before going to see your patient, put a very small amount of carrier oil on your hand, add one or two drops of an essential oil – or one drop each of two (that you think the client may like) – and rub your hands gently together briefly, just to distribute the oils evenly.

1. Take your patient's right hand in yours as if to give a firm handshake (palm to palm – see Fig. 7.1a) and place your left hand over the top of your patient's hand, relaxing your fingers to 'cradle' his or her hand in a sandwich (Fig. 7.1b). While you are holding his or her hand, ask the usual questions, such as 'Did you have a good night?' or 'How is your back this morning?' Your patient is bound to notice the aroma and comment on it. As you explain, you can say essential oils are used for massage too, and if the patient reacts well to the aroma – and he/she shows interest, you can begin moving your left hand over the patient's hand in a stroking movement – even continuing over and around the wrist if the patient appears to like it. Ask if he or she would like the other hand to have a little turn, so that it doesn't feel left out. If the answer is yes please, repeat the 'handshake' on the other hand, then follow steps 2 and 3 below.
2. Gently raise the patient's forearm slightly, leaving the upper arm resting on the bed. Keeping your fingers in complete contact with the arm, begin to move your left hand firmly up the outer side of the lower arm (Fig. 7.1c); turn at the elbow towards the lateral epicondyle, moving your palm underneath the arm and return gently to the wrist down the inner side of the arm (Fig. 7.1d). Turn your hand, bringing it back to the starting point.
3. Repeat the movement a few times, then suggest to your patient that you do the other hand to keep the body in balance.

Once you are confident and the patient is happy about being touched (and for those who already know about the benefits of massage), the following sequences can then be carried out, allowing the essential oils to enter the blood-stream and give the desired benefits.

HAND AND ARM MASSAGE

1. Start with movements 1, 2 and 3 above, repeating three or four times. Where possible, take this stroke right up to and around the deltoid muscle and 'cradle' the whole shoulder, returning via the inner side of the arm, to finish at the wrist.
2. Still holding the patient's hand as in Fig. 7.1a, make large friction circles with the left thumb from wrist to elbow on the upper side of the arm, returning with a single superficial stroke as in step 1. Repeat three or four times.
3. Turn the arm over, leaving the left hand holding the medial side of the patient's hand and placing the fingers of the right hand on the lateral side of the forearm, make friction circles with the right thumb between the radius and ulna as far as the medial epicondyle, returning gently via the lateral side of the forearm to the wrist, with fingers underneath (Fig. 7.2a). Repeat three or four times.
4. Leaving the fingers of both hands over the extensor retinaculum, push the thumbs across the inside wrist firmly in a zig-zag movement, back and forth several times with one thumb in front of the other (Fig. 7.2b).
5. Slide the fingers down until they cover the back of the hand and stroke up the palmar interosseous muscles firmly, using the whole length of each thumb alternately, from finger level to wrist, several times (Fig. 7.2c).
6. Turn the hand over and repeat wrist zig-zags as in step 4, on the dorsal side of arm.
7. Move your fingers down until they cover the patient's palm and stroke firmly between the metacarpals along their full length, right thumb between patient's thumb and first finger (returning via the radial side of the

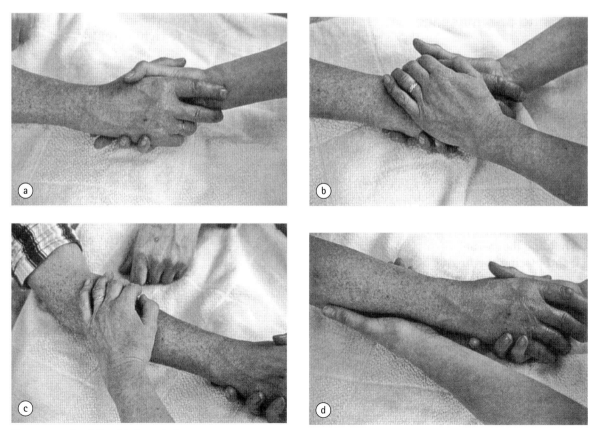

Figure 7.1   (a–d) Handshake technique.

hand) and left thumb between third and fourth fingers (returning via the ulnar border of the hand). Repeat these strokes, this time with your right thumb between the patient's first and second fingers, and the left between the fourth and fifth fingers (Fig. 7.2d).

8. With the fingers of your right hand still supporting the patient's palm make friction circles with your left thumb up the little finger; at the base, turn your own palm uppermost and, using your first finger and thumb, slide down the sides of the finger to the tip (Fig. 7.2e,f). Move to the ring finger and repeat the frictions and return movement. Repeat on the other two fingers, using your right thumb to massage the patient's thumb.

9. Push the fingers of your left hand through your patient's fingers (Fig. 7.2g) and, holding the patient's forearm with your right hand, rotate the wrist slowly and firmly anticlockwise, then clockwise.

10. Smoothly change to the handshake hold and repeat step 1 several times.

To treat the patient's left hand, reverse the directions for 'right' and 'left' in the above text.

FOOT AND LOWER LEG MASSAGE

When massaging the feet, it is very important to hold – and touch – the foot firmly. Many people have a dread of someone touching their feet and in the majority of cases it can be attributed to having had their feet held so lightly that it felt ticklish or insecure – and therefore unpleasant.

1. Place your hands across the dorsum of the patient's right foot at toe level (Fig. 7.3a) and move them firmly up the lower leg to the patella. Separate them towards the lateral and medial sides of the leg, returning gently via these to the ankle (Fig. 7.3b), turning the

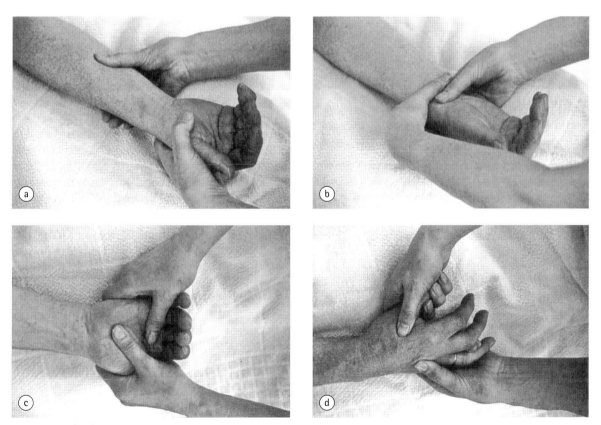

Figure 7.2 (a–d) Hand and arm massage.

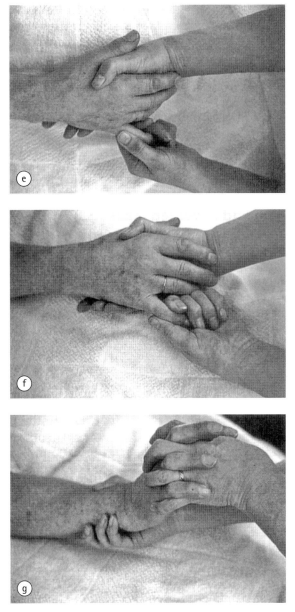

Figure 7.2 (*cont'd*) (e–g) Hand and arm massage.

left hand across the dorsum of the foot towards the wrist of your right hand (Fig. 7.3c,d), squeezing both hands together as they move towards the toes. Lift off your right hand only, replacing it in front of or behind the left hand, ready to repeat the whole of movement 1 (with the sandwich) several times.

3. On the last journey hold the foot firmly in the sandwich for a moment or two, before progressing to the next movement.

4. Turn your hands so that your fingers are underneath the foot and with your thumbs carry out gentle frictions on the metatarsals – as in the hand massage (Fig. 7.3e). The frictions need to be gentle because this reflex area of the foot is often tender, owing to poor lymphatic circulation or bronchial conditions (which the movement can help if done regularly).

5. Bring your fingers back to the anterior surface of the foot and move them towards each malleolus (Fig. 7.3f). Take the first and second fingers, pressing firmly, in a circle behind each malleolus (Fig. 7.3g), relaxing the pressure as you come to the front of the foot. Repeat these circles several times. This movement covers the foot reflex point for the groin lymph and is ideal for relieving lymphatic congestion in the groin and increasing circulation in the legs generally.

6. Turn your hands into the position for movement 1 and repeat this movement (together with the sandwich, as in movement 2) several times, finishing by continuing the squeezing movement until you are no longer in contact with the foot. For the left foot, reverse directions for 'right' and 'left' in the text. Should you wish to increase leg circulation further, ask the patient to bend her knee, placing the foot flat on the bed. Sit on the toes (place a towel over them to protect your clothes from the oil if necessary) and continue as follows:

7. Carry out movement 1 several times, but only from and to the ankle.

8. Slide one hand on to the tendo calcaneus and move it with pressure up the gastrocnemius muscle, following with the other hand, then the first hand again, etc. – about 10 alternate strokes in all (Fig. 7.3h).

9. Repeat movement 5 around the ankle bones.

10. Finish with movement 1.

hands again as you reach the toes, ready to repeat the movement three or four times.

2. When you have mastered this, incorporate the following 'sandwich' into the last part of the movement. As you approach the foot on the return journey, let the fingers of your right hand slide across the instep onto the sole of the foot, meanwhile turning the fingers of the

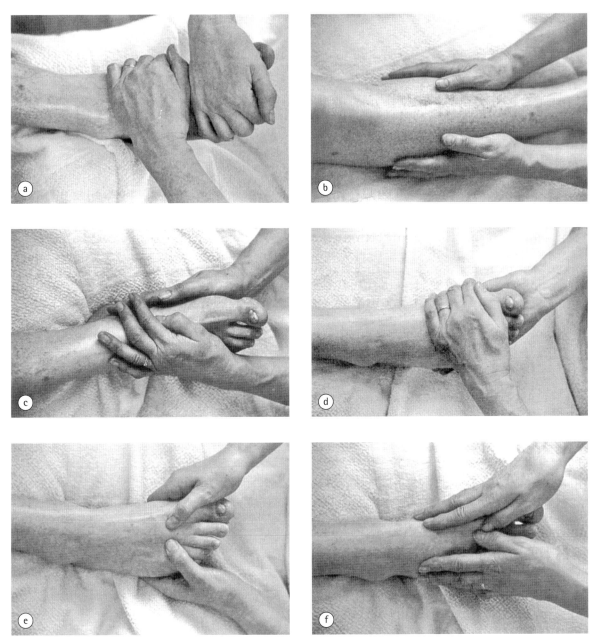

Figure 7.3   (a–f) Foot and lower leg massage.

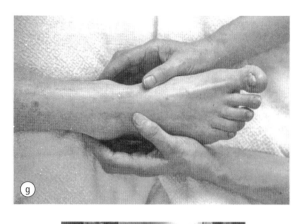

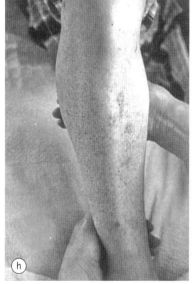

Figure 7.3 (*cont'd*) (g–h) Foot and lower leg massage.

SHOULDER MASSAGE

As a general rule the tensions and anxieties we feel manifest themselves first of all as tension nodules in the trapezius muscle. It is not always apparent as continual pain, but can be felt immediately when someone presses firmly on the precise area of the taut muscular fibres we call nodules.

The best time to give a shoulder massage (unless needed at any time to dissipate a headache) is just before retiring; this not only hastens sleep itself, but ensures a more relaxed body during slumber, which in turn puts the body into a healing mode (see Ch. 8).

If a special back and shoulder massage stool is not available, the best position for the patient to receive a shoulder massage is sitting straddled on a chair with a low back. There should be a pillow over the chair back, on which the arms and head can rest. This position is not always possible, and depends on the age and health of the patient. If it is impractical, the patient may sit normally on a stool or low-backed chair. Then proceed as follows:

1. Your feet should be about 45 cm apart, so that your knees can bend easily for carrying out movements effectively, without strain. Shake your hands to ensure that they are completely relaxed, before placing them gently over each clavicle of the patient (Fig. 7.4a).
2. Take your relaxed hands (you should see spaces between each finger) across the clavicles, cradling each deltoid muscle and across the latissimus dorsi to the base of each scapula – when your wrists will be pointing towards the spine; turn your hands until the fingers almost face one another (Fig. 7.4b) and move firmly with pressure up the back – one hand on either side of the spinal column – until you reach the clavicles again, with your fingers 'draping' over the shoulders as at the start. Repeat this three or four times.
3. Keeping your fingers on each clavicle, make friction movements with your thumbs across the upper trapezius from the neck to the acromion process (Fig. 7.4c). Repeat this several times.
4. Keeping the fingers in the same position, stretch your thumbs down the spine as far as they will go without undue effort. Place them in the spinal channels and make friction circles up the channels as far as you can go without exertion (Fig. 7.4d). Repeat this several times, circling several times on any one spot where you feel tension, before continuing.
5. Move round to the left side of the chair (keeping your hands in contact with the patient), so that the patient's shoulder is directly facing the centre of your body. Your feet should still be about 45 cm apart, as before. Open your hands as shown in Fig. 7.4e and, as you place the 'V' of the left hand at the head of the humerus (level with the acromion process), bend your right knee

(swinging the body to the right) and stroke up the deltoid to the hair line – your fingers will be in front of the shoulder and your thumb behind. As you reach the hair line, swing your body over to the left, bending your left knee, and stroke up the same area with your right hand as your left hand slides off the back of the neck (Fig. 7.4f). This time your thumb is in front of the shoulder and your fingers behind. Continue this alternate effleurage for a moment or two.

6. With your thumb, feel for painful tension nodules in the deltoid muscle. Firmly make friction circles over the knotty tissue with your thumb cushion (Fig. 7.4g). If the thumb tires too quickly, use the full length of both thumbs in single alternate strokes.

7. Repeat the shoulder effleurage described in movement 5.

8. Leaving your right hand on the shoulder, place your left hand on the patient's forehead and, keeping the fingers of your right hand separated from your thumb (as in movement 5), place the 'V' so formed at the base of the neck (Fig. 7.4h). Move firmly up the rotator muscles of the neck, squeezing your thumb

and fingers together as you move towards the hair line. Without lifting your hand from the patient, relax down to the base of the neck and repeat several times.

9. Keeping your hands on the patient, walk round to the back of the chair and repeat movement 2.

10. Without lifting your hands, walk round to the right-hand side of the chair and repeat movements 4, 5, 6 and 7 on the other shoulder.

11. Keeping contact with the patient, walk round to the back of the chair and repeat movement 2, finishing at the base of the scapula with wrists together, and gradually and gently bring your fingertips to the centre and lift off.

FOREHEAD MASSAGE

Standing behind the patient's head, lay your hand across the forehead with the fingertips of the left hand on the right temporalis muscle and the length of the hand lying along the frontalis as in Fig. 7.5a. Move the hand slowly and gently across to the left temporalis (Fig. 7.5b), keeping contact as long as possible until the fingertips are almost on the hair. Before lifting off your hand, place the

---

Case study 7.3 Arthritic pain and mobility – A James – *aromatherapist, UK*

Client assessment
Mrs M, 75 years of age, in general good health, was positive and outgoing. She was very active and did not look or act her age. The pain from her neck and shoulder caused her some problems – as she found it difficult to get comfortable in bed and in the morning she was very stiff.

Intervention
A back massage was suggested, followed by a neck and shoulder massage. She attended the clinic on a weekly or fortnightly basis. The following oils were used for the massage:

- 2 drops *Eucalyptus citriodora* [lemon scented gum] – analgesic, antiinflammatory, antirheumatic
- 2 drops *Piper nigrum* [black pepper] – warming, analgesic

- 2 drops *Zingiber cassumunar* rhiz. [plai] – antiinflammatory
- 7 ml *Prunus amygdalis* var. *dulcis* [sweet almond]

Home treatment: 10 drops of each of the essential oils above were blended into 100 ml of white lotion, which she applied at bedtime and if the pain bothered her during the day.

Outcome
Over a period of 2 weeks there was a great improvement in the mobility of her neck – there was also much less pain. She noticed that if it she did not have her massages regularly her neck and shoulders began to stiffen and her mobility reduced.

After 6 treatments she left a longer interval between treatments – a month to 6 weeks – but continued to use the home treatment prescribed.

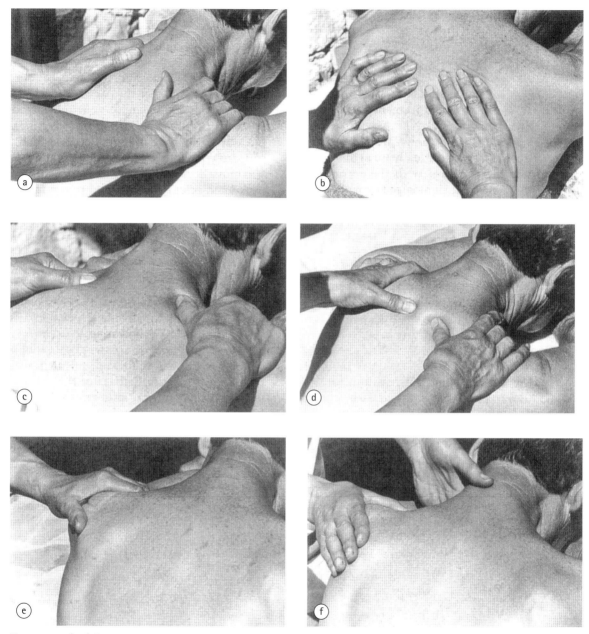

Figure 7.4   (a–f) Shoulder massage.

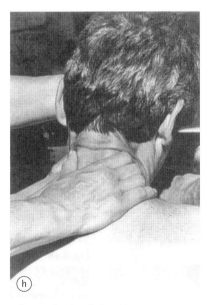

Figure 7.4 (*cont'd*)   (g–h) Shoulder massage.

from stroking the forehead. When executed gently and firmly, massage of the scalp is exceedingly relaxing. If the patient wishes to receive a scalp massage only, gently place under the nose a small amount of the diluted oil you would have selected had you been massaging part of the body. Then proceed as follows:

1. Place the hands on the scalp as shown in Fig. 7.6a and, without moving the fingers through the hair, move the scalp firmly and slowly over the bone beneath.
2. Place the hands as shown in Fig. 7.6b and, once again, firmly and slowly move the scalp over the bone beneath.
3. Move the hands to another position and repeat.
4. Repeat movements 1, 2 and 3 several times.
5. Place the hands as shown in Fig. 7.6c and bring the thumbs and fingers (stroking the scalp all the way) to meet each other at the centre of the scalp (Fig. 7.6d), then gently draw the fingers and thumbs through the hair to the ends.
6. Repeat this movement several times.

SIMPLE BACK MASSAGE

In a hospital situation this should be kept reasonably brief unless it can be carried out on a massage bed of the right height, to ensure the correct posture of the therapist, and prevent backache. The feet should be approximately 45 cm apart, the rear foot facing in towards the bed, the front foot pointing towards the patient's head. Your hip should be level with the patient's gluteus maximus, enabling you to reach the shoulders without strain. To follow the directions given here, it is necessary to stand on the patient's right side.

1. Check your hands are relaxed and use the whole hand, starting with hands on either side of the patient's spine at sacrum level, fingers pointing towards the opposite shoulder (Fig. 7.7a). Use effleurage up the latissimus dorsi muscle (covering as much of the back as possible with your relaxed hands), pushing both hands up either side of the back and around the deltoid (Fig. 7.7b). Return with a superficial stroke right down the lateral sides of the body before bringing the hands back to

fingertips of your right hand on to the left temporalis, laying the length of the hand across the frontalis and moving across to the right temporalis (Fig. 7.5c). Keeping the continuity and rhythm, repeat the two strokes with alternate hands for a few minutes. This stroke can also be done in an upward direction, but teaching may be needed to master this (Figs 7.5d–f).

SCALP MASSAGE

If you have been giving a forehead massage, scalp massage follows naturally. No further oil is needed because your hands will still be lubricated

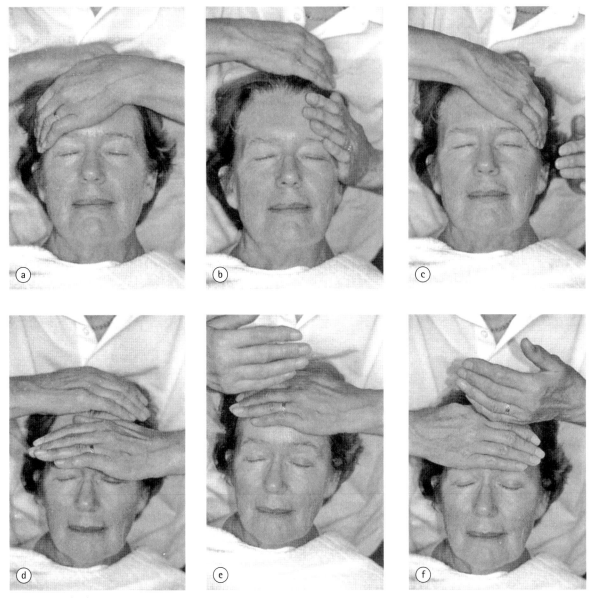

Figure 7.5   (a–f) Forehead massage.

the starting point. Turn the hands and repeat the movement several times.

2. Repeat the same movement, but only around the scapula, several times, finishing with your fingers over the shoulders.
3. Lift up your palms only, leaving your fingers lying over the clavicle and, using your thumbs, make friction circles on the deltoid across the shoulders (Fig. 7.7c).
4. Place your thumbs into the hollow channels on either side of the spine at the hair line, and make small circles there with the pressure on the upward half of each circle. The return journey of the circle should be extended downwards so that the next circular movement will be accomplished a little lower down the back. Extend the return of each circle, until the thumbs are just above the coccyx. Repeat movement 1 several times, then turn to face the patient, with your feet 45 cm apart and the

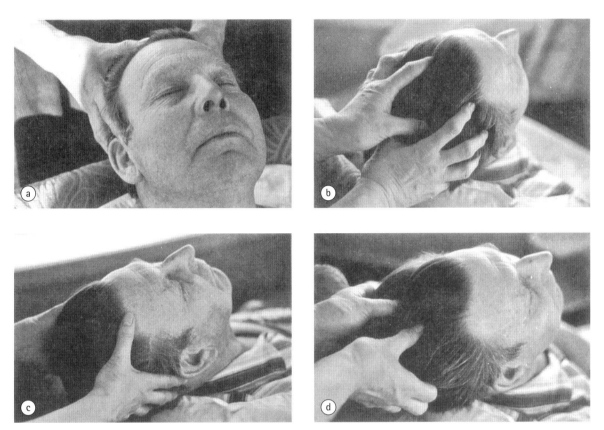

Figure 7.6 (a–d) Scalp massage.

centre of your body opposite the patient's waist line.

5. Place both your hands on the gluteus maximus muscle farthest from you (Fig. 7.7d). Move your left hand towards you, to the right gluteus maximus, with pressure (Fig. 7.7e) on the initial lift. As your left hand returns to the left side of the body, your right hand moves towards you to the right side of the body (Fig. 7.7f,g). As your right hand returns to the left side of the body, your left hand moves towards you again – to the right side. At every move, each hand is directed slightly higher up the body. Continue this two-way movement up to the top of the latissimus dorsi, sliding both hands in a superficial movement down the lateral sides of the back, ready to repeat the whole movement several times.

6. Return to the position required for movement 1 and repeat that movement several times.

7. Using the whole of the length of the thumb and thenar muscle (Fig. 7.7h) push up firmly from the sacrum past the waist level until the thenar muscle is lying in the waist itself. Take your thumb over to the fingers, then turn your hands towards the sides of the body until your fingertips touch the bed. Do not take your fingers around the body, but when your fingertips make contact with the bed allow them to bend as the thenar muscle comes to meet them, making a fist on the bed.

8. Repeat movement 1 several times.

ABDOMINAL MASSAGE

Abdominal massage has been well-documented since the beginning of the 20th century as a natural method of relieving constipation (Hertz 1909). It is also used on people hospitalized for differing reasons such as the elderly, those with

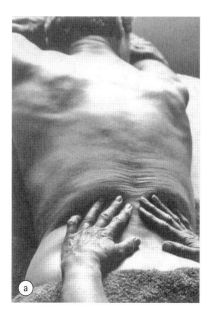

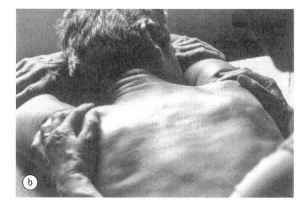

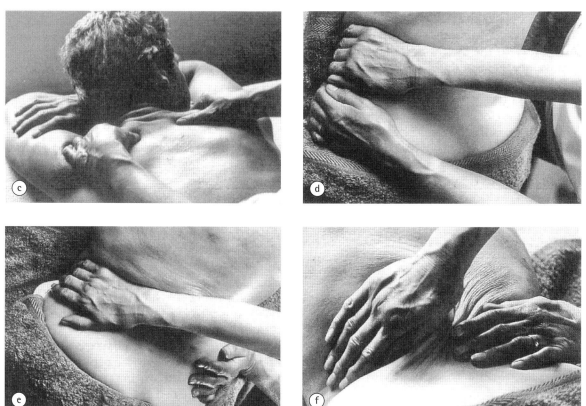

Figure 7.7   (a–f) Back massage.

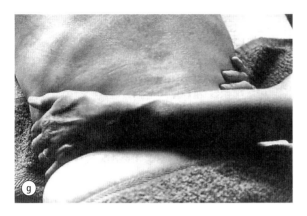

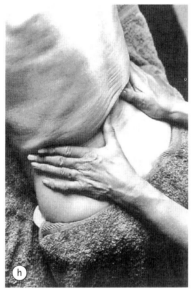

Figure 7.7 (*cont'd*) (g–h) Back massage.

cerebral palsy, Parkinson's disease and those who are HIV positive, etc. (Emly 1993). Movements which follow the peristaltic action of the colon are particularly important.

Stand at the side of the bed and place one hand on top of the other at the top of the patient's diaphragmatic arch (Fig. 7.8a). Check your hands are relaxed and think about your palm when directing the movement. Then proceed as follows:

1. Bring the hands gently down the centre of the body until you can see the patient's navel at the tips of your fingers (Fig. 7.8b). Turn your fingers outwards (Fig. 7.8c) and take them to just under the waist. Lift both hands, keeping full contact and bringing them towards each

other downwards (keeping palms down) to the pelvic bone. With your fingers in the original overlapped position, gently slide up the centre of the body to the sternum. Repeat the whole movement several times.

2. Taking both hands (overlapped) to the right iliac fossa (Fig. 7.8d), move them slowly and gently in a clockwise circle up the ascending colon, across the transverse colon and down the descending colon several times, finishing where you began.

3. Keeping your hands reinforced and fingers relaxed, make small clockwise circles, in one big circle, with your palms, following the colon as in movement 2 (Fig. 7.8e).

4. Place both hands on the far, lateral side of the abdomen (Fig. 7.8f) and perform movement 5 from the back massage above, but gently, with less pressure.

5. Repeat movement 3. For severe constipation, the fingers of the underneath hand may be made into a fist in order to give a slower, more determined stimulus to the colon.

6. Repeat movement 2.

PREGNANCY AND LABOUR MASSAGE

During pregnancy normal massage is encouraged up to the 5th month. As the pregnancy develops, the mother-to-be cannot lie comfortably on her tummy, and the following special techniques show how the massage sequences above can be adapted at this stage.

Back massage is possible if the mother-to-be can be in any of the following positions, whichever she finds most comfortable:

- Semi-prone, often referred to as Sims's position; on the left (or right) side and chest, the opposite knee and thigh drawn up so that it can rest on the bed, the trailing arm along the back (Fig. 7.9a).
- Sitting on the bed with legs in a squatting position, resting the top half of the body on the backrest plus pillows (Fig. 7.9b).
- Sitting straddled on a chair as suggested for shoulder massage above.
- Sitting on a stool facing the side of the bed, resting arms and head on a pillow on the bed (Fig. 7.9c).

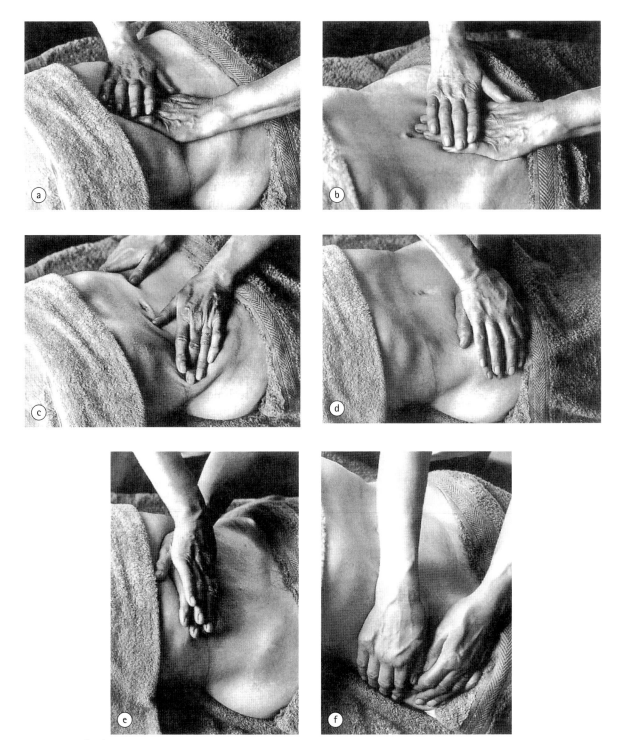

Figure 7.8   (a–f) Abdominal massage.

Leg massage can take place with the patient in a sitting position on the bed, supported by a back-rest and pillows.

Abdominal massage should be very gentle and is excellent for calming the baby and relaxing the mother. Raise the upper half of the body with pillows. Movement 1 has been found to be very effective during a contraction (Fern 1992).

BABY MASSAGE

For ease, the baby will be referred to as 'him' throughout the instructions.

New parents have no difficulty touching, stroking and cuddling their babies and it is a very small step from there to massage. However, as a baby's skin is delicate and rather 'loose', massage has to be gentle. Contact is particularly important for babies, so an excellent way to introduce massage is to sit on the sofa, supporting your back on cushions or pillows (Price & Price 2004). Place a warm soft towel over your abdomen and lay the baby there on his back – head away from you, drawing your knees up towards you to support him. All the following movements can also be done on a baby mattress, covered with a warm towel and placed on a table – this is the best way for massaging baby's back.

Put a little of the selected blend of oils onto warm hands, gently rubbing them together to distribute and warm the oil blend. Then carry out the following movements.

Tummy

Holding one of baby's hands, to make him feel secure – and preventing him from 'thrashing' around (Price & Price 2004) – place the fingers of the other hand gently on his tummy, and using as much of the finger lengths as possible, make gentle but firm clockwise circles around his navel (Fig. 7.10a). Repeat several times.

Scalp and forehead

1. Place the fingers of both hands firmly on baby's scalp, so that it can be moved gently over the bone beneath (Fig. 7.10b). Move the fingers to a different position and repeat.
2. With fingertips on baby's scalp, move the whole length of the thumbs alternately up his forehead several times. Repeat movement 1.

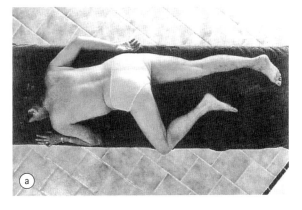

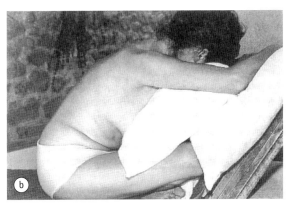

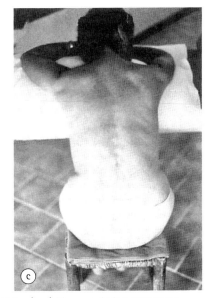

Figure 7.9   (a–c) Massage during pregnancy.

Feet and legs

1. Gently holding baby's right thigh with the right hand, place the left hand fingers on top of his foot – and with as much of the length of the thumbs as possible over the sole of his foot, move in slow circles over the middle area (Fig. 7.10c).
2. Hold baby's foot with the right hand and move the left thumb in circles from ankle to knee, returning lightly (Fig 7.10d). Repeat several times.
3. Gently but firmly take the curved lengths of the left fingers from baby's ankle to thigh, covering as much of the outside of his leg as possible in the one stroke, returning lightly underneath (Fig 7.10e). Repeat several times.
4. Repeat movement 1.
5. Repeat movements 1–4 on the other foot and leg, reversing the hand-hold used.

Hands and arms

1. Placing the fingers of both hands on the back of baby's hand, place the right thumb over his fingers and make circles on his palm with your left thumb (Fig 7.10f).
2. Holding his hand with the right hand, take the left hand gently but firmly up the arm to the shoulder – and around it, returning very lightly on the back of his arm (Fig 7.10g). Repeat several times.

Repeat both movements on the other hand and arm, reversing the hand-hold used.

Back

The back is easier to do on a baby mattress (see above).

1. With fingers and thumbs making a triangle shape (Fig 7.10h), move the whole finger length up baby's back, using as much of the hands as

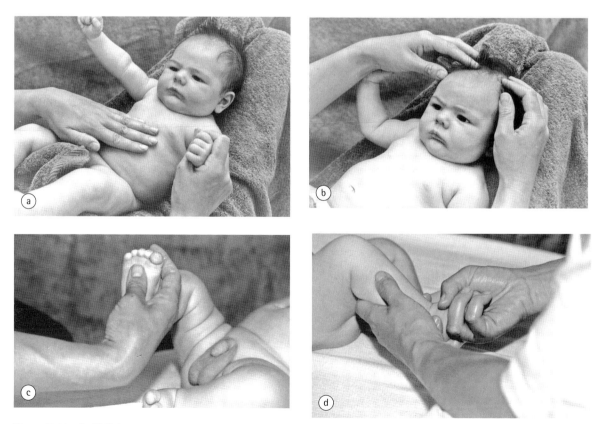

Figure 7.10 (a–b) Baby massage.

possible to 'cuddle' round his shoulders, before returning very gently down the sides of his body. Repeat 4–5 times.

2. Place the hands around the sides of baby's body, with one thumb on each buttock. Making large circles with the flat of the thumbs, move slowly and progressively up his back, with slight pressure on the upward half of each circle. On reaching the shoulders (Fig. 7.10i), take the thumbs right round them, returning very gently down the sides of his body. Repeat 3–4 times.

3. Repeat movement 1.

SWISS REFLEX MASSAGE

This technique was devised by Shirley Price in 1987 while in Switzerland (hence the name) and although based on reflexology points, differs from it.

Reflexology is 'an ancient Eastern technique which makes use of somewhat mysterious connecting pathways or energy flow lines in the body' (Price 2000 p. 43). These culminate in various areas of the body, occurring in the feet, hands, ears and tongue, where reflexes representing every part of the body can be found. Foot reflexes can be

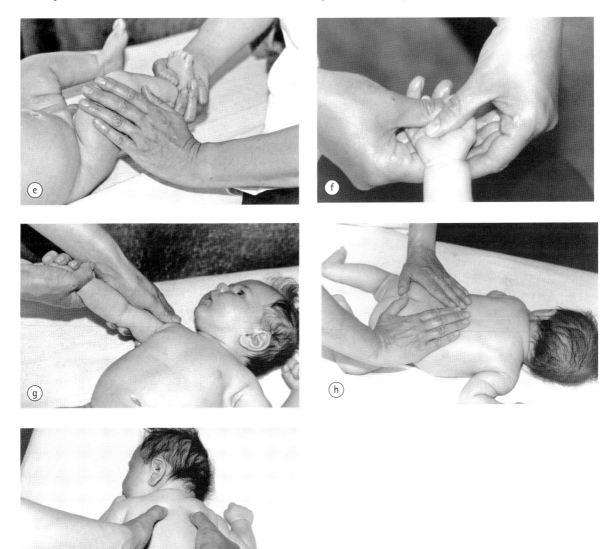

Figure 7.10 (cont'd) (e–i) Baby massage.

used as a valuable diagnostic aid; furthermore, the body can be treated effectively via the energy flow lines through massaging the relevant points with essential oils. As in any professional therapy, it is necessary to undertake an accredited training in order to be able to understand thoroughly the position, significance and interpretation of each bodily system and each reflex point.

Prior to treatment, one must either be aware of the problem areas of the patient, or test each reflex for a reaction.

In a Swiss reflex treatment, reflexes specific to the patient's health are massaged, together with a precise dialogue between therapist and client. A bland cream base is used to which are added essential oils selected by the same method as for an aromatherapy massage treatment. The ratio of essential oil to cream is 30 drops to 30 ml. The treatment is much simpler to learn than are the

techniques involved in reflexology, although knowledge of the location of the representative reflexes is still of primary importance before the treatment can be carried out successfully. As with all practical subjects, attending a practical course is the best way to learn. However, the basic principles are described below.

Swiss reflex treatment involves special client participation, including *daily* self-treatment (or treatment by partner or carer) at home. Without daily treatment, the results are approximately the same as in reflexology or normal massage; however, with daily SRT, positive results are gained much more quickly. Therapists trained in this method by the author before her business passed into other hands – and present students of the Penny Price Academy of Aromatherapy (see Useful addresses, p. 528) – have had some extraordinarily positive results (see Case studies 7.4, 7.5).

Case study 7.4 Arthritic pain – S Price – *aromatologist, UK*

Client assessment
Mrs U, 58, had just recovered from a second attempt at a hip replacement, the healing of which was helped considerably by aromatherapy. Now, she was to undergo an operation to fuse her cervical vertebrae on account of the severe arthritic pain there. She was very anxious about this, as due to the death of her husband she needed to be able to continue driving. She wore a surgical collar, which she hated.

Intervention
Mrs U was given a Swiss reflex treatment, using the following essential oils, added to a 30 ml jar of bland, non-greasy Swiss reflex cream base:

- 10 drops *Rosmarinus officinalis* [rosemary] – analgesic, antiinflammatory
- 4 drops *Origanum majorana* [sweet marjoram] – properties as above
- 8 drops *Juniperus communis* [juniper berry] – properties as above

She was then shown how to massage the same areas herself at home every day – and given the jar of reflex cream.

At the second visit 2 weeks later, no improvement had been made – and it was discovered that the client had been massaging the wrong reflex! This experience indicated the importance of giving the client a marked chart, illustrating exactly not only the sequence of the treatment but also the reflex points to be massaged (on this occasion it had been forgotten!).

2 weeks later, Mrs U was experiencing somewhat less pain and a slight improvement in neck mobility. The improvement continued over the next 2 weeks and at the fourth appointment Mrs A arrived smiling – wearing a collar homemade from firm foam sponge wrapped in a pretty scarf.

Outcome
6 weeks later, with only self-treatment and a visit every 2 weeks to confirm all was progressing well, she arrived without even the silk wrapped foam collar. She had had her appointment with the consultant prior to the operation and he was so amazed at the change in her mobility and the lack of pain, he told her the operation would not now be necessary. He asked her what she had been doing, but unfortunately Mrs U was too embarrassed to say she had been rubbing her big toe!

Case study 7.5 Mining accident – D Moore – *aromatherapist, UK*

Client assessment
Frank had been in a mining accident 19 years previously. A roof beam had fallen on his shoulder, which was damaged, causing a rib to be broken – which had pierced his lung. Apart from being unable to move his arm away from his side, he was having breathing difficulties and when walking could only move his feet 15–17 cm at a time.

He had been under a consultant for the whole 19 years and was becoming progressively worse, rather than better. His wife had heard Shirley Price speaking on the radio about aromatherapy and decided to try this treatment for Frank.

Intervention
When they arrived, it was obvious that an aromatherapy body massage would not be possible – the answer had to be Swiss reflex treatment.

This was given to him twice a week the first week, once a week for 2 further weeks, once a fortnight for the next month, then once a month and eventually once every 2 or 3 months. The oils selected for Frank, in 30 ml of the bland reflex cream base were:

- *Piper nigrum* [black pepper] – analgesic, antispasmodic, expectorant
- *Juniperus communis.* ram [juniper twig] – analgesic, anticatarrhal, neurotonic
- *Boswellia carteri* [frankincense] – analgesic, anticatarrhal, antiinflammatory, expectorant, immunostimulant
- *Lavandula officinalis* [lavender] – analgesic, antispasmodic, calming, general tonic

Frank's wife was taught how to do the daily treatment and they returned in 4 days to check she was doing it correctly – which she was.

After 6 weeks it was obvious she had never missed a day, as Frank could raise his right arm about 10 cm; after another 2 months this had not only increased to 30 cm, but his shoulders and head were half-way to being erect and his feet were able to take steps of around 26–30 cm.

Outcome
After 6 months, he was leaving the centre with his head erect and an almost normal, albeit slow, step. He had proudly shown the therapist how he could lift his arm almost up to his shoulder and was looking forward to the day he could comb his own hair with his right hand again.

METHOD OF TREATMENT

N.B. Having determined which reflexes are in need of treatment, begin always with the solar plexus reflex area (Fig. 7.11a) and finish on the kidney–bladder area (Fig. 7.11b).

1. Apply a very small amount of cream all over the dorsum and sole of the right foot.
2. Carry out foot movement 1 (see p. 175 – but up to the ankle only) and 2, several times, to warm the foot, then wrap in a towel.
3. Repeat these two movements on the left foot and wrap in a towel.
4. Holding the right foot by placing the palm of the left hand over the phalanges and metatarsal of the big toe, begin by massaging the solar plexus reflex area in a circular motion with the whole of the length of your right thumb (Fig. 7.11a) – as firmly as the tolerance of the individual patient will allow (if the patient is highly stressed even gentle stroking will seem painful). The pressure should be just such that the patient feels slight discomfort ('pain'). Maintain this same pressure – and circling – until the client is able to tell you that the 'pain' is no longer evident. If the discomfort is still present after 1 minute, the original pressure was probably too strong and the movement should be repeated with just enough pressure to take the patient to his/her lowest pain threshold.
5. Using the same method as in movement 4, massage any reflex area of which the representative organ is presenting a problem to the patient, e.g. lung area for bronchial problems, digestive system area for constipation (concentrating on the large intestine reflex areas, in a clockwise direction), spinal areas for rheumatism or arthritis (in three small sections

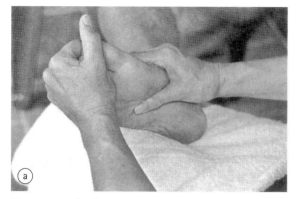 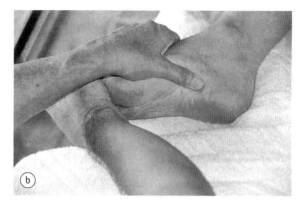

Figure 7.11   (a–b) Swiss reflex massage.

if the whole spine is affected). Change your hand positions when necessary.

6. Placing your right hand across your body and placing it over the patient's toes, massage with the side length of the thumb in a firm circle, following the kidney–ureter–bladder line (Fig. 7.11b) – relaxing the pressure on the return half of the circle.

7. Repeat movements 2 and 3 and re-wrap in the towel.

8. Repeat movements 2–7 on the left foot, reversing 'right' and 'left' in the text.

CARRIER OILS

Vegetable carrier oils constitute the bulk of the material used in an aromatherapy massage. Their function is to 'carry' or act as a vehicle for administering the essential oils to the body and also as lubricants, to make massage movements possible. This section discusses the nature of carrier oils, and details the properties and applications of those more frequently used in aromatherapy.

FIXED OILS

Carrier oils are also known as fixed oils, because they do not evaporate, in contrast to the volatile plant essential oils, which do evaporate. Fixed, carrier oils constitute a different chemical family from essential oils, which is why their properties are so different. Because of their lubricating quality and non-volatile nature they leave a permanent oily mark on paper; essential oils do

not leave an oily mark, although any colour present will leave a stain. All essential oils dissolve easily and completely in fixed oils in all proportions.

Chemically speaking, carrier oils are classed as lipids, which are a diverse family of compounds found naturally in plants and animals. Oils and fats have similar structures, but at room temperature (15°C) fats are solid and oils are liquid. For the detailed chemistry of carrier oils, see Carrier Oils for Aromatherapy and Massage, written by Price et al (1999).

Vegetable oils contain a high level of unsaturated fatty acid units (>80%), which is why they are important for our health. The double bonds are less strong than single bonds and introduce an element of weakness into a compound. Once opened up they can absorb other molecules for transportation elsewhere in the body, and can also facilitate the natural digestive breakdown of the triacylglycerols. However, oils with a high degree of unsaturation are less stable than those that are highly saturated, owing to the weakness of the double bonds; thus they are open to attack by oxygen and moisture, which can lead to breakdown and rancidity.

COLD-PRESSED OILS

Carrier oils used in aromatherapy should, wherever possible, be cold pressed, although this term is a slight misnomer, as the extraction process generates a certain amount of heat – and cooling is normally required. Temperatures are usually maintained below 60°C, however, and in this way changes to the natural characteristics of the oil are kept to a minimum.

Vegetable oils may be refined to meet the particular requirements of large scale users such as the pharmaceutical industry, cooking oil manufacturers, food processors and cosmetics companies. Processing here frequently involves the use of high temperatures and chemicals, when many of the natural properties of the oil are lost, the character is altered and its use in aromatherapy is not desirable. This is the type of oil usually found on supermarket shelves.

Mineral oils are high molecular weight hydrocarbons, with very different properties from those of vegetable oils. They are oily and greasy, with a tendency to clog the pores, and are less able to be absorbed by the skin. They are therefore not suitable nor are normally used in aromatherapy.

TYPES OF CARRIER OIL

There are three broad categories:

- **Basic oils.** These can be used with or without essential oils for body massage and are generally pale in colour, not too viscous and have very little smell. They include sweet almond, apricot kernel, peach kernel (see page 196), grapeseed and sunflower.
- **Special oils.** These tend to be more viscous, heavier and more expensive. They include avocado, sesame, rose hip and wheatgerm. The extra-rich oils such as avocado and wheatgerm are seldom, if ever, used on their own. It is more normal to use them as 10–25% of a carrier oil blend.
- **Macerated oils.** As these have certain additional properties to the oils above, because of the way they are produced, they can be used on their own, although it is preferable to add one or two drops of appropriate essential oils to increase the effect on health conditions. Chopped plant material is added to a selected fixed oil (mostly sunflower or olive), agitated gently for some time, then left for a few days, before filtering. All the plant's oil soluble compounds (including any essential oil compounds which may be present) are transferred to the carrier oil, giving them extra therapeutic effects.

There are more than 20 suitable carrier oils available (see Price et al 1999) – a small selection is detailed below. Table 7.1 gives a more complete list, including particular properties and indications for each.

BASIC OILS

Almond sweet (*Prunus amygdalis* var. *dulcis*)

Sweet almond oil is one of the most used carrier oils; pale yellow in colour, it is slightly viscous and very oily. Apricot kernel (*P. armeniaca*) and peach kernel (*P. persica*) oils are very similar – it can be very difficult to discriminate between them. Their advantage over some other base oils is that they have less of a tendency to become rancid. The unrefined oil has a delicate, sweet smell and a flavour with a hint of marzipan. Sweet almond oil is used in laxative preparations and is said to be effective in reducing blood cholesterol levels (Leung & Foster 1996). It is an excellent emollient and nourishes dry skin; it also helps to soothe inflammation (Stier 1990). Almond oil is beneficial in relieving the itching caused by eczema, psoriasis, dermatitis and all cases of dry scaly skin, and is absorbed slowly through the intact skin (Expert Panel 1983 p. 97). It is said to be non-irritating, non-sensitizing and considered safe for cosmetic use (Leung & Foster 1996) but a few people are allergic to cosmetics containing almond oil, suffering a stuffy nose and skin rash (Winter 1984 p. 49).

Grapeseed (*Vitis vinifera*)

Grape seeds cannot be cold pressed and the oil is produced commercially by hot extraction. If it can be 'rescued' before it is refined, it is suitable for aromatherapy as refining includes chemical processing. The oil is tasteless, almost odourless and as it is very fine (it is used to lubricate watches) it is a very suitable oil for aromatherapy. It is a gentle emollient and leaves the skin with a smooth satin finish without feeling greasy.

Sunflower (*Helianthus annuus*)

Much of the sunflower oil available commercially has been obtained by solvent extraction, so care must be taken to ensure that only cold-pressed oil, which is also available, is used in aromatherapy. Sunflower oil has slight diuretic properties; it is said to aid cholesterol metabolism and may be

Table 7.1 Properties and indications of carrier oils

Fixed oils (*indicates macerated) COMMON NAME / Scientific name	Properties and indications – general														Properties and indications – skin										
	Analgesic (light)	Antiinflammatory	Antipruritic	Arthritis	Astringent	Circulatory	Haemorrhoids	Laxative	Lowers blood cholesterol	PMT	Rheumatism	Sprains/bruises	Varicose veins	Wounds	Acne	Broken veins	Burns	Eczema	Emollient, dry skin	Psoriasis	Scars	Shingles zoster	Sunburnt skin	Sun protection	Wrinkles, mature skin
ALMOND SWEET *Prunus amygdalis* var. *dulcis*		X	X	X				X	X									X	X	X					
APRICOT KERNEL *Prunus armeniaca*		X						X	X									X	X						X
AVOCADO *Persea gratissima*								X				X						X	X						X
CALENDULA* *Calendula officinalis*		X			X							X	X	X	X	X	X								
CARROT* *Daucus carota*		X	X													X	X			X	X				
EVENING PRIMROSE *Oenethera biennis*			X							X	X			X				X	X	X					
GRAPESEED *Vitis vinifera*																			X						
HAZELNUT *Corylus avellana*			X		X	X										X									X
JOJOBA *Simmondsia chinensis*	X	X	X								X				X			X	X	X				X	
LEMON BALM* *Melissa officinalis*																			X						
LIME BLOSSOM, LINDEN* *Tilia europoea*										X															X
MACADAMIA *Macadamia ternifolia*								X																X	X
OLIVE *Olea europoea*			X	X				X	X		X						X	X							
PASSIONFLOWER *Passiflora incarnata*	X																								
PEACH KERNEL *Prunus persica*		X						X	X										X						X
ROSE HIP *Rosa canina, R. mosquetta*														X		X	X				X				X

Table 7.1   Properties and indications of carrier oils (*cont'd*)

COMMON NAME / Scientific name	Analgesic (light)	Antiinflammatory	Antipruritic	Arthritis	Astringent	Circulatory	Haemorrhoids	Laxative	Lowers blood cholesterol	PMT	Rheumatism	Sprains/bruises	Varicose veins	Wounds	Acne	Broken veins	Burns	Eczema	Emollient, dry skin	Psoriasis	Scars	Shingles zoster	Sunburnt skin	Sun protection	Wrinkles, mature skin
ST JOHN'S WORT* / *Hypericum perforatum*	X	X				X					X	X		X			X						X		
SUNFLOWER / *Helianthus annuus*						X			X		X	X													
TAMANU / *Calophyllum inophyllum*	X	X																	X		X	X	X		
WALNUT / *Juglans regia*						X	X												X				?		
WHEATGERM / *Triticum vulgare*						X			X					X					X						X

(Column headers: Fixed oils (*indicates macerated); Properties and indications – general; Properties and indications – skin)

used to counteract arteriosclerosis (Stier 1990). It is expectorant and, as it contains inulin, it may be useful in the treatment of asthma. The oil is beneficial for skin complaints and bruises, and is effective on leg ulcers. It has been reported as being efficacious in the treatment of multiple sclerosis (Anon 1990, Millar et al 1973, Swank & Dugan 1990).

SPECIAL OILS

Avocado oil (*Persea gratissima, Persea americana*) Lauraceae

True cold pressed avocado oil (from the dried pears) is a deep green colour and is comparatively rare. It keeps well but should not be chilled, as precipitation of some useful parts of the oil would occur – it solidifies at 0°C. Occasionally it has a slightly cloudy appearance, occasionally with sediment, which can indicate that it has not been subjected to extensive refining. Refined avocado oil, used by the cosmetics industry, is pale yellow to colourless and bleached; it is widely available but should not be used therapeutically for obvious reasons.

Avocado oil is a good, penetrating emollient – useful for massage, where 10 to 25% is used in a base carrier oil. It is valuable in muscle preparations, has skin healing (Leung & Foster 1996 p. 54), moisturizing, and anti-wrinkle properties and is recommended for dry skins. It has been used in Raynaud's disease (Stier 1990 p. 54). As far as is known, avocado oil is non-irritant and non-sensitizing (Winter 1984 p. 38). The ingested pressed oil is said to be helpful in constipation, liver and gall bladder problems and urinary infections (Price et al 1999 p. 40).

Evening primrose oil (*Oenothera biennis, O. glazioviana, O. nagraceae*)

Evening primrose oil, pressed from the seeds, includes 10% gamma linolenic acid (GLA), which is comparatively rare. This highly unsaturated oil is more reactive and less stable than most other oils. The oil oxidizes on exposure to air and light and is sensitive also to heat and humidity, therefore it should be stored in a cool, dark place. It is thought to be beneficial in the treatment of atopic eczema (Kerscher & Korting 1992, Lovell 1981), although this is contested by Berth-Jones & Graham-Brown (1993). It is known to be useful in the treatment of dry, scaly skin (Price, Price & Smith 1999 p. 73) and to benefit sufferers of psoriasis (Ferrando 1986). The oil improves dandruff conditions and accelerates wound healing (Price, Price & Smith 1999 p. 73); for cosmetic use it is incorporated in anti-wrinkle preparations. Borage oil is sometimes added to increase the level of GLA. When ingested, evening primrose oil is said to control arthritis (Lovell 1981) and Horrobin (1983) claims it is helpful to PMS, though Collins et al (1993) repudiate this claim.

Jojoba oil (*Simmondsia chinensis, Buxus chinensis*)

Jojoba oil is in fact a wax, not an oil; the seeds produce a liquid wax which does not become rancid, giving it a long shelf-life (it will solidify if stored in a refrigerator). It is very stable (indigestible to bacteria) so preservatives (often the cause of allergies or skin irritations) are not necessary. Jojoba contains the antiinflammatory agent myristic acid, making it beneficial for arthritis and rheumatism. It is particularly of use in cases of acne as its molecular structure is similar to sebum; it is used to control the build up of excessive sebum (Anon 1983). It is also used for nappy rash and chapped skin (Bartram 1996 p. 258), psoriasis, sunburn and eczema. Jojoba oil may cause allergic reaction (Winter 1984 p. 154) and contact dermatitis has also been reported (Scott & Scott 1982).

Peach kernel oil (*Prunus persica*)

This oil, usually cold pressed, is chemically and physically similar to almond and apricot kernel oils, though more expensive, due to not being produced in large quantities. It is emollient and nourishing, so is beneficial for dry, sensitive and ageing skins. It is reputed to relieve itching and help eczema (Price, Price & Smith 1999 p. 110). The oil is often used in the cosmetic industry as a substitute for almond oil (Wren 1975) in facial massage oils and skin care creams. Culpeper (1616–1684) tells us that the oil brings rest and sleep when applied to the forehead, and when ingested it is said to relieve constipation and high blood cholesterol (Price, Price & Smith 1999 p. 110).

Rose hip (*Rosa mosquetta, R. rubiginosa*)

Rose hip oil, taken from the seeds within, is a golden-red colour and contains significant amounts of vitamin C. It also contains small quantities of *trans*-retinoic acid, which contribute to its therapeutic properties. Studies in Chile have identified that the oil is a tissue regenerator and has an effect on the skin to minimize premature ageing and wrinkles, also to reduce scar tissue. It is helpful on wounds, burns and eczema.

Wheatgerm (*Triticum vulgare*)

Wheatgerm is a rich orange-brown colour and very viscous. It is seldom used on its own, being commonly employed as 10–25% of the carrier oil mix. Because of its high content of vitamin E, a natural antioxidant, it is added to less stable oils to increase their useful life. The oil is rich in lipid soluble vitamins, and so is good for revitalizing dry skin. It is also said to be useful on ageing skin where its natural antioxidants are an effective weapon against free radicals. The oil is beneficial for tired muscles and should be included in the mix for after-sports massage.

MACERATED OILS

Calendula (*Calendula officinalis*)

Calendula oil is obtained by macerating chopped plant material in sunflower oil and the normal orange-yellow colour of the calendula flowers is reflected in the colour of the oil. Although calendula is sometimes referred to as 'marigold' it is a very different plant from *Tagetes patula* and *Tagetes minuta* [tagetes, French marigold], which are also known as marigold. Calendula extracts have been used to promote healing and reduce inflammation (Fleischner 1985), and it is most effective on broken veins, varicose veins, bruises, etc. Calendula is specifically indicated for enlarged or inflamed lymph nodes, sebaceous cysts and acute or chronic skin lesions (Casley-Smith & Casley-Smith 1983).

St John's wort (*Hypericum perforatum*)

This plant is usually macerated in olive oil, the resulting oil being a deep red colour, owing to the presence of hypericin. An antiinflammatory oil, hypericum is useful on wounds where there is nerve tissue damage and it is also useful for inflamed nerve conditions, hence it is used in cases of neuralgia, sciatica and fibrositis. A 20% hypericum tincture has been used in the treatment of suppurative otitis, and extracts are stated to have been used clinically in Russia to treat infection (Shaparenko et al 1979). The use of hypericum in the treatment of vitiligo (Newall, Anderson & Phillipson 1996) has also been reported, as has its use as an astringent and diuretic (Martindale 1993). Hypericin, the red pigment, is being studied as a possible antiviral agent in the management of acquired immune deficiency syndrome (AIDS) (Abrams 1990, Anon 1991).

SUMMARY

Touch and massage have profound benefits, not only for the recipient, but also for the therapist, and its recent neglect in official health care is slowly beginning to be remedied. This chapter has identified the main benefits, as well as the most important contraindications. It has also provided a basic grounding in simple massage techniques, and suggested some of the more useful massage sequences. Carrier oils comprise the major part of any blend used in an aromatherapy massage and should be selected with care, to augment the effects of essential oils on presenting symptoms.

References

Abrams D I 1990 Alternative therapies in HIV infection. AIDS 4: 1179–1187

Anon 1983 Botanicals in cosmetics. Jojoba: a botanical with a proven functionality. Cosmetics and Toiletries June 98: 81–82

Anon 1990 Lipids and multiple sclerosis. Lancet 336: 25–26

Anon 1991 Treating AIDS with worts. Science 254: 522

Auckett A D 1981 Baby massage. Newmarket Press, New York

Bartram T 1996 Encyclopedia of herbal medicine. Grace, Christchurch, p. 258

Beard G, Wood E C 1964 Massage – principles and techniques. Saunders, London

Berth-Jones J, Graham-Brown R A C 1993 Placebo controlled trial of essential fatty acid supplementation in atopic dermatitis. Lancet 341:1557–1560

Buckle 1997 Clinical aromatherapy in nursing. Arnold, London

Casley-Smith J R, Casley-Smith J R 1983 The effect of *Unguentum lymphaticum* on acute experimental lymphedema and other high-protein edemas. Lymphology 16: 150–156

Chaitow L 2000 In: Field T (ed) Touch therapy. Churchill Livingstone, Edinburgh, p. vii

Collins A, Coleman G, Landgren B M 1993 Essential fatty acids in the treatment of premenstrual syndrome. Obstetrics and Gynaecology 81: 93–98

Culpeper (undated) Culpeper's complete herbal. Foulsham, Exeter, p. 262

Emly M 1993 Abdominal massage. Nursing Times 89(3): 34–36

Expert Panel 1983 Cosmetic ingredient review: 4: Final report on the safety of sweet almond oil and almond meal. Journal of the American College of Toxicology 2(5): 85–99

Fern E 1992 Directorate of Maternity and Gynaecology. Practice Group (Midwifery, Gynaecology and Neonatal Care) Aromatherapy. Midwifery Procedure no. 23, Ipswich Hospital

Ferrando J 1986 Clinical trial of topical preparation containing urea, sunflower oil, evening primrose oil, wheatgerm oil and sodium pyruvate in several hyperkeratotic skin conditions. Medicina Cutanea Latino Americana 14(2): 132–137

Field T 2000 Touch therapy. Churchill Livingstone, Edinburgh

Field T, Scafidi F, Schanberg S 1987 Massage of preterm newborns to improve growth and development. Paediatric Nursing 13: 385–387

Fleischner A M 1985 Plant extracts: to accelerate healing and reduce inflammation. Cosmetics and Toiletries 100: 45

Hertz A F 1909 constipation and internal disorders. Oxford University Press, Oxford

Horrigan C 1991 Complementing cancer care. International Journal of Aromatherapy 3(4): 15–17

Horrobin D F 1983 The role of essential fatty acids and prostaglandins in the premenstrual syndrome. Journal of Reproductive Medicine 28: 465–468

Leung A Y, Foster S 1996 Encyclopedia of common natural ingredients. Wiley, New York

Lovell C R 1981 Plants and the skin. Blackwell, London, p. 255

Martindale 1993 The extra pharmacopoeia, 30th edn. Pharmaceutical Press, London, p. 1378.3

Maxwell-Hudson C 1999 Aromatherapy massage. Dorling Kindersley, New York, p. 41

Mennell J B 1945 Physical treatment, 5th edn. Blakiston, Philadelphia

Millar J H D, Zilkha K J, Langman M J S, Payling Wright H, Smith A D, Belin J, Thompson R H S 1973 Double blind trial of linoleate supplementation of the diet in multiple sclerosis. British Medical Journal 31 March 1(5856): 765–768

Newall C A, Anderson L A, Phillipson J D 1996 Herbal medicines. The Pharmaceutical Press, London, p. 251

Price S 1999 Practical aromatherapy, 4th edn. How to use essential oils to restore health and vitality. Thorsons, London

Price S 2000 The aromatherapy workbook, 2nd edn. Thorsons, London

Price S, Price P 2004, Aromatherapy for babies and children, 2nd edn. Riverhead, Stratford upon Avon

Price L, Price S, Smith I 1999 Carrier oils for aromatherapy and massage. Riverhead, Stratford upon Avon

Sanderson H, Harrison J, Price S 1991 Aromatherapy and massage for people with learning difficulties. Hands On, Birmingham

Scott M J, Scott M J Jr 1982 Jojoba oil (Letter). Journal of American Academy of Dermatology

Shaparenko B A, Slivko B A, Bazarova O V, Vishnevetskaya E N, Selesneva G T, Berezhnala L P 1979 On the use of medicinal plants for treatment of patients with chronic suppurative otitis. Zhurnal Ushnykh I Gorlovykh Boleznei 39(3): 48–51

Stier B 1990 Secrets des huiles de première pression à froid. Self published, Quebec

Swank R L, Dugan B B 1990 Effect of low saturated fat diet in early and late cases of multiple sclerosis. Lancet 336: 37–39

Tattam A 1992 The gentle touch. Nursing Times 88(32): 16–17

Vickers A 1996 Aromatherapy and massage. A guide for Health Professionals. Chapman & Hall, London, p. 6

Wilkinson S 1995 Aromatherapy and massage in palliative care. International Journal of Palliative Nursing 1(1): 21–30

Winter R 1984 A consumer's dictionary of cosmetic ingredients. Crown, New York

Worrell J 1997 Touch: attitudes and practice. Nursing Forum 18(1): 1–17

Wren R W 1975 Potter's new cyclopaedia of botanical drugs and preparations. Health Science Press, Bradford nr. Holsworthy, p. 230

Chapter 8

Aromas, mind and body

Len Price

INTRODUCTION

This chapter explores the connections between a person's thoughts, feelings and immune status, and suggests that the ability of essential oils to affect all these makes aromatherapy worth considering as a truly holistic therapy.

THE IMPACT OF THE MIND AND EMOTIONS ON THE BODY

Throughout the ages, whatever their culture, tradition and background, whether surgeon-barber or medicine worker, people concerned with healing have always been aware that there is a connection between thoughts, emotions and the state of health of the physical body. The following quotation, from an article in the British Medical Journal of 1884, shows accurate observation of the connection between the state of the emotions and physical well-being: 'the depression of the spirits at these melancholy occasions (funerals) . . . disposes them to some of the worst effects of the chills' (Wood 1990a). In modern times this has been recognized not only by psychotherapists and those in psychosomatic medicine, but also in general medicine.

Can a pessimistic outlook influence our immune system directly? The answer must be yes. The way that we assess situations determines our emotional responses to them. Emotions release hormones and hormones can influence immunity. But it is important to realize that this process does not happen (or need not happen) automatically, without our knowing about it. In the last analysis it is the way we think and feel that triggers the immune change

Wood (1990b)

These effects can be real, and changes in blood chemistry have been recorded even when the emotions are conjured up artificially, as in the case of superstition. There is a superstition in the theatre, for example, that playing the part of Macbeth will bring bad luck of some sort, such as ill health. Three thousand years ago the impact and influence of the intangible human mind on the material body had been observed and recorded in the Bible: 'A merry heart doeth good like a medicine; but a broken spirit drieth the bones' (Proverbs 17: 22, King James version).

PSYCHONEUROIMMUNOLOGY

As long ago as 1970 the authors were made aware of the strong influence the mind can have on bodily health; longstanding insomnia problems were overcome and eventually sleeping pills were dispensed with, all by positive thinking. The converse was proved by a female relative, who consistently anticipated adverse negative outcomes to situations and events; they became self-fulfilling prophecies.

In recent years there have been significant advances in the study and understanding of the connections between mind and body. Previously, the psyche, the nervous system and the immune system were studied more or less as independent systems functioning alongside each other but without direct connections. However, a new scientific discipline, known as psychoneuroimmunology (PNI) appeared, and a partial understanding of how the brain and the immune system communicate with each other is developing. They are being looked at now in terms of their intercommunicating system of chemical messengers, their interconnections via nerve tissue and their effects and interactions with one another.

THE IMMUNE SYSTEM

Neuropeptide messengers produced by the immune system and nerve cells, including those of the brain, provide two-way communication between the emotional brain and bodily systems via hormonal feedback loops. The limbic system (hypothalamus and pituitary), the spleen, the adrenal and thymus glands all have nerve interconnections. Thus emotions are capable not only of directing the body but also of receiving and being modified by information feedback from cells in the body.

Adrenalin and cortisol are two of the many chemical messengers whose release can be triggered by negative emotion associated with sudden or long-term stress: these two hormones influence the immune system directly to switch it off (Borysenko 1988 p. 14). Adrenocorticotrophic hormone (ACTH) suppresses pituitary action by stimulation of the adrenal gland to produce adrenalin, which is a stimulator of the autonomic nervous system (ANS). In the wake of research like this, the idea has gradually gained ground that emotional states can translate into altered responses in the immune system: negative thoughts and sad emotions, perhaps resulting from such occasions as bereavement or because of other types of stress, can sometimes lessen the effectiveness of the immune system temporarily. Hence the body puts into physical effect non-material thoughts and emotions – to produce a beneficial healing effect or to inflict self-damage. This idea is echoed by many writers.

THE EFFECT OF THE EMOTIONS ON HEALTH

It has not been possible up to the present for anyone to show a link between a particular emotion and any specific physical disease – 'Pessimism is not linked to any particular disease' (Wood 1990b) – although pessimism or depression amplifies symptoms of pain. It can probably be said, though, that the course and eventual conclusion of nearly all disease is affected by non-physical thoughts, feelings, emotions and attitudes, which are in turn influenced by personality. Studies have confirmed the power of the mind to bring about dramatic changes in the physiology of the body as evidenced in the fight-or-flight response.

Fight–or–flight response

Many thousands of years ago people developed a response to dangerous situations designed to protect the body. This is known as the automatic primary stress response and the arousal system is located in the brain stem. When a person is presented with a threatening set of circumstances, the median hemisphere of the hypothalamus instantly puts into the bloodstream chemical messengers (catecholamines). These, in conjunction with the sympathetic nervous system, trigger a whole array of interconnected reactions – release of steroids, glycogen and adrenalin, faster breathing, increased heart rate, raised blood pressure, dilated pupils and so on – all designed to prepare the body for instant action resulting from the awareness of danger. Today, in modern society, this ancient inbuilt fight-or-flight response is evoked many times, not only in response to short-term acute physical risk (e.g. war, traffic, mugging, etc.) but also to threats such as job security, divorce and money problems. Long-term stress conditions like these make the traditional response inappropriate: not only does it not do any good, it can actually be harmful to the body it is supposed to protect. The high tech, high pressure lifestyle lived by so many people is responsible for many threatening situations, both chronic and acute, and it is now generally recognized that some, if not most, physical problems in our society have a non-physical component in their aetiology. Helen Flanders Dunbar, one of the first researchers in this area, wrote: 'It is not a question of whether an illness is physical or emotional, but how much of each' (Dunbar 1954).

Anticipation stress

Some life events cast a shadow before them. It is known that students are prone to catch colds at examination times and it has also been shown that such times of stress for candidates reduce the efficiency of the immune system. This is due to lowered production of interferon leading to decreased function of natural killer cells. The effects of stress of this kind are popularly recognized in the case of brides-to-be who may catch a 'bride's cold'. Why stress should have the effect of decreasing the body's defences is not clear, and as yet, unexplained. It is noteworthy that some of the more ambitious students suffer a greater reduction in the immune system defences, perhaps because the examination represents a bigger threat to them (Borysenko 1988 pp. 12–16).

Grief

The effect of emotions on health is recognized by the insurance industry. Statistics exist for various stressful situations which make people more prone to accidents and poor health, e.g. divorce, marriage, holidays, death, etc. They show for instance that there are 50% more deaths than would normally be expected in widowers during the first year after the loss of a wife (even though the suicide rate among single men is very high to begin with). Depression following the death of a wife is likely to have an adverse effect on the protective immune system and so on the health of the survivor.

Voluntary stress

While repeated stressful situations may produce ill effects and people may suffer chronic illness as a result, many people joyfully expose themselves to repeated stress with no apparent ill effect, e.g. in sports such as mountaineering, car racing and skiing. This can be explained in the following way: on the one hand, if repeated stress is unwanted and creates unhappiness, then it will have unwanted effects; on the other hand, if the repeated stressful situations are sought and enjoyed, the resultant happiness will bring beneficial effects to the person as a whole. In sporting contexts the euphoria resulting from release of endorphins is recognized, for instance, as 'runner's high'.

THINKING AND HEALING

Using the mind to control pulse rate and breathing, and to bring about general relaxation of the body has long been practised in many different cultures. A few people have mastered the technique to such a degree that they have almost reached a state of suspended animation. This has been documented in people practising transcendental meditation (Benson 1979). In the meditative state the brain waves drop from the β-rhythm to the slower α-rhythm; the blood circulation is diverted more to the brain and vital organs, with less going to the muscles, so that the heart rate is slower, blood pressure is lower and little oxygen is used.

All this is initiated by thought alone, effected via the hypothalamus. Hesse, experimenting on

Case study 8.1 Death and bereavement – M Cadwallader – *nurse aromatherapist,*
Australia

Client assessment

B, a 61-year-old male, was battling severe pain from cancer of the lung and he and his wife were but slowly coming to terms with the fact that his life would not be prolonged.

Intervention

The essential oils used to assist and comfort were put into a 10 ml dropper bottle:

■ 2 ml (40 drops) *Boswellia carteri* [frankincense] – analgesic (to mental pain and fear also), antidepressive, energizing, immunostimulant
■ 2 ml *Chamaemelum nobile* [Roman chamomile] – calming and sedative (easing anxiety, tension, anger and fear)
■ 10 drops *Rosa damascena* [rose otto] – general tonic, neurotonic, balancing and calming to the mind

A few drops of this was applied to the soles of his feet and put on tissue to inhale. 15 drops were put into almond oil for hand, foot and back massages.

The therapist worked closely with him and his family in the hospital setting, his wife carrying a tissue with a drop of rose – she claimed it helped her accept the inevitable.

Outcome

His feeling of relaxation and peace was evident and he claimed he also slept well for a couple of nights after a treatment.

After he passed away – peacefully – the following blend was provided to help the family cope with the bereavement, oils to relieve grief being analgesic, calming, healing and stimulating to the heart and mind:

■ 1 drop *Melissa officinalis* [melissa] – calming, sedative, uplifting to the emotions, a good pick-me-up after shock
■ 3 drops *Origanum majorana* [marjoram] – analgesic, calming, neurotonic, strengthening to the mind
■ 1 drop *Rosa damascena* [rose otto] – cicatrizant, as well as having the properties above
■ 8 ml of lime blossom carrier oil – analgesic, relaxing

This blend was used by the family for self-massage around the neck and shoulders every night and morning. B's mother thanked the therapist, saying that she was sure it had helped her to accept and adjust.

cats in the 1950s, found that when the hypothalamus was stimulated, increased activity or relaxation was produced (Hesse & Akerl 1955). Sometimes, as in the case of people suffering a terminal illness, this mind-to-body effect means that healing is possible even though a cure is not.

Today there is a realization that for optimum healing the sufferer must be fully involved in all stages of the treatment from diagnosis to final cure, and it is generally recognized that all true healing comes from within (as demonstrated by the effectiveness of the placebo). Healing is accomplished by mental and physical routes, with primary roles played by the patient, doctor and nurse, while family and friends take secondary supportive parts. As Plato wrote in the 3rd century BC:

The curing of the part should not be attempted without treatment of the whole. No attempt should be made to cure the body without the soul, and, if the head and the body are to be healthy, you must begin by curing the mind. . . . For this is the great error of our day in the treatment of the human body, that physicians first separate the soul from the body.

TRUST AND PLACEBO

Another well-known example of the effect of thought on the physical body is the placebo effect. This happens when the cure or amelioration of an illness is due either to the patient's trust and belief in a prescribed substance (whether or not the substance in question is passive), or to faith in the healer, or frequently a combination of both. For instance, it has been shown that dummy pain killers are 56% as effective as morphine in the treatment of severe chronic pain (Chaitow 1991). This remarkable and much-used placebo effect is important in all healing. When people are made to feel better, positive healing thoughts, which encourage the healing process, are generated. If an aromatherapy treatment does no more than make people feel better in themselves, it is at least a move in the right direction, for such feelings put the whole person into a healing mode. Positive healing thoughts in the mind can induce healing reactions in the bodily healing processes.

Similarly the efficiency of the immune system is reduced by negative belief and thought. It is not unreasonable to draw the conclusion that we are, in some measure, potentially masters of our own fate so far as our health is concerned, in the sense that immunity from disease appears to be enhanced or diminished by beliefs, and by the environment in so far as it affects our emotions. 'Immunity is to some degree under mental control' (Wood 1990a). Fortunately the human race is intrinsically optimistic, with a will to survive.

WHERE DOES AROMATHERAPY FIT IN?

We must now consider how aromatherapy can play an effective and worthwhile part in the mental–physical sphere of healing. It is established beyond doubt that essential oils can have physical impact in that they are bactericidal, antiinflammatory, antifungal, appetite stimulating, hyperaemic, expectorant, etc. (see Ch. 4 and Table 8.1) and that at the same time they possess properties which can affect the mind and emotions to sedate, calm and uplift.

They are therefore ideal tools for tackling not only physical problems but at the same time mental and emotional states, especially if the essential oils are carefully selected on a holistic basis.

As in all healing situations, another factor to be aware of that may influence the effect of an aroma on human behaviour, mood and health is the placebo effect, the expectations effect.

Table 8.1 Effects of essential oils used internally and externally (from Schilcher 1984)

External application	Internal application
Hyperaemic	Expectorant
Antiinflammatory	Appetite stimulating
Antiseptic/disinfectant	Choleric, cholekinetic
Granulation stimulating	Carminative
Deodorizing	Antiseptic/disinfectant
Insecticide/insect repellent	Sedative
	Circulation stimulating

People's beliefs that odours can influence their mood or health may lead them to perceive such consequences when they are exposed to an odorant and may even help trigger actual effects. The potential for placebo effects is high in an area such as aromatherapy where various essential oils are promoted as having specific beneficial mood and health effects and the individuals using the odorants desire such outcomes.

Knasko (1997)

RELAXATION RESPONSE

When we are safe, in a calm atmosphere, we have the opposite of the stress response, in that tension, blood pressure, oxygen use and so on are all reduced. This highly desirable and very important state has been termed the 'relaxation response' (Benson 1975). It can be brought about by many means, including reading, listening to favourite music, contemplating nature and, indeed, aromatherapy. Spiced apple scent was found to induce EEG responses normally associated with relaxation (Lorig & Schwarz 1988) and a later study showed that other food odours brought about similar results (Lorig 1989). There is a possibility that these results may be due to the individuals associating the odour with food, rather than a direct nervous system effect (Lorig & Schwarz 1988–89).

Inducing the relaxation response

When, during a massage, the touch of the therapist is combined with the mental and physical effects of the essential oils, the client is helped to achieve a temporary separation from worldly worries, somewhat akin to a meditative state. The massage itself induces the relaxation response, which activates the body's healing mode and this, in conjunction with the essential oils, is outstanding for the relief of tension and anxiety, both physical and mental.

Whatever the method of application, it is the feeling of the authors that in many cases most of the healing effect of essential oils takes place primarily through inhalation (see Ch. 5) via the mind and emotional pathways, and that a lesser part of the healing effect takes place via the physical body. There is no doubt that smelling plant volatile oils can affect the mood and general feeling of well-being in the individual. This is especially true when the essential oils are applied with whole-body massage; the physical and mental relaxation achieved over a period of 90 minutes has to be experienced to be fully appreciated. In order to select essential oils to address the mental, emotional and physical needs of the client it is necessary to take the time to identify the cause(s) of the health problem. It is probable that all essential oils have an effect on the mind as well as the

---

Case study 8.2 Panic attacks and vertigo – Kate Stockbridge – *aromatherapist, UK*

Client assessment

A is in his mid-sixties, referred for aromatherapy by a community psychiatric nurse as he had developed panic attacks and vertigo. She felt that aromatherapy would help in relieving his stress and therefore aid relaxation. His problems had arisen as a result of the long term caring, full time, of a relative with Parkinson's disease.

A was physically and mentally tired and not sleeping well. He described himself as having a 'thickness of the head' and 'solid headaches'. Emotionally he was low - and tearful as he expressed his frustration at his condition. His arms and legs had large areas of 'shark's skin' – psoriasis and warts and he complained of coldness and aching in his knees.

Intervention

This was aimed at easing anxiety and depression, promoting sleep, relieving headaches and at the same time, providing warmth and acceptable physical contact.

A was given 6 massage sessions, once a fortnight, remedial massage techniques being used around the patella where there were granular deposits, also around the scapula where there was much tension.

The oils chosen were one drop each of:

■ *Citrus aurantium* var. *sinensis* [sweet orange] – antidepressant, calming, mildly sedative; also recommended for vertigo
■ *Boswellia carteri* [frankincense] – analgesic, antidepressant, energizing, immunostimulant

■ *Origanum majorana* (sweet marjoram) – analgesic, calming, nervous system regulator, neurotonic; also recommended for vertigo
■ 10 ml sweet almond oil – emollient, helps relieve psoriasis
■ 5 ml evening primrose oil – as above

For use in between treatments, A was given a 50 ml lotion containing:

■ 10 drops *Citrus limon* [lemon] – anticoagulant, calming, immunostimulant
■ 5 drops *Boswellia carteri* [frankincense] – analgesic, antidepressant, energizing, immunostimulant
■ 5 drops *Chamamaelum nobile* [Roman chamomile] – antiinflammatory, antispasmodic, calming and sedative, stimulant

This was to be applied twice daily to his shoulders, knees and psoriatic areas.

Outcome

After the first session A was more relaxed, although he still had some tension in the shoulder region. He appreciated the treatments, which relaxed and rejuvenated him.

By the third treatment the discomfort in his head had cleared and he began to feel brighter and more able to cope.

After his sixth and final session he no longer experienced vertigo, the headaches had gone, his skin was much improved and he felt less tense in his shoulders. Emotionally, he was better able to relax at home and felt more positive about the future.

Case study 8.3 Phobias – E Kell – *midwife/aromatherapist, UK*

Patient assessment
J attended the antenatal clinic at the Southern General Hospital in the early weeks of pregnancy and was extremely anxious and agitated. She was suffering from phobias, unable to enter a lift at any time and preferring very light rooms having windows with an open aspect. It became extremely difficult for J to attend the clinic because of her anxiety state and her consultant suggested using aromatherapy.

Intervention
The first consultation took place in the antenatal clinic in a quiet bright room, where, after an initial chat, J relaxed slightly and began to relate to – and trust – the aromatherapist.

She was offered a hand-massage first, which was thought to be less threatening at the outset, allowing her to feel more confident with the therapist. She relaxed very well, so a shoulder and back massage was suggested, with J sitting astride a chair, her arms on a pillow placed on the chair back. The oils were chosen for their emotional effect, being confirmed in Price (2000) – Aromatherapy and your Emotions:

- 3 drops *Lavandula angustifolia* [lavender] – antispasmodic, cardiotonic, calming and sedative, tonic
- 2 drops *Chamaemelum nobile* [Roman chamomile] – antispasmodic, calming and sedative, stimulant
- 1 drop *Citrus aurantium* var. *amara* [neroli] – antidepressive, neurotonic
- 10 ml peach kernel carrier oil

After this first treatment she felt much more able to discuss her fears and worries and counselling was able to take place, after which ways were discussed as to how her partner could help her cope with her fears.

She was given a tape of simple relaxation techniques, such as breathing and visualization, to use daily, together with a blend of the oils above (9, 6, 3 drops in 50 ml peach oil), for her husband to massage into her shoulders every night.

It was decided that it would help allay her fears to continue J's aromatherapy treatments in a labour room, which enabled her to become familiar with both her surroundings and the midwives before she eventually arrived in labour.

In the early stages, J was referred to a psychiatrist, but as she did not wish to take the medication prescribed at that point it was decided to continue with aromatherapy treatments – and her pregnancy progressed well.

When she was admitted to the labour suite, back and leg massages were given, (using the blend above, but with *Myristica fragrans* [nutmeg] instead of neroli. *Salvia sclarea* [clary] and lavender were given to her on a ball of cotton wool to inhale whenever necessary. She progressed well and surprised everyone – including herself – by remaining very calm throughout.

Outcome
Although she needed a forceps delivery, J coped extremely well with this, feeling that aromatherapy had had a great deal to offer her during both pregnancy and labour. She was delivered of a beautiful baby boy and both mother and baby did extremely well.

---

body, although much research needs to be done in this respect: natural unadulterated essential oils have undeniably powerful effects which need to be properly researched and directed.

CHILDREN

The sense of smell becomes important to children with severe learning difficulties (see also Ch. 13) who may have diminished hearing and sight, and essential oils can be used to make their life easier and more friendly. Fragrances have been used on wrist bands to identify carers, each with their own aroma, to identify the child's possessions and to locate areas, rooms and facilities (Sanderson, Harrison & Price 1991). This technique can also be used to make baby sitters acceptable to the child.

THE ELDERLY

Aromas are well accepted in homes for the elderly, where they can create a pleasant atmosphere, either stimulating or relaxing, and some aromas may create an ambience which will bring old memories to the fore, possibly sparking off nostalgic conversation between the residents, with obvious benefits (see also Ch. 14).

GENDER DIFFERENCES

There appears to be a gender difference in the impact on the mind of inhaled essential oils between men and women; it seems that women are the more likely to derive beneficial results.

One study indicating this was the use of *Citrus sinensis* [sweet orange] essence diffused into the waiting room of a dental practice where results of a questionnaire filled in by patients of both sexes showed that sweet orange oil had a relaxant effect compared to non-odour controls. Compared to men, women had a lower anxiety state, more positive mood and higher level of calmness. The typical smell of dental premises, eugenol, was associated with anxiety and fear, but this was masked for women by the orange aroma, lowering their anxiety; for men this was only minor (Lehrner et al 2000).

Another study set out to demonstrate gender effect of odour on pain perception and 20 men and 20 women were exposed to pain by holding a hand in hot water while smelling previously selected odours. Separate analysis for men and women revealed a significant effect of odour on pain perception for women but not for men and when the odour was found to be pleasant women demonstrated a significant reduction in pain perception (Marchand & Arsenault 2002).

Miyazaki, Motohashi & Kobashaya (1992a) investigated the effects on females of inhalation of orange oil (unspecified), *Chamaecyparis taiwanensis* lig. [hinoki] and menthol and found that the speed of performing a mental task was increased and number of mistakes decreased by all three aromas. Profiles of mood state (POMS) scores indicated that depression–dejection, anger–hostility and tension–anxiety decreased after inhalation of the oils while fatigue score tended to increase.

A similar study explored the effects on six male individuals of inhalation of orange oil (unspecified), *Chamaecyparis taiwanensis* lig. [hinoki] and eugenol on the mood of six individuals and POMS were monitored: blood pressure showed a decrease after inhalation of hinoki or orange oils, but a heart rate increase with eugenol. Eugenol was deemed to be unpleasant and scores indicated increase in fatigue, depression–dejection, confusion and anger–hostility and a decrease in vigour score while inhalation of hinoki oil had the opposite effect (Miyazaki, Motohashi & Kobashaya 1992b).

Pleasant smells give pleasure and feelings of self-esteem (Baron 1990, Nezlak & Shean 1990) and the effect on women may be greater because according to Herz & Cupchik (1992) women have more intense odour memories than men.

Note: Following the studies above, it is interesting to speculate why almost all practising aromatherapists and users of aromatherapy products are women and so few men are involved. In addition to these studies it is known (as seen earlier, Ch. 5) that the skin of women is more permeable than that of men to toxic chemicals of similar size to essential oil compounds, and that they can retain more fat soluble compounds in their body and so are affected more (Eisberg 1983). Therefore the overall effects of aromatherapy on women may be more significant than on men hence leading to greater participation by them.

ANOSMIA

If a person is incapable of smelling an aroma, does this mean that aromatherapy will not be effective? There is no definitive answer to this question, but many aromatherapists believe that prolonged use of essential oils will restore the sense of smell in some cases. The authors treated a case of chronic sinusitis (suffered for 17 years), when even after an operation the client was unable to smell his wife's cooking – his main cause for concern! After three treatments he was able to detect *Mentha* x *piperita* [peppermint], one of the essential oils in the mix used (which also included *Eucalyptus globulus* [Tasmanian blue gum] and *Ocimum basilicum* [European basil]). After 6 months he had recovered his sense of smell sufficiently to recognize some of the gastronomic aromas greeting him on his return from work. This is in line with some surprising recent findings which indicate that in both humans and animals possessing specific

---

Case study 8.4   Prolonged temporary anosmia – S Price – *aromatologist, UK*

Client assessment

Mr P had suffered from severe chronic sinusitis for several years, his sense of smell diminishing over the years. After an operation, there was no improvement and not being able to smell was upsetting him. His wife was an excellent cook and he was unable either to smell – or to taste – her cooking. His wife, having heard the therapist on the radio, persuaded him to travel the 60 miles to her clinic, to see if aromatherapy could help him.

Intervention

It was decided to carry out a treatment 'sandwich' once a week – massage of his face, including pressure points, a Swiss reflex treatment on the sinus reflexes of his feet (see Ch. 7), finishing with a repeat of the facial treatment.

Two of the essential oils in the selected blend have extremely strong aromas – yet Mr P was unable to smell them:

- 2 drops *Eucalyptus globulus* [blue gum] – anticatarrhal, antiinfectious, antiinflammatory, expectorant
- 3 drops *Lavandula angustifolia* [lavender] – antiinflammatory, antiseptic, calming

- 2 drops *Mentha* x *piperita* [peppermint] – antiinfectious, antiinflammatory, soothing

After each treatment two spills, with eucalyptus and peppermint respectively, were held to his nose, in the hope of a reaction.

He was also given 20 drops each of the same oils in 50 ml carrier lotion, to apply on his face every morning after shaving, instead of his usual astringent.

Outcome

At the third visit, when the peppermint spill was led to his nose, Mr P let out a delighted yell; 'I can smell mint – it's faint, but it's definitely mint!'

After the next visit, Mr P showed enough improvement for him to visit the clinic only once a fortnight, still using his lotion at home very day.

After 3 months, the visits were altered to once a fortnight – and after 6 months from the commencement of treatment, he had recovered his sense of smell sufficiently to appreciate some of the aromas from his wife's cooking – a happy result for her too!

---

anosmia, the sensitivity to some odours can be restored by repeated exposure to these odours (Holley 1993, Van Toller & Dodd 1992). Nasel et al (1994) in a study noted an increase of cerebral blood flow in humans following inhalation of 1,8-cineole (found in eucalyptus and rosemary essential oils), and a similar result was obtained with an anosmic person.

Not every person can smell every aroma. Unlike vision (where differences between people can be as obvious as the need for spectacles or a white stick), there is no easy means of recognizing differences in the ability to smell. Aromas are made up of individual chemicals and each cilium is equipped with uniquely contoured depressions into which a single aroma molecule can fit, somewhat like a jigsaw puzzle. However, if the appropriate 'docking' depression for the molecule being inhaled is absent, that smell will not be registered.

Only when the molecule is keyed in is a specific signal generated.

Total, specific and temporary anosmia

Anosmia, the absence of sense of smell, can be total (where nothing is smelt at all), specific (an inability to register certain smells) or temporary. Almost everyone suffers from some form of the latter, and probably each of us has about five of these specific anosmias. It is interesting that about 5% of people are insensitive to the sweaty smell notes and, while about 50% of people are anosmic to androsterone, musk is almost universally noticed. Some aromas have exceptionally low detection thresholds (e.g. those of grapefruit and green pepper). It is a fact that there are differences between individuals in the perception of odours, even in young adults, who constitute the most consistent age group (Doty 1991), but these differences are due to more than genetic anosmias, as shown by experiments revealing that repeated exposures can alter detection thresholds (Wysocki, Dorries & Beauchamp 1989).

Temporary anosmia may be caused by colds, rhinitis and sinusitis, and results in a loss of taste. There are four types of taste cells (salt, bitter, sour and sweet) although appreciation of food flavour does not depend solely on these but also on food texture, acidity/alkalinity, hot/cold and the trigeminal nerve, and also chiefly on smell.

Does anosmia, sleep or unawareness negate aromatherapy?

- **Effect of aroma during sleep:** Aromas of essential oils have measurable physiological effects on humans while asleep. Ten participants were monitored every 3 minutes to see whether any physiological changes occurred when they were subjected to 3 minute periods either of air alone or of peppermint odour during stage two sleep. The results revealed conclusively that humans do react behaviourally, autonomically and centrally to the aroma of essential oil of peppermint administered while sleeping. Significant differences in responsivity to odour periods versus non-odour periods were found for EEG, EMG, and heart rate as well as behavioural changes (Badia et al 1990).
- **Awareness:** Odour conditioning and physiological responses can occur even when people are not consciously aware of the odour (Lorig 1989, Lorig et al 1988). Tests by Kirk-Smith & Booth (1990) are interesting to aromatherapists in that they used a fragrance at such a low level as to be imperceptible to the subjects, and found specific mood changes in both men and women rating their own mood compared with a non-perfume situation. In another study, half the subjects were exposed to an aroma and the other half to no aroma while working on stressful tasks. Days later all were exposed to the aroma previously employed and those women previously exposed to the odour reported more anxiety, even though they were not consciously aware of an odour on either day (Kirk-Smith et al 1983).

It may be said from the results obtained in the tests mentioned above that everything points to the fact that inhaled fragrances do have effects on humans even:

- when the aroma is at an imperceptible level, and not noticeable
- whether the subject is anosmic or not
- when the aroma is not being consciously registered
- whether asleep or awake.

Therefore it can be concluded that everyone, anosmic or not, conscious of the aroma or not, awake or not, is likely to benefit from aromatherapeutic treatment.

TRIALS

When the olfactory sense and odours are used therapeutically in clinical contexts they may be working in different ways at the same time. For example, lavender oil may act pharmacologically as a light sedative; it may also be alerting, simply by being there as a stimulus; it may be creating positive feelings because it is pleasant; it may aid recall of past personal situations, positive or negative; and it may have connotations due to social expectations, e.g. connoting health or cleanliness (Kirk-Smith 1995). The placebo effect has to be taken into account when conducting trials using aromas, because the memory, attitude and expectations of the subject may modify the outcome, in addition to any effects of the aroma employed. Although there are difficulties in carrying out trials using aromas, and it can be difficult to assess any results obtained because so many factors other than the aroma may impinge on the situation, aromatherapists should not be deterred from embarking on clinical trials. The use of olfaction in aromatherapy in particular and therapy in general is bound to increase and it is imperative that aromatherapy is put on a surer footing than at present; this can best be done by the thousands of therapists currently in practice. With a little expert help in setting up a simple trial, much useful information could be gained in a relatively short time. Kirk-Smith (1995) in his review of therapeutic processes involving olfaction agrees that further clinical evaluation of olfaction in therapy is needed, but trials involve many skills (therapeutic and scientific), and expectations or perceptions about the odour, as well as pleasantness, must be taken into account when predicting effects. It is not a simple matter to ascribe any reported benefits from the use of an aroma directly to that aroma. As mentioned above, it is imperative that the aromatic materials used in any future trials be precisely identified, otherwise the value of the tests will be diminished.

OLFACTORY PHYSIOLOGY

Speaking at the 12ième Journées Internationales Huiles Essentielles (1993), Professor André Holley of Lyons reported that changes in thinking have occurred about odour reception, following identification of a very large family of genes responsible for coding olfactory receptors (Buck & Axel 1991). Like receptors are grouped together, some specialized for one type of molecule, others more general but with weaker reactions. Considerable advances have also been made in the description of the transduction steps leading from receptor activation by odour molecules to ionic currents generating the peripheral message. Behind this peripheral activity there is a mass of intensely active neurons, involved in such things as memory of odours. Memory is distributed all over the brain, not just in one area, but studies on olfactory memory have revealed new properties of the olfactory bulb in the process of memory storage and it is thought that odour memories probably reside in the olfactory bulb and are modified by other information. Olfactive sensitivity could be dependent on environment.

The nose has two distinct functions, one to condition the air inhaled in preparation for its journey into the lungs, and another to act as the organ of the sense of smell. An average human breathes in about 8 litres of air each minute; this probably means that more than a million molecules are taken in with each breath; and a remarkably low number of some odorous molecules mixed in the air intake can be detected by humans (Engen 1987). People have a very sensitive sense of smell, but have poor perception and have difficulty in describing the quality of a smell because olfactory input is widely distributed in the amygdala and

phylogenetically primitive cortex, without direct projections to the neocortex (Klemm et al 1992).

When essential oils are inhaled, the volatile molecules in the oils are carried by eddy currents to the roof of the nose, where delicate cilia protrude from the receptor cells into the nose itself. According to Bronagh et al (1990) the nasal and lung mucosa are highly efficient at absorbing lipophilic terpenoids. When the molecules lock on to these 'hairs' an electrochemical message is transmitted via the olfactory bulb and olfactory tract to the limbic system (amygdala and hippocampus). This may trigger memory and emotional responses, which can cause messages to be sent via the hypothalamus, acting as relay and regulator, to other parts of the brain and the rest of the body. The received messages are converted into action, resulting in the release of euphoric, relaxing, sedative or stimulating neurochemicals as appropriate. Some researchers believe that subcortical processing yields behavioural responses without conscious awareness of stimuli (Weiskrantz et al 1974). It is worth remembering that the limbic system developed 70 million years ago and that it used to be called the rhinencephalon (from the Greek words rhis = nose, enkephalon = brain).

The limbic system is heavily implicated in the expression of emotion, although whether it generates emotion or merely integrates it is not clear (Stoddart 1990). The body can replace olfactory nerve cells, an unusual feature of human nerve tissue, which serves to underline their importance.

Michael Shipley, a neurophysiologist at Cincinnati University, has demonstrated that fibres from the olfactory nerve carry impulses to two small but significant parts of the brain, the locus ceruleus and the raphe nucleus. Noradrenalin is concentrated in the locus ceruleus and serotonin in the raphe nucleus (Godfrey-Hardinge 1993 personal communication). It is suggested that sedative aromas such as *Origanum majorana* [sweet marjoram], *Lavandula angustifolia* [lavender], *Chamaemelum nobile* [Roman chamomile], *Matricaria recutita* [German chamomile] and *Citrus aurantium* (flos) [neroli] cause stimulation of the raphe nucleus, which then releases the neurochemical serotonin; stimulating aromas such as *Rosmarinus officinalis* [rosemary], *Citrus limon* (per.) [lemon], *Ocimum basilicum* [basil] and *Mentha* x *piperita* [peppermint] will affect the locus ceruleus, which then releases noradrenalin.

The use of essential oil aromas in aromatherapy treatments is not too far removed from intranasal drug delivery in common use today, e.g. steroid inhalers for allergies, peptides and anaesthetics (Chen, Su & Chang 1989). Lavender has been used in the treatment of insomnia (Hardy, Kirk-Smith & Stretch 1995) (see Ch. 14) and lavender consists largely of oxygenated terpenes, which interact with cell membranes to suppress cell action potentials (Teuscher et al 1990), which might account for a sedative effect. Animal tests using 42 essential oils and their components showed linalyl acetate and linalool from lavender oil to have the most sedative consequence (Buchbauer et al 1993), (see Ch. 4); a serum level in line with intravenous injection was produced, possibly owing to ready absorption by nasal and lung mucosa (Buchbauer et al 1991). The use of an essential oil for such a purpose has advantages, as lavender oil:

- does not have unwanted side-effects
- can be used to vary long-term treatment, giving relief from powerful drugs and their side-effects
- masks malodours usually present in psycho-geriatric wards.

Warren et al (1987) patented the use of a fragrance that included nutmeg oil to reduce stress in humans. Subjects were stressed with and without nutmeg oil in a fragrance: with the nutmeg oil the systolic blood pressure was reduced and subjects rated themselves as being calmer with decreased anxiety. Nutmeg oil contains the phenolic ethers myristicin and elemicin, which convert to the hallucinogens TMA (trimethoxyamphetamine) and MMDA (methoxy-methylene-dioxyamphetamine); a higher than normal ambient concentration of the aroma was used.

In their paper on the use of fragrances and essential oils as medicaments, Buchbauer & Jirovetz (1994) draw the conclusion that inter-action between fragrance molecules and receptors in the central nervous system (in combination with reflectoric effects) is responsible for the sedation caused by the inhalation of fragrances or essential oils.

AROMAS AFFECT EMOTIONS

Odours are important in everyday life, though notoriously difficult to describe. We are surrounded – sometimes almost suffocated – by aromas, some natural but many synthetic. There are many natural aromatic messages; e.g. babies are able to recognize their own mothers by the individual odours of the latter, also synchronous menstruation occurs in groups of females. Some messages are imposed; e.g. fragrances are added to almost everything from floor polishes to foods in order to improve sales, buildings may be fragranced to manipulate the working environment, or shops and hotels to invoke a 'feel-good' factor in customers, in airports to reduce apprehension and in cars to reduce traffic stress. These aromas are inflicted on us regardless of our wishes and feelings – like background music – and the short- and long-term effects on people are not always known, since the emotions produced can be strong and unforgettable. The psychosomatic effect of smell is experienced by most people: the unfamiliar mixture of odours encountered in hospitals, for example, can produce a feeling of dread accompanied by physical manifestations such as sweating, nausea and fainting (in visitors as well as patients), and the memory of the smell of school cabbage can affect the appetite throughout life.

The chain of events involving aroma, emotion and physical change, for so long a mystery, is now beginning to be explained scientifically by PNI, as are the special benefits to be derived from the use of aromatherapy (Table 8.2). Essential oils consist of natural molecules and are to be welcomed, at the very least, as a means of introducing a little bit of nature into the mainly synthetic hospital environment. The use of carefully selected essential oils makes good sense therapeutically and financially, for they are simple and inexpensive to use and no costly equipment is required.

CONDITIONING, STIMULUS SUBSTITUTION

Pavlov (1849–1936) showed by experiments with dogs how the secretion of saliva could be stimulated not only by food but also by the sound of a bell which had been paired repeatedly with

Table 8.2   Effects on the emotions mentioned by various authors. The figures indicate the number of mentions

Latin name	Comon name	Anguish	Breathlessness (nervous)	Calming, relaxing	Depression (nervous)	Fatigue (nervous)	Hypochondria	Hysteria	Insomnia	Irritability	Melancholy	Memory loss	Migraine	Nervous breakdown	Nervous system balancer	Nervous debility	Nervousness (excitability)	Nightmares	Sedative	Sleep problems	Sorrow, sadness	Stress	Tinnitus	Vertigo
Aniba rosaeodora (lig)	rosewood	1			2												1	1			1			
Boswellia carteri	frankincense	1		1	4				1	1	1						1	1			1			
Cananga odorata (flos)	ylang ylang	2		1	1			1	1	1	1						2	1						
Carum carvi (fruct)	caraway																							1
Cedrus atlantica (lig)	Atlas cedarwood	1		1					1	1	1						1	1						
Chamaemelum nobile (flos)	Roman chamomile	2		1	2		1	1	1					1	1					1	1			1
Chamomilla recutita (flos)	German chamomile													1										
Cinnamomum zeylanicum (cort)	cinnamon bark			2	3																			
Citrus aurantium var. amara (flos)	neroli	1		1	2				1	1			1				2	1		1				
Citrus aurantium var. amara (fol)	petitgrain	2		2	1				1	1			1					1			1			
Citrus aurantium var. amara (per)	orange bitter	2			2				2	1							2	1	1	1	1			1
Citrus aurantium var. sinensis (per)	orange sweet	2		2					1								1							
Citrus bergamia (per)	bergamot	1		1	1				2	1							2	1	1					
Citrus limon (per)	lemon	2		2					2	1	1		2					2	1					1
Citrus reticulata (per)	mandarin	3		2	1				2	1	1	1					2				1	1	1	2
Commiphora myrrha	myrrh	1		1						1							1	1						
Coriandrum sativum (fruct)	coriander	1		1					1					1		1	1					2		1
Cupressus sempervirens	cypress			2	2				1	3					1		2						1	
Eucalyptus globulus (fol)	eucalyptus	1	1										2								1			
Foeniculum vulgare var. dulce	fennel																							1
Hyssopus officinalis	hyssop	1			1																			
Juniperus communis (fruct)	juniper berry			2					1	1		1		1			1							
Lavandula angustifolia	lavender	4	1	2	3		1	2	2	2				2	1	1	1	4		2	2			2
Lavandula x intermedia Super	lavandin	1								1				1	1			1			1			
Lippia citriodora	verbena	2		1	1													1		2	1	1		
Melaleuca alternifolia (fol)	tea tree													1										
Melaleuca leucadendron (fol)	cajuput			1			1																	
Melaleuca viridiflora (fol)	naiouli	1			3					1		1									1	1		
Melissa officinalis	melissa	2		1	1		1	2	2	1	2			2	1		2	1		2	1	1		1
Menthax piperita	peppermint	1	1		1						2	1	4											1
Myristica fragrans (sem)	nutmeg																		1					
Ocimum basilicum	basil	4			2				1		1	1	3	1			1	1					1	1
Origanum marjorana	marjoram	5		1	2		1	3	2	1	1		4			1	4	1		2	1	1		2
Pelargonium graveolens	geranium	2		1	1				1	1	1			1			3	1			1			
Pimpinella anisum (fruct)	aniseed												2											1
Pinus sylvestris (fol)	pine				2																1			
Ravensara aromatica	ravensara				1				1									1			1			
Rosa damascena, Rosa centifolia	rose otto	1			1				1	1	1							1			1			
Rosmarinus officinalis	rosemary				2	2					1	2	3	1						1				1
Salvia officinalis	sage			1	1	1									1	1								1
Salvia sclarea	clary	1		1	1	1			1	1				1				1	1		1			
Santalum album (lig)	sandalwood	1		1	1			1	1	1	1							1	1					
Satureia hortensis, S. montana	savory	1			3	1								1										
Syzygium aromaticum (flos)	clove bud											1		1										
Thymus serpyllum	wild thyme			2	1																			
Thymus vulgaris ct alcohol	sweet thyme	2		1	1				1	1	1			1				1			1			
Thymus vulgaris ct phenol	red thyme	1			3									1		1				1				1
Valeriana officinalis	valerian	1	1				1	2									2	1	3					
Vetiveria zizanioides	vetiver	1			1																			
Zinziber officinale	ginger				1					1		1					1							

the presentation of food, and came to elicit saliva when presented alone. Here the sound of the bell was the neutral stimulus, which was paired, i.e. associated with, a natural unconditioned stimulus (namely the food), and the response was salivation; after repeated pairings the sound of the bell, previously a neutral stimulus, became a conditioned stimulus.

Classical conditioning, using a visual or an auditory (as above) stimulus, requires many pairings but in the case of olfaction sometimes only one pairing is needed, e.g. conditioning body production of natural killer cells (NKC), fever and cytotoxic T-lymphocytes (CTL) to camphor (see below). This demonstrates the connection between the olfactory and immune systems; this communication is important for species survival (Hiramoto et al 1993). Taste and odour pair easily with illness (therapists should note this); this is useful in some cases but an odour may become associated with an unwanted state or illness. Aversive conditioning using an odour has been used to control overeating and this resulted in a significant loss of weight compared with a control group (Foreyt & Kennedy 1971).

Examples of pairing are:

- Hiramoto et al (1991) paired camphor with fever induction and found that a fever response could be elicited by camphor afterwards.
- In a clinical application, Schiffman & Siebert (1991) found that an apricot fragrance paired with a relaxed state after progressive relaxation later 'triggers' the relaxed state. They claim that this conditioning was particularly useful in the treatment of lower back pain.
- Betts (1994) used olfaction to control arousal symptoms in epileptic seizures, not only in those who experience olfactory auras, but in any patient who has an aura sufficiently long enough to give them time to apply a countermeasure before the major seizure starts. Essential oils employed for this purpose include lavender, chamomile, ylang ylang and lemongrass; rosemary oil is avoided. Betts says that using the autohypnotic technique it is possible to train the patient to associate intense relaxation just with the smell of the oil, so that the remembered aroma is sufficient to act as a countermeasure.

- Ghanta, Hiramoto & Solvason (1987) implanted myeloma cells in mice and 2 days later injected them with PolyIC followed by 4 hours' exposure to camphor. Every 3rd day afterwards they were exposed to camphor again, and these mice had a better survival time than control groups.
- Hiramoto et al (1993) found that injected spleen cells provoke specific CTL. Camphor odour was paired with their injection for 1 hour, and this odour was able to elicit the CTL 1 week later.
- Olness & Ader (1992) paired taste and odour with an anticancer drug in the treatment of an 11-year-old girl who had a severe autoimmune disease. As a result of this pairing, the anticancer drug was needed in only six out of twelve treatments.

A neutral odour can be easily paired with an emotional state, in a single session, so that it will evoke the same emotional state in another circumstance at a later time. This effect appears to be quite strong, and it is not even necessary for the odour to be perceived either during the pairing or when evoking the state; this is likely to be due to olfaction's relative lack of representation in the neocortex (Kirk-Smith, Van Toller & Dodd 1983). King (1988) has similarly paired a 'sea fragrance' with relaxation training, measuring the effects of fragrance alone with forehead EMG (electromyogram). Neither this report nor that of Schiffman & Siebert (1991) above appear to be controlled trials, however, so clinical evaluation remains to be carried out (Kirk-Smith 1995). Rose & Behm (1994) found that inhalation of the vapour from an extract of black pepper serves to reduce the withdrawal symptoms experienced on cessation of tobacco smoking; citral containing essential oils are said to have this effect also.

SEDATIVE/STIMULANT INFLUENCE OF ODOURS

Consider that aromatics, such as incense, were used first as calming agents to induce a state of contentment. This sounds like one of our modern day tranquillizers, however, the aromatic – unlike the pills – is completely safe. As far back as ancient Greece, the physician Galen recommended the use of aromatic herbs against hysterical convulsions.

Burning bay leaves were inhaled by the Oracle at Delphi to induce a trance-like state enabling communication with the gods. Aromatic woods were later burned to drive out 'evil spirits'. Even then, aroma was known to have an effect on the psyche (Lee & Lee 1992).

Over 70 years ago a series of experiments on rats provided confirmation of the anecdotal sedative effects of some oils: when the oils were dispersed in the air the rats took longer to perform tasks (Macht & Ting 1921). The oils used included lavender, rose and valerian. This method is effective (Jirovetz et al 1992) because of the huge area in the lungs available for absorption of airborne oils into the bloodstream.

In the 1920s three papers were published by Gatti & Cayola which looked at the action of essences on the nervous system (1923a), the therapeutic effects of essential oils (1923b) and the use of valerian oil as a cure for nervous complaints (1929) (see also Ch. 4). They noted that the physical effects of the sedative/stimulant action of the oils were achieved more quickly by inhalation than by ingestion, and that opposite reactions could be obtained depending on whether the dose was small or large. The authors' experience confirms this, having found, for instance, that a low dose of lavender is calming and helpful for sleep, but a high dose makes sleep difficult, even impossible.

Since the 1920s further experiments have been carried out and knowledge of the psychotherapeutic effects of essential oils has grown, but nevertheless more research is needed; aromatherapy works but it is necessary to find out how. Some interesting studies which have been published, illustrating calming, stimulating and other effects, are given below.

Many patients undergoing magnetic resonance imaging (MRI), or body scans, find it to be a distressing and claustrophobic situation; this expensive procedure can be aborted by a stressed patient pressing the panic button, wasting a lot of time and money. At the Memorial Sloan-Kettering Hospital in New York, a fragrance (constituents unknown) is used to calm patients receiving whole-body scans. Redd et al (1994) administered bursts of heliotropine (a vanilla-like scent) to patients undergoing this procedure and this reduced recalled anxiety by 63% in those who

liked the smell. The calming brought about was thought to be attributable to the pleasing effect of the aroma, as pleasant conditions make stress more bearable.

Work by Professor Ammen at Tübingen University has shown that rosemary containing 39% 1,8-cineole was refreshing and improved locomotor activity in mice (Buchbauer 1988). According to Dember & Warm of the University of Cincinnati (New Scientist 1991), people do much better in a task that requires sustained attention if they receive regular puffs of an aroma. The test of concentration involved staring for 40 minutes at a pattern on a computer screen and hitting a key whenever the pattern changed very slightly. People generally did well to begin with, but performance eventually fell off and the fragrance effect was likened to a mild dose of caffeine. Peppermint was found to be stimulating, and lily of the valley relaxing.

The effects of peppermint have also been investigated at the Catholic University of America in Washington DC, where changes found in brainwave patterns were associated with alertness. It was also shown that the peppermint aroma enhanced the sensory pathway for visual detection, which allowed the subjects more control over their allocation of attention (Parasuraman 1991). This confirms the traditional use of peppermint oil in aromatherapy.

The aroma of jasmine has been shown to be stimulatory on mental function (Sugano 1989) and to shorten pentobarbital induced sleeping time (in mice) (Kikuchi et al 1989); cis- and trans-phytol were considered the stimulant-like compounds in a solvent extracted oil. The sedative influence of lavender and the excitatory effect of jasmine in humans was confirmed by (Karamat et al 1992). Sugano (1989) also showed that lavender and the compound α-pinene had a sedative effect.

In the early 1990s some patients at the Middlesex Hospital intensive therapy unit (ITU) were assessed for the effects of aromatherapy and massage on post-cardiac surgery patients (see Ch. 13). Foot massage for 20 minutes with and without the use of neroli essential oil on day 1 (postoperative) showed that significant physiological benefit was limited to respiratory rate as an immediate effect of massage. A further follow-up questionnaire on day 5 (postoperative) showed a marked reduction in anxiety compared with a control group using a bland vegetable oil, and indicated a trend towards greater and more lasting psychological benefit (Stevenson 1994).

AROMAS, MEMORY AND MOOD

Schab (1990) found that presence of an ambient aroma during the process of learning words and at the later testing gave a 50% better recall than when an aroma was not present; Smith, Standing & Deman (1992) had a similar result. Another study showing that aromas can influence the way people think and behave was carried out by Baron (1990) where subjects were put in a room that was intermittently fragranced with air-freshener; under these conditions these people set themselves higher goals, were more inclined to negotiate in a friendly manner and were able to resolve conflicts more successfully.

The effects of aromatherapy on feelings of relaxation, alertness, mood, anxiety and electro-encephalogram (EEG) were investigated on 40 subjects using lavender (unspecified) or rosemary (unspecified) essential oil diluted 10% in grape-seed oil inhaled from a cotton swab. The rosemary group had increased alertness (decreased frontal alpha and beta power) and were faster but not more accurate during maths computations. The lavender group performed the maths computa-tions faster and more accurately and the EEG recorded a stronger beta power suggesting increased drowsiness: both groups felt more relaxed and it was concluded that aromas do affect psychological and physiological states (Diego et al 1998).

The effects of *Rosmarinus officinalis* [rosemary] and *Lavandula angustifolia* [lavender] were tested on 140 subjects divided into three groups, one being a control group. Either lavender or rosemary was diffused into a test cubicle prior to the test; laven-der produced a significant decrease in per-formance of working memory and impaired reaction times for both memory and attention-based tasks. Rosemary significantly enhanced the overall quality of memory and the rosemary group was much more alert than the lavender and control groups. Moss et al (2003) concluded that the aroma of essential oils produced objective effects on cognitive performance and subjective effects on mood.

Matricaria recutita [German chamomile] oil has been used to study the effects of olfaction on mood and imaging. When subjects were asked to visualize positive or negative phrases following exposure to either chamomile oil vapour or placebo, the oil significantly increased the time it took for images to be produced, suggesting either that enhanced neural processing was taking place or that the oil was sedative, and also shifted mood rating in a positive direction (Roberts & Williams 1992). These tests did not show whether the chamomile oil was exerting its effect subsequent to absorption through the nasal mucosa and into the bloodstream or because of an entirely olfactory mechanism (Balacs & Tisserand 1998).

PSYCHOPHYSIOLOGICAL EFFECT OF AROMA

There can be no doubt that changes in physio-logical and psychological parameters may be caused by essential oil inhalation, and Miyazaki et al (1991) reported that changes in mood due to inhalation could be measured by using the light reflex of the pupil: they also found that orange oil (unspecified) increased the activity of the parasympathetic nervous system. Miyake et al (1991) used EEG and psychological scoring to examine the effects of inhalation of various oils and found that bitter orange oil increased sleeping time significantly under conditions of mental stress and so was thought to affect the cortex, inhibiting excitement of the central nervous system and causing sedative effects. In psycho-physiological studies of fragrance by Sugano & Sato (1991) it was concluded that lavender, orange and rose would elevate work efficiency and counter the effects of a stressful life: chamomile, jasmine and musk increased beta band micro-vibrations suggesting mental stimulation. Each of these studies demonstrated that psychological and physiological parameters can be changed due to the inhalation of essential oils or their components.

The essential oils used in most of the tests cited in this section were not properly identified; for example, the term lavender may cover oils of widely varying composition from several quite different plants or even a partially reconstructed oil; it is hard to imagine that *Lavandula angustifolia*, the true lavender oil, could consistently be rated as unpleasant, whereas it is entirely possible that *L. latifolia* or *L. stoechas* among others could indeed merit this description; also the ester content of lavenders grown in different regions can vary from 8% to 50%, altering the aroma considerably. It is astonishing that time and money can be spent in research without knowing precisely what materials are being tested and studied, which tends to detract from the value of the whole exercise but this is exactly what has happened in the past. That said, subjective reactions to odours do vary according to personal preference as well as the concentration and aroma make-up; lavender was found to be not pleasant in some tests (Klemm et al 1992, Lorig & Roberts 1990) but to be pleasant in others (Torii et al 1988); there are similar findings with jasmine; all this should be taken into consideration when intending to put essential oils into the air for therapeutic purposes.

Klemm et al (1992) studied the physiological responses of 16 young women to aromas from seven essential oils (birch tar, galbanum, heliotropine, jasmine, lavender, lemon and peppermint); their responses were assessed by EEG (electroencephalogram) recordings from 19 locations on their scalps. Topographic maps were plotted from the amplitude spectra in four frequency bands: delta (1–4 Hz), theta (4–8 Hz), alpha (8–13 Hz) and beta (13–30 Hz). Subjective responses to the odours differed, but the most consistently arousing and strong odours included galbanum, lavender, lemon and peppermint, with heliotropine being classed as weak. The most pleasant odours were lemon and peppermint, while birch tar, galbanum and lavender were consistently unpleasant. EEG map changes occurred in one or more frequency bands in each subject in response to one or more of the odours, and sometimes even occurred with weak odours and when the subject seemed unaware of the odour's presence. The most consistent responses to odours were in the theta frequency band, the odours causing the greatest increase being jasmine, lavender and lemon. All odours used affected the EEG in at least some subjects, and all subjects responded to at least some odours.

It is not clear from studies carried out whether or not personal like or dislike of the odour has a real bearing on the effects of essential oil inhalation. Bulgarian rose, lavender and geranium oils were tested on 48 medical students by spraying a 1% solution into the room and all stimulated neuro-psychic activity; there was an increase in concentration capacity, attention spans and work rhythms with a shortening of reflex times and these effects were independent of personal like/dislike of the aroma (Tasev, Toleva & Balabanova 1969). On the other hand the study by Marchand & Arsenault (2002) (see Gender differences below) came to the conclusion that if the odour was found to be pleasant then mood perception was significantly increased while unpleasant odours significantly decreased mood perception. The authors believe, based on practical experience, that in aromatherapy treatment sessions the client tends to be more relaxed and more ready to accept treatment with a positive outlook if the aroma of the essential oils being used is perceived as being pleasant.

SMELL ADAPTATION

It is a common assumption that the sense of smell, more than other modalities, is readily affected by adaptation as a result of continued exposure to a stimulus. For example, a room one has just entered may have a noticeable odour, but this is no longer apparent after a short while; presumably the odour quickly disappears because receptors fatigue and decrease their rate of firing in the continuing presence of odorous molecules in the mucus (Engen 1982). If the receptors do indeed stop firing, then the question arises of whether aromas can bring about changes in the client in these circumstances. Engen goes on to say that, although olfactory adaptation is apparently commonly experienced, its effect has been exaggerated. He points out that animals using olfactory cues to find a mate would be frustrated if the cue should disappear halfway there. Broad experience in the field of aromatherapy massage says that the aromas are indeed effective throughout the treatment, even though the quality of perception at the end of the treatment may well be different from that at the beginning.

SUMMARY

Great advances have been made in our knowledge of the interactions of the mind, emotions, nervous system and immune system, and there is growing recognition of their combined impact on general health. Essential oils have an effect on everyone and have an important role to play in bringing about a state of relaxation, which can favour healing, and they are effective even during sleep or unawareness of their presence.

Everyone is capable of deriving benefit from aromatherapy.

References

Badia P, Wesensten N, Lammers W, Culpepper J, Harsh J 1990 Responsiveness to olfactory stimuli presented in sleep. Physiology and Behaviour 48(1) (Jul): 87–90

Balacs T, Tisserand R 1998 German chamomile. International Journal of Aromatherapy 9(1): 20

Baron R A 1990 Environmentally induced positive affect: its impact on self efficacy, task performance, negotiation and conflict. Journal of Applied Social Psychology 20: 368–384

Benson H 1975 The relaxation response. Morrow, New York

Benson H 1979 The mind/body effect. Simon & Schuster, New York

Betts T 1994 Sniffing the breeze. Aromatherapy Quarterly 40 (Spring): 19–22

Borysenko J 1988 Mending the mind, mending the body. Bantam, Toronto

Bronagh R C et al 1990 In vivo percutaneous absorption of fragrance ingredients in rhesus monkeys and humans. Food and Chemical Toxicology 28(5): 369–373

Buchbauer G 1988 Aromatherapy: do essential oils have therapeutic properties? In: Proceedings of the Beijing International Conference on Essential Oils, Flavours, Fragrances and Cosmetics. International Federation of Essential Oils and Aroma Trades, London

Buchbauer G, Jirovetz L 1994 Aromatherapy – use of fragrances and essential oils as medicaments. Flavour & Fragrance Journal 9: 217–222

Buchbauer G, Jirovetz L, Jäger W, Dietrich H, Plank C, Karamat E 1991 Aromatherapy: evidence for sedative effects of the essential oil of lavender after inhalation. Zeitschrift für Naturforschung 46c: 1067–1072

Buchbauer G, Jirovetz L, Jäger W, Plank C, Dietrich H 1993 Fragrance compounds and essential oils with sedative effects upon inhalation. Journal of Pharmaceutical Sciences 82(6): 660–664

Buck L, Axel R 1991 A novel multigene family may encode odorant receptors: a molecular basis for odor recognition. Cell 65: 175–187

Chaitow L 1991 Mind your immunity. Here's Health October: 19–20

Chen Y W, Su K S E, Chang S 1989 Nasal systemic drug delivery. Dekker, New York

Diego M A, Jones N A, Field T et al. 1998 Aromatherapy positively affects mood, EEG patterns of alertness and math computations. International Journal of Neuroscience 96(3–4): 217–224

Doty X 1991 Olfactory system. In: Gerchell T V et al (eds) Smell and taste in health and disease. Raven Press, New York, pp. 175–203

Dunbar H F 1954 Emotions and bodily changes, 4th edn. Columbia University Press, New York

Eisberg S 1983 Male chauvinism in toxicity testing? Manufacturing Chemist 3(July): 3

Engen T 1982 The perception of odours. Academic Press, New York

Engen T 1987 Remembering odors and their names. American Scientist 75: 497–502

Foreyt J P, Kennedy W A 1971 Treatment of overweight by aversion therapy. Behaviour Research and Therapy 9: 29–34

Gatti G, Cayola R 1923a L'azione delle essenze sul sistema nervoso. Rivista Italiana delle Essenze e Profumi 5(12): 133–135

Gatti G, Cayola R 1923b Azione terapeutica degli olii essenziali. Rivista Italiana delle Essenze e Profumi 5: 30–33

Gatti G, Cayola R 1929 L'essenza di valeriana nella cura delle malattie nervose. Rivista Italiana delle Essenze e Profumi 2: 260–262

Ghanta V K, Hiramoto R N, Solvason H B 1987 Influence of conditioned natural immunity on tumour growth. Annals of the N Y Academy of Science 496: 637–646

Hardy M, Kirk-Smith M, Stretch D 1995 Replacement of chronic drug treatment of insomnia in psychogeriatric patients by ambient odour. Lancet 346: 701

Herz R S, Cupchik G C 1992 An experimental characterisation of odour evoked memories in humans. Chemical Senses 17(5): 519–528

Hesse W R, Akerl K 1955 Experimental data on the role of the hypothalamus in mechanisms of emotional behaviour. American Medical Association Archives of Neurology and Psychiatry 73: 127–129

Hiramoto R N, Ghanta V K, Rogers C, Hiramoto N 1991 Conditioning fever: a host defence reflex response. Life Science 49: 93–99

Hiramoto R N, Hsueh C M, Rogers C F, Demissie S, Hiramoto N S, Soong S J, Ghanta V K 1993 Conditioning of the allogenic cytotoxic lymphocyte-response. Pharmacology Biochemistry and Behaviour 44(2): 275–280

Holley A 1993 Actualité du mécanisme de l'olfaction. In: 12èmes Journées Internationales Huiles Essentielles. Istituto Tetrahedron, Milano, pp. 21–27

Jirovetz L, Buchbauer G, Jäger W, Woidich A, Nikiforov A 1992 Analysis of fragrance compounds in blood samples of mice by gas chromatography, mass spectrometry, GC/FTIR and GC/AES after inhalation of sandalwood oil. Biomedical Chromatography 6(3) (May/June): 133–134

Karamat E, Ilmberger J, Buchbauer G, Roblhuber K, Rupp C 1992 Excitatory and sedative effects of essential oils on human reaction time performance. Chemical Senses 17: 847

Kikuchi A, Tsuchiya T, Tanida M, Uenoyama S, Nakayama Y 1989 Stimulant like ingredients in absolute jasmine. Chemical Senses 14(2): 304

King J R 1988 Anxiety reduction using fragrances. In: Van Toller S, Dodd G H (eds) Perfumery: the psychology and biology of fragrance. Chapman & Hall, London, pp. 147–165

Kirk-Smith M D 1995 Possible psychological and physiological processes in aromatherapy. In: Aroma 95 One body-one mind conference proceedings. Aromatherapy Publications, Brighton, pp. 92–103

Kirk-Smith M D, Booth D A 1990 The effect of five odorants on mood and the judgement of others. In: MacDonald D W, Muller-Schwarze D, Natynezuk S E (eds) Chemical signals in vertebrates. Oxford University Press, Oxford, pp. 48–54

Kirk-Smith M D, Van Toller C, Dodd G H 1983 Unconscious odour conditioning in human subjects. Biological Psychology 17: 221–231

Klemm W R, Lutes S D, Hendrix D V, Warrenburg S 1992 Topographical EEG maps of human responses to odors. Chemical Senses 17(3): 347–361

Knasko S C 1997 Ambient odour: effects on human behaviour. International Journal of Aromatherapy 8(3): 32

Lee W H, Lee L 1992 The book of practical aromatherapy. Keats, New Canaan CT, p. 125

Lehrner J, Eckersberger C, Walla P, Potsch G, Deecke L 2000 Ambient odour of orange in a dental office reduces anxiety and improves mood in female patients. Physiology and Behaviour 71: 83–86

Lorig T S 1989 Human EEG and odour response. Progress in Neurobiology 33: 387–398

Lorig T S, Roberts M 1990 Odour and cognitive alteration of the contingent negative variation. Chemical Senses 15: 537–545

Lorig T S, Schwarz G E 1988 Brain and odour: I. Alteration of human EEG by odour administration. Psychobiology 16: 281–284

Lorig T S, Schwarz G E 1988–1989 EEG activity during relaxation and food imagery. Imagination, Cognition and Personality 8: 201–208

Lorig T S, Schwarz G E, Herman K B, Lane R D 1988 Brain and odour: II. EEG activity during nose and mouth breathing. Psychobiology 16: 285–287

Macht D I, Ting G C 1921 Experimental inquiry into the sedative properties of some aromatic drugs and fumes. Journal of Pharmacology and Experimental Therapy 18: 361–372

Marchand S, Arsenault P 2002 Odours modulate pain perception: a gender specific effect. Physiology and Behaviour 76: 251–256

Miyake Y, Nakagawa M, Asakura Y 1991 Effects of odours on humans (I): effects on sleep latency. Chemical Senses 16: 183

Miyazaki Y, Takeuchi S, Yatagai M, Kobayashi S 1991 The effect of essentials on mood in humans. Chemical Senses 16: 184

Miyazaki Y, Motohashi Y, Kobashaya S 1992a Changes in mood by inhalation of essential oils in humans I. Mokuzai Gakkaishi 38(10): 903–908

Miyazaki Y, Motohashi Y, Kobashaya S 1992b Changes in mood by inhalation of essential oils in humans II. Mokuzai Gakkaishi 38(10): 909–913

Nasel B, Nasel Ch, Samec P, Schindler E, Buchbauer G 1994 Functional imaging of effects of fragrances on the human brain after prolonged inhalation. Chemical Senses 19(4): 359–364

New Scientist 1991 On the scent of a better day at work. 2 March: 18

Olness K, Ader R 1992 Conditioning as an adjunct in the pharmacotherapy of Lupus erythematosus: a case report. Journal of Developmental and Behavioral Pediatrics 13: 124–125

Parasuraman R 1991 Effects of fragrances on behaviour, mood and physiology. Paper presented at the annual meeting of the American Association for the Advancement of Science, Washington DC

Plato (3rd century BC) The Republic. (transl Lee D) Penguin, Harmondsworth

Redd W H, Manne S L, Peters B, Jacobsen P B, Schmidt H 1994 Fragrance administration to reduce patient anxiety in MRI. Journal of Magnetic Resonance Imaging 4(4): 623–626

Roberts A, Williams J M G 1992 The effect of olfactory stimulation on fluency, vividness of imagery and associated mood: a preliminary study. British Journal of Medical Psychology 65: 197–199

Rose J E, Behm F M 1994 Inhalation of vapour from black pepper reduces smoking withdrawal symptoms. Drug and Alcohol Dependence 34: 225–229

Sanderson H, Harrison J, Price S 1991 Massage and aromatherapy for people with learning difficulties. Hands On Publications, Birmingham

Schab F R 1990 Odors and remembrance of things past. Journal of Experimental Psychology: Learning, Memory and Cognition 16: 648–655

Schiffman S S, Siebert J M 1991 New frontiers in fragrance use. Cosmetics and Toiletries 106(6): 39–45

Schilcher H 1984 Ätherische Öle-Wirkungen und Nebenwirkungen. Deutsche Apotheker Zeitung 124: 1433–1443

Smith D G, Standing L, Deman A 1992 Verbal memory elicited by ambient odour. Perceptual and Motor Skills 74(2): 339–343

Stevenson C J 1994 The psychophysiological effects of aromatherapy massage following cardiac surgery. Complementary Therapies in Medicine 2: 27–35

Stoddart D M 1990 The scented ape. Cambridge University Press, Cambridge, p. 132

Sugano H 1989 Effects of odours on mental function. Chemical Senses 14(2): 303

Sugano H, Sato N 1991 Psychophysiological studies of fragrance. Chemical Senses 16: 183–184

Tasev T, Toleva P, Balabanova V 1969 The neuro-psychic effect of Bulgarian rose, lavender and geranium. Folia Med 11(5): 307–317

Teuscher E, Melzig M, Villmann E, Moritz K U 1990 Untersuchungen zum Wirkungsmechanismus Ätherischer Öle. Zeitschrift für Phytotherapie 11: 87–92

Torii S, Fukuda H, Kanemoto H, Miyauchi R, Hamauzu Y, Kawasaki M 1988 Contingent negative variation and the psychological effects of odour. In: Van Toller S, Dodd G H (eds) 1988 Perfumery. The psychology and biology of fragrance. Chapman & Hall, London, pp. 107–120

Van Toller S, Dodd G (eds) 1992 Fragrance: the psychology and biology of perfume. Elsevier, Barking, pp. 99–101

Warren C B, Munteanu M A, Schwartz G E et al. 1987 Method of causing the reduction of physiological and/or subjective reactivity to stress in humans being subjected to stress conditions. US Patent No. 4671959

Weiskrantz L, Warrington E K, Sanders M D, Marshall J 1974 Visual capacity in the hemianopic field following a restricted occipital ablation. Brain 97: 709–728

Wood C 1990a Sad cells. Journal of Alternative and Complementary Medicine October: 15

Wood C 1990b Say yes to life. Dent, London, p. 60

Wysocki C J, Dorries K, Beauchamp G K 1989 Ability to perceive androsterone can be acquired by ostensibly anosmic people. Proceedings of the National Academy of Science USA 86: 7976–7978

Chapter **9**

Aromatic medicine

Robert Stephen

INTRODUCTION

Aromatherapy has been subjected to caricature. The introduction of the therapy to the UK via the beauty industry has betrayed its seriousness and validity. In the popular mind aromatherapy and massage have become inextricably linked – a link that some have tried to shake off. In the UK, for various reasons – not least being ignorance and fear, aromatherapy has been reduced to a fraction of its potential; to many people it is no more than 'massage with smells'. In order to demonstrate competence as an aromatherapist it remains necessary to be examined in massage as well as in knowledge of essential oils, but aromatherapy exists outside of and beyond massage and it is this area of the therapy that is our focus in this chapter.

Many names have been used for this more responsible aspect of aromatherapy. It was first introduced in Britain as aromatology (Price 2000), although the preferred name is aromatic medicine – which the author of this chapter prefers (aromatologist remains the name for a practitioner of aromatic medicine). 'Aromatic,' because of the sweet odours of essential oils – and also because of their chemistry – and 'Medicine' meaning a curing art that does not involve surgery. The therapy of aromatic medicine is unique to the individual client (in the best traditions of complementary therapies) and is dependent upon a secure knowledge of essential oils and their chemistry on the part of the therapist. There are no reference works at the time of writing that can be cited specifically with regard to aromatic medicine,

Box 9.1   Knowledge over use

Who would attend a university offering a degree in geography if Africa were not included in the syllabus because of political situations? Knowledge of world geography would then not be complete! It is the same with essential oil knowledge; it is incomplete without knowing *all* possible methods of use.

Whether all methods are used or not, is another matter entirely. The important thing is, the knowledge is there, perhaps for use in an emergency, or for self-use.

In the UK, prescribing by mouth is in the hands of the medical profession only; for self-prescription of essential oils by this method (something many aromatherapists do from reading a book), the in-depth chemistry of those oils which can, or cannot, be used, quantities and duration of use, is essential knowledge for all students following an education in essential oils, although not required by many associations.

Surely training schools must take their responsibility seriously to ensure that all graduating aromatherapists have the knowledge necessary for the safe use of intensive treatments and internal use of essential oils. At present, the extra training required to qualify in aromatic medicine and thus become an aromatologist – is only available in two UK schools (see Useful Addresses, p. 528), all candidates having to possess already a qualification and experience in aromatherapy or relevant associated therapy.

although useful information on intensive application and ingestion can be found in several French texts, e.g. Belaiche (1979), Duraffourd (1982) and Franchomme & Pénoël (2001), with massage being very little used (see Ch. 3).

AROMATHERAPY AND AROMATIC MEDICINE

The principal difference, beyond massage, between aromatic medicine and aromatherapy as it is usually practised, is in the method of administration of selected essential oils and in the quantities that are used. Aromatherapy owes its introduction

into the UK to the beauty industry in the mid 20th century, therefore there was, in the beginning, hesitation at applying essential oils in a concentration beyond the minimum dosages and giving them to be ingested.

Thus arose the practice of diluting essential oils into a suitable carrier oil to use with massage, a separate therapy, which has since become known to the French as 'English style aromatherapy'. As the first aromatherapy organization in England was made up mainly of beauty therapists, the beauty therapy code of practice had to be followed, which does not allow the administration of anything by mouth. This was subsequently written into the aromatherapy association's code of practice and into that of every other association to follow. In many ways this was an understandable caution as little was known about the material that was being used. While there are those that hark back to the ancient Egyptians for the origin of the therapy, in truth that which we know as aromatherapy today can look only as far back as the early 20th century for its practice, even if the use of the raw materials can be traced into antiquity. However, confidence in practice has not kept pace with the increase in knowledge. An analogy could be drawn with a top of the range sports car that is only driven at 30 miles an hour to a local shop and back; it is a possible use of the vehicle, but this use does not realize its potential. Similarly, if aromatherapy is only ever used in massage, its potential is only partially realized.

The focus of critical comment on essential oils as used in aromatic medicine (= aromatology) has focused more on the use by mouth than on any other. Although the internal use of oils is taught in depth, the actual use in practice is restricted mainly to digestive conditions. This is, of course, a generalization, which disguises the many different uses and applications in the therapy. Much more commonly used in aromatic medicine is the intensive application of neat oils through the skin, which can be as little as two or three drops or as much as 3 or 4 ml, depending on the situation presented.

Aromatic medicine does not have to be 'heavy' in the use of essential oils, nor does it always have to involve chemically complex blends. One student of aromatic medicine had been suffering from a particular condition and had been self-medicating with a vast array of oils, all selected for good

Case study 9.1   Viral infection – T Birkmyre – *aromatology student, UK*

Client assessment
A middle-aged male, presenting with ME, a history of respiratory problems and a litany of viral infections. There has been a period of major stress and emotional upheaval as a result of the death of both parents in one year. He frequently has a sense of being generally unwell: headaches; sore throat; stiff neck; chest infections – these generally last about 24 hours.

Intervention
Dietary advice was given, especially to reduce dairy intake. Also, a self-administered treatment regime was initiated.

The first course of action was to 'drench' the client with essential oils to boost the immune system, using essential oils that would be antiviral, relieve respiratory congestion and address emotional balance. The essential oils used were:

- 10 drops *Ravensara aromatica* [ravensara] – antibacterial, antiinfectious, antiinflammatory, antiviral, expectorant
- 7 drops *Eucalyptus citriodora* [lemon scented eucalyptus] – analgesic, antibacterial, antiinflammatory, antiinfectious, calming and sedative
- 4 drops *Cinnamomum verum* fol. [cinnamon leaf] – analgesic, antiinfectious, antiviral, immunostimulant
- 7 drops *Eucalyptus stageriana* [lemon scented ironbark] – antiinfectious, antiinflammatory, calming
- 15 drops *Eucalyptus smithii* [gully gum] (excipient) – anticatarrhal, antiinfectious, antiviral, balancing (calming and stimulating)

The first reaction was a sound sleep, followed by waking feeling warmer and exhilarated. There was only one bout of coughing and the nose was less congested, with evidence that the catarrh was breaking up.

His self-treatment regime included a mask for inhalations using:

- 1 drop *Mentha x piperita* [peppermint] – analgesic, antiinflammatory, antimigraine, antiviral, expectorant, mucolytic
- 1 drop *Lavandula angustifolia* [lavender] – analgesic, antiseptic, calming and sedative, tonic
- 2 drops *Eucalyptus smithii* – as above

A few drops each of the essential oils of lavender and peppermint were also to be applied to the scalp to ease head tension.

Outcome
By the fourth day of treatment there was a significant change – especially emotionally. Colleagues were able to see a remarkable difference. The client felt that the pattern of viral disease had been broken. The client was able to secure a new challenging and demanding job through interview.

N.B. Drenching is a means of applying topically a larger amount of essential oil than would normally be used in a classic aromatherapy treatment. No carrier is used. Often an essential oil with a smaller molecular size would be used as an excipient to aid absorption (especially essential oils rich in 1.8 cineol). Once applied the area is occluded to assist penetration.

reason; however, the condition would not improve. When the student telephoned for advice, a more targeted approach was suggested, using a single oil in a small dose, but more frequently. The condition improved (see Case study 9.2).

Any bottle of essential oil carries the warning, 'Not to be taken internally.' Yet in aromatology, use by mouth under certain circumstances is regarded positively. This is

not, as first appears, dangerous or irresponsible, since many medications give warnings to the public and are unavailable to the public in a certain form, yet in the hands of a medical doctor they can be used effectively, safely and confidently. The case is similar with a qualified therapist of aromatic medicine using essential oils. Decrying the use of aromatic oils as medicine can only be given credence if the one who administers such treatment is unqualified, inexperienced and

---

Case study 9.2 Painful throat – J Buick– *aromatherapist (aromatology student)*

Client assessment
The subject is a woman in her mid thirties. The presenting symptom was a very painful throat. There were many other factors that were affecting stress levels. She had, with some knowledge of essential oils, tried to self-medicate. In her panic to effect a cure she had been using very large quantities of essential oil blends, but these were having no positive effect.

Intervention
The treatment recommended involved only one essential oil:

- *Thymus vulgaris* ct. thymol [thyme] – antibacterial, antiinfectious, antiseptic

The method of application was via a gargle. The recommendation was two drops be mixed with half a glass of water once an hour for 12 hours. The rationale was that a single powerful oil administered in an intensive application over a relatively short period would effect the cure that more complex blends could not .

Outcome
After a few hours the pain and irritation had eased. The treatment was continued for the 12 hours, with no side-effects or recurrence.

---

carries no valid insurance to proceed with such a practice. For instance, all bottles carry a warning against using essential oils in the eye; however, a solution properly prepared by a suitably qualified practitioner (supplied after a face-to-face consultation – not sold off-the-shelf) can be used, having due regard to this warning. It is in its use or abuse that any therapy is helpful or harmful.

Historically both aromatherapy and aromatology share the same indivisible root in the development of plant medicine and modern drugs. Aromatherapy was a term coined in the 1930s by a French chemist named Gattefossé and it was not until this point in time that essential oil therapy was separated from mainstream phytotherapy by name. Essential oils were used externally, internally, diluted or neat in those days. Even since that time, in France, the practice of all methods of using essential oils carries on, unchallenged and positively successful, essential oils being administered *per os* by medical doctors and phytotherapists as an effective method for treating disorders of the digestive and excretory systems, thus reaching the problem site by direct route. Internal use by mouth, pessaries and suppositories, plus undiluted (i.e. intensive) topical application (not massage), inhalation and compresses are the most common methods of use practised in France.

METHODS OF USE IN AROMATIC MEDICINE

Some definition of aromatic medicine is needed as distinct from aromatherapy, although the division is, of course, both false and forced. Aromatic medicine is *complete* aromatherapy, properly understood,

Table 9.1 Hierarchy of disease (Gascoigne 1994)

Age	Symptoms/disease manifest
6 months	Eczema
2 years	Whooping cough
5 years	Mucus collection in the middle ear, partial deafness, chronic bowel problems
12 years	Recurrent tonsillitis
19 years	Depression
22 years	Hay fever
25 years	Inflammatory bowel disease diagnosed as ulcerative colitis
25 years	Episodes of indigestion diagnosed as duodenal ulcer
55 years	Onset of tremor, stiffness and rigidity diagnosed as Parkinson's disease

while aromatherapy in England has become mainly massage with essential oils. In truth, aromatherapy should embrace all methods of using essential oils.

Denying internal and intensive use restricts therapists to massage, compresses (which, along with gargling, pessaries, suppositories are also internal, as is massage strictly speaking) and home treatment. Training schools should take their responsibility seriously enough to ensure that all graduating aromatherapists have the necessary knowledge regarding safe use in both intensive treatments and internal use of essential oils, even if not used on clients.

A practitioner of aromatic medicine will begin a consultation with an analysis of the body and lifestyle of the client. This is not dissimilar to an aromatherapy consultation. Due consideration will be given to presenting symptoms, with a closer look at the aetiology of those symptoms.

Gascoigne (1994 pp. 16–22) gives the most accessible introduction to the philosophy of alternative (as it would have been called at that time) medicine, speaking of the physical, emotional and mental levels and how they are affected by illness. Basically, superficial symptoms are manifest at a superficial level and deeper symptoms are the result of issues that are more deeply rooted within that person. When all three aspects – physical, emotional and mental – are combined, then the true aetiology can be explored. This integration of the whole person is vital: it is not possible to treat the whole person if presenting symptoms alone in one of the three areas of the person are treated in isolation. Further, if disease remains untreated with the underlying issues unresolved, the situation worsens. Gascoigne suggests how this can build up over a number of years (see Table 9.1).

While to some this may appear fanciful, in Gascoigne's work there is a logical and demonstrable progression towards this point. On the physical level it makes sense that the common cold will work its way via eczema to asthma and arrive at cancer and AIDS. So too, on the emotional level, irritability through anxiety, via depression, can arrive at a complete absence of feeling. The one weakness in Gascoigne's anthropology is the absence of the spiritual dimension of the person. Doubt, for instance, can be as debilitating as a broken limb for some people and needs to be addressed along with the other aspects of our being.

The practitioner of aromatic medicine has at his or her disposal the whole range of essential oils (not resinoids and absolutes – these are not essential oils, therefore not used), carrier oils and hydrolats. Their use in aromatic medicine is quite distinctive and must not be prescribed or administered without specific training.

ESSENTIAL OILS

Within this book (Ch. 2) a full definition of essential oils and the methods of extraction has been given, together with a breakdown of the primary chemistry of these oils. By way of introducing essential oils for use in aromatic medicine, it only remains to emphasize the quality of essential oils that must be used. In no way and at no time should essential oils be used that are not of the highest quality. Synthetic and modified oils can be dangerous. The essential oil producer (and therefore the distributor) should be able to provide and verify a GC analysis. Indeed, some producers are moving towards 'pharmaceutical' grade oils. These are not different in their chemical constituents, nor in the variations that are admissible – and expected – in a natural product. Simply, it is a level of hygiene and quality control comparable to the production of medical products. Once the grade of the oil is certain, then we may proceed to use them.

The selection of essential oils in the treatment of any client is based on the therapeutic function of the different component parts of the whole oil. This does not mean that the individual components are separated from the whole oil before they can be used, but rather, the balance of the components naturally present is noted in the blend prescribed. A table of the principal component parts and their main therapeutic functions can be found in Chapter 2.

From the chemical analysis of essential oils (see Appendix A(I)) the proportion of each constituent within the whole oil is clear. Each oil used in a prescription is chosen with an awareness of the balance within the oil and noting any contraindications. There are general rules that are applied (for instance, phenols, when used, must always be balanced with alcohols in any blend), but the practitioner is less constrained in the application of the essential oils than an aromatherapist.

Essential oils may be used intensively and applied topically. The number of drops used has to be a therapeutic decision, based on the need of the client and the therapeutic balance of potency and safety within the prescription. In some cases the measure could be in millilitres – in others, single drops. Where aromatic medicine departs from the more usual practice of aromatherapy is that the essential oils may be applied neat to the skin without necessarily using a carrier. These oils will be applied to a specific area and not to the whole body. The use of the essential oil is therefore much more targeted.

The option exists to use the essential oils in a capsule that may then be ingested. Here particular attention needs to be given to the balance of oils used – and ensuring that the chemistry is both effective for the presenting condition and tolerable to the digestive system. After a face-to-face consultation an aromatherapist is free to prescribe appropriately; the prescription is made up for each individual and is unique to that client. There are two further things to note here:

- Ingestion ensures the absorption of all the essential oils used. This gives greater control over a treatment regime than in a traditional massage using a carrier oil or lotion, where only 50% of the essential used is absorbed (Guba 2000 p. 40).
- The carrier oil used as the bulk of the fluid in any capsule can be chosen for the particular therapeutic effect of that carrier. For a detailed description of the benefits and uses of carrier oils, see Chapter 7 and the full work on this subject by the editors of this book (Price, Smith & Price 1999).

Compresses, gargles, diffusers, suppositories, pessaries and massage may all be used also.

Put very simply, once the selection of the essential oils (and carriers, if required) has been made, the practitioner of aromatic medicine, i.e. the aromatologist, is left with the decision of determining which method of application is the most direct and effective – the simplest approach is often the most beneficial.

Safety in using essential oils remains at the heart of practice; it is also at the heart of the debate between practitioners of aromatherapy and prac-titioners of aromatic medicine. Traditional aromatherapists will usually concede that the intensive topical use of essential oils may be sustainable as a practice – but reject internal use; nevertheless these same therapists are using mouthwashes and gargles – some using pessaries and suppositories. It has been a contention for some time that topical use of essential oils becomes internal use (whether diluted or not), in that the essential oil is absorbed through the skin into the bloodstream and then to the rest of the body. In 1877, Fleischer stated that the human skin was totally impermeable to all substances, including gases (Scheuplein & Blank 1971 p. 703). However, by 1945, Valette was able to demonstrate that essential oils do penetrate the skin – and goes on to say:

> Molecules which have passed through the skin's epidermis are carried away by capillary blood circulating in the dermis below. This tends to happen easily because the dermis is more or less freely permeable and the capillaries let small molecules pass through their walls. The most permeable regions of the skin to small molecules, including essential oils and vegetable oils, appear to be the palms of the hands and the soles of the feet, forehead, armpits and scalp.

Balacs 1993, Valette & Sobrin 1963

Each time essential oils are applied to the skin, there is penetration and essential oil molecules are carried into the cardiovascular and lymphatic networks, diffusing into all the organs. Then hepatic sulpho- or glycuro-combination takes place and renal elimination occurs (Byrne 1997 p. 35).

It is most unlikely that any essential oils fail to reach the bloodstream entirely when administered onto the skin; the factors which determine in what quantities they do, and how quickly and in what form are many and complex (Balacs 1992a,b).

Devlieghere (1996) put up a strong defence for the internal use of essential oils at the First Australasian Aromatherapy Conference in 1996. He stated that the anxiety about internal use of essential oils is due to a lack of knowledge, which both the author and the Editors wholeheartedly agree with. It is his contention that ingestion of essential oils may, in some circumstances, be safer than topical application for three reasons:

- **Phototoxicity:** Several essential oils (e.g. bergamot, lime, etc) contain furanocoumarins. The effect is that the essential oils are phototoxic if used topically in combination with UV light. This does not happen when an essential oil is ingested or used under occlusion
- **Allergic reactions:** The risk of allergic reactions is much reduced in ingestion compared with dermal administration
- **Oral toxicity vs dermal toxicity:** Devlieghere, (1996 p. 17), based on the work of Dr Maria Lis-Balchin, Deans & Hart (1995) demonstrated that the LD_{50} (the median lethal dose applicable to 50% of the population) is sometimes safer in internal (oral) administration than topically applied (dermal).

It has become unsustainable on scientific grounds to maintain any opposition to ingestion of essential oils. Not all practitioners should prescribe for use in this way because the majority are not competent: it is the prejudice that needs to be addressed – and the inadequate training.

EVIDENCE OF EFFICIENCY OF AROMATIC MEDICINE

In surveying the literature available, there are a number of case studies, properly presented, which give testimony to the efficacy of aromatology.

EXTERNAL INTENSIVE USE OF ESSENTIAL OILS

In one case of a client with ME, 80 drops (i.e. 4 ml) of a blend of skin-friendly, immune system boosting oils – *Eucalyptus staigeriana* [lemon scented eucalyptus], *Aniba roseodora* [rosewood] and *Boswellia thurifera* [frankincense] – were applied to the client's back each day for a period of 5 days in total. The result was significant improvement, with the client's perception of his own energy levels enhanced. The treatment was enough to start the whole healing process and the path back to a more active and balanced life. While recognizing that there are some who do not accept that ME is a valid disorder, the fact remains that the health of the client was dramatically improved by the intensive application of the essential oils. The

Table 9.2 LD_{50} g/kg values (adapted from Lis-Balchin, Deans & Hart 1995)

Essential oil	Oral LD_{50}	Dermal LD_{50}
Anethum graveolens	4	>5
Boswellia carteri	>5	>5
Cananga odorata forma *genuina*	>5	>5
Cedrus atlantica	>5	>5
Chamaemelum nobile	>5	>5
Cinnamomum camphora (white)	>5	>5
Cinnamomum camphora (yellow)	4	>5
Cinnamomum camphora var. *hosho*	3.8	>5
Cinnamomum verum cort.	3.4	0.7
Cinnamomum verum fol.	2.7	>5
Citrus aurantium var. *amara* flos	4.5	>5
Citrus aurantium var. *amara* per.	>5	>10
Citrus bergamia per.	>10	>20
Citrus limon per.	>5	>5
Citrus sinensis per.	>5	>5
Cymbopogon nardus	>5	4.7
Eucalyptus citriodora	>5	2.5
Eucalyptus globulus	4.4	>5
Foeniculum vulgare var. *dulce*	4.5	>5
Foeniculum vulgare var. *vulgare*	3.8	>5
Jasminum grandiflorum	>5	>5
Juniperus communis fruct.	8	>5
Juniperus mexicana	>5	>5
Juniperus virginiana	>5	>5
Lavandula angustifolia	>5	>5
Lavandula latifolia	4	2
Lavandula x intermedia 'Super'	>5	>5
Matricaria chamomilla	>5	>5
Melaleuca alternifolia	1.9	>5
Melaleuca leucadendron	4	>5
Ocimum basilicum ct. linalool	1.4	0.5
Rosa damascena	>5	2.5
Salvia lavandulaefolia	>5	>5
Salvia officinalis	2.6	>5
Salvia sclarea	5	>2
Syzygium aromaticum flos	2.7–3.7	>5
Syzygium aromaticum fol.	1.4	1.2
Zingiber officinale	>5	>5

effects were lasting and treatment was carried on using normal aromatherapy dilutions in a home treatment regime.

INTERNAL USE OF ESSENTIAL OILS

In a study on the use of peppermint oil for irritable bowel syndrome, the overall assessment of each treatment period showed that patients felt significantly better while taking peppermint oil capsules compared with placebo and considered peppermint oil (unspecified) better than placebo in relieving abdominal symptoms. Patients taking peppermint oil had a lower daily symptom score but there was no effect on the number of bowel actions per day (Drew et al 1984 p. 398).

Valnet (1990) presents many case studies in his seminal work on aromatherapy, among them Mrs F, aged 56, who suffered from deep-seated delirious madness and had been in hospital for many years. She had previously had tuberculosis and had suffered for 3 years from a rhino-pharyngeal infection and chronic bronchitis with persistent fever, which resisted antibiotic treatment. Her general condition was poor. She was treated with trace elements and aromatherapy internally *per os* and by means of suppositories. Her temperature became normal in 3 weeks. These results were consolidated by 20 days treatment each month for 6 months.

Research by Zarno (1994) into the effects of tea tree essential oil on candidiasis produced very encouraging results. She confirms all that is regularly assumed to be true about the essential oil: that it is antiseptic, antifungal and an immuno-stimulant. Zarno recommends 2–3 drops of oil on a tampon for internal application twice a day; 6 drops in a bath and 2 drops in warm water as a gargle for oral thrush to be used after each meal (Zarno 1994).

Research by May (1996), shows the efficacy and safety of capsules containing peppermint oil (90 mg) and caraway oil (50 mg) – both unspecified – when studied in a double-blind, placebo-controlled, multi-centre trial in patients with non-ulcer dyspepsia. After 4 weeks of treatment intensity of pain was significantly improved for the group of patients treated with the peppermint/caraway combination compared to the placebo group. Before the start of treatment all patients in the test preparation group reported moderate to severe

pain, while by the end of the study 63.2% of these patients were free from pain. The pain symptoms had improved in a total of 89.5% of the patients in the active treatment group (May et al 1996).

There are many such clinical uses of essential oils that have demonstrated efficacy, notable among these would be the work of Pénoël. Along with Franchomme, Pénoël has been at the vanguard of much of the experimentation and learning in the various aromatology applications. The total concept of aromatherapy was embraced in England by Shirley Price (therefore necessitating the introduction of aromatic medicine). There were many others in the early 1970s who introduced aspects of aromatherapy; but only the Editors, the Penny Price Academy and the educators, Bob and Rhi Harris, have continued to advocate the holistic approach to the full use of essential oils. Tisserand, in the early days, also advocated this wider use of oils (Tisserand 1977).

EDUCATION

It is worth focusing on what is involved when training for aromatic medicine. While many courses are offered in aromatherapy, ranging from just a few weeks to those recognized by the professional bodies such as IFPA and IFA (see Ch. 16), aromatic medicine is not offered by many training providers in the UK. One of those who does offer training at this level insists on a professional qualification in aromatherapy first, followed by 2 years in practice, thus allowing the would-be practitioner of aromatic medicine time to become familiar with essential oils and to build up their own competence. The student explores the individual chemical components which make up essential oils, their effects on the physiology and pathology of the human being and the potential effects on the psyche. Hazards such as toxicity, skin reactions, etc. are explored in depth. This is followed by an intensive course in the chemistry of essential oils, building on what is known and familiarizing the student with the functions of the chemical components.

The chemistry is a vital part of the training in that this is the element that ensures a firm enough grasp of the required knowledge of essential oils to allow for safe practice. No-one should prescribe for intensive topical application or for internal use

Box 9.2 Uterine tonics

In the latter stage of pregnancy, some practitioners use herbs and essential oils as uterine tonics to prepare for labour. A main herb is *Rubus idaeus*, the leaves of which can be safely taken after the first trimester.

In clinical aromatherapy practice, a number of practitioners recommend internal and external use of eugenol-containing oils in the last 3 weeks of pregnancy as uterine 'tonics' to help uterine tone in readiness for an easy labour. These include *Syzygium aromaticum* and *Cinnamomum verum* fol.

However, an interesting observation is that according to research, eugenol is a powerful inhibitor of prostaglandin production and has been shown to *decrease* myometrial tone i.e. is spasmolytic. Other essential oils said to be uterotonic include those containing *trans*-anethole such as *Foeniculum vulgare* and those containing geraniol such as *Cymbopogon martinii* and *Thymus vulgaris* ct geraniol. Once again, there is evidence that these essential oils act to reduce uterine tone and contraction. Other essential oils with confirmed uterine spasmolytic activity include: *Elettaria cardamomum*, *Piper nigrum*, *Cinnamomum cassia* (cort.), *Origanum majorana*, *Zingiber officinale*, *Curcuma longa* and *Salvia triloba*. These oils thus have a potential role in the treatment of dysmenorrhoea as well as abnormal uterine spasms during pregnancy.

Examples of uterine 'tonic' formulae are as follows:

MDB Editions
Syzygium aromaticum: 30%
Thymus vulgaris ct geraniol: 20%
Citrus lemon: 20%
Rosmarinus officinalis: 20%
Cinnamomum verum (fol.): 10%

Oral dose:
1 drop once per day 3 weeks before labour is due
1 drop twice a day 2 weeks before labour is due
1 drop 3 times per day 1 week before labour is due

Boudoir
Thymus vulgaris ct geraniol: 3 ml
Cymbopogon martini: 3 ml
Syzygium aromaticum: 0.5ml
Vegetable oil: 13.5 ml

6–8 drops massaged over the belly several times a day to stimulate labour if the mother is post-term. Or the same quantity over the lower back every half hour during labour itself.

Thymus vulgaris ct geraniol: 50%
Citrus aurantium ssp *aurantium* (flos): 40%
Syzygium aromaticum: 10%

Oral dose:
1 drop three times per day before meals 3 to 4 days before labour is due.

---

without a demonstrable knowledge of essential oil chemistry.

Whereas in an aromatherapy course full-body massage plays a major role, the would-be aromatologist learns a limited amount of massage, specialized for specific local conditions. Aromatic medicine training is more concerned with accurate assessment, in-depth knowledge of essential oils and treatment using a more prescriptive approach.

Until a few years ago students were expected to have completed a personal study and have submitted a dissertation before proceeding to the final stages of training. This has now changed and the dissertation (working at around a good Master's degree level) remains an option for professional development. It was also the case that a great deal of time was spent on psychoneuroimmunology, in an attempt to understand disease: it was thought that if disease were understood then the treatment would be easier. The emphasis has now changed and, while the understanding of this philosophical aspect still has a place, much more time is spent in developing the practical skills required for this more exacting use of essential oils. While previously students found the course academically stimulating, few had the confidence to incorporate aromatic medicine aspects of the therapy into their dealings with clients. Much more time is now spent with students over the course of their 2 years' training in supervised intensive and internal use of essential oils (the

Case study 9.3 Pressure sore – D Raines – *aromatologist, Portugal*

Client assessment

Alan, a 39-year-old male, fractured and dislocated his fourth cervical vertebra in a rugby accident, which resulted in complete paralysis from the neck down, with no movement of any limbs and confinement to a wheelchair.

Following a friction burn to his right elbow, Granuflex was applied to help heal and protect the area and when this was removed it revealed a grade three pressure sore (around $1^1/_2$ cm in diameter), which was very sloughy with a moderate amount of exudation. It was decided to use aromatic medicine to promote healing.

Intervention

The aim of the intervention was to:

- prevent infection
- reduce inflammation
- create an environment that promotes healing
- encourage formation of granulating tissue
- reduce or remove odour.

Each time the wound was redressed an aseptic technique was maintained. The solution used to clean the wounds was sterile saline 0.9%.

The essential oils used were:

- *Citrus limon* [lemon] – antibacterial, anti-infectious, antiinflammatory
- *Commiphora myrrha* [myrrh] – antiinflammatory, antiseptic, cicatrizant
- *Helichrysum angustifolium* [everlasting] – anti-infectious, antiinflammatory, cicatrizant
- *Melaleuca viridiflora* [niaouli] – antibacterial, antiinfectious, antiinflammatory, antiseptic

The carrier used was *Calendula officinalis*, as it promotes healing and reduces inflammation.

Initially the lemon and niaouli were used to deslough Alan's wound, with myrrh present to encourage granulation. All three oils used at this stage also inhibit infection. The first stage formula was:

- 30 ml calendula with a 10% solution of essential oils – 10 drops myrrh and 25 drops each of lemon and niaouli.

The wounds were cleaned and packed with sterile gauze soaked in the formula. The wounds were dressed twice a day for 2 days, with gauze padding over the top to absorb excess moisture.

After 2 days there was little exudate, minimal slough and good signs of granulation. The 10% dilution was kept but with the balance of oils adjusted to encourage new tissue:

- 30 ml calendula, with 40 drops myrrh and 10 drops each of lemon and niaouli.

To prevent the wound drying out a waterproof dressing (Melolin) was placed over the top, being changed daily.

After a week there were good signs of wound healing.

The third stage of the treatment involved dropping the essential oil ratio to 7.5%, and again changing the balance of the oils used:

- 100 ml calendula, 120 drops (approx 4 ml) myrrh, 25 drops everlasting and 5 drops each of lemon and niaouli.

Outcome

After a further week of treatment the wound was healed, and for gentle maintenance the dilution was reduced to 2.5% on the gauze of a plaster. After a further 5 days the only visible sign to be seen was the pinkness of the new skin.

N.B. Grade three pressure sores involve full thickness skin loss. The break of the skin extends through the dermis into the subcutaneous fat tissue. The sore becomes more than a surface wound and has a crater-like appearance.

---

case studies that accompany this chapter are from students that either the author or the Editors have had a part in teaching).

The effective length of the course is comparable with that of a medical herbalist and yet it is, be-cause of the focus on essential oils (and carriers), more specialized. Those qualified as practitioners of aromatic medicine (i.e. aromatologists) have shown commitment to a demanding and exacting course and will be better therapists as a result (see the Institute of Aromatic Medicine, p. 339, re insurance).

Strong arguments have been presented by some (e.g. Lis-Balchin 1997) against any use of aromatic medicine, even claiming that such is illegal, although this is not the case (Medicines Control Agency 1998 personal communication).

Whether by inhalation, massage, compresses, pessaries and suppositories, intensive application or internal use – essential oils enter the blood circulation. Therefore, there is no sustainable argument that can separate the use of massage from any other use – they may all be regarded as internal use. For this reason, instead of segregating aromatic medicine as a wholly separate study and therapy, it needs to be held under the umbrella of aromatherapy. It is recognized that irresponsible use of oils internally can irritate the stomach lining; however, irresponsible use of any drug will do the same. Aspirin, for example, is known to exacerbate stomach ulcers, and some would suggest that aspirin may even be one of the causes of ulcers. Some essential oils can cause severe irritation of the skin if applied neat in large quantities, but a trained therapist will have been schooled in the chemistry and hazards of the different applications of a particular oil.

While there is a general consensus on safety, there are differing views on the potential hazards of different oils (Ch. 3, Tisserand & Balacs 1995) just as there are different perspectives on the uses of the oils themselves.

Although those who have trained as aromatologists may or may not go on to use the various ways of topical and internal applications that they have been taught, nevertheless, the training raises awareness of these other methods of use, giving deeper knowledge with regard to essential oils and their therapeutic uses than would an 'English style' aromatherapy course.

THE WAY AHEAD

Ideally, in the future (and in accord with the work done by the Foundation for Integrated Medicine) there will be a new approach to training, where all practitioners of traditional or complementary medicine will first undergo a course of study in a foundation module that introduces the principles of the main approaches and gives an understanding of anatomy and physiology (see p. 336). On this foundation will be built a more specialist knowledge in whichever therapy direction that student wishes to go. This may be a long way off – it is not, however, an unrealizable dream.

It may be possible that the rear-guard action fought by those who want to preserve the traditional 'English' usage is driven by a survival instinct. The period of study for the fuller use of aromatherapy (i.e. aromatic medicine) is longer and definitely more scientific; however, it is not an attempt to drive out those who could not manage the academic study yet who are naturally caring.

As with every other discipline there are different thresholds which allow a more comprehensive practice, each level having its own distinctive focus. Massage (with or without essential oils) remains a valid therapy, particularly for stress, but it is not the sum total of aromatherapy. At this present moment the politics advocated by the various camps promoting their particular use threatens to eclipse the one purpose of any therapy, which is to benefit people. Surely the only valid purpose of any therapy is to help people rediscover health and, along with that, a sense of self-worth. If aromatology has some positive contribution to make as an intrinsic part of aromatherapy to this end, then all arguments to the contrary are invalid.

SUMMARY

The benefits and potential of aromatic medicine seem to the author to be clear. It offers a more specific and targeted approach to any presenting conditions. It follows in the best philosophical traditions of complementary therapies. It utilizes a natural product. It is less invasive (as some may perceive it) than a full-body massage. It is clinical and precise.

In a health-care setting, where both time and space are limited, it is possible to offer a treatment and therapy that can be applied without the time consideration of a massage, yet still using essential oils as curative agents. The cost of essential oils used in this focused way is also something that is worthy of consideration, as they are considerably cheaper than most synthetic drugs, yet are demonstrably efficacious.

In private practice, aromatic medicine allows a therapist greater freedom in dealing with each client. The broader spectrum of approaches and the wider understanding of essential oils means that the client can have greater confidence in the therapist.

Perhaps it may be too bold to suggest that aromatic medicine is aromatherapy grown-up?

References

Balacs T 1992a Dermal crossing. International Journal of Aromatherapy 4(2): 23–26

Balacs T 1992b Well oiled pathways: the pharmacokinetics of essential oils. International Journal of Aromatherapy 4(3): 14–25

Balacs T 1993 Essential oils in the body: their absorption, distribution, metabolism and excretion. Proceedings of AROMA 93 Conference

Belaiche P 1979 Traité de phytothérapie et d'aromathérapie. Maloine, Paris

Buchbauer G 1993 Molecular interaction: biological effects and modes of action of essential oils. International Journal of Aromatherapy 5(1): 11–14.

Byrne K 1997 Ingestion of essential oils: food for thought. Simply Essential 26: 34–36

Devleighere G 1996 Oral use of essential oils. Proceedings of the Australasian Aromatherapy Conference.

Drew M J, Evans B K, Rhodes J 1984 Peppermint oil for the irritable bowel syndrome: a multicentre trial. British Journal of Clinical Practice: 394–395

Duraffourd P 1982 En forme tous les jours. La Vie Claire, Périgny

Franchomme P, Pénoël D 2001 Aromathérapie exactement. Jollois, Limoges

Gascoigne, S 1994 The manual of conventional medicine for alternative practitioners. Jigme Press, Dorking, pp. 16–22

Guba R 2000 Toxicity myths – the actual risks of essential oils use. The International Journal of Aromatherapy 10(1&2): 37–49

Lis-Balchin M, Deans S, Hart S 1995 A study of the changes in bioactivity of essential oils used singly and as mixtures in aromatherapy. Journal of Alternative and Complementary Medicine 3(3): 249–256

May B, Kuntz H, Kieser M, Kohler S 1996 Efficacy of a fixed peppermint oil/caraway oil combination in non-ulcer dyspepsia. Arznein-Forsch/Drug Res. 46(II): 1149–1153

Price P A 1998 Aromatology: its history and uses. Positive Health 27: 2714–2716

Price S 2000 The aromatherapy workbook. Thorsons, London

Price L, Smith I, Price S 1999 Carrier oils for aromatherapy and massage. Riverhead, Stratford-on-Avon

Scheuplein R J, Blank I H 1971 Permeability of the skin. Psychological Review 51(4): 702–747

Tisserand R 1977 The art of aromatherapy. Daniel, Saffron Walden, p. 319

Tisserand R, Balacs T 1995 Essential oil safety: a guide for health care professionals. Churchill Livingstone, Edinburgh

Valette G, Sobrin E 1963 Absorption percutanée de diverses huiles animals ou végétales. Pharmaceutia Acta Helvetica 38(10): 710–716

Valnet J 1990 The practice of aromatherapy. C W Daniel, Saffron Walden, p. 237

Weyers W, Brodbeck R 1989 Skin absorption of essential oils. Pharmazie in Unserer Zeit 18(3): 82–86

Williams D G 1996 The chemistry of essential oils. Mycelle Press, Weymouth

Zarno V 1994 Candidiasis – a holistic view. International Journal of Aromatherapy 6(2): 20–23

Zatz J L 1993 Scratching the surface: rationale and approach to skin permeation. In: Zatz J L (ed) Skin permeation: fundamentals and applications. Allured Publishing, Wheaton

Sources

Balacs T 1993 Research Reports. International Journal of Aromatherapy 5(2): 34–36

Bronagh R L, Wester R C, Bucks D, Maibach H I, Sarason R 1990 In vivo percutaneous absorption of fragrance ingredients in rhesus monkeys and humans. Food Chemical Toxicity 28(5): 369–373

Calvery H O, Draize J R, Laug E P The metabolism and permeability of normal skin. Psychological Review 26: 495–540

Hotchkiss S 1994 How thin is your skin? New Scientist 141: 24–27

Schnaubelt K 1989 Friendly molecules: aspects of essential oil constituents and their pharmacology. International Journal of Aromatherapy 2(2): 20–22 and 2(3): 16–17

Webster R C, Maibach H I 1983 Cutaneous pharmacokinetics: 10 steps to percutaneous absorption. Drug Metabolism Reviews 14(2): 169–205

SECTION 3

Aromatherapy in context

SECTION CONTENTS

Chapter **10**

Aromatherapy and primary health care

Christine Stacey and Shirley Price

INTRODUCTION

When the National Health Service made its entry in 1946 Aneurin Bevan did not foresee the monster he helped create. No one would argue with the philosophy – and it does mean that every individual in the United Kingdom is entitled to health care free at source. For many of those with low incomes or with chronic disease it has literally been a lifesaver and advances in medicine have made possible lifespans not envisaged 30 years ago.

Every individual has the right to have care from a general practitioner (GP) – a doctor who has chosen to specialize in what used to be called family medicine. However, as the population has aged and expectations have grown, that family friendly GP is no more; consultations are routinely allocated 10 minutes, in which individuals have to explain their problems, have a diagnosis made and be prescribed treatment. This time-hungry interaction has been shown to be one of the major dissatisfactions that patients have with orthodox care.

It is thought that some benefits that patients derive from massage and/or aromatherapy may be related purely to the lengths of time spent with the therapist, a perspective not available to time constrained GPs (Watson 1997), alongside an increasing desire from consumers to gain greater control over their lives (Doel & Segrott 2003, Saks 2005) and/or a desire for holistic treatments (Douglas 1996, Scott 1998).

Many people with common and chronic ailments are assigned to the primary health care sector by the GP, excluding those where hospitalization is necessary. Ailments treated by aromatherapists can vary from burns, wounds and acne, through maternity (including ante- and postnatal problems) and paediatric care to long-term problems such as multiple sclerosis (MS), myalgic encephalomyelitis (ME), Parkinson's disease (PD).

A trial study and a few case studies are given and further relevant cases can be found in other chapters.

PRIMARY CARE IN THE COMMUNITY

The Health Act of 1999 (the 51st anniversary of the NHS) ended GP fund holding, requiring doctors, nurses, trusts and health authorities to co-operate; it also gave primary care trusts legal status (Gillam 1999, O'Dowd 1999, Smith, Dickson & Sheaff 1999).

Primary health care may be the first level of contact which individuals and families in the community have with the National Health system, bringing health care as close as possible to where people live and work: it constitutes the first element of a continuing health-care process (WHO 1978). The majority of the population never progress beyond visiting their general practitioner; Primary Care or care in the community is considered to be cheaper and more user friendly than the more expensive acute or hospital care. As a result, increasing pressures are brought to bear on GPs to reach targets, rather than concentrate on caring for their patients; patients invariably do not see the same GP each time they visit the surgery and continuity of care is via the computer console and electronic notes. However, the result is that health care is no longer viewed as the primary and sole concern of the GP and successive Government reports have determined that there are 'teams' of providers – different for each patient, depending on their needs.

The team includes practice nurses, those working within a Health Centre or GP premises, midwives and community nurses. Community-based nurses include district nursing teams, health visitors, school nurses, nurses at clinics, family planning nurses and paediatric nurses. Mental health nurses, e.g. community psychiatric nurses, also work in the community and may be based within a Health Centre or GP premises. All make an important contribution to community based health care and when the need arises for a specialist in a particular field, the health care extends to physiotherapists, occupational therapists, etc.

Many in this team of nurses and midwives, who may also be aromatherapists, wishing to introduce aromatherapy to their patients in the community where they feel it can be of benefit, should present the team with a sound policy and guidelines for the use of aromatherapy in their particular field (see Ch. 16), so that direction for this form of treatment can be initiated or approved by the GP or the management to whom the nurse is responsible.

PRIMARY HEALTH CARE COSTS

New contracts mean that the more services that GPs provide for their patients 'in-house' the greater their payment from the Primary Care Trust (PCT) – the potential then for complementary therapies to be integrated should in theory be there. However, regardless of the fact that an increasing number of the population would like to have complementary therapies available (Thomas, Coleman & Nicholl 2003), a lack of credible evidence continues to be the main reason that those who hold the budget in PCTs give for the resistance to commissioning these services (Ernst & Abbot 1998). A total of 62% of PCTs in the United Kingdom do fund some level of complementary care and all but two London PCTs offer a degree of service, although these tend to be from group one of the House of Lords Report (2000), i.e. acupuncture, chiropractic, herbal medicine, homoeopathy and osteopathy (see Ch. 16) (Wilkinson, Peters & Donaldson 2004). Dixon & Smith (2004) state that 50% of patients use complementary therapies without informing their GPs, and approximately 50% of GPs are now encouraging or referring their patients to CAM practitioners.

In 1999 The National Institute for Clinical Evidence (NICE) was established to ascertain from an evidence base which treatments should be NHS funded. The reality has been that patients are now involved in a postcode lottery of whether treatments are funded or not. One of the main reasons given by PCTs for lack of funds to provide new services such as aromatherapy is the massive drug overspend from both the hospitals and primary care, but unfortunately, in order to fund this overspend, money is in fact trawled back from the PCTs to fund the requirements of secondary hospital care.

A great number of patients visit their GP for chronic disease management, which invariably involves a prescription for a drug, whose possible side-effect may require another prescription. Many problems are not solvable by the overstretched GP, requiring interventions other than antidepressants or sleeping tablets. This is a simplistic viewpoint, but it can be argued that if complementary therapies, specifically aromatherapy, were available free at source, there is a potential for reducing the cost of both time and drugs not only at a local level, but also on the NHS at a national level.

AROMATHERAPY AND ESSENTIAL OILS IN PRIMARY CARE

National service frameworks are issued concerning care in the community – for the elderly, mental health, children, coronary heart disease and cancer. These frameworks cover the in-depth way of looking at, investigating and improving the care and working lives of clients and patients (Fleetwood 2005, personal communication).

Although community nurses are concerned with patients who have widely differing nursing needs and are of all ages, 'most of their patients, even as early as 1985 were 65 years and over' (Baly, Robottom & Clark 1987). We have an ageing population and while a significant number are relatively healthy and mobile, an important percentage require increasingly expensive and total care; around 25% of all drugs prescribed are for the elderly, many to treat the side-effects of a main drug. The use of essential oils can help support failing immune systems, alleviate side-effects and counteract the pain and distress caused by chronic disease.

Even though a large number of elderly people still prefer to live in their own homes until necessity places them in a nursing home, hospital or hospice, many live in warden controlled dwellings, residential homes and/or visit day centres for the elderly. On their visits, community nurses/

aromatherapists can use their skills to alleviate any secondary effects being suffered, such as constipation, sleeplessness and anxiety (see Ch. 14).

Many of the common and chronic ailments suffered by people of all ages will be cared for mainly in the primary health sector; multiple sclerosis (MS), strokes not requiring hospitalization, myalgic encephalomyelitis (ME), Parkinson's disease (PD), burns and wound care are only a few of the areas which have been treated by aromatherapists or community nurses in the home. Maintaining and encouraging mobility, lowering the blood pressure, supporting discontinuing smoking – all are possible with essential oils, not forgetting that a dual approach to care is necessary. The significant number of patients who attend for minor illnesses demanding antibiotics is also of concern and can be helped by the use of essential oils, which can not only maintain mobility but also support their mental health (see individual headings below for aromatherapy intervention).

An escalating number of relatively young people have significant osteoporosis with accompanying pain and gradual retreat from activities of daily living. This can result in isolation, causing a considerable percentage of low-grade mental health problems in the elderly.

The physical and empathetic contact with the aromatherapist through massage with essential oils may often be the only physical contact that individual may have, contact which in itself can promote endorphins, enhancing the mood of the patient, which in turn will have an effect on the immune system, improving quality of life (Wilkie, Kampbell & Cutshall 2000).

Also, in modern society, relatives either live a distance away or are unable or unwilling to find time to spend with an elderly or incapacitated relative. Even when there is a loving relationship a near relative may withdraw from physical contact due to a fear of causing pain – this can be counteracted by teaching him or her to deliver a simple massage within their capabilities, with provided blends of essential oils.

USE OF ESSENTIAL OILS

While there are general guidelines as to the properties of essential oils and what effect each oil may have, it is advantageous to use only a small collection, as most patients may be on a significant number of prescribed medications and it is essential not to interfere with their action. Also, although it is known which organic components may exert the general effect required, essential oils are complex substances and 'there is no simple direct relationship between any one of the chemical constituents and the therapeutic effect – or even the hazard – of the whole essential oil' (Price 1990).

Aromatherapy is an art as well as a science and the synergy of an individual oil or a blend works with each individual patient to achieve the aim of improving health.

PAIN AND MOBILITY

Many patients are unable to tolerate non-steroidal antiinflammatory drugs (NSAIDS) and are therefore prescribed increasing amounts of other pain medication, with significant side-effects, frequently requiring further medication to counteract them; these in turn have significant side-effects – thus a downward spiral is initiated. In effect, although difficult to 'prove' for the requirements of NICE, maintaining these individuals in their own homes cuts the state cost of care.

Aromatherapy with the skilful use of essential oils (Doel & Segrott 2004) can help maintain pain at a tolerable level, relieving side-effects such as chronic constipation, tinnitus, dullness of the mentality and drowsiness, etc., which enhances their mood, enables more social interaction, thus allowing them to resume daily activities (ADL).

Although much research is devoted to determining the therapeutic value of isolated active compounds within oils, knowledge which is invaluable when selecting essential oils, aromatherapy involves blending whole, unadulterated oils (see Ch. 3 Part I) for each individual, approaching the patient from a holistic viewpoint. For instance working with an individual who is retreating from ADL due to pain from osteoarthritis, improving low mood has a beneficial effect on the immune system (Yokoyama 2002). This in turn will help regulate the inflammatory response, reducing swelling and pain (Horrigan 2004), allowing the patient to reconnect with life,

live independently and not be a burden on the decreasing financial resources of the NHS.

Essential oils which are both antiinflammatory and analgesic include *Achillea millefolium* [yarrow], *Boswellia carteri* [frankincense], *Coriandrum sativum* [coriander], *Eucalyptus citriodora* [lemon scented gum], *Juniperus communis* [juniper], *Lavandula angustifolia* [lavender], *Melaleuca viridiflora* [niaouli] and *Rosmarinus officinalis* [rosemary]. (See also Ch. 14 on Care of the elderly.)

Lavender, niaouli and yarrow are also hypotensors, should high blood pressure be present also (see below).

HYPERTENSION AND STROKES

There is increasing incidence of cerebral vascular accident (CVA) (more commonly known as a stroke), these appearing to occur more in women than in men – particularly in those with hypertension or diabetes, or in fact any condition leading to atherosclerosis, including smoking and familial hypercholesterolaemia (Ball 1990 p. 189).

The chief aim with patients referred with volatile hypertension is to help the patient to be managed on the lowest dose possible for therapeutic effect, which in turn reduces or eradicates the side-effects of medication, often cited as a reason for non-compliance. Usually, about a third of people who have a stroke will recover with time, though any further strokes considerably weaken the body.

Cardiovascular conditions are managed in primary care mostly by a combination of health education and pharmaceutical support, from both the cholesterol lowering aspect and helping control hypertension, both of which have a significant impact on the costs entailed by the PCT.

ESSENTIAL OIL INTERVENTION

It has been found that cardiovascular conditions can respond to essential oils administered via massage (see Ch. 11) and although it can be difficult to determine whether the massage or the essential oils provide the benefit, early aromatherapy intervention has been found to help even those who have suffered a severe stroke to regain movement in the limbs affected, enabling them to

---

Case study 10.1   Stroke – S Price – *aromatologist, UK*

Client assessment

When the author's (Price) mother-in-law suffered a severe stroke – and fell downstairs – she was taken to hospital. After her return, it was decided to try to lift her mental state (she had been previously very active) and help improve the mobility of her affected limbs with essential oils. Mrs Price also suffered from high blood pressure.

Intervention

Mrs Price was visited every day and the following essential oils were applied in a carrier oil:

- *Rosmarinus officinalis* [rosemary] – circulatory and mental stimulant, nerve tonic and hypotensor
- *Thymus vulgaris* [thyme population] – circulatory stimulant and antidepressive

- *Salvia officinalis* [sage] – circulatory stimulant and neurotonic

These were massaged in an upward direction only, on her arms and legs.

Swiss reflex therapy (see Ch. 7) was carried out on the corresponding reflexes of both feet – plus the throat reflexes, as Mrs Price was unable to talk coherently.

Outcome

She was soon back to her normal daily activities and her speech returned, her doctor remarking on her unusually rapid recovery.

---

return to a level of mobility to help maintain daily activities, thus encouraging independence and reducing costs to the state (see Case study 10.1).

Essential oils, once absorbed, utilize the same methods of transport, metabolism and excretion as pharmaceuticals (Tisserand & Balacs 2002) and as such may have the potential for harmful interaction with prescription medication (Lis-Balchin 1999). They should never be relied upon totally and uniquely for lowering blood pressure requiring medication; however, if any of the following are suitable for treating side-effects, they will also indirectly benefit a hypertensive person.

Hypotensors include *Achillea millefolium* [yarrow], *Cananga odorata* [ylang ylang], *Citrus limon* [lemon], *Lav. angustifolia* [lavender], *Melaleuca viridiflora* [niaouli], *Origanum majorana* [sweet marjoram] and *Rosmarinus officinalis* [rosemary]. Rosemary is a peripheral vasodilator (Mills 1991), the camphor/predominant oil having 'a paradoxical action on the heart: stimulating it if failing, yet dilating the coronary circulation', thus echoing the opinion of Franchomme and Pénoël (2001) that it is balancing for blood pressure – in *low* concentration for high blood pressure and *high* concentration for low blood pressure. It was used therefore in Case study 10.1 even though the patient had high blood pressure.

The most effective oil for promoting the blood circulation and helping to improve mobility of the affected limb/s after a stroke is *Rosmarinus officinalis* [rosemary], for its circulatory and neurotonic properties; others include *Foeniculum vulgare* [sweet fennel], *Thymus vulgaris* ct. alcohol [sweet thyme] and *Vetiveria zizanioides* [vetiver].

N.B. Although *Citrus paradisi* [grapefruit] is a circulatory stimulant, the British National Formulary states that anyone taking calcium channel blockers should avoid eating grapefruit or drinking grapefruit juice, therefore it may be wise to avoid using the essential oil in this instance.

MIDWIFERY AND HEALTH VISITING

The decision to care for antenatal patients is a shared one between patient, midwife, health visitor and doctor, based on need, preference and professional and clinical judgement.

Aromatherapist community nurses are often able to be of help in caring for minor problems not only during pregnancy, but at – and immediately after – the birth, as they are able to visit their patients at home for up to 4 weeks afterwards. In many cases community midwives may go to the hospital when labour is established, to assist with the birth and if they are aromatherapists, can use essential oils in the relief of labour pain.

ANTENATAL CARE

The problems encountered during pregnancy, such as backache, fluid retention, emotional changes, constipation, etc. (see Ch. 12) can all be benefited by essential oils (select from the appropriate problem in Appendix A(II)). Common sense and thorough training in essential oils and their chemistry will determine which oils may be best avoided at certain stages, although a one-off application of, say *Hyssopus officinalis* [hyssop] applied to a bruise or carrying out a mouth rinse with *Myristica fragrans* [nutmeg], *Salvia officinalis* [sage] or *Syzigium aromaticum* [clove bud] for an occasional bout of toothache, although normally contraindicated during the first two trimesters, would be completely without risk to the baby used in these cases.

With dedicated, diligent daily application of the essential oils of *Boswellia carteri* [frankincense], *Lavandula angustifolia* [lavender] and *Pelargonium graveolens* [geranium] from the fourth month of pregnancy, stretch marks can be avoided (Price 2000a), as can also perineal damage (see below).

CARE DURING LABOUR

(See also Ch. 12.)

There is a grey area regarding using *Lavandula angustifolia* [lavender] in the bath when labour begins, although common sense suggests that the proportions normally used (4–8 drops in a bath full of water) are far too dilute to cause any ill effects – it is far more likely that the effects, as proved by Norfolk & Reed (1993), are beneficial. Norfolk & Reed's survey was to determine whether pain relief and relaxation could be achieved without adverse side-effects when partaking in a lavender bath for up to 30 minutes (see Box 12.4).

POSTNATAL CARE

Perineal management is increasingly becoming part of the midwives' role as it is not uncommon for women to experience perineal trauma to some extent during the childbirth process, especially with those having their first baby (Labrecque et al 1994). Essential oils can also be used here.

Many of those qualified in aromatherapy are now advising their clients to massage their perineums from 16–34 weeks onwards with essential oils in a carrier oil, to reduce any future perineal trauma and discomfort, some using essential oils which will also benefit other minor troubles they may have. Preventing tears and other damage saves the midwife from having to suture perineums after the birth. Savings can therefore be made in suture pack costs – both important considerations for the Health Service (Feasey unpublished work 1998).

Avery & van Arsdale are believed to be the first to carry out a study involving essential oils and the perineum. The study, in 1987, involved 29 mothers-to-be who gave themselves a daily massage for 6 weeks prior to the expected date of delivery, and 26 who did not, acting as a control group. Episiotomy and second degree tears occurred in 48% of the first group, compared with 78% in the second group (Guenier 1992). Guenier herself has recommended *Lavandula officinalis* [lavender] and *Pelargonium graveolens* [geranium] to her antenatal groups, with beneficial results.

HAEMORRHOIDS

Should a new mother develop haemorrhoids after the birth, it is possible to help by advocating the use of essential oils in the bath, in a compress or applied in a lotion, *Cupressus sempervirens* [cypress] and *Pelargonium graveolens* [geranium] being two of the recommended oils to use (see Appendix A(II) for others).

PAEDIATRIC CARE

Health visitors have a distinct role within the primary health care team, working across all age groups and young families; for them, children and parents are a priority group (Primary Care Nursing 1997); it is their responsibility to visit every baby born in their area between 10 and 14 days and to monitor the child's health and development until he or she starts school.

When a health visitor who is an aromatherapist calls to see a patient, there may be occasions when

Case study 10.2 Postnatal care – L Reed – *aromatherapist, UK*

Client assessment
A community colleague of the therapist was called out one evening to a client (who was also a medical practitioner) with extremely sore nipples. On arrival, the nipples were cracked, bleeding and extremely painful – made worse by the application of a nipple cream which the client said had caused stinging. The baby was unable to be latched on.

Intervention
First, the community nurse hand expressed the mother and the baby was fed. She then applied the following oil blend on and around the mother's nipples:

- 1 drop *Chamaemelum nobile* [Roman chamomile] – analgesic, antinflammatory, calming, cicatrizant
- 1 drop *Lavandula angustifolia* [lavender] – analgesic, antiinflammatory, antiseptic, antibacterial, calming, cicatrizant, tonic
- 1 drop *Rosa damascena* [rose otto] – antiinflammatory, antibacterial, astringent, cicatrizant, neurotonic, styptic

- 20 ml almond oil – antiinflammatory, helpful to dry skin
- 10 ml calendula – antiinflammatory, astringent, cicatrizant

In the hospital, the above blend is divided into 10 ml small bottles for mothers to use on themselves (in hospital or at home) and one of these was left with this client – with instructions to wash the breasts with warm water just before each feed, applying the nipple oil immediately afterwards.

Outcome
The following morning, when the community nurse revisited, the baby was back feeding on the breast and both client and colleague were surprised by the amount of healing that had taken place.

The mother said that she had felt instant relief as soon as she applied the nipple oil.

N.B. In a small study, the analgesic effects on mothers using the nipple oil blend had a response of 7+ on a scale of 0–10.

Case study 10.3 Juvenile polyart... – M Vanhove – *aromatherapist, Belgium*

An osteopath colleague of the therapist had to treat a 5-year-old child with juvenile polyarthritis. The young girl suffered various inflammations in different parts of her body, and was no longer growing. Her knees were already deformed and she could not walk normally. She was on heavy medication when the aromatherapy was started.

Intervention
Besides the diet changes suggested by the osteopath, massage was given on the therapist's advice, using the following in a 4–5% dilution with the carrier oil:

- *Eucalyptus citriodora* [lemon scented gum] – analgesic, antiinflammatory, antirheumatic
- *Pinus sylvestris* [Scots pine] – analgesic, antiinflammatory, neurotonic

- *Laurus nobilis* [bay leaf] – analgesic (bone and muscle)
- Jojoba carrier – light analgesic, anti-inflammatory, antirheumatic

Intervention
The osteopath visited the girl three times a week to give her a treatment and showed the mother how to massage her on the other days.

Outcome
2 months later the girl had grown by 2 cm and the medication was able to be reduced by 50%. She has not had much pain since, and her behaviour is more positive.

that child, or another member of the family, may have a cold, a bruise, cut or wound, or perhaps a low immune system because of over frequent use of antibiotics (Soulsby Report 1998). With the GP's consent, healing can be assisted by essential oils in these and other areas.

When selecting essential oils for children it is best to keep within a small range, excluding any with a significant percentage of possibly hazardous components such as ketones, phenols and phenolic ethers and aldehydes (see Appendix A(I) and Ch. 2). Aromatherapy for Babies and Children (Price & Price 2004) gives a list of 20 safe oils to use.

The only eucalyptus oil suitable for children is *Eucalyptus smithii* [gully gum]. Although it contains a high percentage of 1,8-cineole, the synergy between components makes it a gentler, equally effective oil as *Eucalyptus globulus* [blue gum] (Pénoël 1992).

Effective, safe methods of using essential oils on babies and children are:

- **Inhalation:** (tissues, vaporizers, cotton tips or balls concealed in the pillowcase or on night clothes).

- **Baths:** The drops of essential oil should always be dispersed first into cream or a base carrier lotion (not oil!) before adding to the bath water, to ensure even distribution with very low concentration. One drop only should be used in a baby bath for babies under 9 months, with 2–3 drops in a normal sized bath being suitable for older babies. For ease of use, 8 drops in total of the selected essential oil/s can be added to 50 ml of base lotion, adding a dessertspoonful of this to each bath (half for babies under nine months) and swishing the water thoroughly (Price & Price 2004).

- **Massage:** The health visitor who is also an aromatherapist – and has obtained permission to do so – can show the new mother how to do a simple massage with essential oils on her new baby, which is of immense benefit to both for bonding – and later, to the child. Massaging baby can also help in the treatment of postnatal depression (Fleetwood 2005, personal communication).

INFECTION

A significant number of patients attend for minor illness demanding antibiotics; however, much research has been done on the antiviral, antifungal and antibacterial properties of essential oils (see Ch. 4) with some interesting yet not widely publicized research into the effect of Melaleucas against methicillin resistant *Staphylococcus aureus* (MRSA) (Caelli et al 2000, Carson & Riley 1995, Carson et al 1995, Carson, Riley & Cookson 1998). A number of essential oils have been found to be effective against *Staphylococcus aureus* – see Table 4.4, where essential oils are listed with their efficacy, supported with references. Two of them *Thymus vulgaris* ct. thymol and *Melaleuca viridiflora* [niaouli] will also boost the immune system, as will *Melaleuca alternifolia* [tea tree] and *Vetiveria zizanioides* (see Appendix B.9).

Upper respiratory tract infections (URTI) are usually viral in origin and will run a recognized course in 7–10 days. However, children or adults who have a lowered immune system due to stress, recurrent infections or due to a pathological condition, may develop secondary bacterial infections. Early intervention with one of the two Melaleucas above and *Bos͏ ͏ ͏eri* [frankincense] or *Citrus limon* [lemo͏ ͏ ͏lation, bath or massage can support ͏ ͏mu͏e system, negating the requireme͏ ͏ ͏ antibiotics, which in their turn confuse the immune system – creating further problems later on.

There is some evidence to support the use of *Ocimum basilicum* var European [sweet basil], as it has the terpene/alcohol/phenol combination suitable for repeated infections affecting the immune system (terpene/alcohol containing oils are suited for normal infections). Sweet basil is also antifungal (Soliman & Badeaa 2002), antiinflammatory (Opalchenova & Obrashka 2003) and analgesic (Moudachirou et al 1999), which properties together – by lessening the pain and inflammation which always accompanies any infection – support the immune system and help the body fight the infection. There is also evidence that essential oils can support prescribed antibiotics when used in tandem (Alexander 2001,

---

Case study 10.4   Tonsillitis – P Price – *aromatologist, UK*

Client assessment

Philip, aged 14, had suffered on and off for several years with tonsillitis, and each time he was given antibiotics, which eventually did not seem to have much effect – his attacks becoming even more frequent. His mother was recommended to the therapist by a community nurse who was just starting a course in aromatherapy so that she could help her patients with chronic problems.

Intervention

The therapist decided to use:

- *Citrus limon* [lemon] – antibacterial, anti-infectious, immunostimulant
- *Eucalyptus smithii* [gully gum] – analgesic, anti-infectious, antiinflammatory, prophylactic
- *Melaleuca alternifolia* [tea tree] analgesic, antibacterial, antiinfectious, antiinflammatory, immunostimulant, neurotonic

3 ml of each were put into a 10 ml dropper bottle for use in the bath (4–6 drops), and 15 drops of the blend were put into 50 ml of carrier lotion for his throat, the latter to be used three times a day.

Outcome

After 4 days Philip's mother reported that her son's symptoms had almost disappeared. She was advised to make sure he kept using the oils in the bath until he had recovered totally – and as a preventative against further attacks.

Two years later, Philip's mother was delighted to report that Philip had had no further attacks – very unusual for him; it confirmed the belief that when the body is helped by the use of natural products to overcome a disorder, then in effect it is made stronger, fitter and better equipped for the environment. By helping the body to heal itself Philip was healthier after the illness than he was previously, because his immune system had been stimulated to deal with further infections that might come his way. Philip is now aged 29 and has had no further problems with tonsillitis.

Opalchenova & Obrashka 2003, Shahvedi et al 2004), thus supporting the synergy theory in Chapter 3.

FUNGAL SKIN INFECTIONS

Prescribed medication, particularly for nail infections, is hepatotoxic and as such has potentially significant side-effects. While the continual use of essential oils may produce sensitivity, they do not have the same potential for serious side-effects, as their metabolism and excretion does not include the first pass through the liver.

There are two main methods of approaching treatment with essential oils:

- The author (Stacey) believes that the pH of the environment can be changed, making it hostile to the mycoses – any essential oil with high alcohol content may have this effect.
- Essential oils such as *Melaleuca alternifolia* [tea tree], *Thymus vulgaris* cts. thymol, geraniol and

linalool [thyme], *Satureia montana* [mountain savory] and *S. hortensis* [garden savory] all have antifungal properties.

Although many essential oils are antifungal, each tackles specific mycoses. Table 4.5 lists essential oils together with the specific effects of each one.

ACNE

Acne can be devastating for young people; it tends to emerge during adolescence, when hormonal changes trigger an imbalance of sebum in the skin, which, if excessive, can lead to blockage of the pores, blackheads, acne and cysts. Stress, such as exams, parents divorcing or moving schools, play their part in this, as do the relevant emotions of anxiety, fear – and even jealousy – which may present themselves in these situations (Price 2001).

A multimillion pound industry provides potions and lotions which purport to 'cure' this condition; however, most of them merely strip the skin of its natural protection (friendly bacteria) and create further problems.

It is imperative when dealing with acne that a holistic approach is taken, checking the diet for unsuitable foods which may be aggravating the condition, such as spicy or fatty foods and dairy products. Only when the whole lifestyle picture has been assessed, can the most suitable and effective essential oils be selected:

- *Pelargonium graveolens* [geranium] is a 'must' for acne as it is has all the required properties, tackling infection, acne, anxiety and stress and helping to reduce fear and jealousy (Price 2000b).
- *Lavandula angustifolia* is antiinfectious, benefiting acne, anxiety and also helping to allay any fear. *Citrus bergamia* [bergamot] and *Citrus limon* [lemon] are antiinfectious, helping to reduce anxiety and also balance the emotions.
- *M. alternifolia* and *M. viridiflora* are both excellent antiinfectious agents and one of these should be used together with one or two of the above, for best results.

SLEEP AND IMMUNITY

While stress (see Ch. 11) is a current buzzword, recognition and treatment remain firmly in the past and it appears that stress-related disease is on the increase (Seaward 2000), two of its major presenting symptoms being fatigue and insomnia. Aromatherapy can support these patients on a variety of levels.

Sleep is a complex, highly organized state vital to health, allowing physical recovery, promoting memory and learning, supporting the immune system and thus promoting health related quality of life (Marieb 2001). Lack of sleep and elevated cortisol levels due to chronic stress upset the circadian rhythm, interfering with the pineal gland and melatonin secretion, resulting in lower CD4 and CD8 cell counts and a body vulnerable to low-grade infection (Dhabhar 2000, Dhabhar & McEwen 1997) which in turn causes more stress. Irwin (2002) identified that continued sleep disturbance affects the immune function, resulting in a threat to health due to the inability to fight off multiple infections. Allowing the body to relax and the release of endorphins may be enough to induce restful sleep, during which the body heals itself. Stress does not have to be emotional; any imbalance whether due to infection or pathology creates further stress – and blending oils which work on both an emotional and physical level can initiate a healing response. Many patients report that after even a single aromatherapy treatment they had their first good night's sleep for weeks or even months, waking up feeling refreshed and with more energy.

Case study 10.5 Acne – C Stacey – *complementary therapist, UK*

Client assessment
C Stacey's son A had malignant acne as a youth, leaving him with chronically diseased lymph glands in his neck. The glands were later a focus for infection and regularly developed into carbuncles with associated fever, anxiety and depression as he retreated from social contact.

Several courses of antibiotics later there was no change.

Intervention
Lavandula angustifolia [lavender] and *Melaeuca alternifolia* [tea tree] were the oils used to help the acne.

Outcome
He now controls the glandular infection himself with a daily wash of the same essential oils. Before the carbuncles start to appear, he applies poultices using the same oils, with the result that he has not required an antibiotic in 2 years.

It could be argued that he could merely have grown out of the condition except that when he forgets, the symptoms recur.

Case study 10.6 Stress and insomnia – J Browne – *aromatherapist, UK*

Client assessment

J, a 46-year-old married lady, had three grown-up children and an 8-year-old daughter. She cared for her mother who was undergoing chemotherapy for her terminal cancer. She tried hard not to cry as she told me that her brother-in-law had just been diagnosed with lung cancer and her daughter had had a miscarriage 4 days before that.

J had been diagnosed with MS 16 years ago, her first relapse leaving her unable to walk for 2 years. However, during a visit to Lourdes in France, 'a miracle happened' and she was able to walk again.

At the moment she suffered with spasm in her legs, poor memory, regular headaches, pain in her neck and shoulders and her sleep pattern was poor.

Intervention

The aim was to improve her sleep and lowered immune response, relieve her headaches and help her to relax. Appointments were made fortnightly.

First visit: the following essential oils were massaged into her back and head, noting that there was a lot of tension in her neck and thoracic region:

- 2 drops *Boswellia carteri* [frankincense] – analgesic, antidepressive, antiinflammatory, cicatrizant, energizing, immunostimulant (all properties recommended for grieving)
- 2 drops *Chamaemelum nobile* [Roman chamomile] – antiinflammatory, antispasmodic, calming and sedative
- 1 drop *Lavandula angustifolia* [lavender] – analgesic, antiinflammatory, antispasmodic, calming and sedative, tonic
- 5 drops *Origanum majorana* [sweet marjoram] – analgesic, antispasmodic, calming, neurotonic (recommended for grief)
- 12 ml jojoba oil – light analgesic, anti-inflammatory

Home treatment: a blend of the oils used was supplied for her husband to massage her back every night before going to bed.

Second visit: J was sleeping much better – but was still uptight, so a neck and shoulder massage was given before massaging her back and legs.

Home treatment: a blend of the essential oils in white lotion was supplied for her to apply to her chest, shoulders and neck morning and evening. She was also shown how to meditate – to be tried for 5 minutes five times a day if possible.

Third visit: J was sleeping well, but still a bit uptight. As the therapist felt she needed to talk, she spent a long time counselling her. J was also a devout Christian, so it was suggested that she also visit a Church minister.

Her shoulders, back and legs were massaged as before with the same blend and J was supplied with the blend in a neat oil mixture, being instructed to put nine drops in her vaporizer and massage one drop into her temples a few times each day.

Outcome

By her fourth visit (i.e. after 8 weeks) J was feeling very much better in herself, and able to cope with her grief. Her muscle spasm was lessening and she was learning to relax more. Because of this, the frankincense was replaced with *Rosmarinus officinalis* [rosemary], for its extra properties to help her muscles and the new blend was given to her in a lotion to rub into her legs every night and morning – and her shoulders, when the blend given to her on her second visit was finished.

J's sister, who lived alone and suffered from osteoarthritis, was looking to her for support; however, the importance of J having time and energy for herself was pointed out – and a form of gentle exercise for her was discussed, choosing swimming, as it was something she could do with her daughter.

By J's sixth visit (3 months after commencing treatment), J had been swimming twice a week. Her memory was better, her headaches were infrequent and she was much more relaxed.

As J was using her essential oil blends regularly at home, an aromatherapy appointment was made for 3 months' time. She thanked me for being there at that particular time with so many things going wrong – she felt that without the aromatherapy, she would have been unable to cope – and may even have had another relapse.

Case study 10.6   Stress and insomnia – J Browne – *aromatherapist, UK (cont'd)*

From the chart that had been filled in at each visit over the 3 months of treatments, it was found that J had achieved the following:

85% relief from anxiety and depression
85% relief from aches and pains
86% relief from stiffness
73% improvement in sleep

78% improvement in mobility
75% improvement in skin condition
90% improvement in relaxation during and after treatment
80% improvement in relaxation for a few days following treatment.

Another significant issue is that these patients frequently visit the GP, but an audit of cases at one London clinic showed that after aromatherapy treatments GP contact was greatly reduced, the number of consultations going down from an average of 27 over 6 months to an average of 11 in the same length of time following treatments.

The list of essential oils which reduce stress is long, but two essential oils which will not only relax patients, but also encourage sleep and strengthen the immune system are *Citrus limon* [lemon] and *Origanum majorana* [sweet marjoram]: see Chapter 11 (Stress) for a further selection.

MULTIPLE SCLEROSIS

Sometimes referred to as disseminated sclerosis, MS is a chronic disorder of the central nervous system; scattered areas of the brain and spinal cord degenerate, the nerve fibres losing their insulating myelin sheaths and their ability to conduct impulses (Wingate & Wingate 1996). Although the cause still remains unknown (Lunny 1997), it is thought that an infection of some kind may be the cause, but no specific virus has been implicated.

Recent research and thinking have identified allergy and food intolerance as playing a significant part in the process of the condition; the major culprits appear to include animal fats and gluten products (Swank 1991, Swank & Dugan 1990) and a few of the trials carried out have indicated that a diet rich in linoleic acid can considerably reduce the severity of the disease (Bricklin 1983 p. 340). MS is progressive but not continuous; symptoms may start with numbness in a part of the body or muscle weakness in a limb, pins and needles, and after weeks or months (or possibly as long as 2 years) of being free from symptoms, these may intensify to shooting pains in the back and spasm in the limbs. Sight and speech can be affected, but the main long-term problems are lack of control of the bladder, leading to urinary infections, and difficulty with walking, often resulting in the patient being confined to a wheelchair (Ball 1990 pp. 201–202).

No allopathic treatment has yet proved to be of value; aromatherapy is not a cure either, but its holistic approach, i.e. consideration of the whole body and state of mind of the patient, has been found to be beneficial, for example, in improving quality of sleep, strengthening muscles and relieving muscle tension or spasm (Mutch 1997). Aromatherapy was able to help a patient in a nursing home who had reached the final stages of the disease and was suffering with persistent pain in both forearms, which 'subsided within two months' (Hulmston 1995). A person suffering from MS was helped by using aromatherapy to boost the immune system, address muscle fatigue, stimulate the circulation and the memory (Donald 1996). The oil chosen to address the latter three conditions was *Rosmarinus officinalis* [rosemary].

Oils common to all three cases were *Santalum album* [sandalwood] and *Pelargonium graveolens* [geranium]; *Cymbopogon citratus* [lemongrass] was used in two of the cases. Lunny (1997) suggests using essential oils which contain large proportions of esters (antispasmodic and calming) and aldehydes (stimulating) in their composition, suitably diluted for massage; the stimulating effects of alcohols and antispasmodic effects of esters may also be valuable in many cases.

POST-VIRAL FATIGUE SYNDROME (CHRONIC FATIGUE SYNDROME, MYALGIC ENCEPHALOMYELITIS)

This disease has only in recent years been accepted by the medical profession as a debilitating and distressing condition. Ball (1990 p.194) says it is thought to be 'a variety of viral encephalitis, occurring both sporadically and in epidemics'. It is known under several names: myalgic encephalomyelitis (ME), chronic fatigue syndrome (CFS) or post-viral fatigue syndrome (PVFS), the latter name being favoured by Wingate & Wingate (1996), who regard the name myalgic encephalomyelitis to be 'a massive overstatement'.

Encephalomyelitis means inflammation of the brain and spinal cord, a serious and sometimes fatal result of infection. ME is an ill-defined collection of symptoms that include aching muscles, lassitude and depression (Wingate & Wingate 1996).

It is true that allopathic medicine has few answers – some orthodox doctors even denying its existence; thus sufferers frequently seek help from natural health-care practitioners.

ME, (CFS or PVFS) manifests itself in varying degrees of severity, including extreme tiredness and lethargy, muscle and joint pains, depression, irritability and diminished coping skills. It is usually accompanied by mild fever, sore throat, tender lymph nodes, headache, sleep disorders, confusion, memory loss and visual disturbances (Encyclopaedia Britannica 1996). According to Bennett (1992 p. 157), although opinions differ as to its cause, it is believed that it may be due to a viral infection compounded by a compromised immune system, this supporting the name post-viral fatigue syndrome. He goes on to say:

> *Experience suggests that nearly all the sufferers have been regular medical drug takers (particularly antibiotics and/or the oral contraceptive pill which are known to undermine the immune system) and that most also appear to have developed* Candida albicans *as a consequence of their drug therapy, aggravated by a diet high in refined carbohydrates.*

There is very little that orthodox medicine can do for a person with ME; however, aromatherapy has had some success with both ME and AIDS by boosting the immune system and raising the spirits.

Symptoms can be helped by an initial selection of immune strengthening and neurotonic essential oils (see Appendix A(II)), selecting from these – wherever possible – oils to treat the presenting symptoms of each individual case. Four oils particularly recommended are *Rosmarinus officinalis* [rosemary], which has neuromuscular action and is neurotonic, *Pelargonium graveolens* [geranium], also neurotonic, *Boswellia carteri* [frankincense] and *Melaleuca viridiflora* [niaouli], both excellent immunostimulants. All four have many other properties which may be found helpful for individual presenting symptoms.

Case study 10.7 ME (chronic fatigue syndrome) – A Wood – *aromatherapist, UK*

Client assessment
Bill, 47, had been diagnosed with ME. His speech was slurred at times, he was totally exhausted and he had a balance problem. After walking about 50 yards, he had to stop because of the excruciating pain in his leg – 'sort of numb and like severe pins and needles'. He also experienced spasm occasionally in his left leg, which gave him great pain.

The therapist persuaded him to try holistic aromatherapy and adjust his eating habits – a low fat diet, fresh fruit and vegetables, no red meat and a reduction in his coffee intake to 2 cups a day and drinking a minimum of 2 pints of water a day. Vitamin C and B complex and vitamin E tablets were to be taken daily. He was also shown some gentle exercises to do daily.

Case study 10.7   ME (chronic fatigue syndrome) – A Wood – *aromatherapist, UK* (cont'd)

Intervention

Bill had 3 treatments each week, concentrating on neuromuscular and lymph drainage massage. The following sets of oils were alternated each week, diluted in almond oil:

Weeks 1, 3 and 5

- *Citrus aurantium* var. *amara* flos.[neroli] – antidepressive, neurotonic
- *Chamaemelum nobile* [Roman chamomile] – antiinflammatory, antispasmodic, calming and sedative, stimulant
- *Pelargonium graveolens* [geranium] – analgesic, antiinflammatory, general tonic, neurotonic
- *Rosmarinus officinalis* [rosemary] – analgesic, antiinflammatory, antispasmodic, decongestant, neuromuscular action, neurotonic, stimulant
- *Salvia sclarea* [clary] – antispasmodic, balancing, calming, energizing to sympathetic nervous system

Weeks 2, 4 and 6

- *Boswellia carteri* [frankincense] – analgesic, antidepressive, antiinflammatory, cicatrizant, energizing, immunostimulant
- *Cedrus atlantica* [cedarwood] – arterial regenerator
- *Eucalyptus globulus* [blue gum] – anti-inflammatory, decongestant
- *Lavandula officinalis* [lavender] – analgesic, antiinflammatory, antispasmodic, calming and sedative, tonic

- *Ocimum basilicum* [European basil] – analgesic, antiinflammatory, antispasmodic, nervous system regulator, neurotonic

Outcome

After the first week, Bill was looking and feeling a lot brighter. He had also felt more relaxed – and had slept like a log.

After the second week, the benefits were showing even more – his speech was much better – not slurred, or slow, except if he did too much and became overtired.

After the third week, Bill returned to work – mornings only – not doing too much, as he found it very tiring. Magnesium tablets were added to the vitamins he was already taking and he was given a blend of antispasmodic oils to massage into his legs at night-time.

After six weeks of part time, sleeping in the afternoons, he returned to work full time, but with a long lunch break.

He no longer needs treatment three times a week, but uses the oils at home every night to help prevent the cramp in his leg. He rests when he begins to feel tired – and has a leg massage or full treatment every now and again, when he feels he needs a boost.

RESEARCH IN A LONDON GENERAL PRACTICE

A large GP practice is presently engaged in small-scale projects looking at chronic fatigue syndrome, fibromyalgia, migraine and *Cannabis sativa* essential oil, and seeking funding and ethical approval for larger studies that might make a difference. The MYMOP self-assessment tool is used to help measure outcomes and to help the patient see the benefits received from treatments. Unfortunately data such as this remains in the anecdotal sphere and as such is not considered evidence. The patients are privileged in that the service is free at source, funded in partnership by University of Greenwich and the practice. Regardless of the increasing evidence base, aromatherapy still appears to be considered a non-essential component of patient care, but hopefully the 'Patient Choice' charter will help somewhat in the argument to fund further interventions such as this, which show the short- and long-term benefits. All patients are referred by the GPs and after 3 years' experience it is often discussed whether aromatherapy intervention would better serve the patient than medication.

PARKINSON'S DISEASE

Parkinson's disease, named after James Parkinson (1755–1824) was described in a paper he wrote in 1817 as 'the shaking palsy'. The disease is due to a lack of a chemical substance, dopamine, needed in the brain to transmit messages to the distal

A project (intended as a preliminary exercise for possible future research) was carried out in 1992 (Price 1993) on three groups of people with Parkinson's disease to determine whether or not essential oils could play a part in improving movement and perhaps increase the time span before administering stronger drugs.

Objective

The objective of the trial was to discover whether daily application of essential oils, without massage, was as effective as using essential oils with regular full-body massage, so that people could benefit without having to receive full-body massage. Group C received the same intervention as Group A, using vegetable oil only, without essential oils.

All participants had to obtain their doctor's permission to take part and be willing to do what was asked of them, especially with regard to home use.

Intervention

The blend of essential oils was identical for Groups A and B – not chosen holistically for each person. The choice focused on lowering stress levels and loosening joints and muscles, with the hope also of relieving insomnia and constipation in those presenting such symptoms. Each group had to use the given mix of essential oils over a 9-month period to validate the results.

Out of the 52 people who volunteered for treatment, 27 completed the 9-month period required for the project (10 in Group A, 9 in Group B and 8 in Group C). The others either found the weekly progress recording difficult (A and C), could not keep up the daily application (B), or had to discontinue due to visits into hospital or changes in medication – which would have falsified the results.

Apart from the undiluted oil for use in the bath (6–8 drops) where this was possible, the oils and/or lotions were mixed at 1.5% concentration and supplied by the authors, to guarantee uniformity. The trial was organized in the following way:

Group A: received a weekly massage from an aromatherapist for 12 weeks, followed by a monthly massage for a further 6 months. The carer applied the same essential oil blend in a lotion base daily in between treatments (every other day during the last 6 months).

Group B: were supplied with pure essential oils for the bath and a lotion or oil based mix containing the same essential oils to be applied daily for 3 months and every other day for a further 6 months.

Group C: received a weekly massage with plain vegetable oil. This was difficult, as the therapists could not be told that there were no essential oils in their mix. As the lack of smell could have made them suspicious, this was overcome by telling them that they were using an extremely low concentration – even though no essential oils were present.

The essential oils selected were:

- *Salvia sclarea* [clary] – relaxant, nerve tonic – to aid general relaxation and relieve anxiety
- *Origanum majorana* [sweet marjoram] – analgesic, antispasmodic, digestive tonic, hypotensor, nerve tonic, relaxant – to relieve muscle pain and insomnia and improve digestion
- *Lavandula angustifolia* – analgesic, antispasmodic, digestive stimulant, hypotensor, sedative – to relax the muscles and relieve pain, insomnia and anxiety

Results

The symptomatic relief between Group A and Group B showed very little difference, which points to the potential of baths and self-application for those who cannot afford aromatherapy treatments.

Group A

7 patients maintained their improvement during the last 6 months when receiving an aromatherapy treatment only once a month.

2 were able to discontinue their medication for insomnia.

2 did not maintain their improvement during the last 6 months, but still felt better than before treatment commenced (beneficial effects of each treatment lasting 4–6 days).

It was felt that fortnightly (if not weekly) aromatherapy treatments would be preferable to monthly intervals.

Box 10.1   Parkinson's disease project (*cont'd*)

Group B

The use of essential oils without massage appeared to give relief in the same areas as in Group A.

A perceived extra benefit of Group A over Group B may be the complete relaxation derived from the massage, with improved circulation as a result (though this was not mentioned in the patient feedback).

Group C

The patients receiving massage (and home care) with a bland vegetable oil found the treatment relaxing, some feeling better generally, although the effects were not lasting. No other noticeable changes were recorded.

The symptomatic improvements experienced by all three groups are shown in Table 10.1.

Table 10.1   Number and percentage of PD sufferers in groups A and B (combined) and group C experiencing symptomatic relief over 9-month trial period

	Groups A and B (combined)		Group C	
	No.	%	No.	%
Anxiety	4	100	–	–
Constipation	5	83	1	33
Cramp	1	50	1	50
Depression	3	75	–	–
Energy lack	4	100	0	0
Insomnia	7	85	2	66
Memory loss	0	0	0	0
Muscular pain	8	100	3	60
Nightmares	2	100	–	–
Rigidity	2	50	–	–
Slurred speech	2	28	–	–
Stiffness	9	100	1	50
Swallowing difficulty	0	0	–	–
Tremors	4	33	1	16
Weak limbs	5	62	–	–

After Price 1993.
Dashes indicate that a person was not asked by the therapist if he/she suffered from that symptom.

muscles (Parry 1997). It is a slow, progressive disorder, usually (but not always) affecting people in later life, though it can occur earlier; it affects the parts of the brain which control movement; the symptoms include trembling or/and stiffness of the limbs, a shuffling walk and difficulty in speaking (Collin 1994). As the disorder progresses, the amount of medication needed increases; this means that more side-effects are evident – and so the vicious circle continues.

The community nurse plays an important part in the life of the patient with Parkinson's disease, providing research-based knowledge of the condition and education on how best to cope with manifestations before they arise. She can also obtain specialist advice and treatment for the patient when appropriate and provide continuity of care, coordinating the various aspects of treatment given by the multidisciplinary team (Livesy 1992).

Many people with PD are turning to aromatherapy to try to lessen the side-effects from their medication: at worst they find their condition remains unchanged; at best they find their mobility increased, their pain decreased and, due to the relaxing properties of the oils selected, they are less tense and anxious and sleeping much better. Also, many side-effects such as constipation can be helped by essential oils (see Box 10.1).

SUMMARY

Conditions which come under primary health care can benefit from aromatherapy, giving the opportunity to reduce side-effects, afford better lives by stress reduction, raise the immune system and above all, lead to a more active life in the community. NHS costs can be cut as a bonus. One of the most rewarding aspects of working with aromatherapy in primary care is that apart from the actual intervention it affords an excellent opportunity for promoting health and well-being to patients.

References

Alexander M 2001 Aromatherapy and immunity: how the use of essential oil aids immune potentiality in four parts. International Journal of Aromatherapy 11(2): 61–66

Ball J 1990 Understanding disease. Blackdown, Devon, p. 189

Baly M E, Robottom B, Clark J M 1987 District nursing. Heinemann Nursing, London, p. 227

Bennett G 1992 Handbook of clinical dietetics. Matthew Price, Stratford-on-Avon

Bricklin P M 1983 Working with parents of learning disabilities/gifted children. In: Fox L H, Tobin D (eds) Learning disabled/gifted children; identification and programming (pp. 243–260). Austin, TX; PRO-ED

Caelli M, Porteous J, Carson C F, Heller R, Riley T V 2000 Tea tree oil as an alternative topical decolonization agent for methicillin-resistant *Staphylococcus aureus*. Journal of Hospital Infection 46: 236–237

Carson C F, Riley T V 1995 Antimicrobial activity of the major components of the essential oil of *Melaleuca alternifolia*. Journal of Applied Microbiology 78(3): 264–269

Carson C F, Cookson B D, Farrelly H D, Riley T V 1995 Susceptibility of methicillin-resistant *Staphylococcus aureus* to the essential oil of *Melaleuca alternifolia*. Journal of Antimicrobial Chemotherapy 35: 421–424

Carson C F, Riley T V, Cookson D 1998 Efficacy and safety of tea tree oil as a topical antimicrobial agent. Journal of Hospital Infection 40: 175–178

Collin P H 1994 Dictionary of medicine. Harper Collins, Middlesex

Dhabhar F S 2000 Stress-induced augmentation of immune function – the role of stress hormones, leukocyte trafficking and cytokines. Brain Behaviour and Immunity 16: 785–306

Dhabhar F S, McEwen B S 1997 Acute stress enhances while chronic stress suppresses immune function in vivo: a potential for leukocyte trafficking. Brain, Behaviour and Immunity II: 286–306

Dixon M, Smith P 2004 Foreword in: Wilkinson J, Peters D, Donaldson J 2004 Clinical Governance for Complementary and Alternative Medicine in Primary Care. Final Report to the Department of Health and King's Fund. Available online cgcam-net@wmin.ac.uk

Doel M A, Segrott J 2003 Self, health and gender: complementary and alternative medicine in the British Mass Media. Gender, Place and Culture 10(2): 131–144

Doel M A, Segrott J 2004 Materializing complementary and alternative medicine: aromatherapy, chiropractic, and Chinese herbal medicine in the UK. Geoforum 35: 727–738

Donald R 1996 Multiple sclerosis; case study. Aromatherapy World. Seeding (Spring): 33–35

Douglas M 1996 The choice between gross and spiritual: some medical preferences. In: Thoughts and styles: critical essays on good taste. Sage, London, pp. 21–49

Encyclopaedia Britannica 1996 Chronic fatigue syndrome (CD ROM)

Ernst E, Abbot N C 1998 Funding complementary medicine research is a 'catch 22' situation. International Journal of Alternative and Complementary Medicine 16(7): 11–13

Franchomme P, Pénoël D 2001 Aromathérapie Exactement. Jollois, Limoges, p. 421

Guenier J 1992 Essential oil obstetrics. International Journal of Aromatherapy 4(1): 6–8

Gillam, S 1999 Trust in the future. Nursing Times 95(13): 57–58

Horrigan C 2004 Aromatherapy in the management and treating of rheumatoid and muscular skeletal autoimmune disorders. International Journal of Aromatherapy 14(3): 110–118

Hulmston N 1995 Case studies: multiple sclerosis. International Journal of Aromatherapy 7(2): 30/31

Irwin M, 2002 Effects of sleep loss on immunity and cytokines. Brain, Behaviour and Immunity 16(5): 503–512

Labrecque M, Marcaux S, Pinarlt J J, Laroche C, Martin S 1994 Prevention of perineal trauma by perineal massage during pregnancy. A pilot study. Birth 21(1): 20–25

Lis-Balchin M 1999 Possible health and safety problems in the use of novel plant essential oils and extracts in aromatherapy. Journal of the Royal Society for the Promotion of Health 119(4): 240–242

Livesy P 1992 Providing a source of support. Nursing Times 88(29): 26–30

Lunny V N 1997 Aromatherapy in the management of multiple sclerosis. Positive Health, March/April

Marieb E N 2001 Human anatomy and physiology, 5th edn. Addison Wesley Longman, California

Mills S Y 1991 The essential book of herbal medicine. Penguin Arkana, London, p. 297

Moudachirou S, Yayi E, Chalchat J-C, Lartigue C 1999 Chemical features of some essential oils of *Ocimum basilicum* L. Journal of Essential Oil Research 11: 779–782

Mutch F 1997 Case studies: multiple sclerosis. International Journal of Aromatherapy 5(2): 40/41

O' Dowd A 1999 New dawn for nurse power. Nursing Times 95(13): 24–25

Opalchenova G, Obrashka N 2003 Comparative studies on the activities of basil – an essential oil from *Ocimum basilicum* L – against multidrug resistant clinical isolates of the genera *Staphylococcus, Enterococcus* and *Pseudomonas* by using different test methods. Journal of Microbiological Methods 54: 105–110

Parry W R 1997 Parkinson's disease. SUR in English (newspaper for Southern Spain)

Pénoël D 1992 Eucalyptus smithii. Lecture notes for Shirley Price International College of Aromatherapy

Price L 1990 Clinical practitioner aromatherapy course notes. Shirley Price Aromatherapy

Price S 1993 Parkinson's disease project. The Aromatherapist 1: 14–21

Price S 2000a Aromatherapy workbook, 2nd edn. Thorsons, London, pp. 233–234

Price S 2000b Aromatherapy and your emotions. Thorsons, London (second edition to be published by Riverhead, Stratford on Avon in 2006)

Price S 2001 Aromatherapy for women. Lorenz Books, New York, pp. 39–41

Price P, Price S 2004 Aromatherapy for babies & children 2nd edn. Riverhead, Stratford-on-Avon

Primary Care Nursing 1997 Nursing opportunities in primary health care. Department of Health, London

Scott A 1998 Homeopathy as a feminist form of medicine. Sociology of Health and Illness 20: 191–214

Seaward B L 2000 Stress and human spirituality 2000: at the crossroads of physics and metaphysics. Applied Psychophysiology and Biofeedback 25(4): 241–246

Shahverdi A R, Fazali M R, Rafii F, Kakavand M, Jamalifar H, Hamedi J 2003 Inhibition of nitrofurantoin reduction by menthol leads to enhanced antimicrobial activity. Journal of Chemotherapy 15(5): 449–453

Shahverdi A R, Rafii F, Tavassoli F, Bagheri M, Attar F, Ghahraman A 2004 Piperitone from *Mentha longifolia* var chorodiatya Rech. F reduces the nitrofurantoin resistance of strains of enterobacteriaceae. Phytotherapy Research 18(11): 911–914

Shahverdi A R et al 2004 Enhancement of antimicrobial activity of furazolidone and nitrofurantoin against clinical isolates of *Enterobacteriaceae* by piperitone. The International Journal of Aromatherapy 14: 77–80

Smith K, Dickson M, Sheaff R 1999 Second among equals. Nursing Times 95(13): 54–55

Soliman K M, Badeaa R I 2002 Effect of oil extracted from some medicinal plants on different mycotoxigenic fungi. Food Chemistry Toxicology Nov 40(11): 1669–1675

Soulsby Report 1998. House of Lords Select Committee on Science & Technology 7th Report. HMSO, London

Swank R L, Dugan B B 1990 The effect of a low saturated fat diet in early and late cases of multiple sclerosis. The Lancet 336(8706): 37–39

Swank R L 1991 Multiple scelorosis: fat–oil relationship. Nutrition 7(5): 368–376

Thomas K J, Coleman P, Nicholl J P 2003 Trends in access to complementary or alternative medicines via primary care in England: 1995–2001. Family Practice 20(5): 575–577

Tisserand R, Balacs T 2002 Essential oil safety: a guide for professionals. Churchill Livingstone, Edinburgh

Watson S 1997 The effects of massage: an holistic approach to care. Nursing Standard 11(47): 45–47

WHO 1978 Declaration of Alma Ata. World Health Organization, Geneva

Wilkie D J, Kampbell J, Cutshall S 2000 Effects of massage on pain intensity, analgesics and quality of life in patients with cancer pain: a pilot study of a randomised controlled trial conducted within a hospice care delivery. Hospice Journal 15: 31–52

Wilkinson J, Peters D, Donaldson J 2004 Clinical Governance for Complementary and Alternative Medicine in Primary Care. Final Report to the Department of Health and King's Fund. Available online cgcam-net@wmin.ac.uk

Wingate P, Wingate R 1996 Medical Encyclopedia, 4th edn. Penguin, Middlesex

Yokoyama M M 2002 Psychoneuroimmunological benefits of aromatherapy. International Journal of Aromatherapy 12(2): 77–82

Sources

Baylac S, Racine P 2004 Inhibition of human leucocyte elastase by natural fragrant extracts of aromatic plants. International Journal of Aromatherapy 14: 179–182

Complementary Medicine 2000 Information pack for Primary Care Groups

DoH 2001 A health service of all the talents developing the NHS workforce – consultation document on the review of workforce planning – results of consultation. DoH, London

Hawkley L C, Capioppo T J 2004 Stress and the aging immune system. Brain, Behaviour and Immunity 18: 114–118

Hori Y, Ibuki T, Hosokawa T, Tanaka Y 2003 The effects of neurosurgical stress on peripheral lymphocyte subpopulations. Journal of Clinical Anaesthesia 15: 1–8

Steele PJ 1998 Profiles of essential oils: a comprehensive reference manual for professional aromatherapists. Ausmed, Adamstown

Chapter 11

Stress, including critical care

Penny Price

INTRODUCTION

This chapter examines the phenomenon of stress in modern life and the natural therapies used to combat it. The role of essential oils in hospital and clinical settings is explored and case studies are given to show how essential oils can be used to beneficial effect.

The chapter also shows the fundamental value of essential oils in intensive care settings and gives examples of their use in different situations. A guide to selection and blending combinations for the relief of stress in all the above situations is given with examples.

The chapter then draws together many referenced applications and ideas to give a wider understanding of the treatment of stress.

DEFINITION

Much research has been conducted into stress over the last hundred years. Some of the theories behind it are now settled and accepted; others are still being researched and debated. During this time, there seems to have been something approaching open warfare between competing theories and definitions. Views have been passionately held and aggressively defended, and what complicates the situation is that intuitively everyone feels that they know what stress is, as it is something all have experienced. A definition should therefore be obvious . . . except that it is not.

The most commonly accepted definition of stress (mainly attributed to Richard S Lazarus (1998)) is that 'Stress is a condition or feeling experienced when a person perceives that demands exceed the personal and social resources the individual is able to mobilize.'

In the last few years the word stress has almost become synonymous with substandard health, assuming such significance that it has now been adopted as a medical term. A recent definition of stress is given by Wingate & Wingate (1996) as: 'Any influence which disturbs the natural balance of a person's body or mind', including 'physical injury, disease, deprivation and emotional disturbance'.

Hans Selye was one of the founding fathers of stress research. His view in 1956 was that 'stress is not necessarily something bad – it all depends on how you take it. The stress of exhilarating, creative successful work is beneficial, while that of failure, humiliation or rejection is detrimental.' Selye believed that the biochemical effects of stress would be experienced irrespective of whether the situation was positive or negative. Since then, a great deal of further research has been conducted, and ideas have moved on. Stress is now viewed as a 'bad thing', with a range of harmful biochemical and long-term effects. These effects have rarely been observed in positive situations.

RESPONSE TO STRESS

According to Selye (1956) there are three stages in the development of the body's response to stress:

1. The initial direct effect of the body exposed to a stressor, bringing about the alarm stage, where:
   - a temporary cessation of digestive juices occurs
   - the respiratory and heart rates increase

   - extra oxygen is transported to the brain and the muscles (in preparation for strenuous action or emotional strength)
   - energy is released quickly from stored fats and sugars
   - extra adrenalin is produced
   - the immune system shuts down.
2. The resistant stage is where the extra oxygen, energy and adrenalin are brought into action to enable the body to cope with this unacceptable situation (expected to be temporary). With isolated occurrences the body is able to rid itself of the stress and the body functions return to normal. However, in the absence of help in or release from the situation, the responses in stage 1 above are continuous and the body tries to adapt itself to the stressor in an effort to reach a balanced state. If the level of stress is prolonged or becomes chronic and is allowed to continue without help, the body reaches the third stage (below).
3. Exhaustion, with reversion to the alarm stage, resulting inevitably in eventual health problems. These may manifest as headaches, inability to sleep, digestive problems, skin disorders, susceptibility to infections, etc. owing to the closing down of the immune responses.

BREAKDOWN

Early on in stage 3, people may become irritable, even aggressive, critical, restless, inefficient, withdrawn, moody and with an uncontrollable urge to cry at the least setback. They may find that coffee, cigarettes or alcohol give temporary relief to their mental stress, or they may take tranquillizing medication, any of which may eventually add to their discomfort.

The combination of several ongoing stressors can result in a nervous breakdown, or what is sometimes termed 'burnout'. The nervous system, influenced so strongly by the mind, is unable to cope, and lethargy, inactivity, apathy and indifference set in. In this state, almost a 'waking coma', nothing seems possible to the sufferer, i.e. there is a breakdown in nervous energy. As the English philosopher John Locke (1632–1704) put it (at the end of the 17th century): 'Though the faculties of the mind are improved by exercise, yet they must not be put to a stress beyond their strength' (Woodhouse 2004).

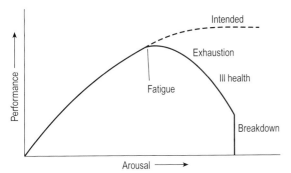

Figure 11.1 The effect of stress on performance.

It is important to be able to recognize the danger signals and find a natural method of combating them, so that severe consequences can be avoided. Figure 11.1 illustrates the relationship of stress to performance: when stress goes beyond a certain level, fatigue sets in and the performance level drops.

A great deal of time and energy is spent on physical fitness but very little effort is put into mental and emotional fitness. There is little doubt that mental and emotional health go hand in hand with certain attitudes to life. People who are happy-go-lucky remain mentally and physically fitter than those who are negative or who have too much stress in their lives to cope with rationally. Lack of stress can be defined as 'a proper emotional balance whereby a full range of responses can be expressed according to the situation – neither too dramatically nor too grudgingly' (Stoppard 1988 p. 73). A person with little stress has a sense of realism about the standards that should be set for oneself, an awareness of strong and weak points and a certain understanding of other people and their reactions to different situations. Dealing with stress means being prepared to take on responsibility for one's own life rather than blaming other people or events.

MODERN LIFE

In all walks of life in the 21st century stress has become a problem. Some years ago, according to O'Hanlon (1998) an estimated 40 million working days were lost each year in the UK as a result of stress; related problems account for more than 6 out of 10 visits to doctors' surgeries.

Stress is an important factor for all health professionals to recognize, both within themselves and in their patients/clients, as the commonly held belief is that emotional and physical stress may eventually lead to emotional and physical dysfunction (disease).

In an attempt to identify and treat stress, health care practitioners need to be able to recognize the symptoms. Since almost everyone suffers from some sort of stress, discernment and discretion are paramount, as most people do not discuss medical stress comfortably. At a common sense level most people would define stress as a 'feeling' which is provoked by any situation which is too much for the person to cope with (Baly, Robottom & Clark 1987 p. 41). However, stress is much more complex than this 'feeling': it is essentially being out of control of your own personal situation, relationships and work environments. During periods of stress, emotions seem out of proportion to what situations warrant, whether uncontrollable, inappropriate or rigidly controlled.

Left untreated, stress can lead to self-destructive or harmful behaviour towards others. Stress related disease is not only on the increase (Seaward 2000), but it has a pathogenic effect on immune function (Hori et al 2003), appearing to exert an effect on the immune system similar to ageing (Hawkley & Capioppo 2004).

FIGHT AND FLIGHT – GOOD OR BAD?

Some of the early research on stress established the existence of the well-known 'fight-or-flight' response. This work showed that when an organism experiences a shock or perceives a threat, it quickly releases hormones that help it to survive.

In humans, as in other animals, these hormones help us to run faster and fight harder. They increase heart rate and blood pressure, delivering more oxygen and blood sugar to power important muscles. They increase sweating in an effort to cool these muscles and help them stay efficient. They divert blood away from the skin to the core of our bodies, reducing blood loss if we are damaged. As well as this, these hormones focus our attention on the threat, to the exclusion of everything else. All of this significantly improves our ability to survive life-threatening events. However, not only life-threatening events trigger

---

Case study 11.1 Severe stress – A de Vos – *aromatherapist, UK*

Client assessment

Sarah, 39, a registered nurse, was recommended by her chiropractor to try aromatherapy for her severe stress. Sarah works full time as a nurse in a palliative care unit. She has two children and her husband was diagnosed with cancer 12 months previously. She was run down and suffered from indigestion, occasional headaches, lack of sleep and neck and shoulder pain.

Intervention

After a holistic assessment, the following essential oils were chosen:

- *Chamaemelum nobile* [Roman chamomile] – antispasmodic, calming and sedative, digestive
- *Citrus aurantium* v. amara (flos) [neroli] – antidepressive, calming, neurotonic
- *Juniperus communis* fruct [juniper] – analgesic, digestive tonic, soporific
- *Lavandula angustifolia* [lavender] – analgesic, antiinflammatory, neurotonic
- *Rosmarinus officinalis* [rosemary] – analgesic, antiinflammatory, carminative, digestive, neurotonic, stimulant to adrenal cortex

She was not sure about using essential oils at home, but made another appointment for a full-body massage.

Outcome

On the second visit, Sarah reported having had a more restful sleep pattern for a few days following treatment – and as she decided she would like to try something at home, she was given 50 ml of base lotion containing 5 drops each of the above oils to rub into her neck and shoulders every night and a dropper bottle containing the same essential oils to use in the bath.

On the third visit, she reported feeling a great deal better and much more relaxed. She was coping better at home and had had fewer digestive problems.

As Sarah recognized the need for relaxation to help with her physical as well as her emotional problems, she decided to continue the aromatherapy treatments as well as treating herself at home.

(Taken from The Aromatherapist 7: 1)

---

this reaction: we experience it almost any time we come across something unexpected or something that frustrates our goals. When the threat is small, our response is small and we often do not notice it among the many other distractions of a stressful situation.

Unfortunately, this mobilization of the body for survival also has negative consequences. In this state, we are excitable, anxious, jumpy and irritable. This actually reduces our ability to work effectively with other people. With trembling and a pounding heart, we can find it difficult to execute precise, controlled skills. The intensity of our focus on survival interferes with our ability to make fine judgments by drawing information from many sources. We find ourselves more accident-prone and less able to make good decisions (http://www.mindtools.com/pages/article).

There is no doubt that much stress today is due to the modern society in which we live – city and motorway driving, environmental pollution,

divorce (which completely changes the traditional form of family life), unemployment, the threat of being mugged or burgled, flying, hospitalization – the list is endless.

HOSPITALIZATION

For many, this is the most stressful thing that could happen to them (Jamison, Parris & Maxon 1987). In hospital, patients lose their identity and become a number, exchanging their daily attire for nightwear and taking on a new role as a 'condition' in a bed (Buckle 1997 p. 165). Even though frequent nursing reassurances may prevent intimidation by the high-tech environment, their state of mind can be calmed further by the use of essential oils (Mullen 2005 personal communication). Stress connected with hospitals is not confined to those who enter as patients, because they are tended by nurses and doctors who themselves are under stress. Aromatherapists working in hospitals often have to treat the staff to help relieve the pressures they are under. Tysoe (2000) conducted a study in three parts to discover the effect on staff of essential oil burners in extended care settings. A questionnaire covering a period of 1 month was followed by a second questionnaire after using lavender oil in burners for a 3-month period. A significant number of respondents (88%) indicated in the first questionnaire their belief that the use of essential oil would have a positive effect on the workplace. Doctors in particular are often unduly stressed, by the very nature and responsibility of the work they do; GPs are no exception. However, some do not give themselves the treatment they prescribe for their patients, often turning to alcoholism and drug abuse, which are both on the increase in the medical profession (Bennett 1987).

The emotions associated with stress can include deep anxiety, depression, desolation, grief, heartache, pain and mental torment. There are various forms and degrees of stress, defined only by each individual's ability to cope with a specific situation. These are normally categorized as belonging to one of two groups – positive and negative stress. Both of these involve a response by the body to internal or external demands made upon it.

Case study 11.2 Drug–induced psychosis – K Stockbridge – *aromatherapist, UK*

Client assessment
Gilly, an 18-year-old girl, was admitted (under Section 3 of the Mental Health Act 1983) to a locked psychiatric ward, due to drug-induced psychosis with schizophrenic symptoms – hearing voices and visual hallucinations.

She had started smoking cannabis at the age of 13 and took Ecstasy from the age of 15. At 17, she began to feel 'out of control' and had a breakdown – being later admitted. Before her admission she had been sleeping on the streets.

When she was referred to the therapist she had been moved to an open ward and was now feeling embarrassed by her earlier behaviour, guilty, ashamed and depressed. She was still feeling anxious and scared of the psychotic symptoms. She was physically run down, had patches of eczema on her face, feet and hands and was suffering from hay fever, PMT and headaches.

Medication – chlopromaxine (antipsychotic drug).

Intervention
The essential oils were selected basically for her depression and anxiety, choosing from these those which would also help some of her symptoms – and boost her self-esteem. Cicatrizant properties are reputed to help heal guilt, while neurotonic and stimulant properties are said to help boost self-esteem:

- 1 drop *Chamaemelum nobile* [Roman chamomile] – antiinflammatory, antispasmodic, calming, cicatrizant, menstrual, stimulant, vulnerary
- 1 drop *Pelargonium graveolens* [geranium] – analgesic, antiinflammatory, antispasmodic, cicatrizant (also to guilt), relaxant
- 1 drop *Rosa damascena* [rose otto] – antiinflammatory, cicatrizant, general tonic, neurotonic
- 1 drop *Salvia sclarea* [clary] – antispasmodic, decongestant, hormonelike, neurotonic

On the first visit Gilly was given a back and shoulder massage, which she enjoyed.

Five days later she had a full-body massage, as she felt more confident about the therapist.

A month went by before the therapist could treat Gilly again, as she had obtained some illicit drugs and become psychotic again.

At this treatment, a hand massage was added to the treatment, as the eczema had cleared.

Treatments were continued on a weekly basis for several months.

Outcome
After her second treatment, Gilly said how relaxed she felt – and her period pains had eased.

After 2 months, she was waiting for Social Services to find accommodation for her. The therapist continued to treat her until she was well enough to be discharged – and for a limited period afterwards, while she settled into the community under the guidance of a Community Mental Health Care Team.

Orthodox medicine offers symptom relief, invariably involving the use of drugs to counteract insomnia, antidepressants for feelings of sadness and/or tiredness and advice that the patient should change his/her diet, take more exercise or even change their lives.

GENERAL COMPLEMENTARY TREATMENT

Of the numerous ways of reducing stress, employing complementary techniques, the following are the most frequently practised in hospitals in the UK and USA:

- **Relaxation.** The Northern View Day Hospital in Bradford has successfully used muscle relaxation techniques combined with a self-hypnosis tape and relaxing music to reduce levels of stress in the elderly (Harrison & Skinner 1992).
- **Counselling.**
- **Reflexology and/or Swiss reflex massage.**
- **Massage (without essential oils).**
- **Therapeutic touch, or the laying on of hands.** This is massage by another name to circumvent some State regulations in America (see Ch. 17) and is used by nurses belonging to the American Holistic Nurses Association as well as by many nurses in the UK (Krieger 1979).
- **Hydrotherapy (often followed by massage).**
- **Laughter.** Worwood (1990) and many others advise patients to laugh as much as possible since it boosts the endorphin level and makes them feel good. Several hospitals in the United States take the physiological effects of laughter so seriously that they have dedicated 'laughter rooms' for patients. Michigan psychologist Zajonc maintains that even fake smiling triggers a reaction in the brain, making a patient feel better (cited in Price 2000b).
- **Essential oils.** A large number of essential oils are stress reducing and to this end can be used independently on a paper tissue, in the bath and in a vaporizer. Also, the effects of massage are enhanced when essential oils are added to the basic massage oil, as discovered by Passant (1990). Patients who have experienced aromatherapy have reported its beneficial

effects in aiding relaxation and reducing stress and anxiety. Sleep patterns have also improved dramatically for those patients who had previously experienced sleep difficulties, as Cannard (1994) found in his trial on elderly people in hospital.

AROMATIC TREATMENT

The main function of aromatherapy as introduced in the 1960s, i.e. with obligatory massage, was to relieve stress. In the beginning, aromatherapists were taught to concentrate only on stress relief, so that the body's own healing mechanism would be enabled to alleviate symptoms brought on by the stress, such as migraines, menstrual problems, eczema, etc. Aromatherapy as practised today combines several aspects of healing which are mutually enhancing. Time is spent observing and listening to the patients, who often unburden themselves of their problems when encouraged by a skilful listener. Simple dietary advice is offered, such as cutting out coffee, tea and caffeinated soft drinks, and relaxing tapes have been introduced by some into their treatments.

CHILDHOOD STRESS

Ill effects due to stress can begin in early childhood, so every client/patient, regardless of age, must be assessed in an endeavour to identify it.

Aromatic medicine, with all its diversity, is an excellent aid toward a peaceful and contented mind-state. Price & Price (2004) state the uses of essential oils for childhood depression and distress, highlighting the fact that the sense of smell, although second to the sense of sight, has always played an important part in the emotional development of the human race.

They go on to say that children can detect articles of clothing that belong to their mother, their father or their siblings. Often when trying to calm a young child at night time, if a parent's garment is put in the cot, the child will snuggle into the garment and feel the closeness of that particular parent. Aromatherapy can also be used to help to develop children's smell receptors to great benefit (Price & Price 2004 p. 12), so that aromas used as above can also be used to put the child at ease with babysitters, childminders, in unfamiliar surroundings and so on.

Infants build up an attachment to 'comfort' objects for the consolation and security they provide. When they are older they verbalize their desire: 'I want to get the smell right' said a 2-year-old boy when asked why he held his teddy bear so close to his nose. The familiar smell of security objects apparently serves as a substitute odour when a loved one is not present (Schleidt 1992 p. 43).

QUIET PLACE

This is a project carried out in a Liverpool primary school which has had a dramatic effect on stressed pupils. The children are reported to love their Quiet Place and there have been great beneficial effects on children with emotional and behavioural difficulties (Wallace 2000).

The Quiet Place has counselling, massage, aromatherapy, therapeutic play and storytelling, as well as music workshops. While different aspects of the room reach different children (and parents), it appears to be the room and its basic aroma that affects the children's behaviour. Spalding (of Liverpool University), measured the children's emotional growth and behavioural disturbance levels and found that Quiet Place children were four or five times better off than an equivalent control group where there had been no emotional interaction.

Odours are as effective at the group level as they are at the individual level. It is not surprising that in deep-rooted human behaviour, our emotional and phylo-genetic sense of smell comes into play. In mammals the smell of the group signals familiarity and security and the same is true for human beings (Schleidt 1992 p. 45).

ADULT STRESS

It must be realized that all human beings require security and a sense of belonging to the wider social framework around them, even from baby-hood, and those who are cognizant of this become more useful to those around and become less prejudicial to those whom it is thought 'should not' suffer from stress. Treatment from an early age is important. An insecure baby will make an insecure child – then adult, if steps are not taken to change the course of emotional behaviour.

Aromatic therapists can take heart and have pride in the fact that the tools of their trade, essential oils, have been well-researched to prove that they are beneficial to the human psyche. Stress can be a learned behavioural pattern, but aromatic treatments can break into that circle to create new learned patterns of calm. This simple fact has been proved by Dr Betts who says that smell responses can be learned to help or enhance a present experience.

Betts (1994) used olfaction to control arousal symptoms in epileptic seizures, not only in those who experienced olfactory auras, but in any patient who had an aura long enough to give them time to apply a countermeasure before a major seizure started. Betts says that using the auto-hypnotic technique it is possible to train the patient to associate intense relaxation with the smell of the oil (see Ch. 8).

MOOD CHANGES

Jellinek & Jellinek (1997 p. 216) cites a study by Warren et al to show that the responses to odour do not have to be taught – the chemical properties of the essential oil have certain psychological effect. In the study 36 test subjects conducted a performance test of 40 minutes duration in which they were exposed to certain optical stimuli and had to react to critical signs by pressing a key. The participants wore masks and were periodically given administrations of peppermint odour, lily of the valley odour, or pure air. In independent tests peppermint had been established as stimulating and lily of the valley as relaxing. The authors' hypothesis was that the stimulating odour would positively affect performance and that the relaxing odour would reduce tension and the feeling of stress. The authors further agreed that stimulating odours might also reduce stress by increasing alertness and the subject's ability to master the task.

After 7 years of experience with the psychological measurement of mood in relation to aroma, Warren & Warrenburg (1993 p. 12) make the following observations:

- Fragrance evoked mood changes are small, but beneficial to our well-being.
- Fragrance can be used to reduce the stress response in humans, but its physiological effects on a non-stressed subject are minimal and difficult to measure.
- Measurement of fragrance-evoked mood changes by psychological methods is feasible and yields intriguing results.

That stress can be dissipated by aroma is clearly demonstrated by Schiffman:

Fragrances may be used to cope with stressful situations throughout the lifespan. Clinical and laboratory studies have shown that certain smells enhance relaxation and reduce stress.

Van Toller & Dodd (1992 p. 57)

CONDITIONING

Personal experience shows that many people experience stress relief when they inhale, or apply a blend of oils that remain the same over a period of time. This is partly due to the creation of a conditioned response – repeated use of a particular aroma for a particular condition will, over a period of time, produce the required response. This is called a 'conditioned reflex' and is used by health professionals the world over. However, it is not a special technique to learn this behavioural response – parents use it every day when putting their children to bed; the same bath routine, a story, a drink, then sleep!

Following the prescriptive theme, Schnaubelt (1998 p.103) says that nervousness, tension and stress call for the sedative qualities of aldehydes, the diverse action of ester compounds on the nervous system and the sympatholytic (calming, dilation of blood vessels) effects of some phenylpropanes (found in oils such as aniseed and fennel). This may mean that essential oils such as *Citrus aurantium* var. *amara* per. [petitgrain], *Citrus bergamia* [bergamot], *Litsea cubeba* [may chang] and *Melissa officinalis* [melissa] (among others rich in at least two of these chemical groups) would suffice to relieve tension and he advocates the neat application of these oils to the temples every day. Interestingly, Schnaubelt is one of the few who do advocate this method of use, the majority claiming inhalation as the most

beneficial route. However, if chemical groups are to be investigated, it would be prudent to include ketones as a possible aid to relieving stress, as they are known to be calming and sedative.

DRUG ALTERNATIVES

In conventional treatment, patients with anxiety who visit their GPs are often prescribed tranquillizers. The effects of these drugs are to repress the individual because the drugs are designed to slow down the body. Gascoigne quotes the figure of 8.5 million prescriptions for anti-stress/depression in the UK in 1989 (1994 p. 360). He goes on to state that the prescriptions given are based on the belief that stress and/or depressive illness is caused by a chemical imbalance in the brain. The difficulty facing the GP in prescribing is that there is no way of determining which chemicals are in imbalance other than by trial and error in the administration of drugs, although the level of thyroxine being produced is now a standard test.

The rationale seems to be that if the thought processes are slowed down then life is easier to cope with. From observation of those who have been treated in this way it seems that it leads to depression born out of the inability to live life from day to day because they lack motivation. Rather than use essential oils to depress the system, it would probably be better to use those oils which are known to be stimulating and invigorating.

Battaglia (2003 p. 481) tells us that aromatherapy provides a valuable alternative to psychotropic drugs and muscle relaxants, which are commonly used in treating anxiety allopathically. He particularly emphasizes the importance of *Ocimum basilicum* [basil], remarking that due to its methyl ether content it soothes, calms and relaxes and is recommended for people with schizoid tendencies. Mojay (1996) says the following:

lavender and melissa both cool the heart and are among the most comforting oils for the mind . . . best employed for anxiety in those who feel oppressed and suffocated.

The claim is also made that geranium oil calms the nervous system and that vetivert restores a sense of stability in those that are anxious.

In 1923, two Italian doctors, Giovanni Gatti and Renato Cayola, published the results of their research into the psychotherapeutic effects of essential oils. This was one of the first tests of this nature to be carried out, and the findings were published in an article entitled 'The Action of Essences on the Nervous System'. In the article, the doctors specifically discuss the possibilities of applying sedative and stimulating plant essences to relieve, respectively, anxiety and depression. Gatti and Cayola did not actually treat or experiment on people suffering from these psychological states; instead they set out to identify sedative or stimulating essences by measuring pulse rate and cardiovascular and respiratory activity before and after the inhalation of each essence. The doctors' recommended oils for anxiety were listed as neroli, petitgrain, cedarwood, chamomile, melissa and valerian (Damien & Damien 1995 p. 150). As is the case with much research, no Latin names are mentioned and therefore some assumptions have to be made regarding the true identification of the essential oils mentioned.

Paolo Rovesti, in the 1970s, practised aromatherapy to treat stress and psychological distress using inhalation techniques. He preferred to use blends rather than single essential oils, thus introducing many variables into his research. For anxiety Rovesti listed petitgrain and neroli with bergamot, cypress, lavender, lime, marjoram, rose and violet leaf (Damien & Damien 1995 p.151).

LIFTING DEPRESSION

There are also essential oils that have been singled out empirically for their effects on the human psyche, such as *Boswellia carteri* [frankincense]. Frankincense has, among its physical properties, the ability to slow down and deepen the breath (Lawless, 1992 p. 99) and others have recognized that it is good for nervous depression (see Appendix A(II)).

Historically, *Melissa officinalis* [melissa] has been used for the longest time as a treatment for depression – Paraclesus calling it the 'elixir of life'. Culpeper said that it 'driveth away all troublesome cares and thoughts out of the mind'. Lawless (1995 p. 173) suggests that on an emotional level melissa is outstanding, having traditionally been

used as a tonic for the heart and a remedy for the 'distressed spirit.' She goes on to say that the oil acts on the vital centre and helps balance delicate or vacillating emotions, which would fit with Schnaubelt's theory that aldehydes are essential for psychological health and well-being, since melissa oil contains around 70% aldehydes (mainly citral).

There are certainly situations in which the following oils may be of use in lifting depression:

- *Eucalyptus staigeriana* [lemon scented iron bark]. Of all the eucalyptus family, *E. staigeriana* appears to have the most profound effect on the emotional level. It is uplifting, antidepressive and has been used extensively in the treatment of ME. The high levels of aldehydes (21–37%) means that although the oil is non-toxic, it can be a mild skin irritant, especially if used neat (there are no reported incidents of such however).
- *Ocimum basilicum* var. *album* [European basil]. Lawless (1992 p. 54) gives basil as an excellent – perhaps the best – aromatic nerve tonic, saying that it clears the head, relieves intellectual fatigue, and gives the mind strength and clarity. This labiate is a popular herb in cooking and has been used widely in all the different medical traditions from antiquity. It is reputed that the phenol content of the oil (eugenol 1–19%) provides the kick-start to the nervous system, although no serious research into this has been published: because the linalool content is relatively high (40–55%), the oil is safe to use.
- *Thymus vulgaris* ct. thymol. Thyme helps to revive and strengthen both body and mind. The phenol (thymol) constituent level stands at 60–80% – but without the balancing alcohols to temper the effect on the skin. When blended with *Ocimum basilicum* [European basil], whose uplifting alcohols complement the stimulating phenols, the resulting blend makes it most effective in the treatment of depressive conditions.

CHOICE OF ESSENTIAL OILS FOR THE EMOTIONS

There are many oils that purport to alleviate stresses and strains: some are from the depths of

Case study 11.3 Stress and depression – P Price – *aromatologist, UK*

Client assessment

Mrs S, who is 48 years old, has a large family and her own business. Although a fair amount of her stress is positive, she had to invest a lot of energy and time into her work. This meant that home life became more of a chore.

She felt tired 'all the time' and did not sleep well – she would fall asleep easily, but the quality was not good. Her nights were disturbed by vivid dreams (she described them as being technicolour, like the movies). Sometimes the dreams were nightmares, in which her business was failing.

Mrs S was losing weight (unnoticed, as it had been taking place over a long time). She suffered from severe headaches, dizziness, disorientation and weepiness. Her whole body ached and as each situation was talked through it became clear that the client was indeed suffering from severe stress and depression.

Intervention

Before selecting the essential oils, time was spent helping the client to re-evaluate and prioritize the daily routines – at home and at work. Unimportant tasks were to be delegated or dismissed. Advice was offered on her eating habits, and she was persuaded to set aside one afternoon a week for leisure. The aim was then to help her to relax, lower her mental stress, have a better quality of sleep and uplift and energize her.

The regime of treatments selected began with a full-body massage once a week. After 1 week the client reported that she felt less stressed, but found it difficult to keep to the lifestyle changes. However, after the third week, the client was noticeably less stressed and looked younger in the face.

Massage treatments every week were not possible for her as she became stressed with the length of time they took from her working day, so she was introduced to Swiss reflex massage, which she enjoyed and found that she could fit the self-treatment in every evening.

With the aims above in mind, equal proportions of the following essential oils were selected for her treatment, in a 5% dilution with hypericum:

- *Melissa officinalis* [melissa] – antidepressant, calming and sedative, choleretic, digestive, tonic
- *Ocimum basilicum* [basil] – digestive tonic, liver stimulant, nervous system regulator, neurotonic
- *Salvia sclarea* [clary] – neurotonic
- *Helichrysum italicum* [everlasting] – hepatic, neurotonic
- *Hypericum perforatum* [St. John's wort, macerated] – said to have antidepressant properties.

The self-treatment was as follows:

- Application – the above essential oils were blended in a 5% dilution with hypericum, which Mrs S was to apply to her neck, shoulders and solar plexus three times a day.
- Bath – the same essential oils were blended in a dropper bottle for use in the bath (10 drops). The client had a bath every morning before work and was encouraged now to spend at least 20 minutes in it so that the oils could penetrate effectively.
- A third dropper bottle was prepared with basil and clary in equal proportions for her to keep in her handbag and for inhalation on a handkerchief or tissue at times of stress or panic.

Outcome

With the self-help treatments and the essential oils, Mrs S began to improve and after 3 months was looking fitter and putting on a little weight.

After 4 months, the self-treatment was reduced to applying the oil blend after the morning bath and reducing the dose of essential oils in the bath to 4 drops.

Rose hydrolat was given to her to drink (a tablespoonful in warm water) at bedtime. She was very grateful and stated that she had not felt so invigorated for a long time. She slowly changed her lifestyle patterns, which she feels she could not have done without the essential oil treatments.

history; some from modern research; some are known by personal experience. The link between the olfactory system and the psyche cannot be underestimated and because of this, it is fairly obvious that pleasant smells will lift the spirit and cheer the soul. 'As far back as ancient Greece . . . aroma was known to have an effect on the psyche' (Lee & Lee 1992).

Odours – and the emotions they produce – are very basic and unforgettable – they are also very difficult to describe. This 'aroma–emotion' reaction appears to take place at a deep level and we are not always conscious of it (see Ch. 8). This places emphasis on the fact that the client should like the smell or have a positive attitude towards it. If the client/patient is not happy with the aroma that has been blended, then every effort should be made to improve it so that the client receives the full psychological benefit from the treatment.

During an aromatherapy treatment, the recipient will be experiencing touch, smell, sound and vision – four of the five senses.

HOLISTIC ESSENTIAL OIL CHOICES FOR BOTH ANXIETY AND DEPRESSION

Up to four different essential oils could be required to treat stress holistically, as their synergy will enhance the total effect. When treating a patient or client holistically, a list should be made first of all essential oils which will benefit anxiety or depression (see Appendix A(II)) – whichever of these is the patient's basic problem. Should any other physical or emotional states also need to be addressed, check if they match any already on the list.

The following oils are balancing for both anxiety and depression and are taken from Aromatherapy and your Emotions (Price 2000b) and L'aromathérapie Exactement (Franchomme & Pénoël (2001):

- *Chamaemelum nobile* [Roman chamomile] – headaches, insomnia, indigestion, irritability, muscle tension
- *Citrus aurantium* var. *amara* (flos) [neroli bigarade] – agitation, insomnia
- *Citrus bergamia* (per.) [bergamot] – agitation, insomnia, indigestion, irritability
- *Lavandula angustifolia* [lavender] – agitation,

headaches, hypertension, insomnia, irritability, muscle tension
- *Lavandula* x *intermedia* 'Super' [lavandin] – agitation, headaches, hypertension, muscle tension
- *Origanum majorana* [sweet marjoram] – agitation, headaches, hypertension, insomnia, indigestion, irritability, muscle tension
- *Pelargonium graveolens* [geranium] – agitation, headaches, irritability, low immunity.

Having selected the required essential oil/s, it is advisable and time saving to make up the blend in a dropper bottle, which should be labelled and used in the method thought most appropriate (see Ch. 5). For stress, the relative proportions of essential oils should be influenced by the aroma preferences of the patient concerned.

Practical example

The method of selecting and combining essential oils described above is illustrated by the following example:

- **Depression, with headaches and insomnia:** *Chamaemelum nobile, Lavandula angustifolia* and *Origanum majorana*. If the immune system is felt to be low, *O. majorana* should be present in the highest proportion in the mix. Should the aroma need adjusting for the client, select any other essential oil from the antidepressive range above or the fuller list in Appendix A(II).
- **Anxiety with agitation, and high blood pressure:** *L. angustifolia* and *O. majorana*.
- **Anxiety with agitation, indigestion and muscle tension:** *L angustifolia* and *O. majorana*.

Should a third oil be desired, one may be selected for whichever symptom is strongest. Consult Appendix A(II) for other symptoms which can be helped with the same oils as those helping to reduce stress or lift depression.

STRESS IN CRITICAL CARE

Many factors need to be addressed when looking after a patient in critical care, including the severe stress experienced by patients and relatives, to say nothing of the possibility of further invasive infections, both of which will respond to essential oils, with or without aromatherapy massage.

However, it is difficult to talk generally about the use of aromatherapy in critical care, simply because the reasons for needing it are many and often sudden, e.g. breathing difficulties, lung viruses (see Case study 11.4), strokes, heart attacks, heart surgery, road accidents, etc.

EFFECT OF SURROUNDINGS

Four decades ago Meyer, Blacher & Brown (1961) suggested that being in a critical care unit (CCU) could be a depersonalizing experience, leading to demotivation, apathy and withdrawal. This is not necessarily true today because the level of attention and expertise given nowadays in most CCUs makes this unlikely. Nevertheless, the acute emotional and psychological trauma patients still endure in a strange and unfamiliar place (often without their loved ones beside them) can leave them with an intense feeling of loneliness and isolation. The CCU can still be a hostile environment to patients who are surrounded by a bewildering array of monitoring and support equipment and subjected to a variety of invasive therapeutic techniques (Waldman et al 1993).

It has been found that a nurse who is able to take the time to touch patients in critical care – holding their hand, even without talking, could establish in a relatively short time an empathetic relationship with them (McCorkle 1974).

In addition, essential oils with and without massage are used generally in critical care units throughout the UK for relaxation, comfort and well-being: massage of even just the feet having been shown to have beneficial effects (Hayes & Cox 2000).

Touch is a very important part of care for any patient, particularly those in critical care. However, massage with or without the use of essential oils would need careful consideration for those patients needing a high level of intensive care, as it could be catastrophic if used inappropriately (Shepherd 2005 personal communication).

LEVELS OF CARE

There has been very little research done in the ICU in relation to aromatherapy over recent years. In some way, this may be due to changes in the way acutely ill patients are treated. In 2000, the Department of Health published the document 'Comprehensive Critical Care', which outlined 'levels' of care for acutely ill patients, grading them from level 0 to level 3.

Most area hospitals have their own codes for levels of care in CCUs; those quoted below are the Department of Health levels 1–3, those in brackets being the level numbers and nurse/patient ratios used at the Royal Liverpool University Hospital.

- Level 3 – (level 4, high critical care patient – 1.5:1 nurse ratio): ICU patients are now classified as level 3 patients and are usually the most acutely ill, with multiple organ failure; they are mechanically ventilated and often receiving potent cardiovascular drugs; they may also need renal dialysis and multiple inotropic support (to maintain heart, circulation function); such patients are severely ill.
- Level 2 – (level 3, average critical care patient – 1:1 nurse ratio): Other, less complicated patients, who would previously have been cared for in ICUs are now classified as level 2 patients and are placed in high dependency units rather than intensive care. Hence, the term intensive care has given way to a more appropriate term – 'critical care patients/units'. Such patients require mechanical ventilation to maintain oxygen levels and function. They will have arterial and central line catheters and multiple infusions, and are usually sedated, fed intravenously and unable to communicate – although some patients will tolerate ventilation and therefore sedation may be reduced. These patients are usually on extensive drug therapy and may have multi-organ failure or sepsis.
- Level 1 – (level 2 – low intensive care/high dependency – 0.5:1 nurse ratio). Patients may be breathing spontaneously and exuberated but need an oxygen mask or CPAP machine to maintain oxygen levels. They may also have a central IV/peripheral line and multiple infusions. Such patients would need very close monitoring and help in caring for themselves. However, they can be helped to wean from a ventilator and remain calm and relaxed by an aromatherapy massage.
- Level 0 – (level 1 – generally ward level care is 0.3:1 nurse ratio). For such patients, aromatherapy would be permitted.

Therefore, while there is a place for aromatherapy with level 0 and 1 (1 and 2) patients, it is not appropriate for level 2 or 3 (3 or 4) patients; complementary therapies in general are not used on these patients. There are exceptions of course and each patient is assessed individually hour by hour. Patients would need to be assessed by a competent nurse/aromatherapist before *any* therapy is given and the patient's consultant must be in agreement (Shepherd 2005 personal communication).

USE OF AROMATHERAPY

Most recorded uses of aromatherapy in critical care are concerned with heart surgery, where the overriding concern of the aromatherapist is patient stress. 'Anxiety can precipitate life-

---

Case study 11.4 Lung virus – E Sonn – *aromatherapist, UK*

Client assessment

The therapist's father, normally fit and healthy, was taken seriously ill overnight with an unknown lung virus. He was rushed to hospital, put on a life support machine and the family was told it was only a matter of time!

After 3 days the therapist realized that if the hospital would allow it, she might be able to help. The consultant was approached to ask if the hospital would allow her to try an aromatherapy intervention. The consultant agreed that she could do whatever was needed.

Intervention

Two drops each of the following essential oils were used in a teaspoonful of grapeseed oil:

- *Eucalyptus globulus* [blue gum] – antiinfectious, antiinflammatory, antiviral, decongestant, expectorant, mucolytic
- *Styrax benzoin* [benzoin] – antiinflammatory, expectorant, sedative, cicatrizant
- *Melaleuca alternifolia* [tea tree] – antiinfectious, antiviral, immunostimulant, neurotonic

This blend was used for the first 2 days for his lung congestion, rubbing it on to his chest at every available time the life support equipment would allow.

The reflex points on his feet were massaged frequently, using Swiss reflex method and the same oils at 20% in a base cream, concentrating mainly on the lung and lymph areas. This was accompanied by gentle music to help relax the mind and balance the emotions. Peace and a wonderful aroma emanated from the room.

The therapist's mother, who was suffering from aching legs, emotional exhaustion and stress, did not go unprotected either. She received a massage using grapeseed carrier oil with two drops each of:

- *Lavandula angustifolia* [lavender] – analgesic, calming and sedative
- *Origanum majorana* [marjoram] – analgesic, calming, neurotonic
- *Rosa damascena* [rose otto] – calming, neurotonic

These three oils are also recommended for apprehension, dread and panic (Price 2000b).

A mix of Bach flower remedies were taken also.

The therapist continued to massage her father in the intensive therapy unit at every available time.

Outcome

X-rays taken on the 4th day showed a slight improvement. The doctors and nursing staff were impressed, and such was their interest that their support increased – along with their curiosity regarding aromatherapy.

Two days later, the following oil was added to help normalize the fluctuating blood pressure:

- *Hyssopus officinalis* [hyssop] – antiinfectious, hypertensor, tonic for general debility

One week later the consultant said that although her father would survive, the oxygen level had to be down to 35% before they could remove him from the life support machine, and this would be a critical phase of his recovery. It could take up to a couple of weeks and at this stage there was a possibility that he would react with panic, fear and irritability.

Case study 11.4 Lung virus – E Sonn – *aromatherapist, UK* (cont'd)

The benzoin and hyssop were replaced at this point with:

- *Rosmarinus officinalis* [rosemary] – mental stimulant (also strengthens the mind and helps relieve fear; Price 2000b)
- *Salvia sclarea* [clary] – neurotonic, (calming to the nervous system)
- Bach flower 'Rescue Remedy' was used between his lips

Outcome

Within 2 hours of being able to be removed from the machine the therapist's father was sitting up and

the medical staff remarked at his speedy recovery. He was removed from the intensive therapy unit within 24 hours and was home within a fortnight, although the prediction had been 8–10 weeks. Once home the massage with essential oils, Swiss reflex treatment and music were gradually stopped. Within 3 months her father was once more to be seen playing golf and swimming a couple of times a week, none the worse for his traumatic experience.

---

threatening arrhythmia and extend infarction areas, if not allayed quickly enough' (Harris 1993). Patients' anxieties have been found to be centred on their personal illness rather than on the hospital surroundings (Herxheimer et al 2000), and though frequent nursing reassurances may prevent intimidation by the high-tech environment, essential oils can calm their state of mind still further.

There may be a role for relatives of critically ill patients to utilize essential oils and aromatherapy to help them cope with their stress as this is a huge crisis in their lives (Green 2005 personal communication).

ESSENTIAL OIL CHOICE

The following essential oils contain sedative properties suitable for use in critical or coronary care:

- all citrus oils – *Citrus aurantium* var. *amara* (flos, fol. and per. [neroli, petitgrain, bitter orange], *Citrus bergamia* [bergamot], *Citrus limon* [lemon] and *Citrus reticulata* [mandarin] – calming and/or sedative in various degrees
- *Chamaemelum nobile* [Roman chamomile] – sedative
- *Melissa officinalis* [melissa] – sedative
- *Commiphora myrrha* [myrrh] – sedative, cardiotonic
- *Lavandula angustifolia* [lavender] – calming and sedative.

INHALATION

Inhalation is a non-intrusive way of using essential oils in critical care, where the interaction between the molecules and the receptors in the central nervous system is responsible for the sedation caused by inhaling the fragrant molecules (Buchbauer & Jirovetz 1994) and there is no need for physical contact with the patient. The higher the level of intensive care needed, the more should inhalation be the method chosen for aromatherapy care – if intervention is permitted at all.

The sedative influence of lavender has been shown by many early research works and was confirmed by Karamat et al in 1992; similarly anxiety and fear can be masked by orange (Lehrner et al 2000). Miyake, Nakagawa & Asakura (1991) found that inhalation of bitter orange oil increased sleeping time significantly under conditions of mental stress. Sugano & Sato (1991) discovered that lavender, orange and rose countered the effects of stress. The authors are concerned that only common names are given for the oils used in most research studies and trials, especially when there are so many varieties for instance, of 'chamomile', 'eucalyptus' and 'lavender'. Full botanical and analytical identification is essential if such trials are to be taken seriously.

MASSAGE

Massage should not be given to level 3 or 4 patients (see above), as it could possibly

Box 11.1   Royal Shrewsbury Hospital: Inhalation

This study was undertaken to try and discover the effectiveness of essential oils in reducing the anxiety level of patients admitted to the coronary care unit – and afterwards in the post-coronary care ward.

Intervention
The method used was inhalation of plant oils from an electric vaporizer over a 4 week period, results being obtained by questionnaire.

Patients were monitored on admission, 12 hours later, and then prior to discharge to the post-coronary care ward.

There were four groups of five people, three of which were given a single essential oil chosen from lavender, ylang ylang and the absolute of jasmine respectively (no botanical names given), the fourth, a control group, inhaling water vapour only.

Results
Of the 14 people receiving essential oils who returned the questionnaire, 71.4% in groups 1–3 experienced a reduction in anxiety and 25% of the control group. All patients inhaling essential oils showed a lowering of blood pressure from their initial admission levels and within 12 hours of the study.

Harris contends that: 'though a significant drop in blood pressure was noted on the majority of patients, this could not be wholly attributed to the inhalation of essential oils'. However, even with such small groups, the results appear to show that some benefit was gained.

(Harris 1993)

endanger those under heavy sedation or on ventilator machines. Massage of the hands or feet is the least intrusive if wishing to use this method when helping to wean people off a ventilator.

RESEARCH TRIALS AND STUDIES

Several trials and studies have been carried out to evaluate the effectiveness of essential oils and massage in the nursing care of patients in critical care units:

- Royal Shrewsbury Hospital (Harris 1993) – inhalation – Box 11.1
- Royal Sussex County Hospital (Woolfson & Hewitt 1992) and Middlesex Hospital, London (Stevensen 1994) – both involving massage of the feet – Box 11.2
- Battle Hospital, Reading (Dunn, Sleep & Collett 1995) – massage on various parts of the body (back, outside of limbs, scalp) – Box 11.3.

TREATMENT OF SEVERE BURNS

Although essential oils have been used with success on severe burns in University College Hospital in 1988, there is no protocol for this – they were used by a consultant who, because he found nothing orthodox to be effective, wished to try the efficacy of essential oils, even though he was made aware that there was no scientific evidence. He said 'what they offer me has been researched – but does nothing; what you have given me has not been researched – yet it works. It is that which interests me!' (Parkhouse 1988 personal communication). However, most critical care units would not allow this *without* researched evidence, of which there is still none, 18 years later. This is a great pity, as the cicatrizant properties of certain essential oils are very powerful, e.g.:

- *Boswellia carteri* [frankincense] – scars, wounds
- *Helichrysium italicum* [everlasting] – burns, open wounds, scars, skin regeneration
- *Lavandula angustifolia* [lavender] – burns, scars, wounds
- *Pelargonium graveolens* [geranium] – burns, wounds.

Two useful oils to vaporize in a burns ward to keep the air antiseptic are:

- *Citrus limon* [lemon]
- *Pinus sylvestris* [pine].

Box 11.2   Royal Sussex County and Middlesex Hospitals: Foot massage

The following trials were set up to see if foot massage with essential oils could lower the blood pressure, heart and respiratory rates of people in critical care.

Royal Sussex Hospital

Intervention
Lavender (botanical name not given) was used.

Two treatments a week were given to three groups of 12 patients each for 5 weeks, observations being recorded at the beginning, end and 30 minutes after each session:

- Group 1: 20 minute massage using lavender in a vegetable oil
- Group 2: 20 minute massage using only vegetable oil
- Group 3: 20 minute undisturbed rest period only

Results
The results showed a consistent decrease in blood pressure, heart rate, pain, respiratory rate and wakefulness in all three groups, the greatest benefits being experienced by group 1, especially in the reduction of the heart and respiratory rates:

Heart rate: group 1 – 11/12 (91.6%); group 2 – 7/12 (58.3%); group 3 – 5/12 (41.6%)

Respiratory rate: group 1 – 9/12 (75%); group 2 – 5/12 (41.6%); group 3 – 16.6%

(Woolfson & Hewitt 1992)

Middlesex Hospital, London

Intervention
Each of the four groups of cardiac patients in critical care was assessed physiologically for heart rate, respiratory rate and blood pressure and psychologically for pain, anxiety, tension before the intervention and 5 days afterwards. Assessments were made of all patients both before and after each session:

- Group 1: 20 minute standardized foot massage
- Group 2: as above, using only apricot oil
- Group 3: 20 minute conversation with a nurse – no tactile input or formal counselling
- Group 4: 20 minute period with routine care – no intervention of any kind

The feet of patients in groups 1 and 2 were massaged once a day, using 2.5% *Citrus aurantium var. aurantium* (flos) [neroli bigarade], chosen for its calming, antispasmodic, antidepressant and gentle sedative actions – in apricot kernel vegetable oil.

Results
Immediately after the intervention, both the respiratory rate and the psychological (pain and anxiety) results showed statistically significant reduction differences between groups 1 and 2 and the control groups 3 and 4.

Even though no difference was seen physiologically at the next measurement period, groups 1 and 2 had statistically significantly better psychological results than the control groups, 3 and 4 at the end of day 5.

(Stevensen 1994)

Conclusion
These two trials show that although massage alone is beneficial, the greatest benefits in all areas tested were achieved when essential oils were used.

SUMMARY

This chapter has examined the phenomenon of stress in modern life, and the role essential oils can play in reducing its effects. A trial project (Gonella 1993), unpublished, clearly demonstrates that massage with essential oils can significantly reduce stress levels in the patients of GPs. The guide presented here to the selection and combination of stress-reducing oils is intended to enable readers to choose and administer appropriate oils for their patients, with a view to achieving similarly beneficial results.

The case studies and trials presented in this chapter clearly demonstrate the efficacy of essential oils in significantly reducing stress levels both in and out of hospital.

Nurses currently using aromatherapy in the critical care units will have little doubt in their minds that it can help relieve some of the stress related to the intensive treatments and procedures their patients are, of necessity, subjected to. It is

Box 11.3   Battle Hospital, Reading: Massage of parts of the body

The following study was carried out to evaluate the effectiveness of aromatherapy and massage in the nursing care of patients in critical care, the protocol being approved by the Research and Ethics committee for the West Berkshire Health District.

Three groups were each given a different treatment: Group 1 receiving a light massage on areas of the body available to the therapist – back, outside of limbs, scalp – using grapeseed oil alone; the same carrier but with the addition of 1% of *Lavandula vera* [lavender] essential oil was used on Group 2 and Group 3 were left to rest for half a hour, with no massage being given. Areas assessed were:

- Behavioural – categorized into a four-point scale
- Physiological – systolic and diastolic blood pressure, heart rate and rhythm, respiratory rates
- Psychological – also using a four-point scale for patients to self-assess their level of anxiety, mood and ability to cope with the present situation.

Results

These showed that the use of essential oils with massage proved to be more effective than massage and rest alone in reducing anxiety.

(Dunn, Sleep & Collett 1995)

important, however, to ensure that we are not so enamoured by aromatherapy that we do not see the potential problems.

Cornock (1998) suggests that . . . 'by being aware of what the patient finds stressful . . . '

(nurses) can, with thought and imagination, find ways to reduce the stressful nature of many of the stressors identified. This in turn may also reduce the stress for nurses because they are actively helping their patients.'

References

Baly M E, Robottom B, Clark J M 1987 District Nursing. Heinemann, London

Battaglia S 2003 The complete guide to aromatherapy, 2nd edn. The International Centre of Holistic Aromatherapy, Australia, p. 481

Bennett G 1987 The wound and the doctor. Secker & Warburg, London

Betts T 1994 Sniffing the breeze. Aromatherapy Quarterly 40 (spring): 19–22

Buchbauer G, Jirovetz L 1994 Aromatherapy – use of fragrances and essential oils as medicaments. Flavour and Fragrance Journal 9: 217–222

Buckle J 1997 Clinical aromatherapy in nursing. Arnold, London

Cannard S 1994 On the scent of a good night's sleep. Trial project. Midland Health Board News January: 3

Cornock M 1998 Stress and the intensive care patient; perceptions of patients and nurses. Journal of Advanced Nursing 27: 518–527

Damien P, Damien K 1995 Aromatherapy scent and psyche: using essential oils for physical and emotional well-being. Healing Arts Press, Rochester, Vermont, p. 150

DoH 2000 Comprehensive critical care: a review of adult critical care services (25 May 2000). Department of Health, London

Dunn C, Sleep J, Collett D 1995 Sensing an improvement: an experimental study to evaluate the use of aromatherapy, massage and periods of rest in an intensive care unit. Journal of Advanced Nursing 21: 34–40

Franchomme P, Pénoël D 2001 L'aromatherapie exactement 2nd edn. Jollois, Limoges

Gascoigne S 1994 The manual of conventional medicine for alternative practitioners: volume II. Jigme Press, Surrey

Gonella 1993 Unpublished work

Harris C M 1993 Is there a benefit to patients in using aromatherapy oils in a coronary care unit? Pilot study results (copies available from The Royal Shrewsbury Hospital)

Harrison L, Skinner R 1992 Relax for health. Nursing Times 88(49): 46–47

Hawkley L C, Capioppo T J 2004 Stress and the aging immune system. Brain, Behaviour and Immunity. 18: 114–118

Hayes J A, Cox C L 2000 Immediate effects of a foot massage in intensive care. Complementary Therapies in Nursing and Midwifery 6(1): 9

Herxheimer A et al 2000 Database of patients' experiences (DIPEx): a multi-media approach to sharing experiences and information. The Lancet 355: 1540–1543

Hori Y, Ibuki T, Hosokawa T, Tanaka Y 2003 The effects of neurosurgical stress on peripheral lymphocyte subpopulations. Journal of Clinical Anaesthesia. 15: 1–8

Jamison R N, Parris W C V, Maxon W S 1987 Psychological factors influencing recovery from outpatient surgery. Behaviour Research Therapy 25: 31–37

Jellinek P, Jellinek J S (eds) (1997) The psychological basis of perfumery. Chapman and Hall, London, p. 216

Karamat E, Ilmberger J, Buchbauer G, Roblhuber K, Rupp C 1992 Excitatory and sedative effects of essential oils on human reaction time performance. Chemical Senses 17: 847

Krieger D 1979 The therapeutic touch. Simon & Schuster, New York

Lawless J 1992 The encyclopaedia of essential oils. Element, Dorset, p. 99

Lawless J 1995 The illustrated encyclopaedia of essential oils. Element, Dorset, p. 178

Lazarus R S 1998 Stress and emotion. Springer, New York

Lee W H, Lee L 1992 The book of practical aromatherapy. Keats, New Canaan CT, p. 125

Lehrner J, Eckersberger C, Walla P, Potsch G, Deeke L 2000 Ambient odour of orange in a dental office reduces anxiety and improves mood in female patients. Physiology and Behaviour 71: 83–86

McCorkle R 1974 Effects of touch on seriously ill people. Nursing Research 23(2): 125

Meyer B C, Blacher R S, Brown F 1961 A clinical study of psychiatric and psychological aspects of mitral surgery. Psychosmatic Medicine 23(3): 194–218

Miyake Y, Nakagawa M, Asakura Y 1991 Effects of odours on humans 1. Effects on sleep latency. Chemical Senses 16: 183

Mojay G 1996 Aromatherapy for healing the spirit. Gaia, London, p. 144

O'Hanlon B 1998 Stress – the common sense approach. Newleaf, New York

Passant H 1990 A holistic approach in the ward. Nursing Times 86(4): 26–28

Price S 2000a The aromatherapy workbook 2nd edn. Thorsons, London

Price S 2000b Aromatherapy and your emotions. Thorsons, London

Price P, Price S 2005 Aromatherapy for babies and children, 2nd edn. Riverhead, Stratford on Avon

Reed L, Norfolk L 1993 Aromatherapy in midwifery. Aromatherapy World (Nurturing, Summer issue): 12–15

Reed L, Norfolk L 1993 Aromatherapy in midwifery. Aromatherapy World (Nurturing, Summer issue): 12–15

Roulier G 1990 Les huiles essentielles pour votre santé. Dangles, St-Jean-de-Braye

Schleidt M 1992 The semiotic relevance of human olfaction: a biological approach, chapter 4. In: Van Toller S, Dodd G (eds) Fragrance: the psychology and biology of perfume. Elsevier Science, Essex

Schnaubelt K 1998 Advanced aromatherapy: the science of essential oil therapy. Healing Arts Press, Rochester, Vermont, p. 103

Seaward B L 2000 Stress and human spirituality 2000: at the crossroads of physics and metaphysics. Applied Psychophysiology and Biofeedback. 25(4): 241–246

Selye H 1956 The stress of life. McGraw Hill, New York

Stevensen C J 1994 Psychophysical effects of aromatherapy massage following cardiac surgery. Complementary therapies in Medicine 2: 27–35

Stoppard M 1988 Every woman's life guide: how to achieve and maintain fitness: health and happiness in today's world. Dorling Kindersley, London, p. 73

Sugano H, Sato N 1991 Psychophysiological studies of fragrance. Chemical Senses 16: 183–184

Tysoe P 2000 The effects on staff of emotional oil burners in extended care settings. International Journal of Nursing Practice (April): 110–112

Van Toller S, Dodd G (eds) 1992 Fragrance: the psychology and biology of perfume. Elsevier, Barking, Essex

Waldman C S, Tseng P, Meulman P, Whitter H B 1993 Aromatherapy in the intensive care unit. Care of the Critically Ill 9(4): 170–174

Wallace W 2000 The gentle touch. Times Educational Supplement 21st January

Warren C, Warrenburg S 1993 Mood benefits of fragrance. The International Journal of Aromatherapy 12: 5(2): 12–16

Wingate P, Wingate R 1996 Medical encyclopedia. Penguin, London.

Woodhouse K 2004. In: Crome L, Ghodse H, Gilvarry E, McArdle P (eds) Young people and substance misuse. Royal College of Psychiatrists, London

Woolfson A, Hewitt D 1992 Intensive aroma care. International Journal of Aromatherapy 4(2): 12–13

Worwood V 1990 Fragrant pharmacy. Macmillan, London, p. 109

www.mindtools.com/pages/article

Chapter 12

Pregnancy and childbirth

Denise Tiran and Shirley Price

INTRODUCTION

Expectant mothers have always been discouraged from using allopathic drugs to treat the symptoms of pregnancy because of the potential adverse effects on the foetus, and some complementary therapies offer a gentler means of achieving optimum well-being during the antenatal period and labour. Reports also indicate an increasing interest among maternity professionals, possibly in response to women's requests, and midwives, obstetricians, GPs and health visitors have found a need to update their knowledge in order to answer questions and provide authoritative advice on complementary therapies.

The use of aromatherapy during pregnancy and childbirth has gained enormous popularity in the last decade and many midwives now incorporate it into their care of women (Ager 2002, Burns et al 1999).

One survey (NHS Confederation 1997) suggested that at least 34% of midwives used one or more complementary therapies in their work, the most notable of which was aromatherapy, as it is easily combined with conventional midwifery practice – especially in the one-to-one situation of labour and delivery care. Aromatherapy and massage offer a pleasant means of returning to the nurturing aspect of caring for essentially well women during pregnancy and labour and enable midwives, partners or birth companions such as aromatherapists to provide more holistic care.

ETHICO-LEGAL AND EDUCATIONAL ASPECTS OF AROMATHERAPY IN MATERNITY

Although 21st century maternity policy emphasizes continuity of care for women, this does not necessarily imply that aromatherapy should be provided only by the midwife responsible for the mother's care. A cooperative team of experienced professional midwives and aromatherapists can enhance the well-being of the mother and add to her overall pleasure and achievement. However, in order to protect the mother and baby, UK law forbids anyone other than a midwife or doctor, or one of these in training under supervision, from taking sole responsibility for the care of an expectant or labouring mother, except in an emergency.

This means that any aromatherapist who is not also a midwife must liaise with the maternity care team and remember that any treatment with essential oils is complementary to normal antenatal, intrapartum or postnatal care, from confirmation of conception until 28 days after delivery, when the legal period of midwifery care comes to an end. Although the majority of aromatherapists work with many aspects of health, giving holistic and individualized care to all clients, there is an argument for specialization within aromatherapy in order to be fully aware of all relevant issues for a particular client group, especially with increasing integration into the NHS. It is vital that an aromatherapist wishing to specialize in maternity care has not only undertaken an aromatherapy course recognized by a leading aromatherapy body, but has also undertaken extra professional education to ensure that she has a thorough working knowledge of pregnancy physiopathology. It is also important that she acknowledge the limits

of her personal practice within the conventional maternity services, and if accompanying a mother for a hospital-based birth, she may be required to produce evidence of adequate personal professional indemnity insurance cover.

Permission will need to be given for the presence of an aromatherapist who is not employed by the Trust and paperwork regarding insurance and potential claims for negligent practice will need to be completed, as above. She will need to confirm her acknowledgement that the midwife and/or doctor retains responsibility in law for the mother's care. In the event of an emergency situation developing, particularly in labour, the aromatherapist must defer to the midwife and/or obstetrician and perhaps discontinue her treatment with essential oils until the emergency has been resolved – if this is considered by them to be in the best interests of the mother.

Comprehensive notes of any aromatherapy treatment must be maintained, but the aromatherapist will need to check with the individual Trust as to whether or not these should be incorporated into the normal maternity notes, or

---

Box 12.1   Issues to consider – physiopathological significance

Would you understand the obstetric significance of the following incidents? Would you know what to do and how it might affect your aromatherapy treatment?

1. An expectant mother coming for one of her regular aromatherapy relaxation massages who, at 32 weeks of pregnancy complains of frontal headache, sickness and blurred vision.
2. A casual question about the baby's movements leads to the 34-week pregnant mother telling you that her baby has been moving around 'even more than normal' for the last 24 hours.
3. A 37-week pregnant client arrives for her next aromatherapy appointment and tells you that she has had a vaginal blood loss the night before.
4. A woman who is 29 weeks pregnant returns to you for her second treatment and informs you that, since last week's session, she has had itching skin on her palms and abdomen.

kept separately. Most expectant mothers carry their own notes for the duration of the child-bearing episode and it may be permissible to add the aromatherapy records to these. However, if the aromatherapist keeps her own notes she should retain these for 25 years, in accordance with the Congenital Disabilities (Civil Liabilities) Act 1976, in case any legal claims for errors at birth are made by the child in the future. Conversely, mid-wives wishing to incorporate the use of essential oils and massage into their practice must be qualified in aromatherapy or be working under the guidance of an aromatherapist. Furthermore, aromatherapy is outside the normal scope of practice of midwives who are regulated by the Nursing and Midwifery Council, unless the necess-ary additional training has been undertaken, in which case, care must be based on current knowledge (NMC 2002a,b). This would ensure that they not only have a comprehensive working knowledge of any essential oils they intend to use, based on available contemporary research evi-dence, but they would be able to apply the aromatherapy theory to midwifery practice. It is not appropriate for midwives to advise women on the use of aromatherapy (or, indeed, any other complementary therapy) unless they have under-taken relevant accredited training to ensure that any information or care given is accurate, safe and up-to-date (NMC 2002a,b). Maternity services, whether NHS or private, usually have guidelines or protocols for practice and midwives must adhere to these, both within the hospital and in the community. Protocols, similar to 'standing orders' for the administration of drugs, may be devised to ensure best midwifery practice and for the protection of mothers and midwives (Tiran 2000). A record of aromatherapy treatment given by midwives trained in aromatherapy can usually be documented in the normal midwifery notes.

INSURANCE

Midwives should have personal professional indemnity insurance cover, although if permission to use aromatherapy within their midwifery prac-tice has been obtained from the employing authority it is usual for the Trust's vicarious liability insurance cover to apply. However, if they provide aromatherapy for mothers on a day when they are not working a midwifery shift, they should check with the local Trust as to whether additional aromatherapy insurance cover is required. Independent midwives are not bound by these protocols unless a woman in their care is transferred from home to hospital for manage-ment of complications, but they should refer to the relevant codes of conduct (see p. 343) to determine that their practice is in accordance with the parameters of midwifery practice. Midwives who have a private aromatherapy practice and wish to use their aromatherapy in the care of pregnant women, should notify the Local Supervising Authority of this intention.

SAFETY ISSUES

There is currently very little direct evidence for the safety of essential oils in pregnancy – and equally, there is a notable absence of any real proof to the contrary. Most antenatal aromatherapy is administered on the assumption that it is safe to use a limited number of essential oils, based on the anecdotal evidence from years of their use by pregnant women, both therapeutically and ingested in foods. There are several misconceptions about whether or not individual essential oils are safe and it is important to put facts and experience into perspective and use currently available knowledge, plus the increasing number of research findings which can be applied to pregnancy. How-ever, studies specifically related to the antenatal period tend to have been done on animals and cannot necessarily be applied to human pregnancy.

This could pose an ethical dilemma about whether or not essential oils should be used at all in pregnancy without sufficient proof – but randomized controlled studies on human preg-nancies are ethically impossible. It is interesting to note that, unlike drugs, essential oils are presumed safe until evidence of risk is available, yet drugs are required to undergo a specific series of tests before use to demonstrate – not that they are safe or effective – but that there is a lack of ill effects from the tests (unfortunately not always evident with hindsight). However, the increasing inte-gration of aromatherapy into maternity care suggests caution rather than complacency; in the event of a claim for negligence being brought, a court of law may consider any theoretical danger of antenatal use of a particular essential oil as being a contraindication to its use – although the dilutions and quantities used are minute compared with tests carried out for toxicity. Nevertheless, it should be standard practice that midwives or aromatherapists administering essential oils to pregnant and labouring women use only those which are considered to be relatively safe, given the dearth of specific proof. It is also fundamental to good practice that aromatherapy midwives and professional aromatherapists apply their knowledge of the chemistry of essential oils to the physiology and potential pathological complications of pregnancy.

There is a certain amount of disagreement amongst therapists and scientists regarding antenatal use of essential oils, but from a clinical perspective, if there is any doubt at all about the safety of any particular oil, given the limited amount of evidence, the aromatherapist should avoid using it when treating pregnant women. Lists of essential oils contraindicated in pregnancy differ from one authority to the next, which emphasizes the need for continual training to ensure that all aromatherapists are practising according to up-to-date information, whether based on experience or research.

Common sense is required to put the latest information and evidence into perspective in order to avoid making inappropriate clinical decisions. For example, where a single research study appears to indicate possible adverse effects in pregnancy, this should be borne in mind, but it should also be balanced against other evidence which may show successful effects. It should also be acknowledged that, while investigations into whole herbal medications may have some relevance to aromatherapy, they should not be taken as absolute, since essential oils are only one constituent of herbal remedies and may not necessarily be the causative constituent of potential dangers.

Many aromatherapists comply with what they are taught prior to registration, i.e. that they should not treat pregnant women 'at all', but this is possibly due to having taken a very short aromatherapy course – or one not recognized by one of the leading aromatherapy organizations –

and is therefore a result of lack of knowledge, confidence and experience – as is seen with the practice of other therapies such as reflexology (O'Hara 2002). An experienced aromatherapist who has the relevant training regarding maternity and aromatherapy can be invaluable in enhancing the care of pregnant and childbearing women. A few simple guidelines will encourage good practice (Box 12.2).

The National Institute for Clinical Excellence (NICE) Guideline on Antenatal Care: routine care of the healthy pregnant woman (2003), states that as there is insufficient evidence for either the safety or efficacy of complementary therapies they 'should be used as little as possible' during pregnancy. Although this is only a recommendation and does not constitute national policy on antenatal care, midwives will need to consider their intentions

---

Box 12.2   Guidelines for good practice when using essential oils for pregnant and childbearing women

- The use of aromatherapy during pregnancy, labour and the puerperium must be *complementary* to normal maternity care.
- Practitioners should have adequate and appropriate education in aromatherapy and pregnancy physiopathology in order to apply *both* theoretical disciplines to practice.
- Practice, where possible, should be based on latest available research evidence, if necessary applying generic principles to the specific area of maternity aromatherapy.
- Maternity–aromatherapy practitioners should limit the number of 'relatively safe' essential oils which they use, rather than administer a wide range for which there may be very little safety data.
- Oils should be administered in as low a dose as is required to obtain a therapeutic effect.
- The number of oils blended together should be kept to a minimum in order to be able to identify the culprit if side-effects occur.
- If there is any doubt regarding the safety of a specific essential oil, practitioners should avoid using it on pregnant women.

regarding aromatherapy use in pregnancy and whether or not they are prepared to defy the Guideline, especially as issues regarding the appropriateness of implementation may be raised by Trust managers keen to be seen to be complying with the NICE Guideline. (N.B. This does not apply to intrapartum or postpartum care, guidelines for which are currently being developed.)

Case in point

A midwife was appointed to implement aromatherapy into a maternity unit. Unfortunately, the midwifery manager who had appointed her left the Trust soon afterwards. Other managers were not as motivated nor as informed about aromatherapy as the previous manager and referred the midwife to the Trust Health and Safety (H&S) advisor, who was not a clinician. This person was aware of the NICE Guideline and also seemed to be under the misconception that aromatherapy *caused* miscarriage and stated that pregnant women would be required to sign a consent form for treatment which expressly stated this. Understandably the midwife was dismayed and concerned and went to great lengths to find research evidence to disabuse the H&S representative of this misinformed belief. She wrote unit policies to protect the women and her own practice, which were ultra-cautious in their parameters, including a stringent list of contraindications and precautions and an extremely limited selection of essential oils to be used. Eventually the H&S representative was satisfied sufficiently to allow the midwife to proceed for a specified time, during which she maintained statistics to present at the end of the trial period. To her relief, the midwife's hard work met with success and, together with positive evaluations from the mothers and staff she was then able to extend the service enough for it to become an integral component of midwifery care within the unit.

EMMENAGOGIC ESSENTIAL OIL USE

Many essential oils are considered to be emmenagogic, although this does not automatically lead to them being abortifacient. Where oils have been reported as causing spontaneous abortion, it has been as a result of ingesting quantities far, far higher (up to 20+ times the amount) than would normally be applied dermally in therapeutic aromatherapy, when maternal hepato- or renal toxicity is a far more likely primary outcome (Balacs 1992). Essential oils generally considered to be abortifacient (such as pennyroyal) are used only in extremely controlled circumstances – and never during pregnancy.

Little is known definitively about the effects on human pregnancy of emmenagogic oils, therefore it is wise to refrain from using them during pregnancy, especially during the first trimester, although they may be safe enough to use in labour, as they are known to stimulate uterine action. Although there is no conclusive evidence regarding the possibility of essential oils 'causing' miscarriage, women who suffer this distressing event tend to look for reasons and may blame their aromatherapy treatment for their loss. Certain individual constituents are claimed to stimulate uterine contractions, e.g. ketones, although this may be dependent on the isomer present in the individual oil (Tisserand & Balacs 1995, Watt personal communication 1996). However, it may be wise to refrain from using essential oils containing ketones, at least during the first trimester, when miscarriage is more common – and particularly in cases of women with a history of preterm labour.

POSSIBLE REACTIONS

ANAPHYLACTIC SHOCK

A few people are sensitive to and can experience anaphylactic shock from ingesting nuts; for example, about 1% of the population are allergic to the benzaldehyde in sweet almonds. Although there does not appear to be any evidence in the professional literature to advocate the avoidance of nut-based carrier oils such as sweet almond or peanut during antenatal aromatherapy or massage, it may be wise to enquire of the mother if she has a sensitivity in this respect. To avoid this uncommon problem altogether, oils derived from seeds or fruit flesh should be used.

BLOOD CLOTTING

The maternal blood clotting mechanism alters during pregnancy, particularly towards term in preparation for labour and the control of haemorrhage, so care should be taken in the last 4 weeks of pregnancy and the early puerperium with any essential oils thought to affect coagulation.

Although there is no research to this effect on the essential oil, it may be as well to avoid *Zingiber officinale* [ginger] during the last month, as this is when the mother's coagulation factors are changing as a prevention against haemorrhage and there is some suggestion that the herb, albeit in large doses, may trigger bleeding (Miller 1998).

BLOOD PRESSURE

Some essential oils are claimed to affect the blood pressure, either by raising or lowering it, although the research evidence is inconclusive. Oils such as lavender have been found to have a sedating effect (Buchbauer et al 1991, 1993; Buckle 1993) which may cause an indirect blood pressure response, but there appear to be very few studies which demonstrate true hypotensor effects, despite the presence of alcohols and sesquiterpenes. On the other hand, many aromatherapy texts continue to identify certain oils which may increase or decrease the blood pressure, suggesting that practitioners should adhere to these guidelines until further evidence is available. For example, oils considered to be hypertensors, e.g. *Pinus sylvestris* [pine] (for others see Appendix A(II)), are best not used on women with a history (in a present or previous pregnancy) of pre-eclampsia – or on those with pre-existing hypertension.

Oils which are thought to lower blood pressure, e.g. *Lavandula angustifolia* [lavender] and *Cananga odorata* [ylang ylang] (others in Appendix A(II)) should not be administered to mothers who suffer significant postural hypotension, fainting in pregnancy or are in labour with an epidural anaesthetic, as the drug used (bupivacaine, which also causes a reduction in blood pressure), may be potentiated by the essential oil. Postnatally, it may also be wise to refrain from using these oils on women who have had a postpartum haemorrhage since severe blood loss leads to a reduction in blood pressure.

DERMAL IRRITATION

Being aware of the essential oils likely to trigger dermal irritation, aromatherapists should carry out a patch test on mothers-to-be where such oils are wished to be used. Although there is no greater risk of skin problems occurring as a direct result of applying essential oils (unless the oils used are adulterated and therefore of inferior quality), therapists should not ignore maternal complaints of itching skin. Due to endocrine effects on bile salts, many women suffer skin irritation (commonly occurring on the abdomen) during pregnancy. Tea tree, which is very frequently adulterated, and has been shown to cause contact dermatitis (Southwell et al 1997), should be avoided – and if an alternative cannot be used it should be applied with care in very high dilution. However, if the mother suffers itching on the palms of the hands or soles of the feet, this could be due to cholestasis, a rare but serious hepatic complication of pregnancy. In this case, medical assistance should be sought immediately.

PHOTOSENSITIVITY

This is not normally a major problem in clinical aromatherapy as any ill effects are thought to be ineffective within 2 hours of administration (see Ch. 3 Part II), but extra care should be taken with pregnant women who have an increased production of melanocytic hormone. This may make them more prone to burning if a minimum waiting period of 2 hours is not observed before being exposed to direct sunlight after the application of certain essential oils (and expressed citrus essences) containing furanocoumarins, which are thought to trigger phototoxicity (Naganuma et al 1985) (see also Ch. 3 Part II). Although most women have a pronounced *linea nigra* in the midline of the abdomen, those who develop chloasma (the butterfly-shaped facial pigmentation of pregnancy) have higher circulating levels of melanocytic hormone and should not apply such oils to the skin on those parts of the body most likely to be exposed to the sun, such as the arms or legs. However, the majority of oils classified as potentially phototoxic tend to be the citrus essences which are otherwise considered relatively safe during pregnancy (see also Appendix B.7).

RUBEFACIENTS

Rubefacient essential oils, e.g. *Eucalyptus globulus* and *Pinus sylvestris* should be used with care during pregnancy as normal physiology causes an increase in maternal core temperature by approximately 1°C due to an increase in circulating blood volume. Although rubefacient oils do not necessarily have a systemic effect, local warming of the skin may make the mother feel uncomfortable.

TERATOGENIC EFFECTS

It is thought that many essential oil constituents are able to pass through the placental barrier and some may have teratogenic effects, although most accounts of possible adverse effects are from studies carried out on mice or rats which have been given systemically toxic doses, which cannot easily be applied to human pregnancy, especially as some studies investigate individual chemical constituents rather than whole essential oils. *Juniperus sabina* [savin oil – rarely, if ever, used], which contains sabinyl acetate, is thought to be abortifacient when administered to mice and rats; Pages et al (1996) investigated rats given *Eucalyptus globulus*, which also contains sabinyl acetate, and found no increased risk of mutagenicity.

Similarly, research on the embryotoxic effects of herbal remedies should not be assumed to apply to the use of essential oils in pregnancy, since whole plant remedies contain numerous other constituents which might affect the developing foetus. However, as with emmenagogic oils, care should be employed, especially during the first trimester when the major organs are being formed. Women are usually cognisant of the need to avoid any potentially noxious substances, including cigarettes, alcohol and drugs, but do not always view essential oils in the same light. This is of particular concern when they purchase poor quality essential oils or aromatherapy blends from popular high street stores and use them injudiciously at home, in the bath, in vaporizers and for self-massage.

CLINICAL USES OF AROMATHERAPY AND MASSAGE DURING PREGNANCY

The use of aromatherapy to relieve specific physiological disorders in pregnancy can also complement the fairly limited number of conventional options and offers mothers, midwives and aromatherapists additional tools at a time when orthodox medications are contraindicated. The selection of essential oils can only be made in conjunction with the individual mother and following assessment of her condition at the time of the treatment, therefore oils suggested below are only a guide. It is to be stressed however that pregnancy is a normal physiological phenomenon and the mother's body should be facilitated to do its own work where possible, thus care should be taken by aromatherapists who are not midwives to ensure that they do not inadvertently interfere with this process, for example, by attempting to use so-called 'hormone regulating' oils.

Although there is an increasing interest in the oral use of essential oils, this remains a controversial method of administration as yet, as insufficient data are available on the rate of and site of absorption within the gastrointestinal tract. In pregnancy, oral administration of essential oils is to be actively discouraged, except on the prescription of a medically qualified aromatherapist, as in France, or an aromatologist working with a medical practitioner, because endocrine effects on the gastrointestinal tract may alter their metabolism in ways as yet not understood.

It is most likely that a pregnant woman seeking aromatherapy and massage will consult a private aromatherapist unless she is lucky enough to be booked for the birth in a district which provides aromatherapy on the NHS, although even this is usually limited to those with the greatest need. Regular antenatal aromatherapy massage can be a very pleasant means of relaxing the mother, enhancing her well-being by aiding sleep and rest, easing physiological discomforts, facilitating foetal growth and giving the mother time for herself.

Massage during pregnancy, using the correct techniques, has been shown to decrease anxiety through a reduction in stress hormones such as cortisol and may contribute to a lower incidence of antenatal, intranatal and postpartum compli-cations (Field et al 1999). Massage enhanced by essential oils can be invaluable in treating conditions such as oedematous ankles, constipation, backache or headaches, relieving anxiety and depression or maintaining blood pressure at acceptable levels in women with a history of essential or pregnancy-induced hypertension. The positioning of the mother for massage should be taken into account prior to treatment, to avoid supine hypotension, especially in later pregnancy, and to prevent discomfort – as in the case of a full bladder.

Care should be taken with the type of massage, avoiding firm sacral massage on any woman with a history in a previous pregnancy of preterm labour, as inadvertent stimulation of the acu-puncture points in the intra-vertebral foramen may trigger uterine contractions. Additionally, there are certain points on the feet which should be avoided, for example, brisk massage of the area between the heel and the inner ankle is contra-indicated in early pregnancy as this is the reflexology zone for the uterus (O'Hara 2002).

For essential oils which are best not used until the last trimester, see Appendix B.2; absolutes, such as *Jasminum officinale* or *J. grandiflora* [jasmine] are not to be used either at this time because of the solvent residue – and the quality; most jasmine oils are hugely adulterated with synthetic jasmone, the component chiefly respon-sible for the well-loved aroma. Although rose otto, the distilled oil of *Rosa damascena* or *R. centifolia*, can be used during pregnancy, the absolutes, like that of jasmine, should not be used until the third trimester, because of the solvent residues which may be left in the end product.

N.B. Oils in Appendix B.3 should be used in low concentration as they may be too stimulating or have an adverse effect on the blood pressure.

USE OF ESSENTIAL OILS DURING PREGNANCY

BACKACHE AND SCIATICA

These two problems are related to the changes in posture as a pregnant woman adjusts to her increasing size and altered centre of gravity, leading to an increased lumbar lordosis. Lower back massage is not always appropriate or desired in pregnancy, although it will relieve the immediate discomfort. However, general back massage can be psychologically relaxing, indirectly influencing the mother's perception of pain and aiding physical muscle relaxation. If the mother is also suffering sciatica, with pain radiating down her legs, care should be taken not to over-stimulate the area, although the use of essential oils in compresses or in the bath if the mother can ease herself in, may be an effective compromise.

A selection of essential oils which will help, because of their analgesic and antiinflammatory properties include: *Boswellia carteri* [frankincense – an effective oil for emotional upsets too], *Coriandrum sativum* [coriander], *Eucalyptus citriodora* [lemon scented gum], *Ocimum basilicum* ct. alcohol [European basil – not exotic basil, whose main constituent is methyl chavicol] and *Pelargonium graveolens* [geranium], the last two perhaps being effective on sciatica – although nerves can be difficult to treat physically.

CARPAL TUNNEL SYNDROME

With this condition, the mother suffers wrist tingling and pain, as well as loss of coordination in her fingers due to oedema around the channel of nerves in the wrist – it can sometimes extend to the arm and shoulder. For these women, massage of the head, neck, shoulders, arms, hands and upper back can be enormously helpful using essential oils such as *Lavandula angustifolia* [lavender], *Boswellia carteri* [frankincense] or *Matricaria recutita* [German chamomile].

CONSTIPATION

This is a frequent feature of pregnancy due to the smooth muscle relaxation effect of progesterone and may be an increased problem in women with irritable bowel syndrome. The best advice is to encourage the mother to double her fluid intake and adapt her diet, although bran is not advo-cated unless she is drinking at least 2 litres of non-diuretic fluid daily. Very gentle abdominal massage (except in the first trimester), combined with suitable essential oils, may be sufficient to

Client assessment

At 28 weeks of pregnancy, B developed severe constipation, with abdominal discomfort, flatulence and nausea, to the extent that she was unable to empty her bowels fully for over 2 weeks. She was referred to the complementary therapy midwife who discussed her diet and fluid intake with her, suggesting that she might try eliminating wheat products for a while, as these are known to trigger gastrointestinal disturbances.

Intervention

At this stage of pregnancy it was not feasible to perform firm abdominal massage, so a 5-minute reflex massage was carried out, concentrating on the arches of the feet and palms of the hands. These areas were massaged firmly in a clockwise direction, using 5 ml of base cream to which were added:

■ 2 drops *Citrus reticulata* [mandarin] – digestive (eupeptic)

■ 2 drops *Citrus paradisi* [grapefruit] – digestive stimulant

Home treatment: The midwife made up a jar of cream with the relevant amounts of the two essential oils for the mother to massage her feet every day, and a small dropper bottle containing 2 ml each of the two essential oils with 4 ml carrier oil for her to use in the bath (10 drops).

The following week the treatment was repeated.

Results

By the third week the mother felt so much better (and had emptied her bowels completely on several occasions) that she cancelled the next appointment.

Her pregnancy progressed normally and she had no further constipation requiring midwifery intervention since she was able to treat herself should the problem recur.

stimulate peristalsis, or if the mother dislikes her abdomen being touched at this time, clockwise massage of the arches of the feet will have a similar effect, working on the reflex zones for the large intestines (see Swiss reflex treatment, Ch. 7). The essences of *Citrus aurantium* var. *amara* [bitter orange] and *Citrus reticulata* [mandarin] can be useful, perhaps combined with the essential oil of *Matricaria recutita* [German chamomile].

HAEMORRHOIDS

Haemorrhoids are an unpleasant form of progesterone-induced varicosities which may be externally protruding; the latter respond particularly well to the astringent properties of the essential oil of *Cupressus sempervirens* [cypress], in either a bath or bidet, applied topically as a compress or blended into a lotion. *Pelargonium graveolens* [geranium] can have a similar effect – and is also analgesic, while *Lavandula angustifolia* may reduce discomfort.

HEADACHES

These are common in the first trimester due to increased blood volume and the progesterone effects on cerebral blood vessels. In the third trimester they may be due to stress or postural problems caused by increasingly heavy breasts, but may also herald gestational hypertension if occurring in the third trimester, especially if frontal and if accompanied by excessive oedema, sickness, visual disturbance and right-sided epigastric pain. Massage of the head, neck, shoulders and upper back using decongestant essential oils such as *Eucalyptus smithii* or *Mentha* x *piperita* [peppermint] would be helpful and generally relaxing oils such as *Lavandula angustifolia* and *Chamaemelum nobile* [Roman chamomile] would also relieve the symptoms. A simple method of use is for the mother to hold the essential oil bottle upside down against her finger and then apply her finger to her temples, behind her ears or/and in the hollows just below the hairline at the base of the skull.

INSOMNIA

Insomnia can be treated with aromatherapy massage, or by advising the mother to apply one drop of *Lavandula angustifolia* [lavender], *Citrus bergamia* [bergamot] or *Citrus limon* [lemon] to a tissue to place under her pillow case (do not apply directly to the pillow, in case of possible eye contact) or relaxing in a bath to which have been added one drop of the same oils or/and *Cananga odorata* [ylang ylang] or otto of *Rosa damascena* or *R. centifolia* for a more exotic aroma.

MOOD SWINGS, DEPRESSION, FATIGUE

Suitable essential oils in a dilution of 1–1½% will act synergistically with the massage to raise the spirits; for example, mood swings or depression may respond to oils such as *Citrus aurantium* per. var. *amara* [neroli] or *Cananga odorata* [ylang ylang]. *Cupressus sempervirens* [cypress], is both calming and neurotonic and the well loved *Lavandula angustifolia* is not only neurotonic and calming, but also balancing (Price 2000). Fatigue can be relieved with *Citrus limon* [lemon] and *Citrus paradisi* [grapefruit].

NAUSEA AND VOMITING

These are two of the earliest symptoms of pregnancy, affecting almost 90% of women, to a greater or lesser degree. Appropriately prescribed aromatherapy can make the difference to 'normal' sickness; the pathological condition of *hyperemesis gravidarum* is more serious and requires hospital admission and intravenous fluid replacement.

Melissa officinalis [lemon balm] and *Matricaria recutita* [German chamomile] are especially effective for morning sickness, other oils to help combat nausea being *Mentha* x *piperita* [peppermint], *Mentha spicata* [spearmint], *Citrus limon* [lemon] and *Zingiber officinale* [ginger]. The chosen oil or

---

Case study 12.2 Hyperemesis gravidarum – L Reed – *aromatherapist/nurse, UK*

Antenatal

Pam had suffered with hyperemesis during all of her previous four pregnancies and had undergone a termination previously because of this condition. She was admitted to hospital for intravenous therapy to correct her electrolyte balance and after several days was discharged.

She was readmitted a few days alter still unable to keep any food down. It was at this time that the therapist was asked whether aromatherapy may be able to help her.

She was offered various oils to smell to ascertain how well they would be tolerated. Those she felt most happy with were:

- *Citrus aurantium* var. *arnara* per. [orange bigarade] – antiinflammatory, calming, digestive
- *C. paradisi* per. [grapefruit] – cleansing, stimulating to digestive system
- *C. aurantium* var. *sinensis* per. [sweet orange] – antispasmodic, calming, stomachic
- *Mentha* x *piperita* [peppermint] – anti-inflammatory, antispasmodic, digestive (nausea)

Lemon was not well tolerated as she associated it with the lemon squash that she had been drinking, which had made her sick.

Intervention
- 1 drop of peppermint oil in a glass of water was to be sipped occasionally when she felt queasy, to settle her stomach
- The orange and grapefruit oils were inhaled from a tissue

Outcome
The following morning she said she felt a bit better; she had also remembered that in the past citrus fruits (apart from lemon) were the one thing that she could eat without feeling or being sick. It was decided therefore that, as soon as she felt able, these were the foods she should try to begin with.

When the therapist arranged to visit her 2 days later, she found that Pam had been discharged, requiring no further admissions.

oils are best inhaled from a few drops placed on a tissue or cotton wool ball, but may also be administered in a light massage if the mother wishes or added to a bath or foot bath.

Zingiber officinale [ginger], not the distilled oil but the whole herbal remedy, has been shown to be statistically significant in its effectiveness in trials on expectant mothers and in cases of nausea from other causes such as motion sickness (Bartram 1995 pp. 198–199) but may actually exacerbate the problem, triggering heartburn (Arfeen et al 1995). Its strong aroma may also increase nausea in some, as many women find that their sense of smell is so pronounced that all odours are anathema.

SYMPHYSIS PUBIS DIASTASIS

This is separation of the bony edges of the pubic rami from the softer cartilaginous joint. This separation is extremely debilitating, sometimes with long-term postnatal after-effects. Massage is not the preferred treatment and will not usually be effective, but judicious use of analgesic essential oils such as *Boswellia carteri* [frankincense] or *Eucalyptus citriodora* [lemon scented gum], *Melaleuca viridiflora* [niaouli] or *Ocimum basilicum* ct. alcohol [European basil], administered as a compress, may be useful. If a mother is suffering from this condition but attends for general relaxing aromatherapy, care should be taken when she gets on and off the massage couch: she should be advised to keep her thighs together rather than moving first one leg then the other, as this would exacerbate the diastasis.

USE OF ESSENTIAL OILS FOR LABOUR AND DELIVERY

Many mothers enquire about the use of aromatherapy in labour and this is where it truly comes into its own for it offers a gentle and pleasant way to reduce pain (Field et al 1997) and anxiety and improve the feeling of general well-being. If used sensibly, essential oils can also facilitate uterine action, reducing the duration of labour and enabling the mother's body to do its own work during this natural human process. Massage with essential oils has an invaluable synergistic and beneficial effect on a

labouring mother. See Box 12.4 and Case study 12.3 for baths.

Women may choose to be accompanied in labour by an independent aromatherapist or they may wish to self-administer essential oils. As the majority of women in the UK give birth in hospital, there are certain issues to be addressed before either of these situations can be allowed. If the mother has been receiving regular antenatal aromatherapy from an independent practitioner it is to be hoped that the aromatherapist will have liaised with the maternity care team before labour to inform them of treatments given. If this is not the case, the mother should discuss her wish to be accompanied by her aromatherapist with her midwife or obstetrician before term, in which case permission will need to be obtained (see p. 270).

If the mother wishes to use essential oils herself during labour she should be encouraged to discuss this with her midwife antenatally, irrespective of the place of birth. If oils are to be vaporized (whether in hospital or at home), this should be carried out with an electrically operated bowl vaporizer or an electrical steam vaporizer, both of which (if in hospital) will require the hospital electrician to check the wiring of the equipment before permission to use it can be given. Although a candle-type vaporizer can be used at home if safely placed, naked flames are not allowed in hospitals due to safety regulations and the presence of oxygen. An alternative is to place safely in the room a bowl of warm water to which essential oils have been added; this may facilitate vaporization and inhalation without the use of vaporizers.

A non-intrusive and safe way in which the essential oils can be inhaled easily by the mother is to place two or three drops on a ball of cotton wool or a tissue, which can be held in her hand and from which she can inhale deeply as and when necessary. This method is particularly useful when contraction intervals become shorter.

Application of essential oils via massage is certainly permissible but the practitioner should be aware that, when the mother is in labour, she may change her mind and decide that she does not want to be touched. She may prefer to inhale the oils by putting a drop or two on a tissue, Q-tip or cotton wool ball, as above, or by holding the essential oil bottle upside down against her finger

---

Box 12.3   Use of essential oils in the labour suite – *Burns, Blamey & Lloyd 2000*

An investigation into the use of aromatherapy in labour was conducted at the John Radcliffe Hospital, Oxford, involving the administration of essential oils to 8058 women (60% primigravidae) in the Delivery Suite from 1990 to 1998 (Burns, Blamey & Lloyd 2000). A small number of nominated midwives undertook a basic aromatherapy course and, with the help of aromatherapists, imparted the necessary information to the remaining midwives in the unit who were not qualified aromatherapists. They were, however, sufficiently educated to administer a designated selection of essential oils for specific purposes, by a designated method, and under instruction, to women in labour; these included pain relief, alleviation of nausea, fear and anxiety and to facilitate uterine action. This meant that labouring women could enjoy the benefits of aromatherapy from the midwife who was already caring for them, enhancing the relationship between the two and maintaining continuity of care, in accordance with the report Changing Childbirth (Department of Health 1993).

Aromatherapy was mainly used in established labour (60%) or in the latent phase (29%).

The oils used – and their reasons for use were as follows:

- *Boswellia carteri* [frankincense] – high anxiety, hyperventilation, hysteria
- *Citrus limon* [lemon] – upper respiratory tract infections, enhance mood
- *Citrus reticulata* [mandarin] – relaxation, enhance mood
- *Eucalyptus globulus* [blue gum] – nasal infection, pain relief

- *Jasminum grandiflorum* [jasmine absolute] – depression, anxiety, assist labour, help expel placenta
- *Lavandula angustifolia* [lavender] – anxiety, stress, headaches, after perineal suturing
- *Mentha x piperita* [peppermint] – nausea, vomiting, headaches, pyrexia
- *Roman chamomile* – mothers with multiple allergies, eczema, anxiety, after perineal suturing
- *Rosa centifolia* [rose absolute] – depression, anxiety, bereavement, to enhance labour
- *Salvia sclarea* [clary sage] assisting contractions, to enhance labour

Although this was not a randomized sample in that women were able to opt in or out of the scheme as they chose, nor was there any control group, save those who declined or who were outside the selection criteria, the 1990–1998 Burns et al study stands alone as the largest clinical aromatherapy trial to date. The essential oils chosen had not been specifically tested for safety prior to use but there was no evidence to suppose that they were contraindicated during childbirth. Furthermore, all the women in the study were observed for adverse effects: the incidence was found to be very low, with less than 1% experiencing minor side-effects, such as skin irritation or nausea, with no negative foetal reactions at all.

Conclusion
The study suggests that aromatherapy has the potential to assist mothers in childbirth, although it is planned to take the work forward by more specific testing.

---

and applying that finger to her temples or the palm of her hand (keep cotton wool and fingers away from eyes).

Relaxing in a bath to which essential oils have been added is also acceptable until the bag of membranes surrounding the baby has ruptured, when it is necessary for the mother to get out of the water to avoid a direct route to the baby's eyes. If she is booked for a water birth it is wise either not to add essential oils to the water at all or to dissolve them first in a dispersant, when they

would be evenly spread throughout the water at an exceedingly low concentration.

Facilitation of uterine action can often be achieved by careful use of essential oils in women who have irregular and inefficient contractions; essential oils in the extremely low dosages of aromatherapy could in no way induce the birth – they can simply encourage the mother's body to do its own work more efficiently.

The Expected Date of Delivery (EDD) is only an approximation, normal pregnancy ending any-

Case study 12.3 Three primigravidae in labour – L Reed – *aromatherapist/nurse, UK*

The following illustrate the use of lavender baths in three primigravidae – at 3, 2 and 5 cm dilation respectively:

Primigravida A

20.05: 3 cm dilated

21.30: Coping quite well

23.15: Persuaded to take a bath with five drops *L. angustifolia*. This was enjoyed but she could not get really comfortable in the bath, so was transferred to a bed after 10 minutes

23.45: 5 cm dilated. Pethidine requested and 100 mg given

00.45: 6 cm dilated; spontaneous rupture of membranes occurred

01.00: A back and gentle abdominal massage were given using one drop each of *C. nobile* and *Chamomilla recutita* and two drops each of *Cananga odorata* and *L. angustifolia*

01.30: Fully dilated

02.54: Normal delivery

Primigravida B

Had made use of TENS (transcutaneous electrical nerve stimulation) machine at home. Admitted to hospital for delivery.

23.30: 2 cm dilated with intact membranes

00.30: Given bath with five drops *L. angustifolia*

02.30: 9 cm dilated; requested additional pain relief. Reluctant to leave the bath, so vaginal examination carried out in the bath. An ARM was performed and Entonox commenced

03.30: Vertex was visible, but progress in the second stage was slow. Advised to get out of the bath

04.30: Transferred to a delivery bed. A gentle abdominal massage was given using two drops each of *C. nobile* and *L. angustifolia* and one drop of *S. sclarea*

05.00: Normal delivery. No other form of pain relief

Primigravida C

Various combinations of essential oils were used for massage in labour. The following were blended (number of drops of each oil in brackets):

- *Chamaemelum nobile* (3), *Lavandula angustifolia* (1), *Salvia sclarea* (3) in 50 ml carrier oil
- *Cananga odorata* (3), *Lavandula angustifolia* (1), *Pelargonium graveolens* (3) in 50 ml carrier oil
- *Cananga odorata* (2), *Jasminum officinale* var. *grandiflorum* (1), *Lavandula angustifolia* (2) in 25 ml carrier oil

The two main aims were:

- to stimulate the pituitary gland and the thalamus to encourage the secretion of endorphins and encephalins to reduce pain
- to utilize the sedative properties of lavender and Roman chamomile to aid relaxation

01.00: 5 cm dilated. ARM performed

01.45: Bath with five drops *L. angustifolia*

02.15: Full dilation confirmed. Urge to push

03.00: Vertex visible on the perineum

03.10: Normal water birth

N.B. The delivery took place in the same bath water, i.e. containing lavender, because it had had over an hour to blend well in the water and either evaporate, or be absorbed through the mother's skin.

---

where between 37 and 43 weeks after the last menstrual period. However, a practitioner who is also a midwife, or an experienced aromatherapist working within a maternity service, may be able to avoid medical inductions of labour in some women who are past their due dates by using emmenagogic oils, but this must be undertaken only with the consent of the obstetrician and be carefully monitored, especially if aromatherapy is combined with the use of prostaglandin pessaries or oxytocic infusions.

POSTNATAL USE OF ESSENTIAL OILS

Newly delivered mothers usually welcome aromatherapy massage unreservedly as it allows them time to themselves for relaxation, as well as relieving the symptoms of the physiological and psychological changes as their bodies readjust to the non-pregnant state and they adapt to new parenthood. At this time, it is nice to let the mother choose the essential oils – to be sure of an

---

Box 12.4   Lavender baths during labour – *Reed & Norfolk 1993*

This trial was carried out by Reed & Norfolk (1993), with the support of the Director of Midwifery Services at Ipswich Hospital – using her practical procedures.

Purpose of trial

19 primigravidae and 19 multigravidae clients took part in a trial to determine whether pain relief and relaxation could be achieved without adverse side-effects, using five drops of lavender (unspecified) in the bath.

Results from questionnaires

Agpar scores:
- 3 women scored 10
- 30 scored 8 or 9
- 2 scored 7 (pethidine given – 150 g and 250 g respectively)
- 1 scored 6 (stale meconium present)
- 2 did not have their score recorded

Deliveries:
- 34 of the 38 clients achieved a normal delivery
- 2 had forceps
- 1 LSCS (failure to progress)
- 1 had ventouse extraction

Additional pain relief given:
- 18 out of the 19 primigravidae clients
- 12 out of the 19 multigravidae clients

Length of labour:
- 8 multigravidae: up to 8 hours
- 5 multigravidae: up to 5 hours
- 2 multigravidae and 8 primigravidae: up to 6 hours
- 4 primigravidae: under 10 hours
- 2 multigravidae: 7–13 hours
- 5 primigravidae: 14–22 hours

Perceived benefits:
- 31 of the clients felt they had benefited from the relaxation effects (2 negative, 5 did not reply)
- 23 clients felt that the baths had given pain relief (7 negative, 8 did not reply)
- 30 clients had enjoyed the experience (1 negative, 7 did not reply)

Conclusion

The good Agpar scores would suggest that 5 drops of lavender in baths present no risks to the baby.

Although it was not possible to assess whether or not labour was shortened by the lavender baths, labour in some clients appeared to progress very rapidly. Progress was better in those clients who:

- used the lavender bath when a 2+ or more dilation was established
- spent more than 30 minutes in the bath.

---

aroma which the mother really likes, regardless of therapeutic effects.

In the first few postnatal days, *Cupressus sempervirens* [cypress] with its styptic properties and *Pelargonium graveolens* [geranium] and *Commiphora myrrha* [myrrh] with both styptic and cicatrizant properties can be used in a vulval wash or in the bidet to alleviate the discomfort of perineal sutures and lacerations. The value of *Lavandula angustifolia* in expediting wound healing has not been confirmed (Dale & Cornwell 1994), but as it is cicatrizant, it should also be of some benefit.

Melaleuca alternifolia [tea tree] is an anti-infectious oil (Carson et al 1996, Appendix A(I)) and can be used for prevention and treatment of wound, chest or uterine infections, as well as the

avoidance of cross-infection in the postnatal ward, although many sweeter smelling oils – and less subject to adulteration – such as the four oils above, which are all antiinfectious, would be equally effective.

A full-body massage to aid general well-being, induce rest and sleep and ease discomfort can be wonderful if time allows, although the breast area should be avoided (except immediately after a feed), to prevent ingestion by the baby while feeding. Gentle head, neck and back massage may assist in alleviating the after-effects of epidural anaesthesia, and facilitating improvement in general mobility, especially if the mother has had a Caesarean section. Although not an essential oil, the absolute of *Jasminum officinale* [jasmine] is often considered to be beneficial in reducing the impact of postnatal 'blues' and preventing depression, and if the mother cannot have or does not want, massage or essential oils, she could be offered jasmine tea. However, the value of jasmine in promoting lactation is controversial since two studies suggest that the flowers may inhibit milk production (Abraham, Debi & Sheela 1979, Shrivastav et al 1988). *Mentha* x *piperita* however, should not be used by lactating mothers as it prevents milk from forming (see Appendix A(I)). *Foeniculum vulgare* [fennel] on the other hand, can help stimulate lactation (Franchomme & Pénoël 2001 p. 382); fennel tea could also be an option.

NEONATAL AROMATHERAPY

The use of essential oils for newly born babies remains controversial, particularly in the light of current guidelines to avoid putting any substance on an infant's skin. However, use of essential oils in the right dosage (0.5%), has been shown anecdotally to be advantageous to overall care, particularly when combined with massage, which has been shown to have a variety of very positive effects on both full-term babies and those born preterm (Field 1995).

Essential oils which are accepted to be relatively safe for use on babies – and also seem to have positive effects on most baby conditions are *Chamaemelum nobile* [Roman chamomile] (indigestion, infantile diarrhoea and sleeplessness) and *Lavandula angustifolia* (colic, flatulence and sleeplessness)

SUMMARY

Aromatherapy is a gentle, relaxing, effective and relatively safe complementary therapy which is fairly easily incorporated into conventional maternity care. However, the legalities of maternity care within the United Kingdom must be remembered and its use must be considered as an adjunct to, rather than a replacement for, normal midwifery and obstetric care, with close communication between aromatherapy practitioners and the maternity care team being maintained. Women should be advised that essential oils are more than simply pleasant smelling, in that they have also a pharmacological action as well as a psychological effect and must consequently be treated with due respect. Although care must be taken to avoid potential ill effects and complications from inappropriate use of essential oils, their judicious, expert use during pregnancy and childbirth can be very beneficial.

References

Abraham M, Debi N S, Sheela R 1979 Inhibiting effect of jasmine flowers on lactation. Indian Journal of Medical Research 69: 88–92

Ager C 2002 A complementary therapy clinic: making it work. RCM Midwives' Journal 5(6): 198–200

Arfeen Z, Owen H, Plummer J L, Ilsley A H, Sorby-Adams R A, Doecke C J 1995 A double-blind randomised controlled trial of ginger for the prevention of postoperative nausea and vomiting. Anaesthesia Intensive Care 23(4): 449–452

Balacs T 1992 Safety in pregnancy. International Journal of Aromatherapy 4(1):12–15

Bartram T H 1995 Encyclopedia of herbal medicine. Grace, Christchurch

Buchbauer G, Jirovetz L, Jäger W, Dietrich H, Plank C, Karamat E 1991 Aromatherapy: evidence for sedative effects of the essential oil of lavender after inhalation. Zeitschrift für Naturforschung C46 (11–12): 1067–1072

Buchbauer G, Jirovetz L, Jäger W, Plank C, Dietrich H 1993 Fragrance compounds and essential oils with sedative effects upon inhalation. Journal of Pharmaceutical Sciences 82(6): 660–664

Buckle J 1993 Aromatherapy: does it matter which lavender essential oil is used? Nursing Times 89(20): 32–35

Burns E, Blamey C, Ersser S, Lloyd A J, Barnetson L 1999 The use of aromatherapy in intrapartum midwifery practice: an observational study. OCHRAD, Oxford

Burns E, Blamey C, Lloyd A J 2000 Aromatherapy in childbirth: an effective approach to care. British Journal of Midwifery 8(10): 639–643

Carson C F, Hammer K A, Riley T V 1996 In vitro activity of the essential oil of *Melaleuca alternifolia* against *Streptococcus* spp. Journal of Antimicrobial Chemotherapy 37(6): 1177–1181

Dale A, Cornwell S 1994 The role of lavender oil in relieving perineal discomfort following childbirth: a blind randomized clinical trial. Journal of Advanced Nursing 19(1): 89–96

Department of Health 1993 Changing Childbirth: Report of the Expert Committee

Field T 1995 Massage therapy for infants and children. Developmental and Behavioral Pediatrics 16: 105–111

Field T, Hernandez-Reif M, Taylor S, Quinho O, Burman I 1997 Labor pain is reduced by massage therapy. Journal of Psychosomatic Obstetrics and Gynecology 18: 286–291

Field T, Hernandez-Reif, Hart S, Theakston H 1999 Pregnant women benefit from massage therapy. Journal of Psychosomatic Obstetrics and Gynecology 19:

Franchomme P, Pénoël D 2001 Aromathérapie exactement. Jollois, Limoges

Miller L G 1998 Herbal medicinals: selected clinical considerations focusing on known or potential drug–herb interactions. Archives of Internal Medicine 158(20): 2200–2211

Naganuma M, Hirose S, Nakayama Y et al 1985 A study of the phototoxity of lemon oil. Archives of Dermatological Research 278(1): 31–36

NHS Confederation 1997 Complementary medicine in the NHS: managing the issues. NHS Confederation, Birmingham

Nursing & Midwifery Council 2002a Midwives' Rules and Code of Practice. NMC, London

Nursing & Midwifery Council 2002b Scope of Professional Practice. NMC, London

O'Hara C 2002 Challenging the rules of reflexology. In: Mackereth P, Tiran D (eds) Clinical reflexology: a guide for health professionals, ch. 3. Elsevier Science, Edinburgh, pp. 33–52

Pages N, Fournier G, Baduel C, Tur N, Rusnac M 1996 Sabinyl acetate, the main component of *Juniperus sabina* L'Herit essential oil, is responsible for the anti-implantation effect. Phytotherapeutic Research 10(7): 438–440

Price S 1999 Practical aromatherapy, 4th edn. Thorsons, London, pp. 55, 70

Price S 2000 Aromatherapy for your emotions. Thorsons, London

Reed L, Norfolk L 1993 Aromatherapy in midwifery. Aromatherapy World (Nurturing, Summer issue): 12–15

Shrivastav P, George K, Balasubramamiam N, Padmini Jasper M, Thomas M, Kanagasabhapathy A S 1988 Suppression of puerperal lactation using jasmine flowers (*Jasminum sambac*). Australian and New Zealand Journal of Obstetrics and Gynaecology 28: 68–71

Southwell A, Markham C, Mann C 1997 Skin irritancy of tea tree oil. Journal for Essential Oil Research 9: 47–52

Tiran D 2000 Clinical aromatherapy for pregnancy and childbirth, 2nd edn. Churchill Livingstone, Edinburgh

Tisserand R, Balacs T 1995 Essential Oil Safety. Churchill Livingstone, Edinburgh

Chapter **13**

Learning disabilities and autism

Elizabeth Walsh, Jane Cummins and Shirley Price

INTRODUCTION

Although ascertaining exact figures is difficult to achieve, it is estimated that autism occurs in around 500 000 people in the UK – that is, an estimated 91 people in every 10 000 (National Autistic Society 2005). About a third of these people have learning disabilities in varying degrees – approximately 210 000 suffer with severe symptoms, with a possible 1.2 million people showing mild/moderate symptoms (DOH 2000a). Valuing people; a new strategy for learning disability in the 21st century (DOH 2001) is founded on the belief that people with learning disabilities are people first.

A learning disability is defined as:

> a significantly reduced ability to understand new or complex information to learn new skills (impaired intelligence), with a reduced ability to cope independently (impaired social functioning) which started before adulthood with a lasting effect on development.

Although much has changed in the past two decades, there needs to be an emphasis on improving their lives and that of their families and carers based on legal and civil rights, independence, choice and social inclusion.

Ascertaining exact figures is difficult, but it is estimated that there are around 210 000 people with severe/profound learning disabilities. This includes 65 000 children and young people, 120 000 adults of working age and 25 000 older people. Some 1.2 million people have a mild/

moderate learning disability (25 per 1000 population).

AUTISM

Autism is a life-long developmental disability, usually occurring before the age of 3 and affecting social and communication skills. There may also be an accompanying learning disability, but whatever their level of intellect they will all have difficulties in processing information and making sense of the world.

There are an estimated 535 000 people with autistic spectrum disorders in the UK, including 117 000 with a learning disability and 417 400 with average or high ability (National Autistic Society).

There are many theories as to what can cause autism, Marshall (2004) stating that 'recent studies strongly suggest that some people have a genetic predisposition to autism, although for some children, environmental factors may also play a role in precipitating it'.

In the past, autistic children who have been labelled 'naughty and uncontrollable' and 'schizophrenic' have often been misunderstood and isolated. The autistic spectrum ranges from those who are impaired severely – needing complete care in a controlled environment, to those who usually have an above average IQ and are known as having Asperger's syndrome (high functioning autism).

Lorna Wing, consultant psychiatrist and autism expert, has said that the problems associated with autism are usually in a triad of impairments:

- social interaction (aloofness, passiveness, lack of understanding, stilted)
- communication (delay and abnormality, mute-ness, literal interpretation, inability to under-stand non-verbal communication)
- imagination (limited understanding of others' emotions).

About 40% of children with autism also have some abnormality of sensory sensitivity (Rimland 1990). Our senses integrate to help us understand everyday experiences. We learn about the world we live in by touching, tasting and smelling, each experience leading on to the next, assisting in our learning and development; those with autism cannot process the information in the same way, often retracting into their own world and losing contact with the world they live in. Professor Temple Grandin (2000), who is autistic, stated, 'the autistic child withdraws because the world is a hurtful place – sound hurts, touch hurts, vision hurts, everything hurts'. Aromas can be over-powering, background noise can be over-whelming and touch can be excruciating. Contending with all three can cause a person to go into hypersensitive overload, leading to sensory shutdown.

VALIDITY OF ESSENTIAL OIL USE

To reach an individual we need an individual remedy and we should look for aromatic sub-stances which will both 'compensate for his deficiencies and will make his faculties blossom' Maury (in Mojay 1996). So it is no surprise that treatment with essential oils and massage can have the most profound effects when treating people with learning disabilities and autism, as well as being a positive experience for both therapist and client. 'Touch and essential oils have been shown to help develop trust as well as ease tension, reduce aggression and improve general health' (Alexander 1993). Aromatherapy can provide a major channel for communication, building up tolerance to touch, encouraging body awareness, promoting relaxation and generally improving health.

While there is little substantive research evidence there does appear to be a consensus of opinion that the use of aromatherapy is positive and that essential oils may alleviate symptoms, be they biologically predisposed or psychologically based.

The choice of oil and the mode of use will be based on the same determinants as for any essential oil but with special attention to the complexity of the individual concerned. This may be to both known and potential medical conditions and include acknowledged contraindications to existing drug regimes and possible side-effects.

TOUCH

People with learning disabilities require the same (and probably more) care, love, touch and atten-

Case study 13.1 Severe agitation – M A Hanse – *aromatherapist, UK*

Client assessment

The therapist had been asked to visit this hospital for mentally handicapped people, to see if aromatherapy had any relevance to severely disturbed, deaf and blind residents with severe mental handicaps.

Frances was a young woman who was very disturbed, giving the impression of being in torment. She continually thrashed backwards and forwards, punching her head with her fists, slapping her head and face, sticking her fingers into her eyes, pushing away any hands that tried to touch her. She ceaselessly thrashed around.

The therapist was told that she refused to let people touch her. Her carers and parents never have the satisfaction of knowing whether she appreciates them as she does not communicate.

Intervention

An electric diffuser was put into the room with the following essential oils:

- *Citrus bergamia* [bergamot] – calming, sedative, tonic to the central nervous system
- *Lavandula angustifolia* [lavender] – calming, sedative

When the therapist entered, Frances at first showed total rejection, then very slowly – after about half an hour – she gradually accepted her presence – and eventually her touch.

The therapist then put 2 drops each of the same oils on her hands – and held Frances on the solar plexus area between ribcage and stomach with the other hand on the adrenals at the back. It seemed that there was a healing calm produced by hands placed on the body, combined with the effect of the relaxing essential oils – the total effect was dramatic.

Outcome

During the last half hour or so of the 2-hour visit, Frances was relaxed and lying back on the bean bag, sometimes with her arms behind her back with a little smile and sometimes giving a gurgling laugh of pleasure. The nurses were wishing that it could have been photographed or better still, videoed, as they had never seen Frances like that. There was a concentration on what was going on in the ward; a focus and a quiet calmness – the nurses said that all the residents seemed more calm than usual.

I believe that there is much useful work that could be done in the area of profound handicaps using essential oils and having the confidence to use hands for communication and hearing.

tion as a person whose illness or disability takes a different form. Terms like 'challenging behaviour' and 'learning disability' have replaced words like 'mentally deficient' and 'backward' and, instead of keeping patients away from contact with the outside world, every effort is made to help them to achieve as normal an everyday life as possible.

It is believed that the lack of positive tactile stimulation could lead to the rocking, hand wringing and head banging that play such a large part in the behaviour pattern of many people with learning disabilities. Touch is a basic behavioural need in much the same way as breathing is a basic physical need and when the need for touch remains unsatisfied, abnormal behaviour will result (Montagu 1986).

Using and developing the sense of touch – holding someone's hand, a kind touch on the arm, a pat on the back or holding someone who is crying, can often convey more easily than words how people really feel (Sanderson, Harrison & Price 1991 p. 11). However, many people with autism can be intolerant to touch, feeling it to be painful – especially a light touch – and a firm pressure is often better. It should be firm enough to stimulate deep pressure receptors. Very light touch should be avoided because it increases arousal and excites the nervous system (Grandin 2000).

Hands are usually the best place to start as they are easily accessible without causing a great deal of stress, and often simply squeezing and holding while applying essential oils will be an adequate treatment. It is important not to force the pace of a treatment, even if progress seems slow.

Children and adults with a learning disability – especially those with a severe/profound delay –

Case study 13.2 Touch sensitivity – S Thompson – *therapist*

Client assessment

Laura, aged 10, has autistic spectrum disorder. She was initially rather defensive about being touched and resisted physical contact by hiding her hands behind her head.

Intervention

Persisting gently, her shoulders and hands were stroked, over her clothes and without essential oil. After a while, she began to tolerate this and to cooperate passively. Essential oil used:

- *Lavandula angustifolia* – relaxing and sedative

After the lavender was introduced, she began to anticipate the activity by initiating and imitating the strokes, and she now sits for up to 25 minutes for lower leg massage.

Outcome

Smiling and sitting opposite with good eye contact, Laura can now choose her own essential oils from a selected group. Her favourite is *Citrus aurantium* var. *sinensis* [sweet orange], which is particularly useful for combating anxiety and nervousness and has an aroma similar to a brand of orange chocolate.

---

have to be touched frequently. Additional sensory impairments with little apparent meaningful communication. and sometimes portrayed as challenging behaviour, may determine the amount of interaction with their carers; in reality these may be outward signs of anxiety, pain, fear, over/under stimulation or the desire to communicate.

Much of the published literature concerning learning disability and the use of essential oils, although mainly anecdotal, uses touch as one of the methods of application. Thompson (2002) concludes that the benefits of using aromatherapy and massage have proved more beneficial than was anticipated, by improving circulation, skin condition, promoting mental and physical relaxation and creating a feeling of being cared for.

COMMUNICATION AND RELATIONSHIPS

Incorporating essential oils into the individual care packages of people with learning disability can help improve communication, enhance relaxation and reduce anxiety. Such people may not have had many valuable experiences and establishing a relationship, which in itself is

---

Case study 13.3 Improving communication – S Thompson – *therapist*

Mark (pseudonym), aged 11, has cerebral palsy and is profoundly handicapped.

Intervention

The following essential oils were used to massage his feet and legs:

- *Lavandula officinalis* – analgesic, tonic
- *Rosmarinus officinalis* [rosemary] – analgesic, circulatory stimulant, decongestant

Outcome

At first he was passive, but gradually began to show signs of enjoyment – in fact, it was noticed that as the session ended, his face became sad.

When his therapist asked him if he wanted more, he moved in anticipation and gave a huge smile of agreement.

He now watches the movements with great interest and is actively enjoying his 'special time'. Because of the rubifacient and stimulation properties of the rosemary, his skin tone is also much healthier.

The manager had seen aromatherapy work in another environment and was very positive in her expectations.

deemed to be therapeutic (Mitchell & Cormack 1998, is an essential component of working within this field. Communication skills need practice and patience – and the willingness to communicate non-verbally (Hollins 2000).

The fact that smell has a direct correlation to human behaviour is accepted (Van Toller & Todd 1988), Engen (1982) suggesting that smell association is a learned behaviour and that application of this theory into practice becomes a useful non-verbal tool in establishing and maintaining links to people and places. If a person with a learning disability can learn that something they perceive as good will happen whenever a particular aroma is present, then the chances of that event happening again – and the associated feeling when the aroma is encountered – will be high. Once established, this principle can be applied to everyday life.

Communication and trust can also be developed in a non-verbal and non-threatening way by using interactive massage, where the emphasis is on encouraging the person to respond and participate, guided by the stages of the Interactive Sequence (McInnes & Treffry 1982).

CONSENT

'It should never be assumed that people are not able to make their own decisions, simply because they have a learning disability' (DOH 2001). Before commencing an aromatherapy intervention, consent should be asked for – if the person is able to give it. If not, provided the treatment is in the client's best interest, it is still possible lawfully to provide treatment and care (DOH 2001) and it can always be discussed with relatives.

Children and adults with learning disabilities are among the most vulnerable people in society. An adult 'may be unable to take care of him or herself or take steps to protect him or herself from significant harm or exploitation' (DOH 2000b). Particular care should be taken to ensure that both children and adults communicate their needs, wishes and feelings in respect of their care and treatment.

Consent, in relation to the child, either directly or through their carer, and inferred refusal by the child's actions must be appreciated by the professional involved. Using essential oils is

therefore not an intervention to be taken without due care and consideration of all the factors involved.

PRESENTATION OF ESSENTIAL OILS

Many of those with autism and learning disabilities are hypersensitive to aromas and as always, any essential oils offered should be dropped onto a spill (the aroma is mostly top notes if inhaled directly from the bottle). If wanting to use a blend of more than one essential oil (never more than two to three), offer the blend, as well as the single oils. Because a person likes the aroma of two separate oils, it does not follow that he/she will like a blend of the same two – the blend must be offered also.

Having selected the essential oils which would be most helpful to the person concerned, the way in which these are presented is of great importance. The aim is to select an aroma which is acceptable to and appreciated by the person for whom it is intended, so time should be taken.

Never offer more than three spills – one at a time, noting the reactions carefully: Did the hand push it away? Was the head averted? Did the person come closer? Did he or she reach out for the hand holding the aroma? The end result will be enhanced when the essential oil favoured by the person is used and the preferred one, on its own – including a blend – should be used first in whatever method of treatment is adopted.

INTRODUCING AN ESSENTIAL OIL

An essential oil can be presented in two ways:

- one drop on a spill or tissue – neat for smelling
- ready mixed in a carrier oil on the back of the therapist's hand. Using the hand sometimes enables the therapist to make physical contact with a client who previously has not been enthusiastic about being touched.

If the diluted method is preferred, small bottles of each essential oil diluted in jojoba oil can be kept for this purpose alone. Jojoba keeps well because it is a liquid wax resistant to oxidation (Price, Price & Smith 1999).

Case study 13.4 Agitation – J Cummins – *aromatherapist/nurse, UK*

Peter (pseudonym) had good verbal communication and understanding, wanting a treatment as he had enjoyed staff massaging his hands. Peter is a young man of large build and when agitated, difficult to calm.

Intervention
Peter's hands and forearms were massaged with the following blend in a carrier oil:

- *Chamamaelum nobile* [Roman chamomile] – calming, sedative
- *Lavandula angustifolia* [lavender] – calming, sedative

He smelt both oils singly and appeared to like them; he also liked the aroma of the two oils together. He rocked throughout his massage – only stopping for very short periods if the therapist moved her position or altered her pressure.

As the weeks progressed, Peter's upper arms and shoulders were included in the massage and his rocking became less during treatments. He indicated that he no longer wanted Roman chamomile and chose *Citrus reticulata* [mandarin] from a small selection of oils.

He became fairly agitated during this particular treatment – trying to touch the therapist's head and upper body, so she reverted to his feet and lower legs, which calmed him.

On discussing his treatment with the manager I was made aware that Peter was 'out of sorts' as he suffered from SAD; as the season was just changing, it often took some time for him to adjust – this is perhaps why he wanted to change his blend.

Outcome
The staff say that he is relaxed for several days after he has had his massage.

Should the person appear to like more than one (or all) of the offered oils, this is not necessarily a sign to blend these together (see above), as a different aroma will be produced, which will also need introducing. Select one of the favoured single oils for the first few treatments, or a blend – already approved – of two or three of the oils on the list (as a 'single' aroma). Should none of the aromas offered gain a positive reaction, rather than change to yet another oil, a drop of *Lavandula angustifolia* can be added to each spill or tissue, and one of these offered again. The blend offered is still a single aroma, but may be more acceptable. Where there is a large number of clients or patients, and time permits, it is useful to keep second sets of both neat and diluted trial bottles which contain *L. angustifolia* together with an equal amount of a single essential oil. A third set using *Santalum album* [sandalwood], *Pelargonium graveolens* [geranium] or another popular oil, such as *Citrus reticulata* (mandarin], in place of *L. angustifolia* is another possibility.

AROMATHERAPY TREATMENT

Both children and adults need to feel loved and to be completely accepted, including the acceptance of any particular physical impairment or negative emotional behaviour. Aromatherapy offers the rare opportunity to develop a professional empathetic rapport with patients, hopefully with the culmination of trust building, sharing and gently guiding the patient towards wellness again (Garnett-Ore 1996). A feeling of being loved will help to increase a person's feeling of self-worth, as will praise when something positive is achieved or the person's hair or other grooming features are pleasing to the eye. Also, 'it is important that tasks which are given should be attainable with short term goals, so that there is early reward, for nothing breeds success more than success itself' (Bischoff 1992).

Respect and care of the profoundly handicapped has changed, more respect and thought going into their care. There is an increasing range of activities on offer, including colour, massage, music, use of symbols, pictures, time lines, etc., all of which can be used on their own, or in conjunction with an aromatherapy treatment. Therapy should be selected where possible on the basis of scientific research but it should be borne in mind that patients have as much right as anyone to enjoy what they do – and all activities need to be planned and monitored for effectiveness (Vlaskamp &

Box 13.1   Learning disability trials

At Grove Park (a school for children with special needs) and a special unit in Wadhurst Primary School, 26 children were given regular massage with essential oils:

■ 20 were able to relax thoroughly (9 of these quite deeply), the other 6 achieving relaxation for short spells of between 2–5 minutes.

■ Within 2 weeks a 12-year-old child who used to whimper when touched was tapping his teacher on the shoulder to request a cuddle and his challenging behaviour was considerably reduced.

■ The leg and arm muscles of one child were fiercely resistant, but since receiving aromatherapy treatment, her hands were no longer tightly clenched and she could open them easily.

■ Since receiving aromatherapy, two girls with cerebral palsy, who always had their fists tightly clenched, opened them and kept them loose most of the time.

■ Other benefits noticed included sleeping more soundly on nights after treatment.

Conclusion

Severely physically disabled children have been loosened up (physically and mentally) by aromatherapy sessions.

Reports from teachers and conversations with parents showed the benefits possible by using essential oils with massage on children with special needs (Holden-Peters 1993).

Nakken 1999). Learning disability nurses are essentially hands on, appearing to choose therapies which reflect this (Wray 1997); thus, for them, massage with essential oils may be a preferred choice. The addition of essential oils to a bland massage oil broadens massage into a therapy which can have profound effects on the mind, thus beneficially affecting the emotional and physical behaviour of the person with learning disabilities.

Many people with autism may have difficulty achieving a relaxed state, but if they are assisted to do so, this can have positive outcomes on mood, anxiety levels and behaviour (Clements &

Zarkowska 2004). An aromatherapy massage is a multi-sensory treatment integrating touch, fragrance and gentle sound to invoke relaxation, warmth and safety, providing the autistic person the opportunity to experience feelings of well-being, an awareness of their environment and a sense of self.

The first session may consist simply of soothing music and discovering essential oils – touch may not come until the second session or so. As people with autism prefer a routine it is better to have the same time and day of the week (if possible) and use the same piece of music (if enjoyed) as, together with essential oils, it can be used as a trigger for relaxation in between sessions during aroused or stressful moments. Disturbances during treatment should be kept to a minimum; this can sometimes be difficult if in a group home setting but all staff and residents should be made aware that therapy is taking place.

The fact that aromas can trigger the memory (Van Toller & Dodd 1988 p. 153) suggests that, on the second and subsequent occasions when the same oil is used, memories of the first occasion are aroused. If these memories are happy ones, treatment will be enhanced each time, building on any therapeutic benefit generated by the first treatment and this has, indeed, been found to be the case (Price 1999).

It is believed that, as with most health problems for which essential oils are used, stimulation and/or relaxation are prime factors in the initiation of the healing process – whatever the health problem. This is particularly evident in the case of those with learning disabilities, where power of communication is considerably increased – and challenging behaviour decreased. The use of essential oils also accelerates any progress being made – and a positive constructive circle is begun, resulting in the person becoming independent in small personal tasks previously attended to by a carer (Sanderson, Harrison & Price 1991 pp. 80–81).

The cost of essential oils compares very favourably with the cost of orthodox drugs, the time devoted to aromatherapy by the staff being the most costly part of the treatment (Hydes 1997).

ESSENTIAL OILS AND MEDICATION

There are certain contraindications for the use of certain essential oils on those with learning dis-

---

Case study 13.5 Communication and agitation – J Cummins – *aromatherapist/nurse, UK*

Norman had no verbal communication and a hearing impairment; when agitated he would rip clothes and furniture to show his frustration.

Intervention

Norman was given weekly massage on his feet using a blend of citrus oils – he always smiled and made pleasurable sounds throughout.

As weeks went by progression was made from feet to legs, then hands and arms and the following two essential oils were added:

- *Santalum album* [sandalwood] – dry, itching skin
- *Zingiber officinale* [ginger] – digestive stimulant (nausea was often a problem)

Outcome

Norman truly enjoyed his massage and staff say they noticed how relaxed he remained for days afterwards.

A blend of oils was made for the staff to use in his bath when he became agitated between treatments.

---

abilities or autism. Many (not all) will take medication for psychosis, chlorpromazine being one; this drug causes photosensitization; however, photosensitizing essential oils pose no problem unless the client is going into direct sunlight or onto a sunbed after the treatment). Beta-blockers are also used to reduce aggressive behaviour, so oils which are noted for their hypotensive action should be avoided. Many people with autism also have epilepsy so careful choice of oils is needed in this area too.

Although laboratory evidence would suggest the use of medication, these have only short-term beneficial effects on self-injurious behaviour. It is interesting to note that Santosh & Baird (1999) suggest medication only when appropriate and only short-term, adding that challenging behaviour is best treated by behavioural therapy. Vickers (1996) suggests that the main role of massage and aromatherapy with disabled children is in the treatment of emotional and behavioural problems.

Self-injurious behaviour (SIB) may result in substantial tissue damage and be perceived as painful to the carer and Hare & Leadbetter (1998) suggest that all incidences of self-injury should be looked into. Essential oils known for their analgesic effects may be considered – or/and those which promote relaxation, thus reducing agitation. A child's perception of and ability to express pain is based on cognitive functioning (Twycross 1998), thus it may be more appropriate to use an essential oil which addresses both issues, lavender (*Lavandula angustifolia*), noted for its calming

properties and its beneficial effect on the skin, being one (Price 2000).

Use of oils containing a high percentage of aldehydes, ketones, oxides, phenols or phenolic ethers may complicate the treatment, so it is recommended that these are not even kept on the premises. There is such a large range of essential oils available to an aromatherapist, that there is no need to include any which may react on the skin or have a possible toxic effect on the nervous system.

Apart from lavender, other essential oils which are both analgesic and calming are: *Cuminum cyminum* [cumin], *Eucaylptus citriodora* [lemon-scented gum], *Euc. smithii* [gully gum], *Juniperus communis* fruct. [juniper berry] *Mentha arvensis* [cornmint], *Pelargonium graveolens* [geranium] and *Ocimum basilicum* [European basil, not exotic].

ESSENTIAL OIL CHOICE

The fact that essential oils have both a direct and an indirect effect does not seem to be in question and research within the field of psycho-neuroimmunology appears to substantiate the mind/body connection (Watkins 1997). However, the lack of credible evidence is a particular issue with this client group and Gaylor (2000) suggests this may hinge not only on ethical issues but also on the diverse nature of the clients and their presenting problems – especially lack of communication skills (Kiernan 1999).

The oils should also be chosen with special attention to the complexity of the person –

Case study 13.6 Nasal congestion – M A Hanse – *aromatherapist, UK*

The therapist had been asked to visit this hospital for mentally handicapped people, to see if aromatherapy had any relevance to severely disturbed, deaf and blind residents with severe mental handicaps.

George was a young man with severe nasal congestion who refused to be touched by anyone apart from two or three staff he knew well. He had been given the usual medication, which did not seem to clear the congestion, and he was keeping others as well as himself awake at night. He had been taken recently to see a specialist in another hospital because the congestion was so troublesome, but he would not let the consultant near him and they had to bring him back unhelped.

Intervention

The therapist selected the following essential oils for sinusitis and catarrh:

- *Eucalyptus globulus* [blue gum] – anticatarrhal, antiinfective, antiinflammatory, decongestant, expectorant, mucolytic

- *Lavandula angustifolia* [lavender] – anti-inflammatory, antiseptic, calming and sedative
- *Melaleuca viridiflora* [niaouli] – anticatarrhal, antiinfective, antiinflammatory, expectorant, immunostimulant
- *Origanum majorana* [sweet marjoram] – anti-infective, expectorant, calming, respiratory tonic

These were put onto a tissue and, while a nurse held them near his face, the therapist worked on his feet, using a Swiss reflex cream containing the same essential oils. Before starting on his feet she chatted to him, very gently touching and stroking his hands. Then she worked on the solar plexus and sinus reflex points.

Outcome

After a while his sinuses started running and he was needing to spit, etc.

The staff were surprised not only at the blockage moving – but at George allowing touch from a stranger.

---

both known and potential medical conditions. Acknowledged contraindications to existing drug regimes and possible side-effects must be take into account, illustrating that the use of essential oils is not an intervention to be taken without due care and consideration of all the factors involved.

The selection of the two or three oils to be presented to each person or child should not be undertaken at random. After the medical details of each case have been studied, oils which will influence the symptoms presented should be pre-selected. From these, two to three oils can be chosen for their relaxing or uplifting properties (whichever is felt to be the effect required). This means that, although the end selection has been made primarily to affect the mental and emotional side of the client, symptoms being suffered, such as constipation, insomnia, rheumatic pain, poor circulation, respiratory disorders, etc. will also be alleviated.

For example, someone who cannot sleep well and who suffers from rheumatism could be offered *Citrus limon, Origanum majorana* and *Chamaemelum nobile* as the selection of oils from which to choose. All three of these would be selected from essential oils beneficial for arthritis and insomnia because they also address mental and emotional problems.

Holmes (1997) considers *Pogostemon patchouli* to be helpful in agitation, irritability, chronic stress and anxiety. As he also suggests it is useful for grounding, it should be a good choice for those out of touch with their bodies and their senses.

SUMMARY

In a world of ever increasing science and technology, every person deserves acceptance and understanding. Using essential oils and massage can help build bridges of communication, add a positive influence to an individual's life and provide lasting relaxation where anxiety and agitation are often commonplace. In spite of the anecdotal nature of aromatherapy's reported successes on people with learning disabilities, including autism, it is clear that it would be worth holding properly conducted trials, especially where the person is an adult, as habits, obsessions and survival techniques have already been ingrained. Not only could more be discovered about the benefits of aromatherapy, but much could be learned about the nature of learning disabilities themselves.

Treating autistic people with aromatherapy can be wonderfully rewarding not only for the client but also for the therapist. When breakthroughs are made they seem huge (even when small!). Flexibility, perseverance and patience are needed by the therapist.

References

Alexander B 1993 The place of complementary therapies in mental health. A user's experience and views. Nottingham Advocacy Group: 3–4

Bischoff L 1992 How aromatherapy can help people with learning difficulties. Treatise; Clinical Practitioner's Diploma. Shirley Price International College of Aromatherapy, Leics

Clements J, Zarkowska E 2004 Behavioural concerns and autistic spectrum disorders; explanations and strategies for change. Jessica Kingsley, London, p. 126

DoH 2000a Framework for assessment of children in need and their families. HMSO, London

DoH 2000b No secrets: guidance on developing and implementing multi-agency policies and procedures to protect vulnerable adults form abuse. HMSO, London

DoH 2001 Valuing people: a new strategy for learning disability in the 21st century. HMSO, London

Engen T 1982 The perception of odours. Academic Press, New York, p. 97

Gaylor M 2000 'Trials and tribulations'. Learning Disability Practice 2(4):14–15

Grandin T 2000 My experiences with visual thinking sensory problems and communication difficulties. www. Autism.org

Hare D J, Leadbetter C 1998 Specific factors in assessing and intervening in cases of self-injury by people with autistic conditions. Journal of Learning Disabilities for Nursing, Health and Social Care 2 (2): 60–65

Holden-Peters P 1993 Grove Park. The Aromatherapist 1(1): 22–24

Hollins S 2000 Developmental psychiatry – insights from learning disability. British Journal of Psychiatry 177: 201–206

Holmes P 1997 Patchouli – the colours within the darkness. International Journal of Aromatherapy 8(1): 18–22

Hydes S 1997 Establishing aromatherapy as a complement to traditional treatment in the mental

health services. Treatise, Clinical Practitioner's Diploma, SPICA, Leics

Kiernan C 1999 Participation in research by people with learning disabilities; origins and issues. British Journal of Learning Disabilities 27: 43–47

Kloth L et al 1990 Wound Healing: Alternatives in Management. F A Davis Company, Philadelphia

Marshall F 2004 Living with autism. Sheldon Press, London, p. viii

McInnes J, Treffry J 1982 In: Sanderson H, Harrison J 1991 Aromatherapy and massage for people with learning difficulties. Hands On, Birmingham

Mitchell A, Cormack M 1998 The therapeutic relationship in complementary healthcare. Churchill Livingstone, London

Mojay G 1996 Aromatherapy for healing the spirit. Gaia Books, London

Montagu A 1986 Touching the human significance of the skin. Harper & Row, New York

National Autistic Society 2005 Day for Autism. 393 City Road London EC1V 1NG

Price L, Price S, Smith I 1999 Carrier oils for aromatherapy and massage. Riverhead, Stratford upon Avon

Price S 1987 The effect of essential oils on the memory. Aroma News 6: 6–7

Price S 1992 Arthritis and rheumatism. Yoga and Health, February: 37/38

Price S 1999 Practical aromatherapy, 4th edn. Thorsons, London, p. 164

Price S 2000 The aromatherapy workbook, 2nd edn. Thorsons, London

Rimland B 1990 Sound sensitivity in autism. Autism Research Review International 4: 1, 6, cited in Attwood T (ed) 1998 Asperger's syndrome. A guide for parents and professionals. Jessica Kingsley, London & Philadelphia

Roulier G 1990 Les huiles essentielles pour votre santé. Dangles, St-Jean-de-Braye

Sanderson H, Harrison J, Price S 1991 Aromatherapy for people with learning difficulties. Hands On, Birmingham

Santosh P J, Baird G 1999 Psychopharmacotherapy in children and adults with intellectual disability. Lancet 354 July 17: 233–241

Thompson S 2002 A fragrant message. Learning Disability Practice 5(5): 15–17

Twycross A 1998 Children's cognitive level and perception of pain. Professional Nurse 14(1): 35–38

Van Toller S, Dodd G 1988 Perfumery: the psychology and biology of fragrance. Chapman & Hall, London

Vickers A 1996 Massage and aromatherapy. Chapman & Hall, London

Vlaskamp C, Nakken H 1999 Missing in execution therapies and activities for individuals with profound multiple disabilities. British Journal of Development Disabilities 45: 99–109

Wing L 1996 The autistic spectrum. A guide for patients, parents and professionals. Constable, London

Wise R 1989 Flower power. Nursing Times 85(22): 45–47

Wray J 1997 Complementary therapies in learning disability: examining the evidence. Journal of Learning Disabilities for Nursing, Health and Social Care 2(1) 10–15

Chapter **14**

Care of the elderly, with particular reference to dementia

Jenny Henry and Shirley Price

INTRODUCTION

Although this chapter is devoted mainly to dementia and its treatment, the specific conditions helped by essential oils also apply to general care of the elderly.

For more than a decade health-care professionals – occupational therapists, physiotherapists, speech and language therapists, podiatrists, nurses and doctors in both hospitals and residential or nursing homes – have realized the benefits of using essential oils to help elderly people, particularly those who have a variety of types of diagnosed dementia. There is also a greater awareness of the need to help those with early onset dementia in a younger age range.

DEMENTIA EXPLAINED

Dementia is a set of symptoms: a decline in memory and thinking which is of a degree sufficient to impair functioning in daily living, present for 6 months or more. This may be accompanied by a decline in emotional control, social behaviour, motivation and/or higher cortical functions (Alzheimer's Society CD). Although attention is usually focused on cognitive deficits, more than 50% of people with dementia experience behavioural and psychological symptoms (BPSD), which are distressing to the patients (Gilley et al 1991) as well as being problematic for their carers (Rabins, Mace & Lucas 1982).

Treatment with neuroleptics has an efficacy of only 20% above placebo – and is often poorly tolerated, having a high risk of adverse events such as parkinsonism, falls and accelerated cognitive decline, as well as a detrimental impact on the quality of life, including activities, well-being and social interaction (Ballard et al 2002).

At the present time there are 750 000 people in Britain with a form of dementia (www.alzheimers.org.uk 2005), although as people live longer – and therefore the elderly population increases – the number of people with some form of dementia will also increase. The importance of the use of our senses cannot be underestimated and with regard to that of smell, researchers in the United States in 1989 discovered abnormalities in cells from the olfactory nerves in the noses of people with Alzheimer's disease (Talame 1989).

About a quarter of people with Alzheimer's disease are found to have Lewy bodies in their brain cells when these are examined after death – they are tiny spherical structures found inside brain cells, which may cause the brain cells to die (Petit-Zeman 1999).

In February 2004 the Alzheimer's Society newsletter refers to new work in Oxford, where Dr Rupert McShane is a consultant in old age psychiatry at the Fulbrook centre. He and his colleagues have found that the sense of smell of people with 'Lewy bodies' in their brains is not as good as that of those without Lewy bodies. Petit-Zeman (2004) informs us that this work involved a detailed series of experiments where ability to detect the scent of lavender while alive was correlated with changes found in the brain after death – and that, in time, a simple 'patient-friendly' smell test (using lavender) could hopefully make diagnosis of dementia with Lewy bodies (DLB) more accurate.

FACETS OF DEMENTIA

People who have diagnosed dementia will have short-term memory loss and will gradually and increasingly become disorientated in time, place and space. Communication becomes difficult due to changes in receptive and expressive ability – and word finding. Changes in perception of taste, vision and sometimes auditory and visual hallucinations lead to changes in behaviour which are distressing not only to the person with dementia but also to the carer and family. These changes in the brain are unfortunately irreversible. It can often be difficult to make a diagnosis, as more than one type of dementia may be involved.

It is essential to assist dementia sufferers to maintain their ability to carry out their own personal skills for as long as possible. When Henry (co-author of this chapter) was working as an Occupational Therapist promoting personal skills in a daily routine – getting up in the morning, going to the toilet, washing, dressing, walking to the dining room and eating breakfast – she found that, for some individuals, a room diffuser in the bedroom, with *Lavandula angustifolia* – in conjunction with music chosen by the patient – would sometimes help to start the day in a relaxed manner, setting the mood for the day, with less evidence of anxiety later on.

The work of Mitchell (1993) showed that any positive impact of essential oils on functional difficulties was maintained, and the increased ratings for wandering represented improved mobility. The wandering was recreational, not aimless, although this might have been associated with an increased desire to be more active.

SHORT- AND LONG-TERM MEMORY LOSS AND REMINISCENCE

Because short-term memory loss is a major symptom experienced by people diagnosed as suffering from dementia, it is essential to learn about their likes and dislikes from their family and friends, in order to understand better each person's personal history. The music used in treatment for someone who habitually plays classical music all day would be different from someone who tunes into 'pop' music. The preferred aroma of soap or aftershave is also personal, relating to lifelong habits – the correct choice of brand, colour and aroma may assist function. Attention to this kind of detail makes for more successful 'person centred care' (Kitwood 1997).

VALUE OF TOUCH AND AROMATHERAPY

The value of aromatherapy when assisting someone with dementia is considerable. Touch and gentle massage of the hands or feet is a 'way in'

Box 14.1   Trial with *Lavandula officinalis* essential oil

A placebo-controlled trial was conducted by Holmes et al (2002) in a long-stay psychogeriatric ward to determine whether aromatherapy with lavender oil is effective in the treatment of agitated behaviour in patients with severe dementia.

The 15 patients met ICD (10 diagnostic criteria) for severe dementia and suffered from agitated behaviour. All had a minimum score of three points on the Pittsburg Agitation Scale (PAS).

Intervention

A 2% dilution of lavender oil was diffused on the ward through an aromastream for a 2-hour period on 5 alternate days, with water alone being used on the 5 days in between and the last day. A PAS score was taken for each patient on all 10 days of treatment.

Results

50% of patients (9) showed an improvement, 33% (5) showed no change and 7% (1) showed more agitation during the essential oil intervention than in the placebo treatment. This last patient was one of three who had Lewy bodies – the other two showed no change.

Conclusion

Although this small study showed that lavender oil administered in an aromastream is of benefit in the treatment of agitated behaviours in severely demented patients, a larger study is clearly required. www.interscience.wiley.com

---

especially when language is diminishing. Although not all elderly people in care want to be touched (McCann & McKenna 1993), touch can be comforting – and in conjunction with aroma diffusion and music will create an ambiance for relaxation and reduction of anxiety. In Henry's experience of over 13 years of working with people who have dementia – and their carers, there was only once a reaction from someone who was clearly not happy to have her hand held and massaged.

The tolerance of someone in the first stage of dementia may be very different from that of a person in the second or third stage. When touch itself has been established, progress can be made to a simple massage, thus avoiding a patient unfamiliar with massage becoming agitated or further confused (Horrigan 1995). The concentration span shortens as short-term memory becomes shorter, therefore the expectation of how long a massage period may last changes.

As early as 1988 Helen Passant, senior nursing sister at the time at the Churchill Hospital Oxford, found that many elderly patients suffering Alzheimer's disease (the most common form of dementia) derived benefit from using essential oils with massage – becoming either more alert, or calmer when anxious or noisy – with the added bonus of enabling the level of conventional sedative drugs administered to be reduced. It was noticed too that the patients' skin became stronger and more resistant to bruising and tissue damage. Both patients and nurses were uplifted, giving the latter a more satisfying role. Passant said that it seemed to open the doors to a closer relationship, 'allowing patients to speak of their dreams and hopes, of their fears and pleasures. To relieve stress and pain on all levels was something I had not thought possible – but it is' (Passant 1990).

The oils she used were lavender, marjoram, geranium, mandarin and cardamom (unspecified – botanical names were not widely in use then). Lavender was also used to promote sleep by using an aroma bath or drops on the bedclothes.

When the use of essential oils became more common, *Melaleuca alternifolia* [tea tree] and *Lavandula angustifolia* were frequently used in baths for skin conditions, the relief of pain, anxiety and agitation.

In Australia, lavender, sweet marjoram, patchouli and vetiver (unspecified) were used in a study carried out on a group of 36 participants, aged 70–90 years, who were divided into two groups. After a period of no massage at all, each group received either base cream – or cream plus essential oils (3.5 ml in 100 g), massaged into their bodies and limbs five times a day for 4 weeks, after which the treatments were reversed for the next 4 weeks. Both groups showed a significant decrease in the average frequency and severity of dementia-related behaviours during their essential oil sessions. However, it was interesting to note that there was also an increased resistance to nursing care in one of the groups, which may reflect the increased mental alertness and awareness caused by the oils (Bowles et al 2002).

CARERS

Carers travel the path of dementia together with the cared for, from its onset to eventual death; this path is very stressful and support is needed for the carer as well as the cared for. Carers who need help with sleep disturbance, anxiety and the stresses of caring can also benefit from aromatherapy, together with safety advice on how to use essential oils at home. Drinking chamomile tea will calm and refresh and a gentle massage given to the carer offers a few moments of quality time and respite, also reducing anxiety and promoting a sense of well-being. Henry has found that a limited 'palette' of oils is often the best approach and less daunting for an already distressed carer. A simple bowl of hot – not boiling – water containing a few drops of oil, or a tissue plus essential oils placed on a radiator, is less expensive than an electric diffuser and safer than using a night-light. Safety must always be paramount so it is sometimes essential to purchase the more expensive types of diffuser.

POLICY AND PROTOCOL

When providing aromatherapy for people with dementia and their carers within the National Health Service, Social Services or the private sector, it is essential to have an approved policy and clear protocols, with an assumption that the aromatherapist is well qualified, registered and insured. In Henry's experience at Newholme Hospital (Bakewell), the consultant verbally referred patients at weekly case meetings. General practitioners referred outpatients for hospital or home treatment, sending a standard referral and/or a letter from the practice. In the hospital, notes of aromatherapy treatment were recorded as part of the patients' multidisciplinary medical records and following treatment a letter was sent back to the referring doctor for their records. The responsibility of referral and medical note recording and its importance are highlighted by Stone (1996).

DOSAGE FOR THE ELDERLY

When determining the dosage of essential oils to be used, the weight, age and health (both mental and physical) of the person should be taken into account (Price 2000 p. 156) and with older people, whose bodily systems have begun to slow down, probably only half the normal concentration of essential oils is needed, i.e. 12–15 drops per 100 ml of carrier oil or lotion. The exact number of drops is rarely crucial (except where internal use is concerned) and is usually given as a range. For patients who need to use the oils over a long period of time, it is best to keep to the lower end of the range. *Eucalyptus smithii* [gully gum] is one of the exceptions to this rule as it is extremely gentle in action and should always be used on the elderly in preference to *E. globulus* [Tasmanian blue gum]. (See Respiratory problems p. 309.)

As in all use of essential oils, synergy within and between essential oils is an important consideration (see Ch. 3). Two oils are always more effective than one, and up to four oils, when selected with knowledge, can be even more so. Each person is an individual, and one essential oil may not have the required effect on everyone – as with drugs, where one type is not necessarily appropriate for each person.

CHOICE

It is essential always to consider that each of us has our own likes and dislikes, especially important to remember when a person with dementia cannot express themselves with ease. Life is made up of choices and it is necessary to allow a person with dementia the dignity of making a personal choice whenever possible. It is not difficult to observe whether someone dislikes the aroma that you are offering. Facial expression and body language will give the clue and when in doubt ask the family or main carer.

Aromatherapy has a great deal to offer the person with dementia, the carers and associated staff.

TREATMENT OF SPECIFIC CONDITIONS

Older people who have dementia experience the physical conditions and health changes associated with old age: cardiovascular conditions, arthritis and circulatory changes – affecting wound healing, etc. – all of which can be helped by the use of essential oils.

ANXIETY

In a biological sense, anxiety is the same as fear (Wingate & Wingate 1996 p. 51). It is the normal response of the body to danger – or the unknown. Anxiety is one of the components which make up stress and the most stressful – and therefore one of the most feared – event in an elderly person's life is to be uprooted from his or her home environment (Jamison, Parris & Maxon 1987) and on arrival in hospital the level of anxiety may rise. Massage and aromatherapy are being seen more and more in the treatment of stress related conditions such as anxiety and are of great value for people who have dementia. Essential oils can also be used in a diffuser (safety must be ensured), and the essential oils chosen from those known to relieve anxiety must also suit the individual concerned, where possible benefiting any other health problem he/she may have.

Many essential oils can relieve anxiety, one of the best – but also one of the most expensive – being *Citrus aurantium* var. *amara* (flos) [neroli bigarade]. For a list of oils to relieve anxiety, look at Appendix A(II), selecting any which are antispasmodic (to release fear), cardiotonic, calming and soothing. In a ward environment *Lavandula angustifolia* can be diffused successfully; it can also be used regularly in an evening bath to alleviate anxiety and promote sleep.

AGITATION AND DISTURBED BEHAVIOUR

Agitation associated with disturbed behaviour is distressing to both the cared for and the carer and is often difficult to deal with. Teaching the carer how to massage the hands and feet of the person he or she is caring for gives much needed physical contact; it promotes relaxation between the two and is particularly valuable when, in an advanced stage of dementia, conversation is limited due to receptive and expressive loss on the part of the person with dementia.

Beshara & Giddings (2002) carried out trials in a long-term care facility in America with a client

group having these problems. A non-randomized sample of five men and five women were exposed to aroma diffusion for several months – and at 1, 3 and 6 months, the frequency of aggressive behaviour in each person was calculated using the target behaviour tracking forms which were generated for the standardized Minimum Data Set (MDS) assessment tool. The chart produced to illustrate the specificity of behaviours over the 6-month trial period showed that some participants demonstrated a marked decrease in disturbed behaviour as evidenced by a 50% decrease in targeted behaviours. Others showed a less significant response but still showed some improvement. The importance of individual preferences in smells and their potential effect on mood and behaviour is highlighted.

Aromatherapy as a safe and effective treatment for agitation in severe dementia was the subject of a double-blind trial carried out by Dr Clive Ballard and colleagues in 2002 (see Box 14.2).

Although *Lavandula angustifolia* is a popular oil, if its aroma is disliked, there are many others which will also help to relieve agitation (see Appendix A(II)).

DEPRESSION AND MOOD CHANGES

People who have dementia may often be low in mood and it is important to be alert to the true signs of depression (Moate 1995). The value of essential oils to assist mood is well-documented. In both a day hospital and a ward, Henry used the essential oils of *Citrus limon* [lemon], *Pelargonium graveolens* [geranium], *Salvia sclarea* [clary sage], *Lavandula angustifolia* and *Origanum majorana* [sweet marjoram] effectively to uplift, calm or balance. However, memory loss (see below) with loss of verbal expression, disturbed sleep, and disorientation occurring as part of the dementia may mask the signs and symptoms of depression.

Touch for caring, massage and essential oils to uplift and calm a mood – with or without music – all are helpful. On one occasion, a patient sitting by the fountain in the sensory garden was calmed by the sound of the water and comforted by the warmth of the sun. By the fountain are pots of melissa, marjoram and lavender and one patient stayed happily in this position for half an hour and was not so restless for the remainder of the day.

Box 14.2 Agitation trial (Ballard et al 2002)

Double blind placebo-controlled trial
Ballard et al conducted a placebo-controlled trial to determine the value of aromatherapy for agitation in people with severe dementia, using _Melissa officinalis_ [lemon balm].

Intervention
72 people with clinically significant agitation were randomly assigned to aromatherapy using either melissa or a placebo (sunflower oil alone) – both blended with base carrier lotion. The blends were applied to the faces and arms of the 36 people in each group twice a day. The results, measured with Dementia Care Mapping, were compared between the two groups over a 4-week period. All but one person completed the trial and no significant side-effects were observed.

Results
A total of 60% (21 out of 35) of the melissa group and 14% (5 out of 36) of the placebo group experienced a reduction in their CMIA (Cohen–Mansfield Agitation Inventory) score, with an overall improvement in agitation (mean reduction of CMIA score) of 35% in the melissa group and 11% in the placebo group.

Conclusion
Aromatherapy with essential oil of _Melissa officinalis_ is a safe and effective treatment for clinically significant agitation in people with severe dementia, and with additional benefits for key quality of life parameters, indicating the need for further controlled trials.

The essential oils of _Citrus limon_ and _Citrus paradisi_ [grapefruit] refresh and help lift both mood and atmosphere. _Salvia sclarea_ and _Cananga odorata_ [ylang ylang] will uplift a low mood.

CIRCULATION

A well functioning circulatory system is essential to good health, so that waste and toxins can quickly be eliminated via the venous and lymphatic systems. Poor circulation is nearly always a problem in the elderly as the bodily systems slow down with age. This slowing down

affects the regeneration of cell tissue, thus all bodily functions are affected, resulting in loss of energy, possible constipation, muscles lacking tone due to insufficient exercise, etc. Firm effleurage towards the heart – in particular on limbs and feet (see Ch. 7) – allows the blood to flow more freely, taking nutrients to all organs and enabling more efficient absorption of waste products, as well as improving the lymphatic circulation to drain away excess fluid and help provide immunological defences (Battaglia 1997 p. 374).

Poor circulation is especially evident in those who have suffered a heart attack or stroke, when massage of the legs and arms – in an upward direction only – can help regain movement in affected limbs. Circulatory stimulating essential oils such as _Rosmarinus officinalis_ should be used in a carrier oil which aids circulation, e.g. hazelnut, sunflower, walnut or wheatgerm (see Ch. 7). For effective essential oils see Appendix A (II).

DIGESTIVE DISORDERS

Currently, the aromatherapy organizations do not allow their members to advocate essential oils internally and their insurance does not therefore cover this activity (unless they are aromatologists and members of the Institute of Aromatic Medicine – see Chapter 9 on page 226). This can be frustrating to many aromatherapists, because complaints involving the digestive system respond much more rapidly to ingestion.

The essential oils suggested for each digestive condition below can be either applied to the abdomen in a carrier lotion or massaged in a clockwise direction into the abdomen with a carrier oil.

Constipation

Many elderly people suffer from constipation, often as a result of medication taken or a poor or over-refined diet. Despite the best efforts of the nutritionists, they can also become constipated owing to the change in environment and daily routine when taken to hospital. As with all health problems, constipation should be treated holistic-ally, endeavouring first to discover the cause, and treatment should include regulating the diet.

Case study 14.1 Movement disability and depression – B Weston – *aromatherapist/nurse, UK*

Client assessment

Mrs P had suffered a severe stroke, leaving her left arm completely paralysed and only partial recovery in her left leg. She had always been very independent and strong-willed, lived alone, and at the age of 89 she still ruled her children with a rod of iron. During her hospitalization, Mrs P had taken her disability very badly, resenting the loss of her independence. She became so depressed – almost suicidal – that she required the assistance of a psychiatrist.

On admission to Weston's nursing home, Mrs P initially settled very well, but after a month became very unsettled and unhappy, realizing she was never going to go back to her own flat. She was angry with her family for forcing her into this decision, and for selling her flat and belongings. Being determined to leave the home, she wandered off, twice falling badly, which resulted in two periods of hospitalization for a fractured pelvis and femur.

The psychiatrist periodically reviewed Mrs P's case, changed the medication to sedate her and relieve her depression. She became very apathetic, and due to the effects of the medication slept 20 hours out of 24, resulting in dehydration, loss of weight, anorexia and incontinence. It was decided to try aromatherapy.

Intervention

Mrs P's mood and behaviour were monitored for 7 days, using the Beck inventory for measuring depression, to see if there was any pattern to her distress and mood. It was noted that she appeared worse in the late mornings and in the evenings before bed. Treatments were therefore given mid-morning and at bedtime.

Daily massage was given to hands, legs and face using 5 drops each of:

- *Melissa officinalis* [melissa] – calming and sedative
- *Lavandula officinalis* [lavender] – calming and tonic to the nervous system
- *Pelargonium graveolens* [geranium] – calming and relaxing

These were added to a 50 ml blend of grapeseed oil and hypericum (restorative to the nervous system).

The same essential oils were used in Mrs P's bath, and periodically placed on her bed linen prior to her returning to it.

Outcome

By the end of 4 weeks, Mrs P was more content and alert; medication had been reduced, and she was eating and drinking well, gaining weight in the process. She has even begun to take outings with her family again and is more positive about the future, planning to enjoy life as best she can.

Constipation is a problem that becomes greater as the path of dementia progresses. Someone with short-term memory will forget that they have already been to the toilet and will continually return unless distracted and assisted. The urge to go to the toilet to open the bowels may be forgotten and not be re-addressed, thus chronic constipation with impaction higher up the colon may develop. The importance of drinking enough water, together with a good diet to aid elimination, cannot be overestimated.

Essential oils can be most effective for constipated patients when used with abdomen massage in a clockwise direction and/or massage of the digestive reflexes on the feet. With the latter, the area to concentrate on is the gastrointestinal tract, located in the soft tissue just below the level of the sesamoid bones and above the calcaneus, on the plantar surface of the foot. If not trained in Swiss reflex treatment or reflexology (see Ch. 7), it is still possible to carry out the following on the soles of the feet.

Using relevant essential oils in a cream base, start with the right foot and massage in large firm circles directed from the lateral to the medial side; the left foot should then be massaged in firm circles from the medial to the lateral side. This directional massage of the colon reflexes, with

---

Case study 14.2 Cerebral infarction and right-sided weakness – P Mullins – *aromatherapist, UK*

Client assessment

An 88-year-old lady came in with a left cerebral infarct and right-sided weakness. She was unable to communicate verbally. She had suffered a previous stroke in the past and was shown to have had hypertension.

The right aspect of the patient's mouth drooped downwards with continual dribbling/drooling when at rest. The position of her jaw hung widely open and was severely affected; there was no attempt to reposition. She had no tongue co-ordination so she could not speak and was nil by mouth. She was flaccid in the facial area.

Intervention

The aim/objective of the treatment was to help tone the muscles in the face and to stimulate sensitivity in the facial area.

This patient received regular face massage with equal quantities of the following at 2% in a carrier oil:

- *Lavandula angustifolia* [lavender] – analgesic, calming and sedative, cardiotonic, hypotensor
- *Citrus reticulata* [mandarin] – calming
- *Melaleuca alternifolia* [tea tree] – analgesic, immunostimulant, neurotonic, phlebotonic

Particular attention was paid to the cheeks, lips, chin (and under the chin) to help stimulate the flaccid tongue, which had no movement.

Outcome

By the 3rd treatment, this patient could move her tongue very slightly with some exercises and managed to swallow some water and thickened juice. She no longer dribbled and managed to keep her lips closed most of the time.

By the 7th treatment, the patient had no dribbling/drooling. She closed her lips together when swallowing and dabbed her mouth when necessary to clear any excessive spillage from her lips. She was also better able to drink fluids as her swallowing had improved.

---

pressure, helps peristalsis, as do movements 2 and 3 of the abdomen massage, carried out firmly and slowly with the heel of the hand, shown in Chapter 7, pp. 185, 186.

Compresses (see pp. 147–148) can also be used, especially on those who are not happy to receive massage.

Several oils are helpful for constipation, the most effective being:

- *Rosmarinus officinalis* [rosemary] (cts. camphor and cineole) – stimulating to a sluggish digestion
- *Citrus aurantium* var. *amara* (per.) [orange bigarade] – digestive (constipation)
- *Zingiber officinale* [ginger] – digestive stimulant

N.B. Ginger is cited for constipation by Franchomme & Pénoël (2001 p. 434) and for diarrhoea by Valnet (1980 p. 135). Like *Foeniculum vulgare* var. *dulce*, it may be a balancing oil in this direction.

Further suggestions can be found in Appendix A(II).

Diarrhoea

This condition can be just as upsetting to a patient as constipation and the following essential oils will be found helpful:

- *Origanum majorana* [sweet marjoram] and *Citrus limon* [lemon] are effective where the diarrhoea is of nervous origin, as they also have tranquillizing effects
- *Melaleuca viridiflora* [niaouli] – also anti-inflammatory
- *Mentha* x *piperita* [peppermint] – also anti-inflammatory and will help against nausea
- *Pelargonium graveolens* [geranium] – also anti-inflammatory and calming

The antiinflammatory oils above are useful where there is colitis or gastroenteritis, whilst *Syzygium aromaticum* (flos) [clove bud], *Pimpinella anisum* [aniseed], *Melaleuca cajuputi* [cajuput] and *Myristica fragrans* [nutmeg] relieve the spasms (Valnet 1980 pp. 95, 101, 114, 161).

A blend which has been found to work well for both enteritis and irritable bowel syndrome, but mostly administered internally, diluted in a dispersant, is equal quantities of *Foeniculum vulgare* var. *dulce* [fennel], *Mentha* x *piperita* and *Piper nigrum* [black pepper].

Diverticulitis (diverticulosis)

Diverticulosis, the harmless presence of small bulges in weak points in the large intestine, exists in most elderly people (Wingate & Wingate 1996 p. 147). It is only when one or more of these diverticula becomes inflamed that chronic diverticulitis can set in and constipation, slight abdominal pain and bleeding may manifest.

The diet should be changed to one rich in fibre, and massage with antiinflammatory essential oils such as rosemary and bitter orange (in Constipation above) would be beneficial. Other antiinflammatory oils which act on the digestive system are:

- *Commiphora myrrha* [myrrh]
- *Chamomilla recutita* [German chamomile]
- *Juniperus communis* (fruct.) [juniper berry]
- *Melissa officinalis*

Indigestion (dyspepsia)

Chronic indigestion can be due to many causes. Common physical reasons, if there is no gastritis or ulcer present, may be eating too quickly, too much – or swallowing air with food. Medication or heavy smoking may also be responsible (Wingate & Wingate 1996 p. 256). In many cases stress can be implicated and this should be treated as well by including relaxing essential oils in the choice.

Abdominal and/or foot massage should be carried out 30 minutes before a meal, using any of the following essential oils:

- *Carum carvi* [caraway], *Citrus aurantium* var. *amara* (per.), *Foeniculum vulgare* var. *dulce* and *Pimpinella anisum* [aniseed] are the most effective
- *Ocimum basilicum* var. *album* [basil] can be added if the indigestion is of nervous origin
- *Origanum majorana* is helpful if gastritis or an ulcer are present
- *Citrus reticulata* [mandarin] and *Rosmarinus officinalis* [rosemary] are useful where there is pain or cramp
- *Citrus limon* (per.) is analgesic and antacid
- *Melissa officinalis* and *Mentha* x *piperita* are often found to be beneficial too

HEADACHES AND MIGRAINES

These can occur for a number of reasons, which are not always apparent, especially in the elderly. Because of this, it is important to make use of the

---

Case study 14.3 Diverticulitis – R Nancarrow – *aromatherapist/nurse, Australia*

Client assessment
Mrs W, in a care home, was unable to open her bowels owing to atrophy of the large intestine – and required admission to hospital every 3 weeks for a colonic washout. Doctors were planning to remove the large intestine, which would have left her with a colostomy.

Intervention
A blend of the following oils was made up in a carrier oil:

- *Foeniculum vulgare* [fennel] – analgesic, antiinflammatory, laxative
- *Piper nigrum* [black pepper] – analgesic, eupeptic

- *Pogostemon patchouli* [patchouli] – antiinfectious, antiinflammatory

The blend was massaged gently into the woman's abdomen in a clockwise direction several times that evening.

Outcome
She had a normal bowel movement the next day.

The massages were continued daily, and an oral operient was taken nightly. The nurses were taught how to do the massages so that no day was missed.

The woman's bowels continued to be opened regularly, thus avoiding the necessity of an operation.

synergy between essential oils and mix two or more together.

The oil most often used is *Lavandula angustifolia*. Equally effective are *Chamaemelum nobile*, *Mentha x piperita*, *Ocimum basilicum*, *Origanum majorana* and *Rosmarinus officinalis*. The choice of oil may depend on the cause, for example peppermint works well on a headache caused by digestive disorders. Inhalation from a tissue (or by other means – see Ch. 5) gives the speediest reaction, though massage of the neck and face, particularly the forehead (using two or three of the above oils in a carrier oil), gives the patient the additional relaxing and soothing benefits of massage (see Ch. 7).

INSOMNIA

Sleep frequently becomes disturbed in people with dementia, which is particularly difficult for carers, who become increasingly tired and stressed. A good quality, refreshing night's sleep is a bigger problem in hospitals than when the patient is at home, especially with the elderly, whose normal sleep pattern may already be erratic (Cannard 1994).

Take care when using lavender, as varieties of both lavenders and lavandins can give very different results. Hospital pharmacists often supply the more camphoraceous *L. latifolia* [spike lavender] rather than the French *L. angustifolia* (Buckle 1992) and Franchomme & Pénoël (2001 p. 392) recommend *L. x intermedia* 'Super' – which they still refer to by its old name, 'Burnatii'

Lavendula angustifolia is the usual, effective (when botanically specified) essential oil used to induce sleep, the effects being enhanced by the addition of *Chamaemelum nobile* [Roman chamomile]. Macdonald (1995) found that 'a few drops of appropriate oils on the pillow helped to induce a peaceful sleep in many patients', implying the use of more than one oil – which Price always believes to be an effective measure.

Mike Hardy at the Old Manor Hospital (Salisbury) used vaporized lavender oil as a nocturnal sedative for elderly patients with sleeping difficulties. Positive observations were made in relation to reduced restlessness, deeper sleep, with more pleasant moods on waking. (Hardy 1991). Further work was carried out at Newholme Hospital (Bakewell) where a multi-

---

Box 14.3   Sleep promotion trial (Wolfe & Herzeberg 1996)

Aim of trial

Wolfe and Herzberg (1996) carried out a trial on two randomly selected patients in 1996 using *Lavandula officinalis* and *Chamaemelum nobile* [Roman chamomile], to ascertain whether they would promote sleep in severely demented patients. One had a history of aggressive behaviour, the other had Alzheimer's disease and was extremely agitated.

Over an initial 2-week period the patients were monitored half-hourly during the night and their sleep and behaviour patterns noted.

Intervention

Each night for the next week (week 3 of the trial) two drops of lavender essential oil were dropped on the bedding close to their heads each night 15 minutes before they retired. During week 4, Roman chamomile was used – and during week 5 a mixture of the two oils was used. During this time the patients were monitored as before. The second period of 3 weeks followed the same pattern of treatment as weeks 4 to 6.

Outcome

This small study gave support to the notion that essential oils can help promote peaceful sleep and a restful night; they may also allow a reduction in dependency on hypnotic medication in demented subjects.

---

disciplinary team of health-care professionals aimed to assess the effect on the number of night time hours patients with severe dementia spent asleep, using lavender in room diffusion (Henry et al 1994).

While other effective oils can be found in Appendix A(II), it is worth mentioning the following:

- *Ocimum basilicum* var. *album* [European basil] – helpful where the insomnia is of nervous origin (Valnet 1980 p. 97)
- *Santalum album* [sandalwood], *Citrus reticulata* (per.) [mandarin] and *Valeriana officinalis* [common valerian] – sleep inducing, due to their sedative and calming effects

Box 14.4   Trial on sleep latency (Miyake et al 1991)

Aim of trial

Using electroencephalogram (EEG) results and psychological scoring, Miyake et al (1991) examined the effects of inhaling essential oils (unspecified) on the sleep latency of humans under conditions of stress.

Oils used

Spike lavender, bitter orange, sweet fennel, marjoram and valerian (unspecified).

The subjects were first given some arithmetic to do, which increased their arousal level. They were then left in relaxed surroundings. The essential oils were presented individually and continuously by an air bubbling system.

Results

Bitter orange oil increased the sleeping time of the subjects significantly. It was thought to affect the cortex, inhibiting the excitement of the central nervous system and causing sedative effects to appear. As a result, the subjects found it easier to sleep even under conditions of mental stress.

■ *Cananga odorata* [ylang ylang] and *Citrus limon* [lemon] – possess sleep-inducing properties and are useful if the aroma of lavender is not liked

The essential oils can be vaporized, used on a tissue, put in the bath or applied in a carrier.

MUSCLE CONTRACTION OF THE FINGERS

In the late stages of dementia contractions of the fingers may occur. This leads to loss of ability to carry out normal activity needed to function, for example, not being able to grip spoons, a comb or a handrail for stability and to prevent falling. It then becomes difficult both to trim the finger nails and keep the hand/s clean and is physically painful for the patient to have his or her hand/s attended to. This can be made easier by soaking the hand first in a small plastic bowl containing warm water and 2 drops each of *Lavandula angustifolia* and *Origanum majorana* [sweet marjoram]. Having some appropriate music playing also helps to distract and calm the patient and enable the hand and fingers to relax (the fingernails may have been digging into the palm, which is both painful and distressing for the patient). The hand can then be dried carefully and massaged to relax it still further, so that the fingers can be gradually extended and the fingernails attended to. *Lavandula angustifolia* is always a stable choice for the elderly, but there are other muscle relaxing and analgesic essential oils – which would allow a change of aroma, for example, *Pelargonium graveolens* [geranium] or/and *Juniperus communis* (fruct.) [juniper berry].

PARKINSON'S DISEASE

Aromatherapy massage can be of great benefit to promote general relaxation and relieve muscular rigidity (Price 2001). In a preliminary trial run by Price (co-author of this chapter) during 9 months of 1992, the following oils, in equal quantities, were used with a good measure of success (100% in the above two symptoms) to give relief to several symptomatic side-effects shown by Parkinson's disease sufferers. Equal quantities of the three essential oils below (Price 1993) were blended together and added at a concentration of 1.5% to either carrier oil for a weekly massage or base lotion for daily application:

■ *Salvia sclarea* (clary) – relaxant, nerve tonic; to aid general relaxation and relieve anxiety
■ *Origanum majorana* (sweet marjoram) – analgesic, antispasmodic, digestive tonic, hypotensor, nerve tonic, relaxant; to relax the muscles, relieve pain and insomnia and improve digestion
■ *Lavandula angustifolia* – analgesic, antispasmodic, digestive stimulant, hypotensor, sedative; to relax the muscles and relieve pain, insomnia and anxiety

Lewy body type dementia is associated with Parkinson's disease and the general use of aromatherapy to alleviate the anxiety and behaviour changes as described above may be considered. Muscular rigidity and changes in gait are a major difficulty and aromatic baths have been found to be beneficial (the use of a specialist hoist for bathing may be needed for safety). Regular

---

Case study 14.4 Flexed fingers – J Henry – *aromatherapist, UK*

Client/patient assessment

An 83-year-old female was experiencing advanced third stage dementia and receiving care in a specialist hospital ward. She was very anxious and had flexed fingers on her right hand, following a small stroke. The flexion of her fingers led to pain when her fingernails grew and cut into her palm. She was even more apprehensive and more anxious when staff attempted to extend and open her fingers to give her necessary care – due to the pain.

Intervention

Anxiety:

- 4 drops *Lavandula angustifolia* [lavender] – calming, sedative, tonic

These were placed on the cartridge of an electric diffuser in her single room, to give her a calm start to the morning (to enable her to get up, go to the toilet, get washed and dressed) and reduce the overall level of anxiety and distress later in the day. As she had been a pianist, her favourite classical piano music was played in the background (Beethoven or Mozart).

Flexed fingers:

- 2 drops *Lavandula angustifolia* – analgesic, calming, tonic
- 4 drops *Melaleuca alternifolia* – analgesic, neurotonic
- Small bowl comfortably warm water

The lady was encouraged to place her flexed hand into the bowl of water and essential oils for a few minutes, when her fingers were helped very gently to uncurl, making it a pleasant, non-fearful experience. After carefully drying her hand, it was massaged with almond oil and lavender, gradually opening the palm – stopping immediately if painful.

Outcome

This allowed the nurse or therapist to cut the finger nails which in turn prevents the pain of her nails cutting into the palm.

The session was finished with a tray of tea for two with biscuits using non-hospital crockery – turning the whole session into a pleasurable experience.

When the room diffuser and music tapes for her anxiety were used on a regular daily basis, the staff commented that the lady was less anxious and brighter in mood (lasting well into the day), thus improving her quality of life.

Addressing the flexed fingers and hand care, also in her single room, with music, room diffusion, the hand soak and massage – followed by tea for two proved successful in lowering both anxiety and pain without confrontation.

---

massage to promote general relaxation will also help stimulate functional ability and regular facial massage can help to relieve the lack of facial expression due to neuromuscular change.

PRESSURE SORES

This is an area where traditional medicine has limited success, and nurses using aromatherapy have been rewarded by the healing which has occurred with the use of essential oils. Cicatrizant oils such as *Boswellia carteri* [frankincense] and *Helichrysum angustifolium* [everlasting], together with a strongly antiseptic oil can be used in a spray with water when the sores are suppurating

– 10 drops in 100 ml water, shaking well each time before spraying the area. *Commiphora myrrha* [myrrh], *Lavandula angustifolia* and *Pogostemon patchouli* are both cicatrizant and antiseptic.

If the skin can be touched, gently apply a little from a mix made from five to six drops of essential oil in 50 ml oil of *Calendula officinalis* (macerated carrier oil), which itself has cicatrizant effects on wounds and persistent ulcers (Price 2000 p. 163–164). Calendula oil will also help to strengthen the skin if the mixture is massaged in gently twice a day. Compresses may be useful (see Ch. 5), but check that the dressing used is non-stick. Passant (1990) frequently used a combination of rose, geranium, lavender and marjoram (all unspecified) in inhalations to calm and comfort her patients before changing dressings (Wise 1989).

The cicatrizant qualities of the resinoid *Styrax tonkinensis* [Siam benzoin] can also play a part in healing.

RESPIRATORY PROBLEMS

The conifer family is chiefly acknowledged in textbooks of materia medica, pharmacology and therapeutics as having expectorant properties (Boyd & Pearson 1946), although there is anecdotal evidence to support the fact that essential oils from other families are reputed to have expectorant properties also.

Elderly people suffering from catarrhal problems, such as chronic bronchitis or asthma, can benefit from a daily application of essential oils in a carrier lotion on to their chest and neck. The thin skin behind the ears also facilitates percutaneous penetration of essential oils.

Eight drops of essential oils in total should be added to 50 ml carrier lotion.

Essential oils which are both anticatarrhal and expectorant include:

- *Abies alba* fol. [silver fir], *Melaleuca viridiflora* [niaouli] – especially in chronic cases and *Myrtus communis* fol.
- *Boswellia carteri* [frankincense] – also antitussive and mucolytic
- *Eucalyptus smithii* [gully gum] – also antiviral (common cold and influenza) and has excellent disinfectant properties
- *Hyssopus officinalis* [hyssop] – also anti-inflammatory and antitussive (suitable only for non-epileptic patients)
- *Mentha* x *piperita* [peppermint] – also anti-inflammatory and useful where there are sinus problems

If any respiratory infection is present, and *E. smithii* is not one of the oils used, add *Thymus mastichina* [Spanish marjoram] and/or *T. vulgaris* ct. geraniol or ct. linalool [sweet thyme] (the latter is both antiinflammatory and antispasmodic).

E. smithii is an excellent preventive measure for winter coughs and colds because it increases the resistance of the respiratory system to infection. It has a pleasant aroma, is inexpensive and can be vaporized daily in the lounge area of the ward, and/or in the ward (or bedrooms, as many of the newer hospitals name the rooms of the elderly or patients with learning difficulties).

RHEUMATISM AND ARTHRITIS

Rheumatism is a vague term which covers various types of conditions associated with pain in the muscles. The two main types are rheumatoid arthritis and osteoarthritis. With rheumatoid arthritis chronic inflammation of the connective tissue around the joints (normally attacking them in symmetrical pairs) is involved, which causes pain, swelling and stiffness, frequently accompanied by weight loss and fatigue. With osteoarthritis (Wingate & Wingate (1996 p. 349) prefer the term 'osteoarthrosis', because there is no inflammation), there is a progressive wearing away of the cartilage, the connective tissue thickens and any fluid which may fill the joint causes swelling, resulting in severe pain and reduced movement.

Pain is perhaps the most important symptom to consider and 'while conventional analgesics give some relief, they seldom give complete or sustained relief' (McDonald 1995). Essential oils have been used successfully for many years to reduce inflammation and pain in the fibrous tissues around the joints (Price 1992), giving increased mobility (see also Appendix A(II)):

- *Origanum majorana* [sweet marjoram], *Pelargonium graveolens* [geranium] and *Juniperus communis* ram. [juniper wood] all have both analgesic and stress-relieving properties; juniper, in addition, is also antiinflammatory (Roulier 1990 p. 268) as is geranium. Juniper also helps to reduce any fluid around the joints
- *Coriandrum sativum* [coriander] and *Melaleuca cajuputi* [cajuput] possess antiinflammatory properties that are effective on connective tissue, thus indirectly dulling arthritic pain (Franchomme & Pénoël 2001 pp. 371, 379)
- for severe pain, *Syzygium aromaticum* (flos) [clove bud], *Melaleuca leucadendron* [cajuput] and *Myristica fragrans* [nutmeg] may have a stronger effect

The most effective method of using the essential oils (diluted for regular use at 1% in a vegetable carrier oil or a base lotion) is to apply them directly to the affected area or with a compress. They can be applied with or without massage, although massage does help to relax the muscles. For a one-off faster effect, applying a few drops of undiluted essential oils is effective on small areas. A warm bath containing essential oils also relaxes the muscles and reduces the pain.

SHORT-TERM MEMORY/REMINISCENCE

Loss of short-term memory yet the ability to remember long term enables the positive use of reminiscence to be made, achieving more relaxed conversation and communication. One must be aware that there may be different reactions, e.g. reminiscent memory may bring tears, although these may be a release rather than distressing (Henry 1993, Henry 2003, Kyle 1998/1999).

The value of aromas is considerable – aroma groups, gardening and the use of sensory gardens can enable people with dementia to respond to familiar smells, textures and tastes. Aromas from the kitchen or other environments open up a wealth of opportunity for reminiscence, e.g. the spices used in Christmas cake and lavender bags used in clothes drawers, new mown grass – many aromas remind people of favourite places. Essential oils such as *Lavandula angustifolia*, *Cinnamomum verum* [cinnamon] and *Pinus sylvestris* [pine] can help stimulate happy memories from the past.

WOUND CARE

Extremely 'paper-thin' skin is relatively common in geriatric patients due to poor circulation, medication, poor nutrition and age, hence skin tears, which can be difficult to heal (Kloth 1990) and wounds are quite common. Nursing professionals in several countries have used essential oils in wound care with success (Kerr 2002), especially in geriatric settings (see p. 330).

Gattefossé and other physicians had remarkable results in the early 20th century with lavender (unspecified) when treating wounds and ulcers, Sassard noting that in all cases, there was a rapid disappearance of pus, a decrease in the number of bacteria, with healing being accomplished 'in a very short time' (Gattefossé 1993). Franchomme & Pénoël (2001 p. 212) tell us that the most spectacular action of oils containing ketones is

---

> **Box 14.5   Trial on wound healing effects of essential oils** (Guba 1998)
>
> ### Aim of trials
> Two studies were undertaken in an attempt to quantify the wound healing effects of various essential oils and aromatic extracts.
>
> ### Intervention
> In each, the blend (Wound Heal Formula – WHF) was applied a minimum of once daily for skin tears, and twice daily for pressure areas and venous ulcers. Generally, the preparation was applied to dry gauze and then taped over the wound.
>
> Other appropriate wound care measures were carried out as usual, such as cleaning with normal saline solution. Nursing staff noted all relevant information on the patient's records, such as initial wound description, with regular updates of treatment progress until healing. The wound healing cream was found to be 'most effective; there was no incident of allergic reactions and in all cases the healing process was achieved in short periods', one nurse saying that 'the standard treatment for pressure areas, such as alginate dressings, generally slough off the necrotic tissue producing a cavity. However, when using the WHF, the necrotic tissue only slowly flaked off, opening up to healthy granulation tissue, with only a small cavity or no cavity at all developing. WHF works without exception on pressure areas.'

---

their power to regenerate and heal cutaneous tissue. *Lavandula officinalis* contains only around 4% ketones, *Lavandula* x *intermedia* 'Super' [lavandin] having from 5–14%.

Helichrysum italicum, containing 15–20% ketones, is a noted cicatrizing agent in wound healing (Franchomme & Pénoël 2001 p. 384). It appears to have only mild neurotoxic effects, with the only potential caution being its use in those prone to epilepsy (Guba 1998) – and that caution would be for ingestion of significant amounts (Guba 2004 personal communication).

Matricaria recutita [German chamomile] has a long history of use in Europe in traditional medicine for its antiinflammatory and healing properties (Weiss 1988).

When selecting a fixed oil for use in wound care, the macerated oil of *Calendula officinalis*, with its antiinflammatory, antiinfectious and cicatrizant qualities is a good choice for wounds (Della Loggia et al 1990, Wichtl 1989), as is also *Calophyllum inophyllum* [tamanu], its effectiveness in wound healing being documented by Daste et al in 1993.

SUMMARY

The older person in today's society expects to live longer and be more active; greater numbers of older people are living into their eighties and nineties, therefore a greater number of people will probably develop a form of dementia. When older people are diagnosed with dementia, Parkinson's disease or other conditions associated with advancing years, the value of aromatherapy can be considerable. We live our lives through our senses. The aroma and specific chemical properties of essential oils used in aromatherapy may be applied to many conditions and aspects of life and care. A myriad of conditions may all benefit from the application of pure essential oils by trained, registered and insured aromatherapists throughout the world. Both carers and cared for benefit from aromatherapy.

References

Alzheimer's Society CD for Primary Care Professionals. Dementia diagnosis and management in primary care (free of charge – see Useful addresses)

Alzheimer's Society web site www.alzheimers.org.uk

Ballard C, O'Brien J T, Reichelt K, Perry E K 2002 Aromatherapy as a safe and effective treatment for the management of agitation in severe dementia: the results of a double-blind, placebo controlled trial with *melissa*. Journal of Clinical Psychiatry 63(7): 553–558

Battaglia S 1997 The complete guide to aromatherapy. The Perfect Potion, Virginia Q, p. 375

Beshara M C, Giddings D 2002 Use of plant essential oils in treating agitation in a Dementia Unit. 10. Case studies. International Journal of Aromatherapy 12(4): 207–212

Bowles E J, Griffiths D M, Quirk L, Brownrigg A, Croot K 2002 Effects of essential oils and touch on resistance to nursing care procedures and other dementia-related behaviours in a residential care facility. International Journal of Aromatherapy 12(1): 22–29

Boyd E M, Pearson G L 1946 The expectorant action of volatile oils. American Journal of Medical Science 211: 602–610

Buckle J 1992 Which lavender oil? Nursing Times 88(22): 54–55

Cannard G 1994 On the scent of a good night's sleep. Trial project. Midland Health Board News January 3rd

Daste A et al 1993 The pacific ocean oils – Tamanu oil l'ami des ingredients. Naturels: 5: 2

Della Loggia, R et al 1990 Topical anti-inflammatory activity of *Calendula officinalis* extracts. Planta Medica 56: 658–659

Franchomme P, Pénoël D 2001 L'aromathérapie exactement 2nd edn. Jollois, Limoges

Gattefossé R M 1993 Gattefossé's aromatherapy. Daniel, Saffron Walden

Gilley D W, Whalen M E, Wilson R S et al 1991 Hallucinations and associated factors in Alzheimer's disease. Journal of Neuropsychiatry 3: 497–500

Guba R 1998 Wound healing. International Journal of Aromatherapy 9(2): 67–74

Hardy M 1991 Sweet scented dreams. International Journal of Aromatherapy 3(2): 12–13.

Henry J 1993 Dementia – aroma groups improve quality of life in Alzheimer's disease. International Journal of Aromatherapy 5(1): 27–29

Henry J 2003 Aromatherapy for people with dementia. In Essence 2(3): 23–25

Henry J, Rusius C W, Davies M, Veazey-French T 1994 Lavender for night sedation of people with dementia. International Journal of Aromatherapy 6(2): 28–30

Holmes C, Hopkins V, Hensford C et al 2002 Lavender oil as a treatment for agitated behaviour in severe dementia: a placebo controlled study. International Journal of Geriatric Psychiatry 17: 305–308

Horrigan C 1995 In: Rankin-Box D (ed) The nurse's handbook. Churchill Livingstone, Edinburgh

Jamison R N, Parris W C V, Maxon W S 1987 Psychological factors influencing recovery from out-patient surgery. Behaviour Research Therapy 25: 31–37

Kerr J 2002 Research Project – using essential oils in wound care for the elderly. Aromatherapy Today 23 September: 14–19

Kerr J 2004 The use of essential oils in healing wounds. International Journal of Aromatherapy 12(4): 202–206

Kitwood T 1997 Evaluating dementia care booklet. Bradford Dementia Group, School of Health Studies, University of Bradford

Kloth L 1990 Wound healing: alternative in management. Davis, Philadelphia

Kyle L 1998/1999 Aromatherapy for elder care. International Journal of Aromatherapy 9(4): 170–177

McCann K, McKenna H 1993 An examination of touch between nurses and elderly patients in a continuing care setting in Northern Ireland. Journal of Advanced Nursing 18: 838–846

McDonald E M 1995 Aromatherapy for the enhancement of the nursing care of elderly people suffering from arthritic pain. The Aromatherapist 2(1): 26–31

Mitchell S 1993 Dementia – aromatherapy's effectiveness in disorders associated with dementia. International Journal of Aromatherapy 5(2): 20–23

Miyake Y, Nakagawa M, Asakura Y 1991 Effects of odors on humans (1): Effects on sleep latency. Chemical Senses 16: 193

Moate S 1995 Anxiety and depression. International Journal of Aromatherapy 7(1): 18–21

Passant H 1990 A holistic approach in the ward. Nursing Times 86(4): 26–28

Petit-Zeman S 1999 All about dementia. Mental Health Foundation Booklet

Petit-Zeman S 2004 Sniffing out dementia? Alzheimer's Society Newsletter, February 8th

Price S 1992 Arthritis and Rheumatism. Yoga & Health Feb: 37/38

Price S 1993 Parkinson's disease project: is aromatherapy an effective treatment for Parkinson's disease? The Aromatherapist 1(1): 14–21

Price S 2000 Aromatherapy workbook, 2nd edn. Thorsons, London

Price S 2001 Aromatherapy for women. Lorenz Books, London, pp. 90–91

Rabins P V, Mace N L, Lucas M J 1982 The impact of dementia on the family. Journal of the American Medical Association 248: 333–335

Roulier G 1990 Les huiles essentielles pour votre santé. Dangles, St-Jean-de-Braye

Stone J 1996 Complementary Therapy Health Service Journal (January) 26–27

Talamo B 1989 Nature. Reported in the New Scientist 11th March 1989: 35

Tisserand R 1989 Olfactory aid to Alzheimer's diagnosis. International Journal of Aromatherapy 1(4): 3

Valnet J 1980 The practice of aromatherapy. C W Daniel, Saffron Walden, p. 135

Weiss R F 1988 Herbal medicine. Arcanum, Göteborg, p. 24

Wichtl M 1989 Herbal drugs and phytopharmaceuticals. CRC Press, Boca Raton, pp. 118–120

Wingate P, Wingate R 1996 The Penguin medical encyclopedia. Penguin Books, London, p. 39

Wise R 1989 Flower power. Nursing Times 85(22): 45–47

Wolfe A, Herzeberg J 1996 Can aromatherapy oils promote sleep in severely demented patients? International Journal of Geriatric Psychology 11: 926–927

Chapter 15

Palliative and supportive care

Sue Whyte, Elaine Cooper and Shirley Price

INTRODUCTION

Palliative and supportive (P & S) care differ in philosophy from curative strategies in that they focus primarily on the consequences of a disease rather than on its cause or specific cure. Thus the approaches are holistic, pragmatic and multi-disciplinary, with very little distinction between palliation and support (National Council for Hospice and Specialist Palliative Care Services 2000). This chapter gives an insight into palliative and supportive care, together with the use of essential oils. With the help of aromatherapy, hundreds of people have enjoyed a quality of life better than they might otherwise have experienced, with even better prospects for the future.

DEFINING CARE AND SUPPORT

Total, active care of patients and their family begins from the time the diagnosis is first suspected and continues after death with care of the family in bereavement. It is needed the moment a patient no longer responds to curative treatment, when the best quality of life for them and their families becomes the most important issue. In itself, palliative care neither hastens nor postpones death; it merely recognizes a patient's right to spend as much time at home as possible, and pays equal attention to physical, psychological, social and spiritual aspects of care wherever the patient is (World Health Organization [WHO] 1990).

WHO went on to say that death should be regarded as a normal process, although those aspects of care – psychological and spiritual – should be given to patients so that they can come to terms with their own death as fully and constructively as possible. Relief should be provided for pain and other distressing symptoms, so that they have an improved quality of life until death – if this is expected. P & S care does not see the patient in isolation, but as part of the family unit and a support system must be in place to help families cope during the patient's illness and their possible bereavement. The carers themselves are regularly facing the reality of death, bringing them face to face with their own mortality, and they are therefore able to empathize with patients.

NEGATIVE LANGUAGE

When a person has a disease that is no longer curable, many people, including health-care professionals, describe the person as being terminally ill and any care they may require is described as terminal care. These are negative terms, focusing on death rather than life; they are also vague and ambiguous – who knows how long a life the person has left? There is a rapidly growing number of people in well-developed countries who are living for several years with 'a terminal illness' such as cancer, yet lead useful lives that are reasonably satisfactory to them. This is why words such as 'terminal', 'end of life' and 'care of the dying' were – and still are – considered to be unsuitable. What has come to be called palliative and supportive care has sprung from the pioneering work of Dame Cicely Saunders and the modern hospice movement. Care is tailored to each individual patient, changing as their needs change, so the word 'terminal' is irrelevant, as there is no demarcation line.

PROVISION OF CARE

P & S care requires the expertise of a care team whose members are drawn from different quarters – doctors, nurses, physiotherapists, occupational therapists, social workers, clergy, counsellors, complementary therapists and so on, but not forgetting the patient and his or her family, who play an important part.

Aromatherapists need to be aware of the necessity of interprofessional communication with the rest of the care team, especially if they notice any changes in the patient's condition. The aromatherapist is part of a team, even when working independently and must keep them informed of his/her part in the patient's care.

Referrals for aromatherapy may come from the patient themselves, a family member or health professional. Where patients are seen will depend on the particular setting in which the therapist is working and how the service is organized, and may be any of the following:

- the aromatherapist's own private treatment room
- the patient's own home
- an inpatient setting, singly or shared with other patients
- an outpatient setting in an individual room or one shared with other patients e.g. waiting for or receiving chemotherapy treatment.

Palliative care supports carers as well as the patient, so referrals may be made for the carer in some services.

DISORDERS INVOLVED

Although the philosophy and principles can apply to any client group, P & S care is aimed primarily at people with specific disorders. Notably, these include:

- cancer
- infection with human immunodeficiency virus (HIV) and acquired immune deficiency syndrome (AIDS)
- degenerative neurological disorders such as motor neurone disease (MND), multiple sclerosis (MS) and Parkinson's disease
- disorders that occur only in childhood, e.g. cystic fibrosis and Duchenne muscular dystrophy
- various genetic and congenital disorders.

Where cure is not an option, care is focused on helping them through the difficult times ahead of them, supporting them while learning acceptance and coping, and maintaining optimum independence with the best quality of life possible.

The above diseases all have the following characteristics in common:

- An increased likelihood of fear, psychological, social and spiritual distresses.
- Unpredictable symptoms, which are always changing and can be very distressing. There will be good days and bad days, which can add to the frustrations and stress of the patient, family and carers.
- A lack of understanding of these disorders by some health-care workers and by society in general, can unwittingly contribute to the person's distress.
- Life-threatening, with shortened life expectancy – often quite significant, and the last phase of the illness probably being relatively short.
- A 'life' pattern which can fluctuate quite markedly both in the individual and from person to person, e.g. there may be periods of remission, exacerbation or stability, or there may be a slow progressive decline; never-theless, people may also appear fit and well with little or no change to their way of life.
- The rate and manner of decline can fluctuate and varies considerably from person to person. There will come a point where the condition of the person leaves no room for doubt that death is likely to occur in a matter of hours or days rather than weeks.

PHYSICAL SYMPTOMS

The following symptoms relate to many of those occurring in P & S care, all except perhaps those with an asterisk being able to be alleviated or helped by essential oils. The essential oils which may be used for the individual symptoms can be found in Appendix A(II).

- pain
- nausea and vomiting
- muscle spasms – rigidity – weakness – loss of control* – difficulty in swallowing* – dribbling of saliva – attacks of choking*
- impaired speech*
- weight loss – poor appetite – loss of interest in food
- loss of bladder control
- reduced mobility – reduced dexterity
- mouth problems – sore – dry – ulcerated – infected
- breathing problems – panic attacks
- impaired sensation* – reduced/increased/altered

Case study 15.1 HIV/AIDS – A Barker – *aromatologist/nurse*

Client assessment
A is in the last stages of full-blown AIDS. He cannot cope with baths or massage due to the onset of Kaposi's sarcoma. Added to this there is evidence of infiltration of the nervous system, due to the virus which has at this point become phagocytosed by the macrophages, allowing these cells to cross the normally impervious blood–brain barrier. The options open to the team were very limited, but not beyond helping. There needed to be a way to get the oils into the lymphatic system in order to stimulate the growth of T-helper cells and white blood cells.

Intervention
The essential oils (in a carrier lotion) were applied to the main lymph nodes, i.e. armpits, thorax, groin area – a rather unorthodox way, but it was necessary to adapt to the needs of the client.

10 drops each of the following oils were used:

- *Citrus limon* per. [lemon] – antianaemic, antiviral, immunostimulant
- *Thymus vulgaris* ct. alcohol [sweet thyme] – antiviral, immunostimulant, neurotonic
- *Melaleuca alternifolia* [tea tree] – antiviral, immunostimulant, neurotonic
- 30 ml base carrier lotion

The lotion, applied twice a day in a thick smear, was easily absorbed into the skin/lymph node areas without any difficulty, such that A was soon able to apply the lotion himself.

At the time of writing his T-helper cell count is rising, he is stable and coping well with the applications.

- epileptic fits, usually associated with brain tumours
- feeling tired all the time – no energy – feeling weak
- swollen limb(s)
- joint contractures
- skin problems/lesions
- generalized level of impaired body function.

PSYCHOLOGICAL SYMPTOMS

The aromatherapist should be aware of the problems and issues that can arise psychologically – and here again, essential oils can be of great help, as aromas are known to affect the mind (Gati & Cayola 1923, Lee & Lee 1992). Price's book, Aromatherapy and Your Emotions (2000) deals with all emotional aspects, essential oils to help many of these being found in Appendix A(II) of this book.

Psychological symptoms can include:

- shock and disbelief at the diagnosis
- anger and frustration with delays in diagnosis, appointments and failure of treatment
- anxiety and fear of pain and other distressing symptoms
- fear of death itself
- distress and anxiety
- tense, depressed, anxious and panicky, but not able to say why
- feeling helpless and no longer in control
- confusion, including disorientation (usually associated brain tumours).

Case study 15.2 Brain tumour – J Maher – *aromatherapist, Australia*

Mrs B, a lady in her 50s, had had a brain tumour removed, but still had a malignant tumour level 4 growing deep into the middle of the brain. She had received 6 weeks of radium treatment and was on a lot of medication. She had been a healthy hard-working lady, the first symptoms of her disorder being loss of balance and migraines – which she did not normally suffer. On visiting the doctor, he immediately did tests and referred her to a neurosurgeon. They operated – a shock to both herself and her family. Her daughter contacted the therapist a few months after her mother's operation.

Client assessment
Mrs B was partly paralysed down the left side and was using a walking frame. Circulation and lymph were poor, she had a broken sleep pattern due to arm and leg twitches, her general health was not good and she was having seizures at least once a week – increasing as time went on. She became dehydrated easily and had a very itchy scalp where her hair was growing back and the skin was very dry. The physiotherapy treatments (up to 3 times a week), to exercise the partly paralysed limbs, made her very tired, so they were cut to once or twice a week.

Intervention
Treatments were given twice weekly using the following:

- *Boswellia carteri* [frankincense] – analgesic, antidepressive, immunostimulant
- *Citrus limon* [lemon] – antiinflammatory, calming, immunostimulant
- *Lavandula angustifolia* [lavender] – analgesic, antiinflammatory, antiseptic, balancing, calming and sedative, neurotonic
- 10 ml carrier oil – 80% almond oil, 5% avocado, 5% calendula – to help her dry skin

Outcome
She found she was more relaxed after treatments – not only helping to give her a better quality of sleep, but also stopping the nervous twitching of her arm and leg.

The doctors ceased both physiotherapy and aromatherapy for a period of 1 month, after which time, they found the tumour had spread and seizures were becoming more frequent. The doctors then suggested she recommence aromatherapy treatments, as she had commented how much they had helped her feeling of well-being. Also, it had been found that during the course of treatments, not only had the seizures been of shorter duration and less violent; but she had experienced less pain.

Behavioural changes can occur some of which may be personality changes, or out of character and some of which may be able to be helped with essential oils:

- marked fluctuations in moods
- becoming clinically depressed
- withdrawing from people – not talking about their illness – keeping loved ones at a distance
- low morale – 'can't be bothered . . .', 'what's the point . . .', etc.

IATROGENIC EFFECTS

Apart from the physical symptoms which may be suffered (detailed above), symptoms resulting from or relating to the treatment include:

- nausea and vomiting – 'the thought/sight of food makes me feel sick'
- fatigue
- diarrhoea/constipation
- hair loss
- hot flushes and hot sweats
- mouth feels dry/sore or has a nasty/metallic taste
- 'things smell and/or taste different'
- weight loss
- neuropathy (altered sensation in extremities e.g. pins and needles, reduced feeling, tingling pains etc.)
- sleep disturbances
- confusion/disorientation
- skin problems: dry/thin/papery/marks, tears or bruises easily/sore, etc; from the effects of radiotherapy
- surgical wounds/pain and discomfort/convalescence

AROMATHERAPY INTERVENTION

A person is more than just a collection of cells. S/he is a social being with a mind and spirit as well as a body. As in the synergy of essential oils, the synergy of the whole person is greater than the sum of the parts. Each is interdependent, with spirituality pervading all and giving meaning to life.

Social problems and issues arise from changes and adjustments that have to be faced in relationships and daily life, whether they are temporary or permanent, and aromatherapists need to be aware of the social implications of advanced diseases and adapt their treatments to meet these changes, especially those carried out in the patient's home, as these require a great deal of knowledge and skill.

Many books and articles have been written about how aromatherapy and massage can help reduce stress, anxiety and tension – both muscular and psychological as well as other problems (massage in the context of P & S situations is discussed below). It also helps restore self-confidence, raise self-esteem, encourages a positive attitude, allays extreme agitation and restlessness, lifts mood, raises morale and promotes a general sense of well-being. Pain and other symptoms such as sleep disturbances, breathing problems and panic attacks have been helped, largely due to the vicious circle being broken. This has a two-fold effect:

1. It helps the patient cope more effectively with their illness and day-to-day problems.
2. It reduces stress, therefore pressure on the immune system is lessened. Evidence from various studies discussed and cited by Tavares (2003) in the National Guidelines is encouraging as it supports the anecdotal evidence that aromatherapy and massage can indeed:
   - reduce anxiety, tension, depression and other psychological symptoms;
   - reduce perception of pain, pain, nausea and other physical symptoms;
   - help relaxation;
   - improve mobility, tiredness, function, ability to return to paid employment and overall quality of life

(Corner et al 1995, Downer et al 1994, Grealish et al 2000, Pan et al 2000, Wilkinson et al 1999).

However encouraging this may be, there are some issues, which will be discussed later, of which the aromatherapist needs to be particularly aware (see 'What the aromatherapist needs to know', below).

SPIRITUALITY

Being confronted with his or her own mortality often makes a person turn inwards and question his/her innermost thoughts, beliefs and values in an attempt to make sense of what is happening.

The less a person is able to do physically, the more time he/she has for thinking, which can lead to much anguish and torment. Aromatherapy treatment may afford help in spiritual care, bringing comfort and peace to distressed patients in the form of deep relaxation. They may then be able to focus on their own spirituality. Essential oils which could help here are those which are both uplifting and soothing, analgesic and/or tonic to the heart, relieving any fears: *Citrus bergamia* [bergamot], *Lavandula angustifolia* [lavender], *Ocimum basilicum* [sweet European basil] and *Origanum majorana* [sweet marjoram] (Price 2000 pp. 138–142).

PAIN

How severely the patient perceives/feels a physical symptom and how well it is coped with depends to a greater or lesser extent on the interaction between the social, physical, psychological and spiritual aspects. A good example of this is pain. According to Twycross & Lack (1984) the perception of pain is modulated by the patient's mood and morale, the meaning of pain to the patient and the fact that pain may remain intractable if mental and social factors are ignored.

Pain is a warning of actual or potential tissue damage. It elicits an arousal and an emotional response, and is modified by mental state and emotions (Marieb 1998). Most people with pain usually become anxious about the possible implications; this leads to muscle tension and muscle tension increases the pain that increases the emotional response, and so on, each perpetuating the other into a vicious circle that can become a spiralling process (McCaffery & Beebe 1989).

Several essential oils are analgesic (Appendix A(I)), including, *Lavandula angustifolia* [lavender], *Origanum majorana* [sweet marjoram] and *Boswellia carteri* [frankincense] – the latter would help ease mental pain also (Price 2000 p. 121); the use of these together with a massage has been found to be most beneficial. Where massage is not an option, a compress or inhalation can be employed.

From observing, listening and talking to patients over many years, Whyte believes that the principle of the pain spiral may apply to other physical symptoms the patient may experience. Similarly, a person's general outlook on life will contribute to his/her mood and confidence; the coping strategies

---

Box 15.1   Pain

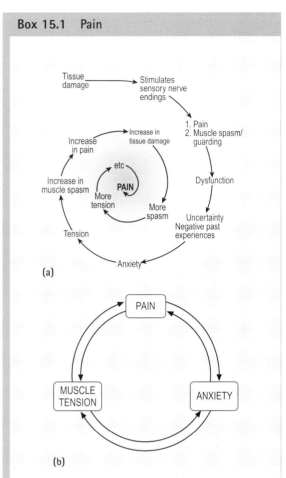

(a)

(b)

Figure 15.1   (a) The pain spiral; (b) the vicious circle (after McCaffery & Beebe 1989).

Factors that affect a person's tolerance to pain include:

Threshold lowered	Threshold raised
Other symptoms/discomfort	Relief of symptoms
Insomnia	Sleep
Fatigue	Rest
Anxiety	Sympathy
Fear	Understanding
Anger	Companionship
Sadness	Diversional activity
Depression	Reduction in anxiety
Boredom	Elevation of mood
Introversion	Analgesics
Mental isolation	Anxiolytics
Social abandonment	Antidepressants

(Twycross & Lack 1984)

they use – and their personality – do not usually change because they are ill, although they may subsequently. The effects of the close, subtle interplay between the physical, psychological, social and spiritual aspects should never be underestimated. Any negative factors in the person's life will lower their tolerance level to symptoms whereas positive ones raise it. Most people when they feel 'down in the dumps', find everything seems to be worse; likewise, when feeling 'full of the joys of spring', they can cope with anything. Illness is no different. However, even the most cheerful and positive of people can be knocked off balance and succumb to physical symptoms that nothing seems to ease. For example, feeling sick all the time, which is made worse by the sight, smell and sometimes even, just the thought of certain things, can be a major problem for some patients by making them more anxious and distressed. Anything that will interrupt the vicious circle or spiral of events must give them some benefit – and aromatherapy can – with uplifting and balancing oils such as *Pelargonium graveolens* [geranium] and *Origanum majorana* [sweet marjoram], which are also analgesic.

WHAT AN AROMATHERAPIST NEEDS TO KNOW

Because of the complex nature of the disorders and therapeutic interventions used, an aroma-therapist should have some understanding of the problems and issues the patient may be facing and any special needs he/she may have. An in-depth knowledge of anatomy and physiology is required and a basic working knowledge and understanding of the particular disease(s), their treatments and the physical, social, emotional, mental and spiritual effects both have on the patient. Without this knowledge the aromatherapist will be unable to make a thorough assessment in order to make the best choice of essential oil(s) and method of treatment.

Cancer, HIV/AIDS, MND etc. are not in themselves a contraindication to aromatherapy or massage. The approach to treating clients or patients with these disorders should be no different from that taken with other clients – the principles are the same.

If in doubt, don't treat the patient without discussing the situation with an experienced aromatherapist working in palliative care, nursing or medical staff. In many cases the doctor or nurse will have limited understanding of the use of massage and essential oils unless the practice of aromatherapy is well established in the service. There is however a growing number of specialist aromatherapists who have worked in palliative care for many years. *'Above all else, do no harm'* (Hippocrates).

Case study 15.3 Cancer of the mouth – S Lewis – *aromatherapist, UK*

Client assessment
CN, 28, lives with her parents. She was very depressed and stressed due to having cancer of the mouth and jaw and had a great deal of residual tension and pain in the neck from intensive radiotherapy and an operation. She also suffered from headaches, insomnia, congestion of the lungs, painful joints, sinusitis and poor circulation. She was referred by the consultant for aromatherapy as a support therapy.

Visualization and meditation techniques were discussed and support from the clinical psychologist was suggested and accepted. Her diet was fair but under the circumstances an appointment was arranged with the dietician for extra help and advice.

Intervention
It was decided to massage CN's back, neck, and shoulders, arms and hands, together with a gentle scalp massage – at weekly intervals.

First visit: after a thorough consultation, the essential oils chosen were:

- 2 drops *Boswellia carteri* [frankincense] – analgesic, anticatarrhal, antidepressive, anti-infectious, cicatrizant, expectorant, immunostimulant

---

Case study 15.3   Cancer of the mouth – S Lewis – *aromatherapist, UK (cont'd)*

- 2 drops *Citrus aurantium* var. *amara* fol. [petitgrain] – antiinfectious, antiinflammatory, balancing, calming
- 1 drop *Juniperus communis* fruct. [juniper berry] – analgesic, antiseptic, soporific
- 15 ml grapeseed with a little wheatgerm

She was given the same essential oils (6, 6 and 3 drops respectively) in 50 ml base lotion with which to massage her neck, shoulders and abdomen every evening.

Second visit: CN had enjoyed using the lotion at home and felt that aromatherapy not only gave her something pleasant to look forward to, but gave her the feeling of being able to help herself.

Third visit: During the massage CN broke down and cried for a long time. She was counselled

afterwards and said she felt as though a weight had been lifted from her shoulders. More lotion was prepared for home use.

Outcome

Fourth visit: CN was much brighter, not so tense and felt as though she had turned a corner. She had also been seeing the psychologist.

Fifth visit: CN was sleeping a little better and felt more relaxed. Her joints were less painful and she had progressed well.

It was decided that CN would continue her aromatherapy treatments now at one month intervals, with a whole body massage, interspersed with short treatments as and when necessary.

The above case is taken from The Aromatherapist 6(1): 20–21.

SOURCES OF INFORMATION

Theoretical knowledge and general information can be obtained from reading medical and nursing textbooks of which there are many and some are not too detailed. Organizations such as CancerBACUP, Macmillan Cancer Relief, Bristol Cancer Help Centre and the Multiple Sclerosis Society produce booklets, audio-cassettes and video tapes that give information on the disease and its treatment. Many provide a telephone help-line and information service and some run courses and workshops for professionals working in this particular field.

Having obtained the information it needs to be assessed to determine the course of action to take. For example, are there any contraindications and/or cautions to aromatherapy or massage *per se*, or only to particular oils or particular aspects of their application.

MASSAGE AND ESSENTIAL OILS

Confusion exists in many people's minds concerning the use of massage with those who have cancer. Books and courses often say that massage is contraindicated in cancer, yet massage and

aromatherapy are two of the most popular and frequently used therapies in P & S care (Lewith et al 2002, Macmillan Cancer Relief 2002). This paradoxical situation has arisen because many believe that massage can spread cancer cells through the body by stimulating the lymphatic and vascular circulation. Breathing and normal physical activity also stimulate the flow of blood and lymph, and patients, if they feel well enough, are often encouraged to take physical exercise. Massage would appear to be safe as long as it is gentle and pressure avoided over tumour sites and lymph glands (Holey & Cook 2003, McNamara 2004).

CONTRAINDICATIONS TO MASSAGE

- Unexplained lumps, bumps, swelling or area of heat – these may be disease related and need to be discussed with patient's doctor – massage of hands or feet may be offered if unaffected.
- Areas where there is unexplained pain, especially over bones, as this may indicate spread of disease to the bone especially in cancer – if used with great care, light or holding touch can be very comforting.
- High fever/infection/sepsis as there is a risk of spreading infection, making the patient

feel worse – light, holding touch can be comforting.

- Areas of the body receiving radiotherapy – and for up to 5 or 6 weeks afterwards, as the skin is extra sensitive after treatment. However, massage with essential oils (*Melaleuca viridiflora* [niaouli] is one) is recommended, to strengthen the area before treatment (Franchomme & Pénoël 2001).
- A limb or foot where deep vein thrombosis (DVT) is suspected or recently diagnosed – there may be general swelling of the part with redness and pain. People with advanced cancer are more susceptible to DVT, especially when they are frail, ill and have reduced mobility (Johnson et al 1999); use gentle massage only.
- Skin lesions, rashes, recent scar tissue, a red, painful and inflamed patch could indicate cellulitis.
- Avoid massaging over stoma sites, catheters, medication patches, TENS machine pads, syringe driver cannulae and tubing or any other medical device.

Although Tavares (2003) suggests that muscle spasm, rigidity and pain are contraindicated, especially if neurological in origin, the authors would like to say from the experiences of therapists they have trained that it depends entirely on the type of massage given. Cramp can be excruciating and can be successfully alleviated with *gentle*, *light* massage and essential oils. A professional and knowledgeable aromatherapist would apply an essential oil blend with light effleurage, as is necessary in many health areas, without having to contradict the method altogether.

Use massage with caution in the following circumstances:

- Presence of petechiae on the skin (pin-prick bruising, which indicates a low platelet count); use gentle stroking, or light holding touch only, unless working in a specialist area and able to discuss this with the medical team (Tavares 2003).
- Limbs or areas with lymphoedema, when direction and pressure (lack of) are important. Without previous experience, it may be best to work in conjunction with a lymphoedema nurse specialist or physiotherapist (Tavares 2003).

- Possible side-effects of radiotherapy, which can be delayed and include sore skin, fatigue and local effects depending on site of irradiation, e.g. neck area may result in sore, dry mouth and difficulty in swallowing; the stomach area, digestive disturbance.
- Avoid radiotherapy entry and exit sites for 3–6 weeks; effects on the skin are dose-related.
- Patients may be frail, or suffering side-effects of treatment (see above) which need to be taken into account, e.g. massage should be modified in relation to the duration of treatment, pressure used and the area of the body to be worked on.

Nevertheless, there is almost *always* something one can do with aromatherapy. For example, as a preventative against skin damage in radiotherapy, niaouli can be used beforehand (with a spray if necessary) to lessen the harmful effects on the skin (see above).

Also, compresses, topical applications or inhalation can all be used when massage is not appropriate. If a patient attends expecting aromatherapy it is important that they receive some form of treatment, providing it is safe and likely to give benefit.

USE OF ESSENTIAL OILS

Generally speaking, in the context of aromatherapy, essential oils may be considered safe, as they are only used in low concentrations. However, where a boost is needed, the careful clinical application of a higher concentration of oils has proved safe and effective.

Although there is no conclusive evidence that some oils have oestrogen-like properties, it is probably preferable to err on the side of caution in their use with patients who have oestrogen dependent tumours (Tisserand & Balacs 1995). Oils should be used with caution on patients who experience nausea and vomiting or respiratory problems see 'Cautions' below), because these patients are very vulnerable physically, mentally and emotionally. If there is doubt about the significance of any symptoms and signs found during consultation, the safety of using essential oils or massage, the aromatherapist must discuss this further with the other professionals on the team.

Case study 15.4 Bowel cancer – L F Cox – *aromatherapist, Hong Kong*

Client assessment

A patient who had been admitted with a suspected bowel obstruction was vomiting heavily – over 2 litres a day. He had had a laparotomy and was found to have bowel cancer, which necessitated a further operation. The operation itself had no complications and the patient recovered.

Three or four days after the operation, the patient started having diarrhoea, producing almost 3 litres a day. To begin with, the doctors thought it was due to the patient fasting for some time and having intravenous fluid. He was therefore started on a liquid diet, gradually progressing to a soft diet. The patient tolerated the diet plan very well for 4 days, with no complaints of nausea or vomiting, but the diarrhoea did not subside and he continued passing 3 litres of faecal fluid every day. Following this, the doctors changed the diet back to intravenous infusion and the patient was given total parenteral nutrition (TPN) in order to give his bowels a rest and cease the diarrhoea. The TPN feed was carried out for another 3 days with no improvement in the patient's frequent diarrhoea and he was put back on a normal diet. By then it was more than 10 days since his operation.

The primary nurse accepted the suggestion that aromatherapy be tried; permission was also granted by the patient and his wife. Due to the surgical operation body massage was not possible, so Swiss reflex therapy was carried out every day.

The reflex massage cream was prepared with the following:

- *Chamaemelum nobile* [Roman chamomile] – anti-inflammatory, antispasmodic, calming, digestive
- *Eucalyptus globulus* [blue gum] – antibacterial, antiinflammatory
- *Lavandula angustifolia* [lavender] – analgesic, antibacterial, calming and sedative, tonic
- 30 ml Swiss reflex base cream

Outcome

After the first session the patient said that he had had a good sleep and after six daily sessions said that he had not felt so well for a long time.

The amount of faecal fluid gradually reduced from day to day – and by the 6th day it was down to 900 ml. Everyone was very pleased with the result.

The therapist then changed her duty rota, so was unable to treat him for a week. When she returned to work the patient's diarrhoea had returned to 3 litres a day.

The treatments were recommenced – three times a day – during which time an improvement was evident to the primary nurse. However, the patient was discharged – and about 9 months later he was readmitted, dying soon afterwards.

A nite-lite vaporizer with a naked flame is not permitted in hospitals, but may be encountered in the home. In this case, it should be placed in a safe position and never be left unattended.

CONTRAINDICATIONS VERSUS ADVANTAGES

Never forget that the purpose is to bring a net gain to patients. Weighing up any contraindications vs. potential benefit is important – for example, the fact that an essential oil given to relieve nausea (below) may at a later date bring on this same feeling – via association – needs to be balanced with the fact that the oil is relieving nausea at a distressing time for a patient:

- Nausea and vomiting may be contraindicated if there is likely to be a problem – and a similar smell may be encountered in the future. The likelihood is reduced if a blend of 2–3 of the less common aromas are used.
- Take account of the effect the aroma might have on other patients in the room.
- Some diseases and/or their treatment can alter a person's sense of smell and taste and as result, some essential oils may be disliked.

- Seizures and epileptic fits can be precipitated by smells – check with staff or family if this is a possibility.
- Skin allergies or sensitivities. Patients undergoing palliative chemotherapy often have increased skin sensitivity – if in doubt do a patch test first.
- Be aware of patients with asthma or other respiratory conditions; essential oils can bring relief and are extremely beneficial.

TREATMENT

If aromatherapy is not suitable, an explanation should be given as to why, along with possible alternatives or an appropriate referral. If relevant, the treatment plan and its aims should be discussed with the patient. After obtaining consent, the choice of oils and the method of application is determined by taking into account any contraindications, cautions and precautions there might be for particular oils or application, whether general or specific, as well as the client's preference. For example, because of skin sensitivity or a change in sense of smell, the patient may prefer a carrier oil only. Although carrier oils too have therapeutic properties, some may cause skin sensitivity in some people, thus it is vital that therapeutic quality is obtained.

It may be an idea to make your own cross reference chart, not including oils which are not appropriate for use in palliative care. Then, the problems to be addressed should be identified in order of priority from the patient's point of view – to a maximum of three. Select 2–3 oils which are common to the three problems, using a maximum combined total of 4 drops in 10 ml of vegetable carrier oil (relevant to the patient's skin condition) – less if the patient is receiving palliative chemotherapy.

Test the aroma on the inside of the patient's wrist, trying a different ratio of the oils or changing one if disliked – a very rare occurrence!

If essential oil(s) is/are to be inhaled or used in a vaporizer, a drop of each should be placed on a tissue or Q-tip to verify its acceptability to the person concerned.

Decide which method of application is best suited to the patient's needs and preferences, for example, with an aromastream or tissue as an air freshener or deodorizer for a patient with a stoma or fungating tumour is a good idea, whereas massage is more beneficial for cramp or muscular pain.

If massage is selected, decide on which part of the body to work and what kind of massage is to be given – light pressure/gentle holding/stroking etc. The patient may be too frail or feeling too ill to tolerate more than a foot or hand massage, and back massage would not be possible where radiotherapy is involved, as lying on one's front could cause pain or the turning over be too stressful.

CHANGES AFFECTING TREATMENT

The aromatherapist needs to be familiar with situations which may occur when treating a patient – even though some may be rare. He/she needs to know what action to take and who to inform should there be any change in the patient's condition – the aromatherapist may be the only person who has an opportunity of seeing changes in parts of the patient's body normally covered with clothing, such as skin lesions or swellings. Consultation with the professional team will decide what changes need to be referred, whom to notify when necessary and what advice to give patients who report a change in their condition:

- recurrence of pain
- nausea and/or vomiting
- breathlessness or other breathing problems, severe panic attacks or choking
- epileptic fit or other form of seizure (usually associated with brain tumours).

Rare occurrences are:

- haemorrhage: this can be via the mouth – from coughing or vomiting, from the stomach, from the nose, the vagina, the rectum or from the site of a stoma
- pathological fracture – usually associated with bone metastases of cancer
- spinal cord compression occurs in 5–10% of people with cancer (Doyle et al 2003, Falk and Fallon 1997) and is a neurological emergency. Symptoms may be present for weeks or may occur suddenly and include pins and needles, sensory loss and weakness – usually in the

lower extremities – starting in the feet and moving upwards. If this remains untreated paralysis will ensue, so urgent medical advice should be sought.

Without distancing themselves, aromatherapists should be able to support the patient through any distressing emotions that may arise. They should also be aware of other available options for support and the means of referral. Those who work in P & S care, including aromatherapists, may need support themselves and some form of supervision of this may be available, although varying quite considerably.

The therapist at all times should recognize and acknowledge his/her limitations and those of aromatherapy and know when to refer a patient.

PREVENTING CROSS INFECTION

As a result of their diseases and/or treatments, a patient's immune system is often highly compromised, making him/her more vulnerable to infection. This is more likely to occur when patients are debilitated. Equally the patient him/herself may be a source of infection that can be passed to others. As blood and all body fluids are potentially infectious, it is incumbent on therapists to make themselves familiar with universal infection control procedures if they are likely to be working in an environment such as a hospital or hospice, where they may come into contact with patients' body fluids. Similarly, if they are likely to be giving treatments to people with infections such as methicillin-resistant *Staphylococcus aureus* (MRSA), they should seek advice on local infection control procedures. If an aromatherapist is in good health with good energy levels, and follows a high standard of hygiene and infection control practices, the risk of cross infection is minimal.

To prevent cross infection, the aromatherapist should follow good basic hygiene practices at all times. The most important practice of all is the thorough washing of hands before and after treating a patient – even if gloves have been used – and the judicious use of essential oils, many of which have been proved to suppress *S. aureus*.

Box 15.2   Aromatherapy in a UK NHS supportive and palliative care service

This service began in 1993 when Elaine Cooper, an aromatherapist trained by the author (S Price) approached the NHS trust in the town where she lived about introducing aromatherapy into the day hospice as part of the palliative care service. Today Walsall NHS Trust has an example of 'best practice', meeting the NICE guidelines for supportive and palliative care. This service now offers complementary therapies (aromatherapy being the most popular) as an integral part of palliative care across the whole health economy in Walsall.

The aim is to:

- provide one seamless and equitable service across the whole of palliative and supportive cancer care
- ensure therapies are delivered effectively and appropriately so as to bring most benefit to patients
- allow the patient and carer the chance to receive aromatherapy and other complementary therapies without charge, in an NHS health-care environment
- ensure audit and evaluation is carried out effectively
- provide education relating to complementary therapies

The aromatherapy service provides treatments such as massage and compresses and also a valuable prescription service where essential oils and aromatherapy blends are supplied to patients to aid symptom control.

The main reasons for referral are anxiety and tension, fear and panic, pain, insomnia, skin problems such as dry skin or pruritus, mouth problems such as *Candida* or ulcers and to aid relaxation and quality of life.

In the 12-month period 2004–2005 the clinical caseload for this service has been on average 80–100 patients at any one time with over 1000 treatments delivered to patients. Funding is currently via the Primary Care Trust and Macmillan Cancer Relief.

Box 15.2   Aromatherapy in a UK NHS supportive and palliative care service (*cont'd*)

Education is vitally important in the service, with training and presentations being delivered to medical and health professionals at regular intervals. These have proved successful with one GP giving money to the service, others offering rooms in their practice for the service to outreach. It sounds wonderful but has had its sceptics and many problems along the way, but the success of the service lies with the determination of lead therapist Elaine Cooper and the team of health-care professionals in Walsall who have made this happen. The service structure consists of a complementary therapy committee which reports to the palliative care strategy group, a lead therapist, several paid therapists and a group of volunteer therapists.

The town's 'Hospice Appeal' has a school of aromatherapy where students are trained, some of whom will work within the service and others in the outside community. All profits from the training go to the hospice appeal so aromatherapy benefits everyone – even financially. Penny Price and Dr Robert Stephen have given considerable help and support regarding the Hospice aromatherapy course.

This service is an excellent example of how aromatherapy can be fully integrated into the NHS system and become the norm. Both palliative patients and health-care staff have more treatment choices and thus a quality health-care package is delivered.

ESSENTIAL OIL RECIPES

The following information is based on Cooper's experience over more than 10 years of using essential oils in supportive and palliative care in an NHS integrated service:

Mouth ulcers due to chemotherapy or disease in the mouth

5 ml *Calendula officinalis* macerated [calendula]*
2 drops *Commiphora myrrha* [myrrh]**
Apply a drop directly to the mouth ulcer using a cotton bud 3 times a day.
*Calendula extracts are used to promote healing and to reduce inflammation (ESCOP, Fleischner 1985, Price, Smith & Price 1999).
**Myrrh contains a high proportion of anti-inflammatory and slightly analgesic sesquiterpenes and antiseptic alcohols.

Candida in the mouth

1 drop *Aniba rosaeodora* [rosewood]* in water – use as a mouth rinse 3–5 times a day.
*Rosewood contains up to 90% alcohols, which are antifungal, antiseptic and free from irritation.

Vaginal *Candida*

3 drops *Aniba rosaeodora*
2 drops *Lavandula angustifolia* [lavender] – use frequently in the bath
Use in white lotion for direct application.

Malodour due to discharging or fungating wounds

Vaporize *Thymus vulgaris* ct thymol or ct linalool with *Eucalyptus citriodora* [lemon scented gum] or *Citrus bergamia* [bergamot] with *Lavandula angustifolia*.
As an alternative or addition to vaporization place a few drops of oil on a pad and place over the top of any wound dressings.

Pruritus (skin itching)

The author's (S Price) soothing balm, containing *Santalum album*, *Lavandula angustifolia* and *Mentha* x *piperita*.

In 10 years Cooper says she has not found anything better than this blend and uses it extensively for pruritus associated with liver disease and jaundice. It often gives more relief than any

---

Box 15.3   Wound care for palliative patients in Belgium – S Sarazin

General Hospital Middelheim, Wilrijk, Antwerp, Belgium

Wound care protocol: Prepare all material necessary for an aseptic wound care. Explain wound care to patient; respect privacy; place in relaxing position. Nurse to check nursing file, use a mask if respiratory infection present, wash hands.

Black wounds

Black wounds indicate necrosis or dead tissue. Necrosis does not allow wound healing. Moreover it is a possible breeding ground for micro-organisms and therefore for infection. To stimulate the wound healing the necrosis tissue should be removed.

Superficial black wound with little suppuration:
To help soak off necrosis apply compress soaked in 10 ml St John's wort oil with 5 drops *Lavandula angustifolia* (mix A).

With symptoms of infection:
■ apply mix of 10 ml honey with 5 drops *Lavandula angustifola* (mix B) or 5 drops *Melaleuca alternifolia* (mix C) and leave on 15 minutes
■ rinse off with sterile water
■ apply compress using mix A

Superficial black wound with much suppuration:
■ rinse wound with sterile water
■ apply mix C and leave for 15 minutes
■ rinse off with sterile water
■ apply a compress soaked in mix A above

Deep black wound:
■ rinse wound very thoroughly with sterile water
■ apply special bandage for deep wounds soaked in mix A above
■ fix compress over the bandage

Yellow wounds

Yellow wounds contain debris (dirty material from tissues), fibrous and superfluous wound suppuration.

The yellow fibrous secretion presents ideal conditions for micro-organisms and thus for infection. Therefore the wound must be cleaned.

Superficial yellow wound with little more suppuration:
■ rinse the wound with sterile water
■ apply compress soaked with mix C above and leave for 15 minutes
■ rinse off with sterile water
■ apply compress soaked in mix A above

Deep yellow wound:
■ rinse wound very thoroughly with sterile water
■ apply special bandage for deep wounds soaked in 10 ml St John's wort oil with 5 drops of *Melaleuca alternifolia*
■ apply compress soaked in mix A above
■ apply extra compress when necessary

Red wounds

The red aspect springs from the formation of granula tissue. These wounds are free from debris.

Superficial red wound with little/more suppuration:
■ apply one or more drops of undiluted *Lavandula augustifolia* to the wound (using a medical glove)
■ apply dry compress and bandage

Deep red wound:
■ apply special bandage for deep wounds soaked in mix A above
■ rub wound-edges with undiluted *Lavandula angustifolia*
■ fix dry compress over bandage

Erythema and purple colour of the skin:
Apply 10 ml almond oil with 5 drops *Lavandula angustifolia* gently to vulnerable skin.

---

prescribed medication with patients frequently saying it is the best relief they have had. The excellent effect is well known in our area with Macmillan nurses, Hospice nurses and palliative care consultants all requesting it be provided for their patients.

Anxiety and panic

When patients are experiencing severe anxiety and panic there are many calming and sedative essential oils to choose from, such as *Chamaemelum nobile* [Roman chamomile] *Cananga odorata* [ylang

Case study 15.5 HIV positive – J Burnett – *aromatherapist, UK*

Client assessment

Steve, 37 years old, was diagnosed HIV positive in 1996. He developed *Pneumocystis carinii* infection, pneumonia and various other infections early in 2001. Aids Support had been asked by the patient's consultant if any help was available – and had recommended aromatherapy.

Steve was very depressed, angry and unable to handle his own sense of helplessness. His whole body was covered with atopic dermatitis. He was unable to walk because of pain in his legs and ankles – he scratched constantly – his legs, ankles and bottom being scratched raw.

Intervention

It was decided to massage his back, arms and hands with the following essential oils:

- *Chamomilla recutita* [German chamomile] – anti-inflammatory, cicatrizant, (also to help his impatience and irritability)
- *Citrus bergamia* [bergamot] – antiinfectious, anti-irritant, calming, cicatrizant, tonic (also to help his depression, anger, fear and weariness)
- *Lavandula angustifolia* [lavender] – analgesic, antiinflammatory, antiseptic, calming, cicatrizant, tonic (also to help his anger and depression)
- *Pelargonium graveolens* [geranium] – analgesic, antiinfectious, antiinflammatory, relaxant (also to help anger)
- *Santalum album* [sandalwood] – antiinfectious, decongestant and moisturizing to skin, general tonic (also to help repressed anger and fear)

He was also given the same mixture to apply to himself daily (to relieve the itching and help combat the dermatitis) and a blend to use in the bath.

Outcome

One week later: the skin on his legs was much improved (Steve was applying the oil up to six times a day), so the same massage sequence was carried out.

After 2 more weeks, his temperament seemed to have improved (his mother's comment). His skin was much better but the pain and swelling in his feet were considerable, so juniper was added to the blend to help reduce the oedema:

- *Juniperus communis* fruct. [juniper] – analgesic, diuretic

This was gently applied to his legs and feet and a few juniper drops were added to his mixture for him to apply himself.

After another 2 weeks, he stated he generally felt much better and had managed to walk a little. His skin had continued to improve and he was applying his blend regularly.

By the next treatment, his skin was much better; his ankles were still red and itchy but he was no longer scratching. He was feeling generally a lot better and had been away for Christmas. His legs were less painful and he was managing to walk a little more.

Treatment continued successfully through the early months of the following year, the skin problem erupting again only when he was taken into hospital in May, just before he died.

---

ylang], *Citrus aurantium* var *amara* per. [orange bigarade] and *Eucalyptus citriodora* [lemon scented gum] (also see Appendix B.9). The patient can be asked to choose from a small selection of single oils, and/or a couple of blends of 2–3, the aroma they find the most pleasing.

Patients can be given a 10 ml bottle of the chosen oil blended in a carrier to use themselves on pulse points during periods of anxiety. If they feel a panic attack pending they can inhale the

neat essential oil from a tissue. Over the years many, many patients have claimed a reduction in anxiety, panic or fear simply by inhaling their chosen oil. Over a period of 18 months, Cooper has been working closely with a clinical psychologist in oncology and palliative care in the primary care trust where she works, with referrals requesting 'to aid relaxation and reduce anxiety with aromatherapy' and there have been some outstanding results with some of the patients.

Essential oils chosen most frequently are *Rosa damascena* [rose otto] *Citrus aurantium* var. *amara* flos [neroli], *Boswellia carteri* [frankincense], *Lavandula angustifolia* and *Chamaemelum nobile* [Roman chamomile].

Pain (localized)

Massage with analgesic essential oils brings its own benefits but if massage is not advisable, the application of essential oils in a lotion – or with a compress or spray – can bring a reduction in pain.

Factors to be considered, which may be contributing to the pain include inflammation, tension, swelling or nerve involvement etc. A significant reduction in pain in patients can be achieved by using the following:

Chamaemelum nobile [Roman chamomile], *Lavandula angustifolia* [lavender] and *Citrus aurantium* var. *amara* (fol) [neroli], all containing esters, which are generally regarded to be antiinflammatory, antispasmodic and calming, which makes them very useful for pain.

Pogostemon patchouli [patchouli] and *Commiphora myrrha* [myrrh] may also be antiinflammatory, and *Lavandula angustifolia* [lavender] and *Zingiber officinale* [ginger] are useful for their analgesic properties.

Box 15.4   Aromatherapy statements from Walsall

The following is a collection of statements obtained from health professionals and patients regarding aromatherapy.

An increasing number of patients undergoing chemotherapy and other cancer treatments would benefit from aromatherapy and I feel this is an integral part of comprehensive cancer care.

Consultant Radiotherapist & Oncologist (Birmingham and Walsall)

A small number of the patients under my care with malignant disease have so far had the benefit of aromatherapy and have without exception found it to have a positive effect on their well-being. Such a result is consistent with some of the more scientific studies which have been conducted and I have no doubt that the service is both popular and worthwhile.

Consultant Haematologist (Walsall)

(This consultant funded the furnishing for the complementary suite at the hospital)

There is no doubt that provision of aromatherapy to Walsall patients has provided great benefit. Many have had pain improved and anxiety reduced.

Consultant in Palliative Medicine (Wolverhampton and Walsall)

Since the aromatherapy service began some years ago, it has provided an invaluable service for patients all over the Walsall area. Speaking of my own sector of Walsall I can assure you that many many patients have derived comfort, relaxation and alleviation of symptoms.

General Practitioner (Walsall)

Complementary therapy which in my case means aromatherapy, is time out for me, space away from the medical rigours of my treatment, and an opportunity to relax and let some of the tension go; it's a treatment that's focused on me and my needs and not the disease. It helps me get through the chemotherapy when I have something of such value to look forward to.

Palliative cancer patient and senior manager in the NHS (Walsall)

Whatever you did with the aromatherapy treatment was a miracle, I had the best night's sleep for months and continued to sleep better for several days, the pain reduced considerably and I have not needed to take so much morphine since.

Palliative cancer patient (Walsall)

Elaine M Cooper MIFPA LIAM January 2005

Where there is pain combined with anxiety or depression, a blend of *Boswellia carteri* and *Commiphora myrrha* have been found to be most helpful.

The following essential oil blend has been found to be useful for frequently presenting symptoms in lung cancer – shortness of breath, discomfort, upper body tension, potential infection and coughing:

> *Pinus sylvestris* [pine], *Cedrus atlantica* [cedarwood], *Boswellia carteri* [frankincense] and *Melaleuca viridiflora* [niaouli]

The essential oil blend alone can be used in inhalation; it can also be put into a carrier oil for gentle upper body massage or into a lotion as a chest rub. Using these methods, patients have frequently reported less upper body tension and discomfort, easier breathing and a feeling of control. Having something to use themselves which is not a medical intervention and for which they have a choice appears to empower the person.

SUMMARY

With its popularity continuing to grow, aromatherapy is one of the three most frequently used complementary therapies provided by hospices and palliative care units in the UK – the other two being massage and reflexology (Macmillan Cancer Relief 2002, Wilkes 1992).

The effects of caring touch should never be underestimated and the shared experience between the giver and the recipient is to their mutual benefit. This is an aspect that can be of benefit to the patient, partner, family and the carer. The aromatherapist could teach a simple massage technique to one or more of these people – even the patient, to give them an opportunity of giving and receiving caring touch. It can be a transforming experience as so often the loved ones feel helpless in not knowing how to show they care, or are frightened of 'doing the wrong thing'. Similarly the patient often feels s/he is giving nothing in return for the love and care shown him/her and being able to participate in a simple massage can make a world of difference. Aromatherapy massage and therapeutic touch are pleasant, non-clinical experiences that can be of great benefit to sufferers and their carers.

The use of essential oils can also provide another clinical tool in health-care practice giving both health-care professionals and patients another choice along the healing or therapeutic pathway.

References

Corner J, Cawley N, Hildebrand S 1995 An evaluation of the use of massage and essential oils on the well-being of cancer patients. International Journal of Palliative Nursing 1(2): 67–73

Downer S et al 1994 Pursuit and practice of complementary therapies by cancer patients receiving conventional treatment. British Medical Journal 309: 86–89

Doyle D, Hanks G, Cherny N I, Calmank E (eds) 2003 Oxford Textbook of Palliative Medicine, 3rd edn. Oxford University Press, Oxford

Falk S, Fallon M 1997 ABC of palliative care: emergencies. British Medical Journal Dec; 345: 1525–1528

Franchomme P, Pénoël D 2001 L'aromathérapie exactement. Jollois. Limoges, p. 304

Gatti G, Cayola R 1923 L'azione della essenze sul sysema nervosa. Rivista Italiana delle Essenze e Profumi 5(12): 133–135

Grealish L, Lomansney A, Whiteman B 2000 Foot massage. Cancer Nursing 23(3): 237–243

Holey E, Cook E 2003 Evidence-based therapeutic massage: a practical guide for therapists. Churchill Livingstone, Edinburgh, pp. 263–268

Johnson M J, Walker I D, Sproule M W, Conkie J 1999 Abnormal coagulation and deep vein thrombosis in patients with advanced cancer. Clinical and Laboratory Haematology 21: 51–54

Lee W H, Lee L 1992 The book of practical aromatherapy. Keats, New Canaan, CT, p. 125

Lewith 2002 Complementary cancer care in Southampton: a survey of staff and patients. Complementary Therapies in Medicine 10: 100–106

Marieb E 1998 Human anatomy and physiology, 4th edn. Addison Wesley World Student Series

McCaffery M, Beebe A 1989 Pain, clinical manual for nursing practice. Mosby, London.

Macmillan Cancer Relief 2002 Directory of complementary therapy services in UK cancer care. Macmillan Cancer Relief, London

McNamara P 2004 Massage for people with cancer, 3rd edn. The Cancer Resource Centre, Wandsworth, London

National Council for Hospices and Specialist Palliative Care Services 2000 Draft National Plan and Strategic Framework for Palliative Care, June 2000

Pan C X, Morrison R, Ness J, Fugh-Berman A, Leipzig R M 2000 Complementary and alternative medicine in the management of pain, dyspnoea and nausea and vomiting near the end of life. A systemic review. Journal of Pain Symptom Management Nov; 20(5): 374–387

Price L, Smith I, Price S 1999 Carrier oils for aromatherapy and massage. Riverhead, Stratford-on-Avon, p.45

Price S 2000 Aromatherapy and your emotions. Thorsons, London

Tavares M 2003 National guidelines for the use of complementary therapies in supportive and palliative care. Cited in The Prince of Wales Foundation for Integrated Health and The National Council for Hospice and Supportive Care Services, May 2003.

Tisserand R, Balacs T 1995 Essential oil safety guide, a guide for health care professionals. Churchill Livingstone, Edinburgh

Twycross R G, Lack S 1984 Therapeutics in terminal cancer. Churchill Livingstone, Edinburgh

Watkins A (ed) 1997 Mind–body medicine: a clinician's guide to psychoneuroimmunology. Churchill Livingstone, Edinburgh

WHO 1990 Cancer pain relief and palliative care. A report of the WHO Expert Committee. WHO Technical report series 804.

Wilkes E 1992 Complementary therapy in hospice and palliative care. Sheffield Trent Palliative Care Centre and Help the Hospices

Wilkinson S, Aldridge J, Salmon I, Cain E, Wilson B 1999 An evaluation of aromatherapy massage in palliative care. Palliative Medicine Sep; 13(5): 409–417

SECTION 4

Policy and practice

Chapter 16 (Part I)

Aromatherapy in the UK

Penny Price and Shirley Price

INTRODUCTION

Part I of this chapter shows how professional aromatherapy has developed (and is still developing) in the UK – from simple beginnings to being the model for many other countries to follow (see Ch. 17). It reports the current situation within the field of complementary medicine and aromatherapy in particular, giving details of the relevant associations which have been set up to look after the interests of aromatherapy and the therapists who practise it, especially with respect to standards of education and legislation regarding the use of essential oils. There have been increasing demands that complementary therapies (and therefore aromatherapy) should become regulated and observe similar ethical and practical constraints to those of orthodox medicine and this is discussed.

Chapter 16 Part II discusses issues relevant to most health professionals – physiotherapists, occupational therapists, those who work in mental health etc – and also aromatherapists. A model set of policies and protocols are proposed for the professional practice of aromatherapy in UK health-care settings.

AROMATHERAPY DEVELOPMENT

Since arriving in Britain in the late 1960s via the beauty therapy industry, aromatherapy has greatly expanded into health, in (and out of) hospitals, doctors' surgeries and complementary health centres. Two people well known throughout the world and considered by many to be somewhat responsible for its advancement from the 1980s are Robert Tisserand and Shirley Price, educators and authors of several text books on the subject. Both helped instigate the first purely aromatherapy association in Britain.

By the 1990s, more and more physiotherapists, nurses and midwives were attending accredited courses and other countries of the world were (and still are) keen to follow the 'British way' – some, at first, through beauty therapy and others directly into the world of health (see Ch. 17).

Educational standards have improved immensely over the last 10 years and different associations and bodies have been set up to deal with subjects such as the quality of essential oils, self-regulation of the therapy, an umbrella body for the many aromatherapy associations, EC legislation, etc.

Previously little used, hydrolats, during the last decade, have become a valuable additional tool for aromatherapists and the first English book on the subject, 'Understanding Hydrolats' (Price & Price 2004) has been published by Elsevier.

It is now imperative that an aromatherapist, whether in nursing or private practice, is trained in the volatile chemical constituents making up essential oils and their possible effects on the human organism. With the increase in use of hydrolats and the fact that one of the possible uses of these is by mouth, the importance of this knowledge is underlined.

Aromatherapists are now showing an interest in studying advanced clinical aromatherapy (aromatic medicine/aromatology), first introduced in the 1990s by the Editors and now offered at two aromatherapy schools in the UK. Although this involves intensive application to the skin and the use of hydrolats by mouth to fight bacterial and viral infections as well as chronic conditions, graduates of advanced clinical aromatherapy courses do not necessarily practise all methods on their clients. Such courses, however, do provide complete and full training in aromatherapy methods of use, ensuring that essential oils are used safely and with understanding for intensive skin applications, gargles, pessaries and suppositories (most aromatherapists use these methods at the moment without any training).

The Editors sincerely hope that aromatherapy schools already teaching to a high standard will soon include aromatic medicine in their syllabus (see Ch. 9).

REGULATIONS

PRACTICE OF AROMATHERAPY

Unlike some other European countries (see France and Germany, Ch. 17), non-medically qualified practitioners of complementary and alternative therapies in the UK are, at present, free to practise under common law, irrespective of their levels of training or clinical competence.

The UK adopted the European Medicines Law in 1994 and complementary and alternative medicine (CAM) practitioners in most other European countries are required to be medically qualified before they can practise.

AROMATHERAPY PRODUCTS

There are longstanding provisions in UK legislation, principally in Section 12(1) of the Medicines Act 1968 which permit unlicensed herbal remedies to be supplied to individual patients under certain conditions. The Medicines & Healthcare Products Regulatory Agency (MHRA) regulates medicinal products and has consistently confirmed that Section 12(1) applies to aromatherapists and allows them to sell on essential oils for a medicinal purpose under certain conditions.

A remedy specifically formulated to benefit a health problem can be labelled as such for any client after a face-to-face consultation with an aromatherapist (under S12(1) of the Medicines Act 1968); however, no claims can be made on any bottle to be sold to the public without such a consultation first.

The European Union has already brought in legislation regarding the use of essential oils through several directives which have been transposed into UK law and include the Cosmetics Products (Safety) Regulations 2004, the General Product Safety Regulations 2005 and the Medicines (Traditional Herbal Medicinal Products for Human Use) Regulations 2005.

Medicinal claims are not permitted under any circumstances on products for sale directly by manufacturers and traders to the public or consumer, although there is no single regulatory framework for aromatherapy products; consequently these products must be classified according to the most appropriate regulatory framework. Since the retail supply of essential oils and aromatherapy products is not subject to the Medicines Law it is likely to be subject to the UK 2004 and 2005 regulations above – or other applicable legislation. Further information can be found on the Aromatherapy Trade Council (ATC) website.

The Traditional Herbal Medicinal Products Directive (THMPD) requires the registration of all herbal products under a simplified registration procedure. These must have a continuous traditional medicinal use of 30 years, including at least 15 years within the European Community. Details are available on the Medicines and Healthcare Products Regulatory Agency's (MHRA) website (see Useful addresses). The MHRA has confirmed that any product not classified as a medicine should not be affected by the Directive and at the moment essential oils may continue to be sold under the current regulatory regimes of Cosmetics and General Products (Baker 2003a).

European cosmetics legislation was recently amended (the 7th Amendment), primarily to eliminate animal testing; it was also extended, to include 26 chemical substances which have been identified by the EC as important causes of contact-allergy reaction. 16 of these occur naturally in essential oils commonly used in aromatherapy (component names are on the ATC website – see Useful addresses, p. 528). As of March 2005, if a product contains one of these fragrance chemicals in excess of 0.01% (wash-off) or 0.001% (leave-on), it must be included on the label (ATC 2004). The Directive also requires cosmetic products to be labelled with a period of minimum durability according to the stability or shelf life of the product in its unopened state. Products with a minimum durability of more than 30 months must carry an open jar logo and an indication of how long they may be safely used once opened. The European cosmetics legislation has been transposed into UK law by the Cosmetic Products (Safety) Regulations 2004 and an excellent Guide

to the Regulations is available on the DTI's (Department of Trade and Industry) website at www.dti.gov.uk

EDUCATION

WHICH COURSES?

To ensure that there is always the choice of routes for trainees, clarity in standards needs further publicity – there are many occasions nowadays where a therapist has undertaken a course at a local centre, only to be told afterwards that the qualification is not recognized and needs significant updating.

Serious trainee aromatherapists are faced with a minefield of options: where to train and to which standard. While there are many schools offering adequate training there are plenty more that are not, and the trainees can sometimes find that they are not able to be employed in certain clinical situations just because they have chosen the 'wrong' course.

It seems incredible that in this age of improving standards, these appear to be measured against peripherals rather than competency in therapy. Even after the intervention of Prince Charles, the academic importance and relevance of aromatherapy is not taken as seriously as it could be and 'aromatherapists' are literally being churned out who are only really capable of very basic treatment to help relieve minor stress or to improve the skin. The academic therapist is tarred with this brush and the very name 'aromatherapist' can be more of a patronizing term than a compliment. Training has to be serious and if private education can provide this then steps need to be taken to ensure the security of the future of such establishments.

HOUSE OF LORDS REPORT

In November 2000 the House of Lords Select Committee on Science & Technology Committee published a report on complementary and alternative therapies (CAM), which called for more evidence based research, tighter regulation of therapies and practitioners and more reliable information, so that the public could make informed choices regarding their health care. The training and qualification of therapists is a key issue in policy development and the House of Lords report identified the need for all complementary therapies to develop a sound system of regulation and accreditation.

In response to this, the government urged the representative bodies within each therapy to unite to form a single body for regulating their profession (DoH 2001) in the best interests of patients and the wider public, as well as potentially enhancing the status of individual professions (Tavares 2003). It also urged CAM regulatory bodies to put in place codes of practice to limit claims made by practitioners, and to ensure that their members recognize and follow them.

One of the principal requirements of modern health care provision can be summed up by the term 'evidence based'. It is no longer sufficient for any therapeutic approach simply to rely on a long history of use, or popularity, or widespread availability, to justify its continued acceptance. Evidence of both safety and efficacy, of all forms of therapeutic intervention is now required (Field 2003).

The Report classified therapies according to their evidence base and level of professional organization in relation to regulation (see Part II and Table 16.1).

TRAINING

Professional training in aromatherapy is carried out by private training schools, colleges of further education and universities, most of the latter offering aromatherapy only as part of their CAM courses and no degree course offers aromatic medicine (see Ch. 9) as part of the curriculum.

One or two universities have had their aromatherapy section validated by an aromatherapy association (see Associations below), while most of the others comply with National Occupational Standards (NOS – see below). The development of NOS was started by the Aromatherapy Organizations Council (AOC) before it was dissolved in 2003 to create one new body – the Aromatherapy Consortium (AC), so that the whole profession could work together on structure and policies for a UK regulatory body for aromatherapy (also started by the AOC).

The AC's Aromatherapy Education Working Party (AEWP) has finalized the new Core Curriculum, which was unanimously ratified by the whole profession in March 2005. The document can be downloaded from the AC website and lists all the requirements, including anatomy and physiology, contact hours for each module, learning outcomes and the teaching qualifications and experience required for a tutor.

The elements common to all therapies and hoped to be covered in the curriculum are:

- basic anatomy, physiology and related pathology
- fundamentals of orthodox medical diagnosis and guidelines for patient referral
- complementary and alternative therapies (CAM) and their potential uses, including the principles of assessment and practice
- holistic models of health care
- professional ethics
- therapeutic relationship
- impact of social, cultural, economic, employment and environmental factors on health
- counselling skills
- principles of quality management and audit
- organizational skills, including record keeping
- technical skills ranging from prevention of cross infection to information management.

Eventually, once curricula are standardized and everyone is teaching to the same level, the ideal would be an educational system where every would-be complementary practitioner has to study the necessary basics – whatever therapy is eventually to be practised, and only after this is the chosen complementary therapy studied – in depth. Uniformity in the basic skills required by all complementary practitioners would then be ensured. It would also simplify the study of further therapies, not only saving repetition of certain modules in each discipline studied, but enabling the extra time thus gained to be spent on more in-depth knowledge of the therapy in question, so that this will be practised efficiently and knowledgeably.

Human beings have an interdependent relationship with plants, depending on them for oxygen, food and energy: the human and plant ecosystems rely intimately on each other, and are part of the whole which is life itself. As we know, essential oils have been proving their ability to influence human health on physical, emotional and mental levels. It is this emotional dimension that confirms aromatherapy as an art, and lifts it up from a mere interaction of plants and human chemicals (Eccles 1997).

As both herbal medicine and aromatherapy use the extracts from plants, it would seem to the Editors that the two subjects should be amalgamated and taught as one, which would then make aromatic medicine a valid practice for aromatherapists. Whether or not this will ever happen is a moot point.

NATIONAL OCCUPATIONAL STANDARDS

Aromatherapy was one of the first complementary therapies in the UK to have these Government-recognized educational standards – in 1998, with Skills for Health, in terms of qualifications and what constitutes a practitioner.

The purpose of developing NOS for health care was to improve continually the quality of services for all who receive care. They are competence based, covering the practice of aromatherapy and the important principles and values involved. Government funded aromatherapy courses are required to meet NOS standards and are checked by the AC. NOS are not qualifications, but are used to create syllabi, for which The AC Core Curriculum will be a guide; this does not restrict or limit schools from including more in-depth training to make their courses more attractive to prospective students.

The aromatherapy section of degree courses in complementary therapies must comply with the minimum competences as laid out in the NOS, although one, Wolverhampton, has had their aromatherapy section validated by the International Federation of Professional Aromatherapists.

As more research is done it becomes even more imperative that aromatherapists (and particularly those studying complete Aromatic Medicine) understand the chemistry behind the oils and the relationship (if any) between these and the effects of the oils on the body. In addition holism, the theory that a complex entity, system, etc. is more than merely the sum of its parts, has still to play a major part in aromatherapy treatments for the scientific application to be truly successful.

HELPING THE PUBLIC SELECT THERAPIES AND THERAPISTS

There exists at the moment an overabundance of different representative bodies in most complementary therapies. This can be confusing to the public, who have no way of knowing which therapies are safe and appropriate in the circumstances of their particular condition or what qualifications and level of skills an individual therapist in any one discipline possesses (Integrated Health Care 1997 p. 5). To help patients, the Prince of Wales Foundation for Integrated Health has published a Guide for Patients, which suggests questions to ask a practitioner in order to check his/her qualifications and experience.

The AC is developing the national register set up by the AOC, which will show registered therapists who have trained to National Occupational Standards (NOS), and are nationally recognized as competent (Preen 2004 personal communication). The public has access to this also, giving two ways in which they can be directed to a knowledgeable and competent therapist.

USE OF ESSENTIAL OILS IN HOSPICES AND HOSPITALS

The University of Exeter survey, as long ago as 1997, revealed that, from the number of members from complementary therapy associations working in the NHS, up to half were from aromatherapy, healing and reflexology associations. 'Aromatherapy and reflexology are popular with nurses and this is likely to account for much of their involvement' (University of Exeter 1997 p. 60).

With the degree of responsibility and accountability applicable to the practice of aromatherapy in hospitals today, it may now be the time for nurses suitably qualified in aromatherapy to declare to be an aromatherapist first and foremost – as did the following writer:

I am an aromatherapist first and foremost. All too often I hear the same cry – 'I am a qualified nurse using aromatherapy' . . . We should be proud of our profession in the use of essential oils and not need to use another profession as a crutch . . . If we are insecure with our training and wish to hide behind the apron strings of another profession, this is not acceptable to either discipline; in fact, the one will strangle the other.

(Barker 1994)

Barker goes on to say that we are competent and appropriately trained professionals in our own right, and do aromatherapy and aromatic medicine a great disservice by tagging it on to another discipline to give it credibility when it is already a valid system of medicine.

Several hospitals are now funding nurses on aromatherapy courses, many of these being run specifically for the nursing profession and consultants. As a result, GPs, since the mid-1990s, have a much more sympathetic and cooperative attitude towards aromatherapy than when the Editors came into the profession in the 1970s. The medical profession are now more willing to listen seriously to claims of the positive and sometimes dramatic effects that essential oils can have on people's overall health (see Ch. 4). A number of private therapists also now work in conjunction with their local GP on minor health problems which can be helped by essential oils. A major breakthrough occurred in 1993, when GPs were empowered to refer patients to complementary therapists for treatment on the NHS, provided that the GP concerned remained clinically accountable for the patient.

There have been many clinical successes in hospitals where essential oils have been used and the results of projects and trials (albeit not of rigorous research standard, which is very difficult in the case of essential oils) have led to a greater willingness to listen and to utilize aromatherapy in hospitals and community care. The change in status of NHS hospitals in 1990 may have been a contributory factor to the increase of complementary therapies being practised in health care.

Self-governing status for NHS hospitals – NHS Trusts – was created in the 1990 NHS and Community Care Act. These were set up to manage hospitals and other NHS services. Since 1990 all providers in the NHS have opted for NHS Trust status and there are no longer any hospitals which are directly managed by Health Authorities (Farrer 1997 personal communication).

AROMATHERAPY ASSOCIATIONS

While aromatherapy is affiliated with many multidisciplinary complementary therapy bodies such as the Institute of Complementary Medicine (ICM) and associations such as Embody and others, there are three self-governing associations (two affiliated with the umbrella body below) dedicated solely to aromatherapy, providing codes of ethics and practice and high educational standards which are so respected that they are followed in many countries of the world (see Ch.17).

THE AROMATHERAPY CONSORTIUM (AC)

The AC is the emerging regulatory body for the UK aromatherapy profession and voluntary self-regulation should be in place by 2006, together with policies, standards and procedures. It is envisaged that the Consortium will then become the Aromatherapy Council. This will operate a single national register of aromatherapists in the UK of aromatherapists conforming to NOS standards and accepting the Code of Ethics, Disciplinary Procedures and continual professional development (CPD) guidelines set out. This will form the basis of voluntary self-regulation of the UK aromatherapy profession, but the profession will also explore the benefits of statutory regulation for the future, especially as aromatherapists use essential oils as an integral and fundamental part of their work and legislation on the trade is ever changing.

The AC has united the aromatherapy profession, having nine associations (including complementary and alternative medicine associations) who are members.

THE INTERNATIONAL FEDERATION OF PROFESSIONAL AROMATHERAPISTS (IFPA)

The IFPA (a limited company and registered Charity) was launched in April 2002 as a result of the International Society of Professional Aromatherapists (ISPA – formed in 1990 by the Editors) and the Register of Qualified Aromatherapists (RQA – formed in 1991 by

G Mojay) joining together. Joined also by some members of the IFA (below), the IFPA has quickly established itself as a significant force in the world of aromatherapy and is now the largest professional aromatherapy organization in the United Kingdom, its total membership in December 2005 being 2614 (2424 of these in the UK). It promotes high standards of education and professional training and accredits schools here and abroad, as well as the aromatherapy section of several universities, including Napier, Wolverhampton, Thames Valley and Huddersfield. The IFPA:

- offers a quarterly in-house journal 'In Essence'
- offers a comprehensive insurance and legal package
- has regional groups both in the UK and overseas
- holds annual conferences
- works closely with other organizations, especially the Aromatherapy Consortium (see above), to regulate the aromatherapy profession.

THE INTERNATIONAL FEDERATION OF AROMATHERAPY (IFA)

The IFA was the first independent aromatherapy organization to be established for professional aromatherapists, its membership in December 2005 being 1662 (around 600 of these in the UK). It was originally formed in the UK in 1985 by 10 aromatherapists, including the Editors, to act as an independent representative body for the profession of Aromatherapy and is a registered charity. The IFA:

- offers a quarterly journal, The Aromatherapy Times
- offers comprehensive insurance
- has regional groups both in the UK and overseas
- holds annual conferences
- has set up branches in Australia and Singapore.

THE INSTITUTE OF AROMATIC MEDICINE (IAM)

The IAM is an umbrella group for both aromatherapists and those who practise intensive application of essential oils and/or use essential oils and hydrolats *per os*.

Comprehensive insurance is offered at all levels of qualification, and includes home practice (see below).

The IAM is not in itself a training organization, but rather an accrediting body for courses in the UK and worldwide. The range of competence covered is unique to the UK.

The IAM:

- is committed to supporting organizations and therapists to the highest level of training and at the most professional level of service; it offers support and advice to all members and associates:

  Associate Membership (AIAM), with insurance, is open to aromatherapists in the first year of practice.

  Membership (MIAM), with comprehensive insurance, is open to aromatherapists with one or more years in practice.

  Licentiate Membership (LIAM), with additional insurance for intensive application and use by mouth, is open to practitioners of Aromatic Medicine (aromatologists) who can demonstrate a thorough and adequate training.

- Fellowship (FIAM) is an advanced qualification (UK Master's degree level) offered by the IAM, details of which can be obtained from the Registrar.

THE AROMATHERAPY TRADE COUNCIL (ATC)

This is the UK Trade Association for the aromatherapy essential oil industry. Founded in 1993, the ATC's mission is to promote responsible marketing of genuine aromatherapy products and also safe usage of essential oils by consumers. To this end, it has established a Code of Practice for product labelling and packaging and publishes Guidelines on the Regulation, Labelling, Advertising and Promotion of Aromatherapy Products to assist those setting up in business, e.g. it will review labels and promotional material prior to printing to ensure they comply with the complexities of the law. It has a policy for the random testing of its members' oils.

The ATC represents the interests of manufacturers and suppliers in the trade at legislative forums where decisions are made which affect the industry (see Regulations above); it advises its membership and the public alike on ever-changing legislation and its likely effects on the industry.

The ATC works closely with the Aromatherapy Consortium and other organizations to ensure the needs of the profession are served appropriately by the aromatherapy trade.

RESEARCH

Research in the UK can be viewed on the links page of the AC website and also on The Essential Oil Resource website, which provides scientific information about essential oils, is fully searchable and available on-line by subscription (see Useful addresses, p. 528). See also COST B4 in Appendix C.

Chapter 16 (Part II)

Aromatherapy within the National Health Service

Angela Avis and Shirley Price

DEVELOPMENT OF COMPLEMENTARY THERAPIES

Many health-care professionals are exploring the potential therapeutic use of a range of complementary therapies, which are not only gaining in popularity with the public (Ernst & White 2000, Thomas, Nicholl & Coleman 2001) but are finding a more substantial place in health care (Peters et al 2002).

1995 – almost 40% of GP partnerships in the UK referred their NHS patients to CAM therapists where they felt it would be of benefit (Thomas, Nicholl & Coleman 2001).

1997 – a survey conducted by the Research Council for Complementary Medicine said that about 75% of the public were using complementary therapies through the NHS.

1999 – in a BBC Radio 5 Live survey, 74% of the public said they would choose these therapies if they were available on the NHS (Ernst & White 2000).

This increasing interest among the general public (Ong & Banks 2003) and health-care professionals in CAM therapies such as aromatherapy, has encouraged its use more and more within palliative care, nursing and midwifery.

Aromatherapy is a multiple therapy embracing touch, massage and the administration of essential oil remedies – not to mention the accompanying pleasing aroma, which may be partly responsible for it being possibly the most popular complementary therapy which nurses wish to study. There have therefore been increasing demands that, in the best interests and safety of patients and clients, complementary therapies should become regulated and observe similar ethical and practical constraints to those of orthodox medicine.

The House of Lords Report (2000) classified therapies according to their evidence base and level of professional organization in relation to regulation (see Part 1 and Table 16.1).

Regarding nursing and midwifery, the Report identified Group 2 as covering those therapies most often used to complement conventional care. It was felt that the therapies mentioned in this 'comfort' category gave appropriate help and support to patients, in particular in relieving stress, pain and alleviating the side-effects of drug regimes.

Although there was concern about the lack of scientific evidence – as measured by random con-trolled trials (RCTs) – the Report recognized that there was a growing body of qualitative research. The therapies most frequently used by nurses and midwives, such as massage, aromatherapy and reflexology, come within the 'comfort' category. The most recent RCN survey in 2003 confirmed that these are still the key therapies used within clinical practice.

The House of Lords Report also encouraged the regulating body, Nursing and Midwifery Council (NMC) and the Royal College of Nursing (RCN) to collaborate in making familiarization of CAM a part of the pre-registration nursing and midwifery curricula, which would enable nurses and mid-wives to have some insight into the choices that their patients or clients make and to offer knowledgeable support. The report went on to suggest that these bodies should provide specific guidance on appropriate education and training for nurses and midwives who wish to integrate therapies such as aromatherapy into clinical care.

INTEGRATING AROMATHERAPY INTO CLINICAL CARE

When considering the integration of any comp-lementary therapy into clinical care there are key principles of professional practice. These involve the following and can be found in policies that have already been developed:

- patient-centred care – identifying the patient's needs or problems and the subsequent outcome of care
- appropriate choice of therapeutic intervention
- identification of the parameters of practice
- pinpointing the evidence supporting integration
- identification of the appropriate integration model
- ensuring education and training needs that will provide safe and effective practice
- development of effective evaluation strategies and on-going development needs that will sup-port a sustainable service.

A policy for integration, based on evidence (Richardson, Jones & Pilkington 2001) and a valid audit process is essential, otherwise it is difficult to see how nurses and midwives can argue for CAM integration into clinical practice, especially

Table 16.1 Therapies classified according to their evidence base and level of professional organization in relation to regulation

Group 1 Professionally organized alternative therapies	Group 2 Complementary therapies	Group 3 Alternative disciplines
Acupuncture	Alexander	3a Long
Chiropractic	technique	established
Herbal medicine	Aromatherapy	and traditional
Homoeopathy	Bach and other	systems of
Osteopathy	flower remedies	health care
	Massage	Ayurvedic medicine
	Reflexology	Anthroposophical
	Healing including	medicine
	Reiki	Chinese herbal
	Hypnotherapy	medicine
	Shiatsu	Traditional Chinese medicine
		3b Other alternative disciplines
		Crystal therapy
		Dowsing
		Iridology
		Kinesiology
		Radionics

Categories of CAM disciplines (House of Lords Report 2000).

as therapies are often used as a result of enthusiasm on the part of one or two nurses or midwives. A number of Trusts have already allocated time and effort to developing policies and it is by such work that standards are defined and patients are assured of care that is safe, appropriate and effective. The appropriate therapy is often determined by the nature of a particular clinical area. The area of cancer and palliative care is one in which national guidelines on the integration of complementary therapies have been published by the Prince of Wales's Foundation for Integrated Health (PWFIH) (Tavares 2003) and offer a wealth of information, including models of good practice.

As there is no national strategy to collect data, professionals have to rely on publications in journals that describe the use of complementary therapies within the various health fields. A small proportion of these are based on research projects but many are anecdotal.

NURSING AND MIDWIFERY COUNCIL (NMC)

CODE OF PROFESSIONAL CONDUCT

Nurses, as professional and accountable practitioners, have to take into account both the NMC Code of Professional Conduct (CPC) (2002a) and the Guidelines for the Administration of Medicines (2002b), since these documents govern all nursing activities. Some of the information on specific circumstances, safeguards, policies and procedures needed to provide treatment or care appropriate to each area of practice would be applicable also to aromatherapy practitioners; the relevant points will be brought into focus for the purposes of this chapter. The addition of the word 'aromatherapist', inserted by the author (Price), appears in order to show that the stated codes of conduct or guidelines for the administration of medicines apply also to this discipline.

The shared values of all the United Kingdom health care regulatory bodies are that, as a registered nurse, midwife or health visitor (or aromatherapist), you are personally accountable for your practice. In caring for patients and clients, you must:

- respect the patient or client as an individual
- obtain consent before you give any treatment or care

- protect confidential information
- co-operate with others in the team
- be trustworthy
- act to identify and minimize risk to patients and clients.

Both aromatherapists and nurses should be prepared to acknowledge any limitations in their knowledge and competence and decline any duties or responsibilities unless able to perform them in a safe and skilled manner. Be sure to have suitable insurance cover specific to the use of essential oils. RCN members are covered when working as a nurse; however, if cover is required when working independently it can be obtained from one of the professional aromatherapy or aromatic medicine associations on becoming a full member. The International Federation of Professional Aromatherapists (IFPA) and the Institute of Aromatic Medicine (IAM) also insure student aromatherapists during their time of study.

Many practitioners of different disciplines do not regularly update their knowledge. This is unwise since updating is of paramount importance, especially in a world where ideas and accepted behavioural patterns are changing fast. The practice of nursing and complementary therapies takes place in a context of continuing change and development.

The NMC Code of Professional Conduct (2002a) states that as a registered nurse, midwife or health visitor you must:

- protect and support the health of individual patients and clients
- act in such a way that justifies the trust and confidence the public have in you
- uphold and enhance the good reputation of the professions.

GUIDELINES FOR THE ADMINISTRATION OF MEDICINES

With respect to the above, nurse, midwife, health visitors and aromatherapists using essential oils, whether for baths, inhalations, topical application (including compresses), suppositories, pessaries and/or massage, should accept that they are administering medicines. Therefore, some of the NMC guidelines indirectly apply to them, emphasizing yet again the need for professional training or supervision. The NMC expects that, in this area of practice as in all others, practitioners (including aromatherapists) will have taken steps to develop their knowledge and competence and that all registered nurses, midwives and health visitors must recognize the personal professional accountability which they bear for their actions.

Medicinal preparations are prescribed by a physician or nurse (since 1992), checked and dispensed by a pharmacist and administered by a nurse. An essential oil prescription is prescribed by a competent aromatherapist or aromatologist and administered by that practitioner, or by a nurse suitably trained in the method of administration; in ideal circumstances the prescriber should not be the dispenser and the dispenser should not administer (Farrell 1994 personal communication).

When administering medication against a prescription written by a registered medical practitioner or another authorized prescriber, the prescription should:

- be based, whenever possible, on the patient's informed consent and awareness of the purpose of the treatment
- be clearly written, typed or computer-generated and be indelible
- be dated and signed by the authorized prescriber
- not be for a substance to which the patient is known to be allergic or otherwise unable to tolerate
- clearly identify the patient for whom the medication is intended
- clearly specify the substance to be administered, using the generic or brand name (in the case of aromatherapy, the scientific plant name/s should be used), together with the strength, dosage, timing, frequency of administration, start and finish dates and route of administration.

The NMC states (p. 6) that there is no legal barrier to dispensing – except under exceptional circumstances; however, this must be in accordance with a doctor's written instructions. Any health professional should be able to justify and be accountable for any action taken.

Some nurses, midwives and health visitors, having first undertaken successfully a training in complementary or alternative therapy which involves the use of substances such as essential oils, apply their specialist knowledge and skill in their practice. It is essential that practice in these respects, as in all others, is based upon sound principles, available knowledge and skill. The importance of consent to the use of such treatment must be recognized. So, too, must the practitioner's personal accountability for her or his professional practice (NMC 2002a).

AROMATHERAPISTS AND NURSES WORKING IN THE NHS

Work to support the regulation of therapies such as aromatherapy, massage and reflexology is presently underway (see Education in Ch. 16 Part I). As it is vitally important that the use of any therapy, such as aromatherapy, is always in the best interests and safety of the patients and clients, each health-care professional must act within the code of conduct of their professional body, for example, the NMC Code of Professional Conduct (2002a), points from which are stated above, requires that nurses and midwives must be convinced of the safety and relevance of any therapy chosen and be able to justify its use. They should also act in accordance with the policies and protocols set by the particular hospice or hospital in which they work. These should be achieved without compromising or fragmenting existing areas of practice and care. Collaboration is also part of professional practice, hence the need to discuss the use of CAM with members of the multi-disciplinary health team caring for the particular patient.

In some areas of the NHS, services are being developed that include therapies such as massage and aromatherapy, especially within palliative and cancer care, where aromatherapists are either employed or work as volunteers (Wilkinson 1995). Patients can either be referred by other health-care professionals or have direct access to aromatherapists – and a full assessment is undertaken to determine an appropriate treatment regime. Where nurses use essential oils within their nursing practice, their primary employment is as nurses, and they are therefore governed by the

Nursing and Midwifery Council's code of professional conduct.

The emphasis is on protocols that demonstrate safe and effective clinical decision making, for example, where midwives use essential oils to support women in childbirth (Burns, Blamey & Lloyd 2000) at the John Radcliffe Hospital in Oxford:

Two midwives who were qualified aromatherapists led the initiative in the early 1990s. The reaction of the women who experienced essential oils in the delivery suite was so positive that a decision was made that all women who delivered their babies in the unit would have access to the use of essential oils for symptom management. A basic training programme was set up so that all midwives on the unit could offer women the use of a prescribed range of essential oils under the supervision of trained aromatherapists. The midwives understood that this training did not qualify them as aromatherapists but provided the knowledge to use essential oils appropriately and effectively within midwifery practice.

If they move to another hospital their training may or may not be accepted. This will be dependent on the policy of that hospital and on the type and range of care that is offered on that unit. This innovation is part of the policy cycle at the Oxford Radcliffe NHS Trust and has recently been updated in 2005. The midwifery education package has been refined and developed. Other complementary therapy initiatives in the Trust are able to move forward coherently within the policy development framework.

Polices are framed somewhat differently where independent aromatherapists are employed by the NHS or are volunteers within a service. For example, at St Ann's Hospice in Manchester, emphasis is placed on establishing a register of therapists with specific qualifications and the establishment of a training and supervision programme that supports aromatherapists to work with patients who have complex clinical and psychological needs.

There are various examples of policies already in place relating to the integration of complementary therapies, and health-care professionals must work within any given constraints – however frustrating.

POLICIES AND PROTOCOLS

Written polices and protocols are designed to provide a framework of consistency and continuity which is particularly important during any change of personnel. Once recorded, policies become the means for providing legal indemnity.

- **Policies** – state clearly what is expected of staff and cover issues which the organization considers important for the delivery and management of the integration of complementary therapies.
- **Protocols** – are the step-by-step methods for achieving policy statements. A policy statement records 'what the rule is and to whom the rule applies'. In order that health-care professionals are able to abide by the rule, protocols should indicate clearly 'what must be done and by whom'.

POLICIES

- **Operational policies** are those for the day-to-day management and practice of individual therapies, including expectations of therapists.

Developing policy is not an overnight task. The minimum period from planning to ratification is usually 2 years and many have taken as many as $4\frac{1}{2}$ years . . . stamina is needed!

Learning from the experience of nurses who have been involved in the development of policies, here are a few tips:

- Talk to the right people.
- Know the organizational structure that you are working in.
- Know who is on your side.
- Have some idea of the scope of the policy from the beginning.
- Keep the document simple.
- Not too much detail – people won't read it.
- Also too much detail can hem you in.
- Keep your options open.
- Detail is more appropriate at the clinical protocol level.
- Don't have unreal expectations.
- Be pragmatic because there will have to be compromises.

- Make sure that firm review dates are built into the system to keep the document alive – not something that just sits on the shelf.
- Keep up-to-date with national developments.
- You will need to be ready to become the 'expert'.

It won't happen overnight – so be prepared for the long haul. Neither will it necessarily be a smooth path – there will be many times when you think the way has been blocked. This is when you need to be able to think laterally and be flexible about what you want to achieve.

Because of the differing organizational cultures there is no one template that can be used. However, a review of existing policy documents would suggest that the following headings might be taken as core requirements:

- **Title of policy** – needs to communicate clearly what the policy is about.
- **Identification of aims of the policy** – tells people what the document will cover.
- **Definition of terms used within the policy document** – sometimes this is presented as an appendix.
- **Identification of objectives that can be evaluated and measured** – this will describe the outcomes that are hoped to be achieved.
- **Identification of what will be covered by the policy** – sometimes the reality is that only a particular aspect or technique of aromatherapy will be used and this needs to be defined.
- **Reasoning behind the use of aromatherapy** – this will include clinical information and any relevant research or evidence of efficacy.
- **Identification of who should deliver the aromatherapy treatment** – sometimes this involves setting up a register of available practitioners.
- **Definition of competency to practise** – this will include a description of the aromatherapy knowledge and skills needed to practise in a particular clinical area.
- **Identification of educational criteria to determine competent practitioners within a particular clinical area** – this may include the identification of specific aromatherapy training courses.
- **Identification of lines of accountability** – this may include medical authorization.

- **Safety issues** – this will include contra-indications and risk assessment.
- **Informed consent** – there will be clear guide-lines about how and when this is obtained.
- **Documentation to be used within the clinical area** – ideally this should be based on multi-professional collaboration.
- **Equity of access** – do all the patients in a particular clinical area have equal access at any one time to suitably trained aromatherapists?
- **Environmental issues** – providing peace and privacy, etc.
- **Methods of evaluation** – what tools will be used to audit and evaluate the service?
- **Financial considerations** – (a) who should pay for essential oils used and (b) is the aromatherapy to be carried out within the existing contract of the practitioner or will there be additional hours and payment?
- **A timetable for the review of the policy** – this must be stipulated.

This list is not exhaustive and there is a useful chapter in the Nurses' Handbook of Complementary Therapies by Denise Rankin-Box and Maxine McVey (2001) that has some extra ideas. Also, Tavares (2004) has produced a very comprehensive guide for writing policies, procedures and protocols for the use of complementary therapies in supportive and palliative care. It contains several examples of policies – some relatively simple – and there is also an example of a therapist's contract from the Cavendish Centre in Manchester.

DRAFT PROTOCOL FOR THE USE OF ESSENTIAL OILS

A draft example of a protocol for the use of essential oils by nurses at St Gemma's Hospice, Leeds is included in Tavares' guide and is divided into the following headings:

- **Preamble** – describing the situations for the use of essential oils, e.g. to help mask offensive odours or to help patients enjoy a better sleep.
- **Electrical diffusers** – explanation of diffusers and some precautions to be observed when using them.
- **Choice of oils** – a limited range of oils is used, under the supervision of a nurse aromatherapist.

These include bergamot, grapefruit, lemongrass, lavender and sandalwood (author [Price]'s note: Latin names should be used to ensure correct variety or chemotype is used each time).

- **Method of use** – three different methods of application are described: aromastream, aromastone and via a tissue or external dressing. There is detailed instruction on how to proceed, depending on the method used.
- **Documentation** – there is some discussion about where the treatment should be recorded.
- **Storage** – instructions about how and where the essential oils should be stored.
- **Advice** – this section reminds staff that if they have any queries, they must consult the complementary therapy co-ordinator for the unit, who is also a qualified aromatherapist.
- **Accidents and adverse reactions** – instructions about how these should be reported.

At the bottom of the protocol is a section for the date when it will be ratified and a date for review. There is also information about who is responsible for the review.

An interesting issue that falls within policy development is that of informed consent. Because aromatherapy is not part of mainstream health care it is important that explicit consent is obtained from the patient, who must understand not only the potential benefits but also the limits of a treatment. Any safety issues must also be highlighted. Many units are producing leaflets explaining the services offered, making sure patients have access to the information before they arrive, so that they can raise any concerns during the initial assessment.

As can be seen, policy development for the integration of aromatherapy within the NHS is a complex process. While there is undoubted enthusiasm within many health-care professions, the development of policy is most often 'guarded' by the medical establishment. Obviously all health-care professionals understand the need to base any care on evidence and wish to provide a service to patients which is responsive to needs, as well as being appropriate and effective. For many, the use of essential oils adds another dimension to care, to complement often harsh orthodox regimes – and to enhance a patient's quality of life. Unfortunately the preoccupation of the medical establishment with random-controlled trials means that qualitative research methods which, for example, explore patient outcomes, are denigrated. Winning the support of medical colleagues is part of the complex process.

The practical approach would be that use of essential oils be limited to a relatively small range of therapeutic interventions within appropriate clinical settings, which should be fastidiously evaluated. The evaluation should then be published so that success is well-documented and will build a foundation from which the use of essential oils can be appropriately spread throughout the health service.

SUMMARY

Part I of this chapter has shown the great steps that have been taken towards self-regulation of aromatherapy in the UK and the current legislation situation directed by the European Union. Part II has demonstrated how policy and practice guidelines can be put into practice and it is to be hoped that more health provision agencies will follow the lead already made in the UK where appropriate.

References

Aromatherapy Trades Council Newsletter 2004 European Legislation Update – July 2004: p. 2

Baker S 2003a Update on European legislation. In Essence 2(3): 10–12

Baker S 2003b The role of National Occupational Standards (NOS) in UK aromatherapy education and training. Information sheet

Burns E, Blamey C, Lloyd A 2000 Aromatherapy in childbirth: an effective approach to care. British Journal of Midwifery 8(10): 639–643

Department of Health 2001 Government Response to the House of Lords Select Committee on Science and Technology's Report on Complementary and Alternative Medicine. CM5124. The Stationery Office, London

Ernst E, White A 2000 The BBC survey of complementary medicine use in the UK. Complementary Therapies in Medicine. 8: 32–36 (data provided by ICM Research Ltd)

Field T 2003 Touch therapy. Elsevier, London, p. vii

House of Lords Select Committee on Science and Technology 2000 Complementary and Alternative Medicine. HL Paper 123. November. The Stationery Office, London

Integrated Health Care 1997 A way forward for the next 5 years? The Foundation for Integrated Medicine, London

Nursing and Midwifery Council 2002a Code of Professional Conduct. Nursing and Midwifery Council, London

Nursing and Midwifery Council 2002b Guidelines for the Administration of Medicines. Nursing and Midwifery Council, London

Ong C-K, Banks B 2003 Complementary and alternative medicine: the consumer perspective. The Prince of Wales's Foundation for Integrated Health, London

Peters D, Chaitow L, Harris G, Morrison S 2002 Integrating complementary therapies in primary care. Churchill Livingstone, Edinburgh

Price L, Price S 2004 Understanding Hydrolats. Churchill Livingstone, Edinburgh

Rankin-Box D, McVey M 2001 Policy development. In: Rankin-Box D (ed) The nurse's handbook of complementary therapies. Ballière Tindall, London

Richardson J, Jones C, Pilkington K 2001 Complementary therapies; what is the evidence for their use? Professional Nurse. 17(2): 96–99

Royal College of Nursing 2003a Complementary therapies on nursing, health visiting and midwifery: guidance on the integration of complementary therapies into clinical nursing practice. Royal College of Nursing, London. Publication code 002 204

Royal College of Nursing 2003b In Touch; Newsletter of the Complementary Therapies in Nursing Forum. Royal College of Nursing, London: Autumn

Tavares M 2003 National Guidelines for the Use of Complementary Therapies in Supportive and Palliative Care. The Prince of Wales's Foundation for Integrated Health and National Council for Hospice and Specialist Palliative Care Services, London

Tavares M 2004 Guide for writing policies, procedures and protocols. complementary therapies. In: Supportive and palliative care. Help the Hospices, London

The Prince of Wales's Foundation for Integrated Health (PWFIH) (2003) Setting the agenda for the future. The Prince of Wales's Foundation for Integrated Health, London

Thomas K, Nicholl J, Coleman P 2001 Use and expenditure on complementary medicine in England: a population based survey. Complementary Therapies in Medicine 9: 2–11

Wilkinson S 1995 Aromatherapy and massage in palliative care. International Journal of Palliative Nursing 13(5): 409–417

Sources

Avis A 1999 When is an aromatherapist not an aromatherapist? Complementary Therapies in Medicine. 7(2): 116–118

Corner J, Cawley N, Hildebrand S 1996 An evaluation of the use of massage and essential oils on the well-being of cancer patients. International Journal of Palliative Nursing 1: 67–73

Currie L, Morrell C, Scrivener R 2003 Clinical Governance: an RCN resource guide. Royal College of Nursing, London

Department of Health 1995 The Policy Framework for Commissioning Cancer Services. The Stationery Office, London

Department of Health 1997 The New NHS, Modern Dependable. The Stationery Office, London

Department of Health 1998 A First Class Service: quality in the new NHS. The Stationery Office, London

Department of Health 1999 Clinical Governance: Quality in the new NHS. The Stationery Office, Leeds

Department of Health 2000 The NHS Cancer Plan: a plan for investment, a plan for reform. The Stationery Office, London

Hudson R 1996 The value of lavender for rest and activity in the elderly patient. Complementary Therapies in Medicine 4: 52–57

Luff D, Thomas J 2000 'Getting somewhere'. Feeling cared for: perspectives on complementary therapies in the NHS. Complementary Therapies in Medicine 8: 253–259

Mackereth P 2001 Supervision and complementary therapies. In: Rankin-Box D 2001 The nurse's handbook of complementary therapies. Ballière Tindall, London

National Institute for Clinical Excellence 2004 Guidance on Cancer Services: improving supportive and palliative care for adults with cancer. The Stationery Office, London

Rankin-Box D (ed) 2001 The nurse's handbook of complementary therapies. Ballière Tindall, London

Russo H 2000 Integrated healthcare: a guide to good practice. Foundation for Integrated Medicine, London

Sanderson H, Harrison J, Price S. 1991 Aromatherapy and massage for people with learning difficulties. Hands-On Publishing, Birmingham

Semple M, Cable S 2003 The new Code of Professional Conduct. Nursing Standard. 19(17) No 23: 40–48

Shuttleworth A 2003 Protocol based care. Nursing Times Publication, Emap Healthcare, London

Tiran D, Mack S (eds) 2000 Complementary therapies for pregnancy and childbirth, 2nd edn. Ballière Tindall, London

Chapter **17**

Aromatherapy worldwide

Len Price

INTRODUCTION

The practice of, and knowledge in aromatherapy varies widely across the globe. In some countries, such as France, phytotherapy (which includes aromatology – see Ch. 9) is an established branch of medicine for which essential oils may be prescribed by the doctors concerned, usually for use by application to various parts of the body – although without massage, and very often orally, per rectum and vagina, compresses, gargles or in a diffuser. In other countries, such as Portugal, aromatherapy is in its infancy, and is practised in hospitals using mainly massage, and on a voluntary basis, by aromatherapists and interested nurses.

This chapter examines aromatherapy use within the health-care systems of 21 countries, representing a range of different stages of development, implementation and styles of practice.

The following headings are used for each country as far as the information allowed:

Aromatherapy development
Regulations
Essential oils
Education
Use of essential oils in medical establishments
Associations
Research

EUROPE

BELGIUM [S Sarazin]

Aromatherapy development

It is not clear exactly when aromatherapy came to Belgium, but it appears to have started with the sale of essential oils in health shops. Although some herbalist courses have been given to shop owners, most of them know too little about them to give useful information to the clients.

Some beauty colleges teach a little aromatherapy.

Regulations

There are no laws governing either essential oil use or aromatherapy training and as it is not a recognized medical or paramedical discipline, it is not available on health insurance.

Essential oils

There is a general lack of information on essential oils, especially regarding quality and safety issues. Essential oils are subject to the new herb regulations and need to be noted for oral use in preparations, although some are not allowed for this use any more. Non-oral use is regulated by the new European Cosmetics law.

Essential oils are used mostly in massage, baths, and in a vaporizer, the most popular treatment being baths and the least popular, massage.

Education

There are no set standards for training and most courses consist only of about 4–20 hours, with a few longer ones of approximately 40 hours. Most of the courses offer a qualification, although the teaching is not to the standard of accredited schools in the UK.

Nurses usually obtain their training from courses which teach several complementary therapies – and therefore acquire only the basics in aromatherapy.

There are no academies or schools which give a proper professional training in aromatherapy, apart from Morgaine netfirms, who give workshops and training in massage, chakra's and aromatherapy.

Use of essential oils in medical establishments

Although aromatherapy and phytotherapy are not well accepted in most hospitals, a few do use them. For example, the nurse-unit for palliative care at St Camillus in Antwerp uses aromatherapy for physical and psychological purposes and also during the dying process. In 2000, essential oils began to be used in palliative care at Middelheim hospital in Wilrijk, where the head-internist (oncologist) approved a protocol for wound care and the use of aromatherapy and *Lavandula angustifolia* and *Melaleuca alternifolia* have been used with very good results – (see Ch. 15).

The majority of elderly care centres and palliative care centres use aromatherapy for massage, relaxation and in a bath, particularly with demented patients.

Associations

Although there is no association yet for aromatherapists, a research association exists, which also has a branch in Japan.

Research

Belgium has a Natural Aromatherapy Research and Development association (NARD).

CROATIA [Z Jezdi]

Aromatherapy development

Essential oils have been part of Croatian tradition for many years – as part of herbal and traditional medicine and the making of candles and aromatic substances. Both production and sale of essential oils have expanded over the last 10 years, people using them now as a form of self help.

Some private firms and a few public open schools run aromatherapy courses.

Regulations

There are no laws as yet regarding the use of essential oils or the practice of aromatherapy.

Essential oils

Essential oils are imported mainly from France and Germany, some shops putting their own label on them. Although the Institute for Public Health checks the quality of essential oils, there is no law regarding quality.

Education

A registered nurse, Zrinka Jezdi, who trained at the Shirley Price International College of Aromatherapy before Shirley Price's retirement, was the first aromatherapist to open a school in Croatia – *Aromavita*. The school runs two in-depth aromatherapy courses, both having been accepted by the Croatian Ministry of Education and Science. Qualified aromatherapists can start a business legally – recognized by the government as National Classified Employment in branches of human medicine. This status was achieved through the valuable work done by the principal of the school above.

The *Aromavita* school offers two levels of education:

1. **Aromatherapist**: This involves 24 hours per week over 6 months (370 hours) and includes anatomy and physiology, practical and holistic aromatherapy, massage, the chemistry of essential oils and aroma cosmetics. Each student must complete in addition 6 case studies, 3 of which have to concern patients from a health establishment.
2. **Aromatherapy specialist**: This course is over 12 months for 2 days a week, one for theory and one working in homes for the elderly and private houses, plus every third weekend – 960 hours in total, which includes 450 hours' practical work, 40 on holistic aromatherapy and 50 on kinesiotherapy. The chemistry of essential oils, pharmacognosy and phytotherapy, together with production and cultivation of medicinal plants take up 150 hours. 60 hours are spent on anatomy and physiology, pathology and pathophysiology. Only those who have completed some form of health education first, or have taken first level aromatherapy above, can apply for this course.

Each student is given practice in wellness centres and must also have 200 hours of practical work in a private clinic, home for the elderly or home nursing, completing 10 case studies, plus 3 cases on handicapped children and 10 on their own clients.

[N.B. The editors were impressed with the clinics they visited.]

At the end of 2004, the school had 200 aromatherapists and 15 aromatherapy specialists.

Use of essential oils in medical establishments

Some special hospitals integrate aromatherapy into their work and have a department for aromatherapy; the Varadinska hospital for rehabilitation is such a one, where short courses are run for nurses and physiotherapists. Private clinics are also beginning to have a department for aromatherapy, as it becomes more and more popular.

Associations

An association to be called the Croatian Society of Professional Aromatherapists is in the process of being formed (2005). The society hopes to be connected with the International Federation of Professional Aromatherapists (IFPA) in the UK.

Research

There is no known research on essential oils taking place at the moment.

FINLAND [A Saarenheimo]

Aromatherapy development

Aromatherapy started with a general surge in interest towards complementary medicine at the beginning of the 1980s. Beauty therapists led the way by inviting an English aromatherapist to teach them how to use essential oils in skin care. In 1984 a beauty/aromatherapist, Taina Maisala, started teaching aromatherapeutic massage at Frantsila herb farm and natural medicine training centre, with Virpi Raipala-Cormier. By the middle of the 1990s several natural medicine institutions were offering aromatherapy training, although only two colleges now provide comprehensive aromatherapy programmes.

The public is learning about aromatherapy through aroma- and other therapists, magazines, books and courses held for home users. As a result, the use of essential oils is steadily growing. As a rule, aromatherapists work as private practitioners in their own therapy rooms or in the spas.

Regulations

There are no direct laws governing the use of aromatherapy, but there are several which apply indirectly to the use of essential oils, such as the laws regarding cosmetics and medicine.

Education

The private colleges have harmonized their programmes with respect to each other – and to be compatible with international trends. The aromatherapy part of the curriculum includes in-class training in essential oils and full-body massage, documented case studies, clinical practice, exams, essays and a thesis about a subject related to aromatherapy. A basic curriculum of orthodox and natural medicine is mandatory for all. The non-medical students take courses in anatomy, physiology, pathology, neurology, psychology and psychiatry. In addition, all students are required to take two or more modules of natural medicine: phytotherapy, nutrition, natural supplements, etc.

In 2003, a working group set up by the Ministry of Education comprising members of orthodox medicine and a few prominent aromatherapists agreed on guidelines for teaching aromatherapy to massage therapists, assistant physiotherapists, foot specialists and beauty therapists. The guidelines include treatment protocols and lists of recommended essential oils for the different disciplines.

Use of essential oils in medical establishments

There is no aromatherapy training within the medical establishments and nurses wishing to study this subject attend one of the private institutes teaching aromatherapy. If they then want to use their skills as an aromatherapist, they must do it outside the medical establishment, in their own private practice – in the role of a therapist – not as a nurse.

However, although aromatherapy is not practised in hospitals as yet, its use in hospices seems to be on the increase, where the methods of application vary: aromalamps are popular as mood enhancers, but massage is the most popular form of therapy, given as full- or part-body treatments, with the clients' permission – and that of their superiors. Some residential homes for pensioners may be using aromatherapy as the interest grows.

Associations

There are two aromatherapy associations in Finland:

Suomen aromaterapeutit ry, with membership which is independent of training establishments.
UMG-Aromaterapiayhdistys ry, which is an association formed by one of the colleges for its own qualified students.

Neither association has arranged insurance for its members – practising aromatherapists are expected to obtain their own liability insurance.

Research

No scientific research has being done specifically on essential oils and aromatherapy, although the University of Helsinki has carried out some small scale research concerning essential oils.

FRANCE [R Harris]

Aromatherapy development

The profession of aromatherapist does not really exist in France, the use of essential oils in body massage, as practised in the UK, only being known since the 1990s. Essential oil use is generally included with medical herbalism (phytotherapy), and hundreds of medical doctors, pharmacies and some analytical and bacteriological laboratories are involved in aromatology (aromatic medicine) and phytotherapy. Different plant extracts (tinctures, gelules) and essential oils are prescribed orally and/or as pessaries and suppositories – and occasionally to be applied externally, when they usually involve much higher concentrations than used in the UK – around 5–10% dilution. Body massage is not used.

Although doctors who have followed a course of natural medicine (médecine douce) may practise complementary therapies alongside allopathic care, it is illegal for a non-medical person to practise any therapy having a therapeutic effect without a licence – even if working with the support of a medically trained person. Nevertheless, a massage therapist, kinésithérapeute (physiotherapist), is allowed to practise aromatherapy English style legally – and the word 'massage' is reserved only for these therapists.

It would probably be an equal task to establish the profession of aromatherapist in France as it would be to convince the UK medical profession of the value of intensive and internal use of essential oils (aromatology/aromatic medicine). What is needed is a change in the educational and legal systems to enable people who are neither medically trained, nor massage therapists, to receive full aromatherapy training so that they can practise professionally.

Regulations

Essential oil use for therapeutic purposes is largely the domain of the doctor, veterinarian, dental surgeon and doctor of pharmacy.

In French law, massage is to be carried out exclusively by masseurs (physiotherapists) holding a State recognized diploma. The Syndicat National des Masseurs-Kinésithérapeutes Rééducateurs (SNMKR), jealously guards the physiotherapist's monopoly of massage and regularly challenges practitioners and aestheticians through legal proceedings.

Even though an aromatherapist, masseur or wellness practitioner is appropriately trained elsewhere in the European Union, they do not have an automatic right to practise within France; aestheticians may practise only face massage – for beauty purposes, even though their state approved training included body massage techniques.

Numerous practitioners have attempted to continue their work using a different name for their therapy, for instance: 'practicien de toucher' (touch practitioner), 'modelage', 'toucher therapeutique', 'effleurement tactile', 'technique manuelle anti-stress' – all terms describing their work; however, they are skating on thin ice with regard to the law.

The Association Soutien Massage Bien-Etre (ASMBE – well-being massage) was recently formed in response to a court case against Joel Savatofski, taken to court for promoting and giving seated massage to drivers in an autoroute stop, to refresh and relieve tension. This case was one of the few success stories, as on-site massage did not come under the massage monopoly held by kinésithérapeutes.

Despite these obstacles and risks, hundreds of non-medical natural therapy practitioners work in France, reflecting the enormous public demand for 'softer' alternatives to allopathy. It is hoped that with increasing collaboration between countries in the European Union, the French legal system will become more flexible.

Essential oils

Several hundred pharmacies stock a range of therapeutic quality essential oils – the rest stocking standardized oils, health food stores and many open markets in the south of France also selling essential oils. Not all essential oils are available to the general public – since 1986, mugwort, wormwood, cedar, hyssop, sage, tansy and thuja are restricted to prescription only. Fennel, star anise and aniseed oils are also restricted, due to their potential use in the illegal making of alcoholic drinks such as Pastis. Because the botanical names are not specified, there is often confusion and frustration within the essential oil industry.

The majority of aromatherapy practitioners obtain their essential oils by mail order direct from French laboratories, thus having access to GC/MS analyses for the oils they buy. The perception that it is easier to access quality essential oils in France than many other countries is not necessarily true.

Education

Complementary training for doctors, pharmacists and other health-care professionals varies in depth and duration and as aromatherapy is recognized as a branch of phytotherapy (herbal medicine), studies usually include other forms of herbal extracts as well as essential oils.

Bobigny University, Faculty of Medicine, Paris

This is the main centre for the study of natural medicine, where two university courses are offered:

- A 3-year diploma (252 hours) on medical herbal practice. Doctors following this teaching are called naturothérapeutes, to distinguish them from naturopaths, i.e. those who are not medical doctors.
- A 2-year diploma (196 hours) in herbal advice and information – open to osteopaths, kinésithérapeutes (massage therapists), midwives, nurses, pharmacy assistants, etc.

Other natural medicine studies, including naturotherapy are also available. However, naturopaths, like osteopaths, are not legally allowed to practise – though many do.

Montpellier University

Two phyto-aromatherapy courses are offered:

- 2 years, involving six weekends, or
- 1 year, involving two blocks of study totalling 10 days.

Only doctors can practise legally with this diploma.

The Institut Méditerranéen de Documentation d'Enseignement et de Recherche sur les Plantes Médicinales (MDERPLAM)

This Institute, also in Montpellier, offers aromatherapy training for non-medical personnel. The study period is over 3 years, of which three weekends (24 hours) involve aromatherapy training. The Editors taught here for several years.

The Lyonnaise School of Medicinal Plants

Two training options are offered, principally to doctors and paramedic personnel, although open to all:

- Applied aromatherapy – over three weekends.
- Herbalism (Herboristerie) – over 3 years.

Distance learning

The concept of learning via correspondence is well established and accepted within France. A more recent trend is that of offering training in phyto-aromatherapy by e-learning – principally open to medical personnel.

Hippocratus is a leading college offering this form of learning, involving 300 hours of study over 2 years, leading to a diploma in phyto-aromatherapy and medicinal plant advising.

Use of essential oils in medical establishments

Aromatherapy is largely conducted in general practice by a doctor 'aromatologue' (aromatologist), who may also be a homoeopath and/or acupuncturist. Treatments vary from an 'allopathic' approach, using essential oils as medicaments (like drugs), to a more holistic approach, where doctors trained as naturotherapeutes analyse all lifestyle elements of their patients. A prescription, which may contain both essential oils and herbal extracts, is given, consisting of capsules or solutions for oral use, suppositories or pessaries for rectal or vaginal insertion and/or preparations for application to the skin. The approximately 40-minute consultation with an aromatologist (2005) costs from 30 to 90 euros and in most cases, part of the prescription cost can be recovered from the French health insurance system.

The majority of illnesses for which essential oils are successfully prescribed in France – and thus reduce recourse to antibiotics and other medicaments – are infectious or inflammatory in nature. Others include allergies, immune dysfunctions, rheumatology, dermatology, gynaecology and hormonal imbalances, viral diseases. cardiovascular disease, digestive disturbances, urinary disorders, nervous, psychological and sexual dysfunctions, including genital problems. They are also used in emergency situations involving burns, wounds, external trauma, etc. where no placebo or psychological effect can be said to intervene – thus providing confirmation of their efficacy. Much attention is paid to the health of the liver, so the prescription is often accompanied by dietary or other measures to support its healthy function.

Several laboratories carry out aromatogram testing (see Ch. 4), making up prescriptions on site according to the test and using oils from the same batch. The cost of aromatogram testing is not reimbursable.

Research

In France, there is a considerable amount of essential oil research conducted, which unfortunately does not all get published in the international scientific press. Most of the work focuses on the antimicrobial, antiinflammatory and 'active cosmetics' aspects of essential oil activity.

GERMANY [E Zimmerman, Dr D Wabner and M Hoch]

Aromatherapy development

Aromatherapy became known in Germany in the 1980s and although growing fast, there is still a fairly low level of knowledge about essential oils, e.g. few pharmacists are aware of the different chemotypes of thyme.

The use of essential oils is more evident in the south, with aromatherapy courses being better attended there than in the north.

Many health food stores sell essential oils, some firms educating the staff concerning their use. Workshops are available, mainly directed at nurses, heilpraktikers (natural medicine practitioners), physiotherapists, doctors and pharmacists.

Regulations

Aromatherapy can only be practised legally by doctors and heilpraktikers. A few doctors use essential oils in their own practices; nurses and occupational therapists work as aroma-care therapists offering 'wellness' and preventative treatments.

Essential oils are considered to be under household law as 'objects for improving the odour of rooms' and not as medicines, which come under pharmaceutical law. Aromatherapists and nurses have to accept that they are treating their patients with a room deodorant (even though the oils may have been selected for a health problem).

No medicinal claims can be made on essential oil labels and the European Union has produced many restrictions regarding their use, with special labels for oils containing more than 10% hydrocarbons; these carry the warning: 'bad for one's health' (even lavender). Cosmetic companies have to show the contents of so-called sensitizers on the label. Estragol and safrol cannot be ingredients of cosmetic substances, the content of methyl eugenol having been reduced to 0.0002% in leave-on products.

Essential oils

Essential oils are available in all pharmacies, although most stock only those standardized according to the German pharmacopoeia (DAB) – mostly of poor quality. However, some pharmacies, essential oil companies and many health shops, tea shops and markets stock good, sometimes high quality, authentic, genuine oils and mixtures.

Lay people are not aware of the possible hazards which can be caused by using the cheap – and therefore obviously adulterated – oil of tea tree available in supermarkets, which has caused both minor and severe irritations in those using it.

Education

There are hardly any aromatherapy schools in Germany and courses are of different lengths. The big aromatherapy companies, such as Primavera Life, offer essential oil education for everybody, two companies only for pharmacists.

As there is no set training or general policy for nurses using essential oils, most acquire their knowledge from weekend workshops and aromatherapy books. However, a few midwifery and nursing schools include some instruction on aromatherapy in their curricula and several workshops are available:

■ *AIDA* (Aromatherapy International) follows a British curriculum, offering a certificate after examination and also holds courses for care workers, including doctors and midwives.
■ The Augustinum clinic in Munich offers training in cooperation with AIDA for employees from the health professions.
■ The Munich *City Institut für Pflegeberufe* (Institute for Nursing Care) provides a yearly 4-month seminar (80 hours) on aromatherapy in care, in cooperation with NORA-International, with a written exam and certificate.
■ *The Technical University of Munich* with NORA-International provides a weekly 2-hour lecture over two semesters for medical and science students.

There are three levels of training in the use of essential oils:

1. **Aromatherapy**: for doctors and state approved naturopaths (includes ingestion of essential oils).
2. **Aroma-care**: for health professionals (nurses, midwives, physiotherapists).
3. **Aroma counselling**: for all other professions; this therapy is called aroma culture (not aromatherapy) and the qualification is that of aroma counsellor or aroma expert (not aromatherapist).

Use of essential oils in medical establishments

From Freiburg to Munich essential oils are in regular use in around 5–10% of the hospitals and hospices by enthusiastic well trained nurses. However, most doctors, not being conversant with their healing properties, hear about their esoteric effects in the press (without scientific background), making it difficult for nurses to convince them of their pharmaceutically active components.

Many freelance midwives use essential oils in their work outside hospital; nurses within a hospital are allowed to use them to alleviate minor conditions such as dry skin or headaches, but must have permission from the doctor in charge if they wish to use them for more serious medical conditions. They must keep an up-to-date written progress report of the essential oils used, how often and how many drops; treatment changes and improvements must also be recorded.

Conditions treated include: anxiety, depression, difficult breathing, headaches, pneumonia, digestive problems, all kinds of infections, insomnia, burns, scars, wounds, ulcers, postoperative intestinal atony and *Candida albicans*. Essential oils are also used in terminal illness, pregnancy and birth, endocrinology and psychocancer therapy and with patients in psychosomatic wards.

Since 1995, essential oils have become a fundamental part of nursing and health care in Stiftsklinik Augustinium – a clinic with departments for cardiology, pneumology, angiology, nephrology, and metabolic diseases. Aromatherapy intervention is carried out with the doctors' cooperation; it is documented and standards and protocols have also to be followed.

Nurses trained in aroma-care can apply essential oils using gentle stroking (effleurage) without having a recognized qualification in massage. Other methods include inhalation, sponge baths (in cases of fever), compresses, foot and hand-massage and foot baths for pain control. High concentration of oils and mixtures are used for wounds and after an operation, sprays being used for decubitus ulcers (bedsores).

Associations

Forum Essenzia
Set up in 1991, this association gives workshops which emphasize the necessity of using quality essential oils for therapeutic purposes.

NORA-International (a branch of the Natural Oils Research Association, UK)
Established in Germany in 1996, this association has worked within essential oil information and research, with lectures, seminars and congresses, manuscripts, papers, scientific investigations, studies and even television features.

Research

Research was carried out at Kiel University in 1996 to compare the analgesic effects of *Mentha* x *piperita* versus paracetamol (acetaminophen) on people with tension headaches. It was found that 10% of peppermint oil in ethanol had the same effect as 1000 mg of paracetamol, leading to the development of Euminz, a special commercial roll-on for forehead and neck.

At Munich Technical University Prof. Dietrich Wabner is working in cooperation with the dermatological department at Biederstein clinics and NORA-International on several aspects of essential oils, including quality control, physiology of essential oil producing plants, use of essential oils against hospitalization and oil-mixtures possible against neurodermatitis in children.

ICELAND [M Birgisdottir and S Sigurdsson]

Aromatherapy development

Aromatherapy was introduced into Iceland in 1989, essential oils being imported in quantity to Reykjavik in 1992. By the mid-1990s essential oils were used more in people's daily life, as the number of practitioners began to increase. Courses at first were intermittent and very basic, but the introduction of more advanced courses enabled a faster growth, especially in areas of nursing. Most aromatherapists either have their own practices or join complementary health centres, those who are midwives and nurses using their new found therapy in their hospitals. Although insurance is available for clinical work, there is none specially for aromatherapy.

Incidentally, unlike most countries, aromatherapy did not start with the beauty therapy profession, although it is beginning to be included in beauty therapy syllabi.

Regulations

There are no laws governing essential oils or aromatherapy practice at the moment but the Ministry of Health has assured the profession that this is in process. In the meantime, people trading essential oils have to fulfil the same requirements as those for other oils used externally, such as sun oils, etc.

Essential oils

Essential oils from many different sources are on offer in Iceland from various importers and private bodies importing small quantities (see Useful addresses, p. 528).

Education

The *Nuddskóli Islands* (Icelandic School of Massage), opened in 1993, includes aromatherapy in its practical studies, using essential oils for common ailments and to help prevent illness. Before being accepted for the aromatherapy course, non-medical students first have to complete a course at a multidiscipline school, *Armulaskoli*, whose course includes basic health studies as well as 20 hours on essential oils The methods by which essential oils enter the body, blending, carriers, how essential oils came to western countries – as well as assessing a client prior to treatment are all part of this pre-qualification course. (Nurses wishing to enrol at the Icelandic School are exempt from this.)

After completing an 800-hour course at the Icelandic School of Massage, of which 60–70% is aromatherapy, students work in a clinic for 968 hours before receiving their massage and aromatherapy degree.

Lífsskólinn School started teaching aromatherapy in the late 1990s, with professional aromatherapy lecturers. The school teaches anatomy, physiology and pathology as well as aromatherapy massage.

Use of essential oils in medical establishments

Nurses caring for elderly people have shown great interest in aromatherapy, taking it into their hospital work. In the University Hospital of Iceland aromatherapy and massage is accepted as a 'side' therapy to be given only if asked for by nurses or doctors. It is used for people with all kinds of dementia, particularly those who are very agitated or difficult to communicate with. These patients receive massage with essential oils on their shoulders, feet and hands, with positive results. Patients in the geriatric area are treated by an aromatherapist trained at the Norwegian branch of the Shirley Price International College of Aromatherapy.

Associations

At the moment there is no aromatherapy association, although preparation for one is already underway (2005).

Research

Although the existence of research on essential oils is not well known, Sagamedica have been doing research on Icelandic plants for therapeutic use for at least 10 years.

NORWAY [G Fosstvedt]

Aromatherapy development

Aromatherapy was introduced to a few beauty therapists in the late 1970s by Arnould Taylor, Eve Taylor and Shirley Price and in the early 1980s, because people had become increasingly open to alternative methods of health and healing, aromatherapy soon became known as an appealing and effective way of treating stress related problems, with not only professionals, but also lay people attending courses.

Over 80% of the population (male and female) have now tried complementary therapies, having been helped by the government decision in 1995 to allow complementary therapies (including aromatherapy) in hospitals, should patients wish to receive it.

At the end of 2004 there were 12 schools offering diploma courses and 240 practising aromatherapists belonging to the NNH (see below).

Regulations

Practitioners of complementary therapies are now allowed to treat all patients, including those with cancer and diabetes. However, they are encouraged to obtain the doctor's written permission/ acceptance, and to communicate with him/her when necessary. It is emphasized that the aim is to support conventional medical treatment, to stimulate the immune system and to enhance well-being and quality of life.

Regarding marketing, the kind of health problems being treated can be mentioned, diplomatically, although no results can be claimed.

Essential oil of tea tree can only be sold in pharmacies.

Education

The *Norsk Aromaterapiskole* (NAS) was the first school to specialize in aromatherapy (1982), followed by the Norwegian branch of the *Shirley Price International College*; later several others appeared and lectures were also given to midwives and children's nurses.

Educational training varied in all complementary health areas – from a 2–3 day workshop to training taking 1 or 2 years – the educational group of the NNH (see below) took this in hand.

Currently, schools belonging to the NNH give 230 compulsory hours of theoretical and practical training, with 30 massages to be accomplished outside the school. Practical and theory exams in aromatherapy, plus anatomy, physiology and pathology have to be taken before a certificate will be given. Some schools offer advanced courses of medical aromatherapy, psycho-aromatherapy, aromatherapy for women's health, aromatherapy for babies and children, aromatherapy and cancer care – to mention only a few.

Use of essential oils in medical establishments

Aromatherapy is not used in hospitals in any organized way, but some hospitals will allow – and often encourage – patients to have aromatherapy if they so desire. From 2005 there will be a 'green room' for complementary therapists at a cancer ward in Ålesund, although patients have to make their own arrangements, as therapists are not employed by the hospital. These new green pavilions are to be opened now in several hospitals.

Quite a few institutions for multi-handicapped children, youths and adults have been using essential oils beneficially in diffusers, massage and baths for some time.

Outside hospital settings, a number of medical doctors encourage their patients to consult aromatherapists for problems such as fibromyalgia, headaches, rheumatism, muscular pain and stiffness. Although the majority are still ultra sceptical to ideas differing from their training, there is a growing interest in less harmful medication, especially for nervous and hormonal problems.

A few teachers teach the oral use of essential oils and hydrolats, which is such a valuable – and in many cases, indispensable – method (requiring much extra knowledge), although therapists cannot prescribe this to patients.

Associations

The Norske Aromaterapeuters Forening (NATF)

This was formed in 1989/90 to establish professional identity, set rules and standards for education and practice and to make the benefits of aromatherapy known to the public.

The Norske Naturterapeuters Hovedorganisasjon (NNH)

This umbrella organization was formed in 1995 to cater for complementary therapies, e.g. reflexology, aromatherapy and kinesiology, the largest professional group being aromatherapy – the Aromaterapifaggruppen.

The NNH has successfully influenced the health authorities, and is presently establishing a suitable common curriculum and common exam so that all complementary schools can gain official recognition.

The NNH is also working to establish a distinction between *aromatherapy* as a serious complementary treatment system, and *aroma massage*, as practised by beauty therapists using ready-made blends and semi-natural commercial products.

Research

In 2000 the National Centre of Research of Complementary Medicine (NAFKAM) was formed at the University of Tromsø for the scientific study of natural medicine, from homoeopathy to healing, including essential oils and aromatherapy.

In 1993, an academic research foundation, Rogalandsforskning, asked a student from the aromatherapy Biomedisinsk Senter in Stavanger to organize a clinical study of the general stress reducing and health and energy enhancing effects of aromatherapy on 30 people working in professional health care. Over a period of 6 months the subjects received a $1\frac{1}{2}$ hour treatment twice per month. The same number of people had free aerobic training, while another 30 had nothing.

Results: the aromatherapy group all reported more energy both at work and in their private lives than the other two groups.

Inspired by the good results, Trondheim University carried out a similar study, again, with convincing results. The test clients reported significant reduction in aches and pains, less irritability, greater feeling of flexibility, endurance and ability to take constructive action. They all felt more fit, physically and psychologically/mentally.

In 1994, a research project was carried out on 1200 employees in Stavanger, working on a North Sea platform. The aim was less absence from work due to bad health, by having weekly $\frac{1}{2}$ hour aromatherapy treatments. The results showed that aromatherapy gave major health benefits physically and psychologically.

Two systematic scientific studies have been carried out by two psychologists; one, by Tor Magne Hansen (University of Trondheim) in 1998, was a practical research project on the psychological evaluation of aromatherapy This showed clearly that people with professionally related muscular pains and problems (mainly restaurant employees, etc) experience a significant improvement with both short- and long-term use of essential oils compared to the control group. The other (University of Oslo 1995) was a thesis, by Selvåg, Holm and Thune. The 135-page study describes the effects of essential oils on various psychological/psychiatric problems. Although the results are very promising, more research and better testing methods are felt to be needed.

In Stavanger in 2002–2003, 400 council employees were given $\frac{1}{2}$ hour aromatherapy treatments once a month. 99% of the participants were very positive, which led to all 7000 employees being offered aromatherapy for a whole year. The results were so positive that the council decided to continue this free offer.

PORTUGAL [D Raines]

Aromatherapy development

Aromatherapy arrived in Portugal during the 1990s, mainly through its use in beauty salons and spas. The majority of these practitioners have trained outside the country, as aromatherapy is not taught as part of the beauty therapy curriculum in colleges. Unfortunately, Portugal still uses the word 'alternative' when referring to therapies which are complementary in the UK.

Although there is much interest from the Portuguese community, as yet there is no real acknowledgement from the powers that be as to its efficacy.

It is very difficult for practitioners of aromatherapy to obtain insurance, as the UK associations do not insure those members practising outside the UK. The only way forward is to set up a Portuguese branch of a UK aromatherapy association and have it accredited in Portugal, although the process would be slow and costly. Reflexology is only just on the verge of getting professional accreditation, having already taken 2 years, despite the support of the UK Association of Reflexologists.

Regulations

Aromatherapy is considered to be neither legal, nor illegal. Basically, no one minds what an aromatherapist does, as long as there are no complaints. Health shops are allowed to sell essential oils because they are seen to be for external use only. There does not appear to be any legislation regarding their sale or quality.

Many of the bureaucratic problems and narrow mindedness in government relate back to the dictatorial regime, which lasted 46 years and only ended in 1974. During this time, the health service was only available to those who could pay. The poor masses were kept in check while the wealthy were kept happy. As a result, it would suffice to say that Portugal is behind Britain by about 20 years.

Education

Aromatherapy training for both non-medical people and nurses is very basic – most people probably attending only a one weekend workshop.

Unfortunately, there are no real professionals to train students to a minimum standard and the best practitioners learn abroad. Despite this, the Portuguese are really thirsty for knowledge and willing to take longer courses.

Use of essential oils in medical establishments

Aromatherapy is not generally accepted in hospitals because it is seen as an alternative form of medicine, although some hospitals and doctors are open to most things if it can ease someone's suffering. There may be occasional use of essential oils, especially in terminal illness, where alternative methods are acceptable.

Aromatherapy is offered in some private clinics and the occasional single unit in palliative care, although hospices as such do not exist at present. In the south there are outpatient oncology units, where people simply sit on a chair whilst receiving a treatment.

Oncology hospitals, mainly in the north, are using a few complementary therapies as part of the voluntary sector, but unfortunately aromatherapy is not one of them as yet.

Associations

There are no aromatherapy associations. However, there are many foreigners living in the country who have trained abroad and are affiliated to their own associations – for example the International Federation of Professional Aromatherapists (IFPA).

Research

There is no research being carried out in Portugal at present regarding any alternative therapy.

REPUBLIC OF IRELAND [C Courtney]

Aromatherapy development

Complementary therapies are very popular in Ireland, aromatherapy having been introduced not long after it came to the UK. Some GPs will recommend their patients to have an aromatherapy treatment for stress related illnesses but these recommendations are normally made on a personal level where the GP knows the therapist and/or the therapy.

Public health nurses (the equivalent of health visitors) and nurses in various areas of specialty are showing a great interest in training, although the majority of aromatherapy is carried out in private practice at present.

Regulations

Because there is now such a huge interest by the general public in complementary therapies the Minister for Health at the Irish Department of Health and Children started the process of regulation of complementary therapies. A working group was set up in 2003 to look at ways in which complementary therapists can be self-regulated, as this would benefit the general public. The report, which will be produced after much discussion with the interested organizations and therapists, should be finalized in 2005 and will lead, over time, to agreed standards of practice, levels of training, etc. – which can only benefit all concerned.

Education

The accredited training offered in Ireland is either from the UK International Federation of Professional Aromatherapists (IFPA) or from the International Therapy Examination Council (ITEC). No special training is offered by hospitals to nurses. Nurses train privately, then bring their skill to the hospital. On occasions hospitals will pay for training.

There are two IFPA accredited schools in Ireland, the *Obus School of Healing Therapies*, Dublin and the *Body Wisdom School*, Sligo. Both principals were trained by Shirley Price.

Use of essential oils in medical establishments

The situation is comparable to the UK in that each hospital needs to discuss the introduction of aromatherapy with its Board of Management and Department of Nursing.

Aromatherapy is used and recommended in maternity hospitals, hospice care, nursing homes, cancer support units and some AIDS clinics. Many hospices and hospitals are offering posts to nurses who are also trained in aromatherapy, making aromatherapy available to patients in long-term and terminal care. This move is an acknowledgement of the benefits of aromatherapy in general health care, and together with self-regulation, will see it more widely available through the health service over the coming years. There is very positive feedback coming from the patients themselves and their families of the tremendous benefits these treatments have for the well-being of the patients.

Aromatherapy is being practised in several hospices and hospitals, among them Tullamore General Hospital, O'Connell Court in Cork (a residential unit for sufferers of Alzheimer's disease), the St Patrick's Hospice in Cork and the Bons Secours hospital, where aromatherapy is mainly available in the maternity unit. Establishments in Dublin, Limerick, Tipperary and Galway, providing psychiatric services for people with learning difficulties, are all using aromatherapy, with great benefit to patients and clients.

Much teaching has also been carried out throughout the country within the North Eastern Health Board, with particular emphasis on the Disability and Psychiatric Services. The calming effects of essential oils have been particularly noticed here on clients with aggressive behaviour and tea tree oil has been used to good effect to irrigate wounds which were MRSA (methicillin resistant *Staphylococcus aureus*) positive, all swabs being negative to MRSA after treatment.

Associations

The Republic of Ireland has no associations of its own, aromatherapists joining UK associations on qualifying.

The inauguration of the Irish branch of the International Society of Professional Aromatherapists (ISPA) in 1996 was a major step forward for the therapy. This association is now called the International Federation of Professional Aromatherapists (IFPA) which no longer has official branches, but is in the process of setting up overseas regional groups.

Research

As with the UK and other countries Ireland lacks research. This is an area that aromatherapy as a profession worldwide needs to address. It needs to be added to training courses so therapists leave courses knowing how to carry out research, how to record findings and most of all, with a commitment to research.

SWEDEN (as in 1999)

Despite being introduced in the early 1980s, aromatherapy is still not very widespread in Sweden, where not many complementary therapies are practised. Perhaps because there is no tradition of natural or complementary medicine, the health-care system does not completely accept or apply complementary therapies. Nevertheless, many nurses and people working with the elderly, children or handicapped people, are beginning to show a great interest in aromatherapy, even though they cannot use it in their work. Aromatherapists are not yet allowed in the hospitals to work, not even on their own clients who may be in there.

Regulations

Aromatherapists outside the hospital work with classical aromatherapy, mostly massage and skincare. They are subject, along with other complementary practitioners, to a law called 'the quack's law'. This law states (together with other items) that:

- It is forbidden to treat patients within the state health-care system unless permission has been sought and obtained.
- Children under 8 years of age may not be treated, although discussions are now taking place with a view to raising this age limit.
- Venereal diseases and illnesses which may occur during pregnancy may not be treated, neither may diseases such as cancer, diabetes and epilepsy.
- All treatments must be on a face-to-face basis with the client.

If any of these laws are broken, a fine or a term in prison will be enforced. Not being knowledgeable about the laws is not acceptable as an excuse.

The laws surrounding complementary therapies are tightening up every year and therapists are finding it hard to work within the very limited space left to them. It appears to be a question of politics and the feeling is that the government wishes to see complementary therapies and products banned completely from the market.

One reason for this may be that there was no great demand for other therapies (there being no tradition of complementary medicine in Sweden, and the health-care system functions exceptionally well). This is changing slowly, albeit with difficulty, mainly because state health care has become so expensive and does not always bring the desired health benefits. The population is now demanding the right to choose its own form of medicine.

Associations

There is one aromatherapy association in Sweden, the Swedish Aromatherapy Association, which was founded in 1992. It monitors the schools and their educational levels and also has a close relationship with companies selling essential oils. It is hoped that this kind of cooperation will advance the use and knowledge of aromatherapy.

SWITZERLAND [G Furrer and B Bernath-Frei]

The following relates to the German part of Switzerland and is comparable to aromatherapy as practised in Germany. In the French part of Switzerland the approach is similar to that found in France, having a more medical approach, based on the knowledge of the chemistry of the oils. In the French region, it is common to use essential oils internally.

Aromatherapy development

Aromatherapy was first known in 1985/6, when well known aromatherapists from other countries, like Valerie Worwood, Shirley Price, Martin Henglein and Suzanna Fischer-Rizzi were asked to teach here; the first aromatherapy shop (Farfalla) was founded at the same time. Although in principle aromatherapy has begun to be accepted in hospitals, where treatment is carried out only by nurses, it is difficult to introduce. Some doctors use essential oils in their private clinics.

Except in certain cantons (e.g. Appenzell), the term therapist is reserved for those in a profession approved by the Federal Government, such as

doctors and certified naturopaths. In aromatherapy therefore there are two distinct professions:

1. **Aromatherapist**: Those with medical qualifications – i.e. doctors and naturopaths.
2. **Aromatologist**: Those without medical qualifications, although receiving the same training as aromatherapists.

Regulations

There are strict legal restrictions on the practice of natural therapies in Switzerland, similar to Germany, and it is expected to be a long fight before State approval of aromatherapy is granted. The legal use of essential oils depends on what they are to be used for and how they are used. They are allowed to be used in general nursing for caring purposes – following necessary guidelines, but if a nurse wishes to use essential oils to cure – or to heal – then he or she needs authorization from a doctor or the leading nurse of the station.

Essential oils

Essential oils of a very high quality have been sold in Zurich since 1985 (see Useful addresses, p. 528). Today there are about four or five reputable retailers and unfortunately, many who sell low quality, adulterated oils.

Education

Outside the nursing profession, training in aromatherapy is available mostly through German schools, each having its own training standards, though everyone would like to see a nationally recognized training in aromatology for non-medical people. However, Farfalla have started to organize training in essential oil use.

Long-term education in aromatherapy and aromatology is offered by one or two schools, e.g. *Woodtli Schulen*, with Martin Henglein and the *Schweizer Schule für Aromatherapie*.

Basic training is offered by several organizations, mainly in conjunction with well-known aromatherapy teachers.

Regarding insurance, the biggest health insurance companies have applied a standard for therapists set by the Erfahrungs Medizinisches Register (EMR) in order for them to be covered. Any therapist requiring insurance has to show a minimum of 150 hours of medical training plus at least 105 hours of aromatherapy training. Without the EMR standard, most health insurance companies will not pay for client treatments.

Regarding education in the nursing profession, a lot of changes are underway in order to meet international standards and the first of two health care school training centres has started its programme at the beginning of 2006.

Use of essential oils in medical establishments

Although no official guidelines for nurses using complementary therapies in a hospital setting have been written as yet, there is an increasing interest, particularly among nurses, in the possible benefits of aromatherapy, with some hospital patients requesting treatment. In most hospitals using aromatherapy, a nurse-standard is applied, i.e. how essential oils can be used in certain applications/situations.

The Swiss professional association of nurses (SKB) originally laid down national principles of procedure and basic rules for establishments in which aromatology sanctioned by doctors is allowed. For example: nurses must possess minimal technical knowledge (e.g. HöFa 1) and be able to justify nursing procedures using essential oils; knowledge must include risks and limitations as well as potential benefits. The patient or relatives decide whether or not therapy with essential oils is undertaken.

Apart from disinfection of rooms, personal hygiene and hair care, essential oils are used for fear, anxiety, confusion, giving comfort to the dying and physical problems such as colds, disturbed sleep, fevers, mycosis, pain, relaxation and skin problems, including burns and wounds. They are also used for aspects of pregnancy and labour.

The most common method of application is inhalation (vaporizer, handkerchief, steam); other methods are baths, compresses, dressings and swabs, massage and frictions, using neat oils and blends. Washing with hydrolats and/or diluted essential oils is used for fevers, and cold compresses with 3% peppermint oil are used on the forehead for headaches, based on a study by Prof. Göbel from University Kiel/Germany. The basic rules for the use of essential oils include:

- No synthetic oils to be used, as they may cause side-effects such as headaches and nausea.

- Essential oils should always be diluted before use (neutral liquid soap, honey, cream, vinegar, vegetable oils, etc.). Exceptions are swabs in mycosis.
- Essential oils, although natural, are not innocuous. Risks include sensitivity, irritation and possible toxic effects.
- Essential oils should never be brought into contact with the eyes.
- Oral application is the exclusive domain of medically trained aromatherapists.
- A sensitivity test on the skin inside the elbow should be carried out on those with known allergies before each application of a new oil. If the area turns red or itches after 24 hours, care should be taken.
- Care should be taken if a homoeopathic remedy is being taken, because of possible interferential action.
- Descriptions of how to store essential oils correctly, and where they can be ordered.

The use of aromatherapy depends to a large extent on the level of acceptance of the medical staff.

Hospitals in the Canton of Bern successfully carry out fever washing for general well-being, reduction of fever and healthy sweating in adult patients. The mix used is 1 drop each of bergamot, eucalyptus, lavender and mint (unspecified) emulsified with a dispersant in lukewarm water. For genital and thrush-like ailments, 1–2 drops each of lavender and tea tree are used.

Local massage or compresses with essential oils are also offered/applied to ease insomnia, fear, stress and general pain.

Although aroma lamps cannot be used in hospitals, electric aroma stones or absorbent stones saturated with essential oils are used to help anxiety and sleeplessness, etc.

Some psychiatric clinics use aromatherapy regularly and successfully for generalized fear-syndrome, psychotic symptoms, depressions, and borderline as well as burn-out syndromes.

The first hospice to use aromatherapy was in Zürich in the 1990s, permission having being given to use essential oils in any external form, with guidelines being written in 1994.

Associations

No association gives standards of training for aromatherapists – each school has its own.

VEROMA

This is a Swiss association formed by a German aromatherapist and teacher, although there is little activity within it at the moment.

Forum Essenzia

This is a German association, which is a little active in Switzerland. This association networks with other aromatherapists and members receive a magazine twice a year with information about new studies and experiences.

Research

Some studies have been made by Professor Reinhard Saller (in cooperation with his German colleagues) concerning tea tree oil for mycoses, bacterial and viral infections.

Studies have been carried out with regard to HIV-positive patients (results not yet known).

REST OF THE WORLD

AUSTRALIA [R Guba and T Dunning]

Aromatherapy development

Aromatherapy is at an exciting stage in Australia, with increasing cooperation between complementary and conventional practitioners, holding great promise for aromatherapists.

Aromatherapy is one of the most popular complementary therapies, widely used in nursing practice. Although it still has application in beauty care, there is an increasing focus on its use in aged and palliative care and midwifery. Some aromatherapists are employed by aged care facilities, although most are in private practice and contract services to individuals or health service providers.

Regulations

In 2003, the federal Minister for Health appointed an expert committee to report on complementary therapy use. Although the Minister has not yet responded, there are likely to be some changes affecting aromatherapy education, practitioner regulation and the labelling of products.

The Australian government does not currently have the power to regulate complementary therapy practice except for Traditional Chinese Medicine in the State of Victoria. Others are not expected to be regulated unless posing potential harm to the public; in most states, they are self-regulated through their relevant professional associations.

Conventional medicines and essentials oils are regulated through the Therapeutic Goods Association (TGA), under Listing and Registration. Under Listing, no therapeutic claims can be made for any route of administration – inhaled, ingested, topical applications, etc. Listed products have to make a lower level of therapeutic claim, as they would not require a prescription – and are considered safe for general use. Any claims made must be supported, but do not require to establish efficacy, because they are for 'self-limiting' conditions – muscle pain, etc. Although there is no guarantee to the public of any benefits of listed essential oils, listing indicates that they are relatively safe if used according to directions.

Registration may require expensive research studies, as the products are for the treatment of specific disease states – comparable in a sense to prescription medicines, thus perhaps having a higher risk factor.

Essential oils

Reputable companies guarantee the composition and purity of their products. Nevertheless, it is possible to buy 'essential oils' with no guarantee of purity or composition, as not all essential oil companies apply to have their oils listed or registered, primarily because adulterated oils are less costly and easy to pass on to those with little or no background in aromatherapy.

Education

A number of colleges offer their own aromatherapy training courses, those wishing to be accredited by the Australian National Training Authority (ANTA, a government body) having to meet their standards.

Education curricula include theoretical and clinical hours as well as self-directed home study and there is an increasing focus on competency-based aromatherapy education.

A plethora of short aromatherapy courses over a few hours, days or a week have materialized in the past few years, reflecting the growing popularity of aromatherapy. Nurses are major participants in these courses and although important professional development programmes, they are insufficient for autonomous aromatherapy practice. The issue of inadequate training is a major concern – an area to be addressed in the report to the Minister for Health.

A number of aromatherapy-specific policies/guidelines for nursing practice have been developed and these include position statements by the Royal College of Nursing, Australia and the Australian Nursing Federation. Nurses using aromatherapy are regulated through the nurse regulatory authorities in each state, which issues licences to practise nursing, not aromatherapy. However, nurses have a duty of care under their professional standards and codes to practise at the level of their knowledge and competence – and this includes aromatherapy.

Use of essential oils in medical establishments

Aromatherapy is widely used and accepted in aged care facilities, largely because of the Federal Government's 1997 policy reforms and subsequent accreditation standards for aged care facilities. In aged care essential oils are used for environmental fragrancing, to promote sleep, reduce wandering behaviour, manage 'sundowner's syndrome' reduce anxiety and stress and care for wounds, especially skin tears.

They are primarily used in vaporizers, on linen or clothing, compresses and/or in massage. In some facilities, 53% of residents have aromatherapy treatments routinely. Some facilities purchase the essential oils used, but in others aromatherapists or individual patients supply the oils. Although not widely used in acute care, aromatherapy is accepted in some coronary care units, maternity and neonatal care, mental health and palliative care.

Associations

Aromatherapy is self-regulated through the two main aromatherapy associations in Australia:

The International Federation of Aromatherapy (IFA)

This branch of the UK IFA was the first association to be formed in Australia – in 1988. Continued professional development (CPD) is a requirement of membership.

The International Federation of Professional Aromatherapists (IFPA)

Many Australian aromatherapists possess qualifications from this UK association, which, before it changed its name from 'Society' to 'Federation' in 2002, had a branch in Australia. There is no IFPA branch at the moment.

The Australian Aromatic Medicine Association (AAMA)

As well as holding full aromatherapy courses, the AAMA has held post-graduate courses in aromatic medicine (the internal and intensive use of essential oils) since 1990. Although education in these methods of use is essential to an aromatherapist, they are not yet widely accepted or applied in Australia. A full training course in aromatic medicine is to be accredited with ANTA and offered through a new registered training organization (RTO). Continued professional development (CPD) is a requirement for membership of the AAMA.

Nursing associations which include aromatherapists

A number of nursing complementary therapy associations exist, for example, the Complementary Therapy Special Interest Group (CTSIG) and the College of Holistic Nurses (CHN), aromatherapists making up a significant number of their members. These bodies hold regular meetings and national conferences, as do the IFA and the AAMA. Attendance at these forums contributes CPD points to both nursing and aromatherapy professional associations.

There are State nurse regulatory authorities in many of the Australian states and their Nursing Services website lists them all.

Australian National Training Authority (ANTA)

ANTA is a government body responsible for setting standards for tertiary education, in this case, competency-based training standards for schools under the Technical and Further Education (TAFE) scheme.

Research

Since the establishment of the Office of Complementary Medicine a number of complementary therapy research units have been established, although most do not research aromatherapy practice. However, much laboratory-based research is into the chemical constituents and properties of essential oils, leaving aromatherapy practice still largely based on anecdotal reports, traditional use and inadequately described case reports.

Individual aromatherapists and The Aromatherapy Research Group (TARG) are conducting some quality aromatherapy research which can be directly applied in patient care. Examples of aromatherapy clinical research include Guba's and Casey and Kerr's works in wound care, Bowles et al's work in aged care, Dunning's work with people with diabetes and Dunning and James' work in rehabilitation.

In the last few years a large amount of data is being generated about the chemical composition of a range of unique Australian essential oils, particularly their antibacterial properties, primarily in Charles Stuart University.

CANADA [M Mitchell]

Aromatherapy development

Although it is not known exactly when aromatherapy first appeared in Canada, essential oils have been available in health stores – and one or two schools have been teaching aromatherapy – for several years.

Regulations

At the moment, British Columbia is the only Provincial Government to recognize aromatherapy as a distinct profession and has granted Occupational Title Protection to the members of the British Columbia Alliance of Aromatherapy (BCAOA – see associations below) with the exclusive right for its members to call themselves Registered Aromatherapists (RA).

Regarding labelling, in 1996, the Canadian Cosmetic, Toiletry and Fragrance Association (CCTFA) started working with Health Canada officials to develop and implement mandatory ingredient labelling for cosmetics and personal care products, including aromatherapy products.

Education

Aromatherapy is available at different levels; from basic weekend workshops to courses of 200 hours or more. An advanced aromatherapy diploma can be gained by attending further in-depth programmes. Approved diplomas are licensed through the Ministry of Education in Ontario, Canada, entitling the successful therapist to use the letters RAHP (Registered Aromatherapy Health Practitioner) after their name.

Many schools teach the standard programme of aromatherapy such as that offered at the *International Certified Aromatherapy Institute* (ICAI), 200–220 hours of aromatherapy (National Association of Holistic Aromatherapy approved – see United States). Around 40 hours of this is bodywork, the rest, theory and case studies, approved by the Canadian Examining Board of Health Care Practitioners (CEBHCP). This latter is a private non-profit, federally chartered organization promoting health-care programmes of complementary medicines, including aromatherapy, for which it has set professional qualification standards, providing a forum for the development, exchange, and dissemination of knowledge and skills appropriate to professional aromatherapists. Having established a Code of Ethics, Conduct, and Practice, the Board recognizes institutions which meet their standards, offering practitioners who have graduated from any of the approved aromatherapy programmes the right to use the letters CAHT (Certified Aromatherapy Health Therapists).

Aromatherapists can apply for a business licence, allowing them to practise in their own area – depending on the Government bylaws of that area. To receive this holistic business licence and practise as an alternative health-care provider, aromatherapists must prove that they belong to a complementary health-care organization, which can then supply them with an Errors and Omissions/Malpractice insurance. If a number of aromatherapists group together, an association may gain a smaller insurance fee than that of an individual practitioner.

Use of essential oils in medical establishments

Community hospitals within the Fraser Valley Health Authority in British Columbia have spa-like therapy rooms, in which both patients and their families receive alternative therapies such as aromatherapy privately. The interior health authority hospitals there also have carts containing aromatherapy lotions, blankets, CD players, etc. and a special environment is provided for the patient to use them. These are the only hospitals known in Canada which accept aromatherapy at the moment although it is offered in many private clinics.

There is no knowledge of aromatherapy being practiced in hospices.

Associations

The British Columbia Alliance of Aromatherapy (BCAOA)
Registered in 1999, this organization is dedicated to establishing aromatherapy in the Province of British Columbia. The BCAOA has applied for government registration under the Health Act of British Columbia.

The British Columbia Association of Practicing Aromatherapists in British Columbia (BCAPA)
Formed in 1995, this association supports all practising aromatherapists, also educating the public in the benefits of aromatherapy. The BCAPA has a stringent code of ethics and a high standard in professionalism and continuing education.

The Canadian Federation of Aromatherapists (CFA)
This organization was established in 1993 and is a voluntary federally chartered, non-profit association, which is sponsored by contributions, donations, fund raising events and membership fees, some of which are spent on promoting aromatherapy.

The International Aromatherapists and Tutors Association (IATA)
Established in 1995, this is a government registered non-profit association to implement safety standards in aromatherapy, their highest priority being the safe use of essential oils. It is responsible for the development and use of carefully researched tuition materials from aromatherapy teachers in Britain.

Research

There does not appear to be any research on essential oils or aromatherapy at the moment.

CHINA [Yu Wing Zheng]

Aromatherapy development
Around 1990, the concept of aromatherapy was being accepted by some people. It was first brought to mainland China by the family of a Taiwan businessman who established a factory in mainland China – and through their discussions on the basic application of essential oils and the promotion of its possibilities, aromatherapy began to spread. Having first appeared as skin care, beauty salons started using essential oils in face and body massage, which are now the most common forms of use.

Young women (18–25) went to Europe and America to study and experience essential oils for themselves, then spread their knowledge to other young women in mainland China via forums and websites, etc. As herbalism was already well-known, young people accepted aromatherapy very easily.

Shirley Price's 'Aromatherapy Workbook' was published in Chinese in 1998, and in 2004, Patricia Davies' 'Aromatherapy A–Z' and Marguerite Maury's 'Guide to Aromatherapy' were imported in English, which limited readers. There are few aromatherapy books in Chinese, so knowledge is via newspapers, magazines and/or the Internet. Some large aromatherapy websites have been established which include the translation into Chinese of references in English to help the progress of others.

Lack of professional knowledge of essential oils is the biggest stumbling block to the development of aromatherapy and because it is not easy to get this, some users with little knowledge are profiting from the great interest shown in the subject.

Aromatherapy has been identified by the Shanghai Vocational Training Orientation Centre (SVTOC) as an area for growth, an agreement being made recently with the International Federation of Professional Aromatherapists (IFPA) to develop aromatherapy training British-style.

Regulations
Many people – including the government – classed aromatherapy with beauty and hairdressing and as some practitioners were without professional knowledge, some errors occurred in the use of

essential oils, affecting some of the clients' health adversely. Because of this, the government planned the introduction of an 'Aromatherapist Qualification Standard', which came into force at the end of 2004. Aromatherapists have to follow these recommendations published by the government to ensure that aromatherapy progresses in the right direction.

Education

The basis for all professional courses follows the syllabi of two British and one American association:

The International Federation of Aromatherapy (IFA)
Training in China was originally done by an English aromatherapist – one of her trainees from Taiwan is now training by distance learning.

The International Federation of Professional Aromatherapists (IFPA)
This organization now has an agreement (see above) with the SVTOC in Shanghai, which was the result of 3 years' work by an IFPA accredited school based in Singapore.

The Penny Price Academy, accredited by the above associations, began distance learning courses in mainland China (the Academy already runs courses and has a school in Taiwan which uses, and exports to mainland China, Penny Price essential oils). These courses emphasize the UK training standards.

There are also a few schools which run short-term training.

The National Association of Holistic Aromatherapy (NAHA
This organization is based in the USA.

Associations

At the time of writing, there is no Chinese professional association for aromatherapy.

Research

In January 2004, Shanghai JiaoTong University and the XinJiang Plant Technology Development Company together established 'Shanghai JiaoTong University – XinJiang Aroma Technology Universal Research Center' to improve the research of aromatic materials, because at the moment, research is based more on the raw materials used in perfumes with very little on aromatherapy.

ISRAEL [G Hauser]
Aromatherapy development

Aromatherapy, introduced in the late 1980s, is now producing many dedicated practitioners. Many CAM colleges are offering training programmes, mainly in traditional Chinese medicine (TCM); aromatherapy is taught together with naturopathy and/or herbal medicine studies.

Health insurance was not mandatory until 1995, although 96% of the population was insured before the National Health Insurance Law came into effect. Citizens can become a member of one of three health funds, which have also opened CAM clinics, offering treatments for members at a reduced fee, aromatherapy coming under the heading of massage.

There is no group complementary medical insurance system for practitioners, only private brokers.

Nurses, birthing coaches, midwives and physical therapists are studying aromatherapy courses on their own initiative and then introducing it individually and unofficially into their professional settings.

Regulations

There are no regulations in Israel regarding either essential oils or the practice of aromatherapy. People are free to treat whoever they wish, even after only a 2-day course.

Essential oils

At the moment, importers can label essential oils as they wish and most have no botanical name/variety/source of oil or contraindications – though some suppliers will take this in hand when new labels are printed. Oils imported from Germany are sold in local health shops, another supplier (who has also written the first aromatherapy book in Hebrew), supplying the beauty therapy industry.

Education

A non-profit organization is presently being established by principal aromatherapy teachers from the major CAM colleges, to set standards for curriculum development and bring about a self-governing body to monitor them.

Haim Schloss College

This is the only specialist college in aromatherapy, the principal having been involved with essential oils since 1988. The college offers professional training to health-care practitioners only. Aromatherapy is not taught together with massage – and internal use of essential oils is part of the syllabus. The total number of teaching hours over 2 years is 352, which includes a comprehensive chemistry curriculum. A qualification in anatomy and physiology (A&P) is mandatory.

Reidman International College for Complementary Medicine

Reidman College is the only Israeli College accepted into the European Association of Naturopaths and represents universities from around the world. The college has five main study centres and teaches aromatherapy as part of the naturopathy syllabus.

The aromatherapy section has 80 academic hours, a student wishing to study only aromatherapy having also to take an anatomy and physiology course. It is hoped to introduce, in addition, a special course in essential oil chemistry.

Genesis College of Complementary Medicine

This college was founded in 1982 and, as in all other colleges/schools, TCM is the main subject taught. Aromatherapy is taught together with naturopathy, the aromatherapy section running for 112 hours over 1 year. It can also be studied separately. There are no requirements to study anatomy and physiology.

School of Complementary Medicine, Tel Aviv University

This is a new college, where aromatherapy is a year long course of 28 3-hour sessions (84 hours) and is taught in conjunction with reflexology. It is affiliated to both the university and Ichilov hospital and is gaining a good reputation due to its high standards of training.

Use of essential oils in medical establishments

Major hospitals in Tel Aviv, the central region and Haifa have established CAM centres on their campuses, although they are not officially financed or recognized by the hospitals themselves.

Aromatherapy was first introduced via a workshop to Hadassah Hospital School of Nursing and Midwifery in June 2004. The hospital has now officially requested a list of basic essential oils for use in the delivery rooms.

Associations

The Chamber for Complementary Health Professions (CCHP)

This is a self-governing umbrella body representing the eight major CAM disciplines practised, each having its own organization and setting its own standards. The chairperson is setting up a dialogue with the Ministry of Health so that practitioners can be recognized and receive a licence after completing a training period of 2–3 years. As soon as aromatherapists have formed their own self-governing body (which is presently underway), aromatherapy will be included in the CAM organization.

The Israel Aromatherapy Association

This organization is in process of being formed (as of 2005).

Research

The Natural Medicine Research Unit (NMRU) at Hadassah aims to provide evidence of the efficacy, safety and biological mechanism of complementary therapies, although as yet no studies have been done specifically on essential oils.

The Neve Ya'ar agricultural research centre at Galilee researches wild aromatic and domestic plants. The Aromatic and Medicinal Plants section is researching the introduction, acclimatization and breeding of new aromatic crops, together with the biosynthesis of essential oils in aromatic plants:

- factors affecting essential oil yield, content and composition; breeding, selection and introduction of wild plants from the Middle East as peculiar sources of essential oils with biological activities;

- allelopathy: essential oils as allelochemicals – mode of action and their potential as bio-herbicides;
- sweet basil: breeding of high-quality varieties resistant to Fusarium wilt;
- vetiver for soil stabilization.

The centre is keen (together with UK scientists) to research essential oils for aromatherapy.

JAPAN [A Ikeda]

Aromatherapy development

Aromatherapy officially arrived in Japan in 1985, when 'The art of aromatherapy' (Robert Tisserand) and 'Practical aromatherapy' (Shirley Price) were published in Japanese; holistic aromatherapy was then brought from the UK. 'Aromatherapy for babies and children' by Shirley Price and Penny Price was published in Japanese 2005.

The popularity of aromatherapy increased greatly during the 1990s, with related products being widely available all over the country; by 2004 the aromatherapy population (including those under 20 years of age) was huge. Many people have started using essential oils as household cleansers, as artificial detergents are considered bad for both health and nature.

Large sections in bookshops are dedicated to aromatherapy and magazines frequently feature aromatherapy as an essential part of the modern lifestyle. There are around 200 aromatherapy schools, over 250 aromatherapy shops and five aromatherapy periodicals.

Regulations

There is no clear regulation for aromatherapy, although there are government licences for acupuncture, moxa therapy, and shiatsu massage. In the early days, it was thought that UK style aromatherapy massage was illegal if practised professionally without having this licence, so serious therapists became doctors or acupuncturists in order to be able to practise therapeutic aromatherapy.

Others created a system of non-professional, 'do-it-yourself' aromatherapy, mainly concerning skin care and essential oil blending for basic family massage. This had particular appeal in Japan, leading many to become aromatherapy teachers, rather than becoming massage therapists. This, together with the re-launching of UK aromatherapy massage and sorting out of regulations, no doubt accounts for the great expansion of the aromatherapy industry.

There is no independent body to regulate the quality of essential oils – each aromatherapy association sets its own standards. However, a committee from the Aromatherapy Association of Japan (AAJ) has established standards for essential oil trading and quality control, including safety, with a code of ethics for essential oil traders. By August 2004, 29 essential oil brands had qualified for these standards.

Essential oils

Essential oils are widely available – in one up-market department store in Tokyo, the huge aromatherapy area is manned by well-educated (including legal issues) shop assistants who hold qualifications from one of the associations below. Stocks are impressive too – including *Lavandula angustifolia* oils from at least five different countries.

The 3rd of November, a national holiday 'Cultural Day' is now also an 'Aromatherapy Day' to celebrate aromatherapy culture. Four leading associations – AAJ, JSA, JHMS and Forum Essenzia Japan (see below) – set up the scheme, supported by the Ministry of Environment and the Foreign Embassies of essential oil producing countries. A trade fair, 'Aroma Week', was launched across Japan in 2004. The one in Tokyo took up two floors of a department store, with 23 free seminars/workshops on one floor and an aromatherapy trade show on another, with essential oils from all over the world.

Education

As the first aromatherapists were trained in the UK, British associations and standards were well known. After a few years, several Japanese associations were set up, each with their own standards of training and qualifications (see below), many running courses approved by UK associations (see Ch. 16).

The AAJ (see Associations below) has started a Schools Education Project (SEP), sending out qualified instructors to educate 12–15-year-olds in the safe use of essential oils, since when there has been an increase in the number of young people using essential oils.

Use of essential oils in medical establishments

Clinical aromatherapy practice has increased substantially since the 1990s, when some hospitals and medical practitioners started using essential oils, especially in obstetrics practice and terminal care. Childbirth is not covered by the national health service, thus, without the limit of state budgets, aromatherapy quickly found its way in.

Dr Yukari Miyoshi introduced aromatherapy to the Ida municipal hospital in Kawasaki in the early 1990s, establishing the Kawasaki total care centre (including a palliative care unit) in 2000. The hospital has practised clinical aromatherapy since 1986.

The Obitsu sankei clinic, where patients can enjoy aromatherapy treatment, has succeeded in combining modern medicine and holistic medicine; the Akasaka Tameike psychiatric clinic has established a complementary therapy room and herbal shop.

Associations

Several aromatherapy associations have been set up since 1990s but there is no inter-organizational council and each association sets its own individual qualifications.

The Aromatherapy Association of Japan (AAJ)

The AAJ was founded in 1996 and since 2005 is a government recognized non-profit organization. It is the biggest association and by July 2004 had 17 170 individual members and 148 company members, including cosmetic giants such as Shiseido and Kanebo, as well as aromatherapy schools, shops, essential oil distributors, medical doctors and any individuals interested in aromatherapy.

The association provides four levels of qualifications, including a general qualification (Aromatherapy kentei), which can be taken by members of the general public who wish to possess enough basic knowledge to use essential oils safely under Japanese law. Although this is not a professional qualification, over 38 000 people have passed this examination.

The AAJ also have three levels of professional qualifications:

- Aromatherapy Advisor: for shop assistants, to give them knowledge of handling essential oils;
- Aromatherapy Instructor: for those who wish to teach 'self-care' aromatherapy;
- Aromatherapist: for massage therapists who wish to practise holistic aromatherapy.

This association started research in the 1990s into regulations and legislation, finally finding a way to protect the status of holistic aromatherapists. As a result, the holistic aromatherapist qualification set up in 1999, which included an insurance scheme, significantly increased its popularity.

The Japanese Society of Aromatherapy (JSA)

The JSA was founded in 1998 by doctors, nurses, midwives, dentists, pharmacists, acupuncturists and dieticians in order to advance aromatherapy in the medical field.

The Japanese Holistic Medical Society (JHMS)

The JHMS is a non-profit organization founded in 1987 mainly by medical doctors, nurses, dentists, acupuncturists, psychotherapists, counsellors, social workers and patients. It has 2200 members and promotes holistic medicine, including aromatherapy.

The Japanese Aromacoordinator Association (JAA)

The JAA was founded by an ayurvedic doctor and promotes holistic health using essential oils. The number of its members is expanding as its aromatherapy correspondence course attracts many students from the suburbs.

Forum Essenzia and the Natural Aromatherapy Research and Development

These are German and Belgian associations respectively which have branches in Japan.

Research

The Journal of Aroma Science and Technology, published by Fragrance Journal Ltd., is dedicated to aromatherapy research, and leading aromatherapy associations each have their research team.

Aromatherapy research has also become a common theme among universities and company laboratories:

- Honorary Prof. Shizuo Torii, Toho University, is a founder of research involving a physiological study with CNV brain waves, using essential oils (Fragrance Journal 77: 16–20, 1986).
- Dr Yoshihiko Koga, Kyorin University is famous for his research study on 'Using lavender in palliative care' (Aromatopia 15: 24–27 03/1996)
- Mr Motoyuki Iwahashi, working in a technology development centre in Shimizu corporation, has carried out a study on environmental use of essential oils (Aroma Research, Extra issue no.1, 2000).

KOREA (as in 1999)

Complementary therapies already established in Korea are oriental systems of herbalism, acupuncture, and related techniques. The first form of Western natural therapy to be practised was aromatherapy, introduced by Dr Oh, who trained in Canada. There is no licensing system established yet for professional aromatherapists, but the use of essential oils in the aesthetical field, including skin care shops, has recently started to become popular and aromatherapy is expected before long to be one of the most popular natural therapies in Korea.

Essential oil use

The general public can already buy essential oils in herb shops and department stores and use them to reduce stress, nervous tension and other small daily problems. Aromatherapy treatments they have experienced were considered to be positively beneficial to various conditions. The main medical applications of essential oils are neuropsychiatric disorders including: depression, anxiety, headaches and migraines, insomnia and general stress, together with respiratory infections, skin problems and cardiovascular disorders. The clinical methods used are inhalation and massage (particularly combined with meridian acupoint massage). Clinical data and results from experimental studies have been accumulated from a few hospitals, including some using EEG, EAV, Doppler and thermographic devices.

Use of essential oils in medical establishments

Although several medical doctors are responsive to aromatherapy, most are still slightly sceptical.

Nevertheless, despite the fact that it is not widely used in Korean hospitals, there are a few doctors who are interested enough to attend workshops and seminars, most of which are organized by the Institute of Naturopathic Medicine in conjunction with the Korean Aromatherapy Association.

Associations

The Korean Association of Naturopathic Medicine was established in January 1997 and over 100 medical doctors are now members. Apart from monthly academic meetings, the association runs various seminars and workshops where naturopathic modalities like aromatherapy, homoeopathy, hydrotherapy, chiropractic and qi (chi) energy medicine are introduced. As a result, the Korean Aromatherapy Association was founded, its members (who are not allowed to prescribe essential oils internally) being mainly medical doctors and beauty therapists.

NEW ZEALAND (as in 1999)

There has been a great increase of interest in aromatherapy during the last 10 years, especially among nurses and various health institutions, who are now accepting aromatherapy programmes. Books such as 'Aromatherapy for Health Professionals' are a great asset and resource, certainly helping to increase the professional profile.

A survey revealed that most of the essential oils used in health institutions were of high quality. Two purchased oils with certificates of authenticity, others being purchased from reputable suppliers who gave guarantees of quality.

Education

Because of the increased demand and recognition for adequate training, a 2-year full-time diploma in professional aromatherapy was offered at *Manawatu Polytechnic*, which has developed over the last 4 years from an initial 250-hour course to one of 1200 classroom hours, the course naturally including a far greater number of essential oils than the six used in the hospices. In the North Island, students attending an aromatherapy training course at one polytechnic are accepted for periods of clinical placement in a local health-care institution.

Basic training covers massage and diffusion techniques, extraction methods, safety precautions and a detailed study of a minimum of six essential oils – it is considered sensible to use only a few oils at that level.

The Te Omango hospice and the Mary Potter hospice in Wellington have their own in-house basic training programme, which includes safety issues, in-depth study of eight oils, using and cleaning the vaporizers; basic massage techniques for feet, hands, neck and shoulders, keeping records of treatments and a holistic approach to health. At the Mary Potter, treatments are under the supervision of the consulting aromatherapist, who makes up the oil blends for each client and administers, monitors and evaluates the programme.

The New Zealand Register of Holistic Aromatherapists (NZROHA) was a founding member of the NZ Charter of Health Practitioners Inc. and has developed a syllabus and examination structure which is currently awaiting approval by the NZ Qualifications Authority, a government body, before it becomes operative nationally.

Essential oil use in medical establishments

Rest homes, hospices and centres for people with disabilities enthusiastically offer aromatherapy as a complementary therapy, supported by medical staff.

Expenditure on health care has been reduced, making it difficult to find funds for aromatherapy supplies. In some cases the authorities have approved payment from general funds; in others the oils are chosen and donated by the aromatherapist. Sometimes donations are made towards the purchase of essential oils by patients or their relatives.

Protocols are in place in two instances and are being formalized in others, where currently the programmes follow established formal guidelines and those of the New Zealand Register of Holistic Aromatherapists (NZROHA), the professional body of aromatherapists in New Zealand.

Conditions treated include nausea, insomnia, respiratory problems, digestive problems, wound management, sleeping problems, terminal illness, skin problems, poor circulation, muscular pain and anxiety and depression. In one institution the aromatherapist has used lotions containing *Leptospermum scoparium* [manuka] with success in cases of chronic skin problems; *Melaleuca alternifolia* [tea tree] in cream base has also been found to be efficacious.

Use of diffusers in rooms with lavender to enhance sleep is common among the institutions, the range of treatments including baths, foot baths, massage of hands, feet, backs, necks and shoulders. Regarding safety, all places surveyed used only electric oil vaporizers to diffuse essential oils.

Associations

New Zealand Register of Holistic Aromatherapists (NZROHA)

New Zealand is very fortunate in that it has only one professional body for aromatherapy, which means that there is some degree of consistency in training.

The Register was formed in 1993, originally as a support group for aromatherapists and to inform the public of the benefits of consulting an aromatherapist. It has set professional standards for all those who wish to become members, who also have to abide by the Code of Ethics and Code of Practice.

A quarterly magazine 'Sharing aromatherapy' is produced, which contains a list of trained aromatherapists throughout the country.

SOUTH AFRICA (as in 1999)

The field of complementary health care in general – and aromatherapy in particular – has grown considerably over the past few years.

In terms of recognition of the profession, a great deal of work has been done over the past 10 years.

Essential oil use in medical establishments

At the nursing college attached to Groote Schuur Hospital, a large government-funded teaching hospital in Cape Town, the increasing interest among nurses is shown by requests for lectures to post-basic students.

The Association of Aromatherapists of South Africa (AAOSA) is very active within the community, running successful voluntary services within hospice and hospital situations through its Aroma Care Plan, as well as in other areas where nurses and aromatherapists are using essential oils independently of the association, e.g.:

- At St Luke's Hospice, Cape Town, where Aroma Care therapists first began working at the beginning of 1993, the demand for their services has grown considerably. Here, all aromatherapists in the Aroma Care Plan are required to do the hospice counselling course before having contact with the patients, after which weekly visits are made to St Luke's, working on the wards and in the day care centre, where a number of patients come specifically for aromatherapy. Many of them come for massage of oedematous limbs, and some for the easing of specific aches and pains associated with bone metastasis. Shoulder massage is of great relief to those suffering from lung cancer and the associated dyspnoea and many come just for the benefits of the touch therapy itself.
- In Groote Schuur Hospital, these therapists provide a weekly aromatherapy service in the haematology unit, for patients receiving chemotherapy and radiotherapy, (mainly for the treatment of leukaemia and other bone marrow diseases). This service has become increasingly valued by doctors and nurses, the weekly aromatherapy treatments being considered to be positively beneficial, helping to reduce stress levels and muscular tension as well as providing relaxation and a feeling of well-being. Sessions consist mainly of foot and hand or back and shoulder massage.
- A weekly service is provided within a centre for people living with AIDS and HIV.
- At a school in Cape Town for children with cerebral palsy, therapists achieve exciting results with both mobile and wheelchair-bound children of all ages up to 18 years. Teachers and physiotherapists have commented on the reduced limb spasticity and reduced anxiety rate following sessions.
- In Kwazulu Natal, aromatherapists work with patients on a daily basis at the Highway Hospice.
- In Gauteng, aromatherapists are carrying out a pilot study on aromatherapy and stress management in a group of police volunteers.

Associations

The Association of Aromatherapists of South Africa (AAOSA)
This was formed in 1991. One of its main aims is to inform and educate the public regarding the use of essential oils.

TAIWAN [G Chan]

Aromatherapy development

Apart from Traditional Chinese Medicine, the popular complementary disciplines are acupuncture, reflexology, osteopathy, shiatsu and chi-kon (meditation of mind for relaxation good circulation and physical exercise). Aromatherapy joined these around 1990, its development relying principally on private cosmetic companies selling essential oils of various brands, and independent individuals interested in natural personal care. The beauty industry is one of the biggest businesses in Taiwan and at first, 'borrowed' the aromatic characteristic of essential oils to attract consumers – completely ignoring their holistic therapeutic benefits. The key obstacle to development was that most Taiwanese could not manage the English language, thus limiting access to information.

Fortunately, some independent users discovered the beneficial aspect of aromatherapy by studying abroad. One or two aromatherapy books were translated into Chinese, including Shirley Price's 'Aromatherapy Workbook' in 1998, with her book 'Aromatherapy for the Emotions' published in 2005. Nowadays, there are many Chinese aromatherapy publications available on the bookshelf, most of them translated from overseas, others written by Taiwanese aromatherapists.

Regulations

So far there are no policies or regulations regarding the sale, method of use or storage of essential oils; they are simply treated as commercial commodities related to health care.

Essential oils

Many shops sell essential oils and related products, mostly imported from Europe, Australia, UK and the USA. These are of differing qualities, labelling being incomplete and some being standardized or adulterated (one containing a high percentage of isopropyl alcohol). Many do not indicate safely and correctly how to blend and use them for improving health and many businessmen sell poor quality or diluted essential oils at a very low price, to attract consumers. This practice is detrimental to both the consumer and the aromatherapy industry, since consumers cannot assess the quality unless they have participated in an aromatherapy seminar; poor quality oils may also have given little benefit, resulting in a negative view regarding their effectiveness. Fortunately, some quality essential oils are now being imported and sold in Taiwan and China.

The main methods of use are by application, massage, vaporization and inhalation. Owing to the wet and hot climate of Taiwan, elderly people frequently get muscle aches, arthritis and influenza, many also suffering with sinus and lung problems as a result of air pollution. All of these can be helped by essential oil mixes.

Education

During the 1990s, people went to England or Australia to study aromatherapy, returning to promote the knowledge they learned, and at the turn of the century a few universities and private training schools began to offer aromatherapy courses, many inviting members from the International Federation of Aromatherapy (IFA) and the International Federation of Professional Aromatherapists (IFPA) to lecture. In 2004, one of these schools has become a branch of the IFPA accredited *Penny Price Academy* in the UK. The syllabus covers anatomy and physiology, massage, chemical profiles and effects of essential oils and applications of use.

One school, the *Institute of Aromatherapy*, established in 1996, was invited in 2000 to lecture in hospitals and schools, as well as being invited by the Ministry of Education in Taiwan to give an aromatherapy seminar–workshop for professors and teachers from national universities.

Use of essential oils in medical establishments

Recently, the Taiwan Palliative Care Hospice has offered a range of supporting services, including aromatherapy, for its patients, either sending

medical staff to receive professional training or employing professional aromatherapists. The treatment procedures include massage, washes and swabs, compresses, gargles and mouth washes, ointments, room fragrances, inhalation, baths and ingestion. Although mainly dedicated to terminal cancer patients, the service will be extended to other patients due to the positive feedback from patients and their families.

Associations

There is as yet no independent national organization, association or society for aromatherapy. Each school works individually, some having their own association, but there is no national accreditation. It is to be hoped that with the rapid growth of interest in education, an independent association to represent all schools will be formed in the near future.

Research

There is no known research on essential oils as yet.

UNITED STATES OF AMERICA
[E Cristina and P Conrad]

Aromatherapy development

Aromatherapy appeared first in the state of California in the mid-1980s, where many companies selling essential oils were housed. The first world conference on aromatherapy was held in Los Angeles in 1990, followed by one in New York in 1994, several now being held in different states.

Health care is paid for privately and only a few insurance companies cover complementary therapies, making it difficult for hospitals to provide these services. However, due to an increasing awareness in the health field of the therapeutic and financial value of complementary forms of medicine, the insurance situation should improve.

Nurses belonging to the National Association of Nurse Massage Therapists (NANMT) were among the first to introduce aromatherapy into mainstream hospitals and many leading healthcare institutions now use aromatherapy to promote patient healing. The Massachusetts State Board of Nursing was the first to write aromatherapy into its nurse practice act, followed by 25 other State Boards following their example.

Nurses in several hospitals have now written – or are writing – protocols for the use of aromatherapy in their facility. Clinical aromatherapy is therefore rapidly gaining popularity, with widespread use by nurses throughout the whole country – and the medical profession is beginning to show some acceptance.

Education

As there are many bogus accreditation claims in the aromatherapy education industry, it is important for potential students to know that the only legitimate accrediting bodies in the United States are those approved by the US Department of Education. *The Australasian College of Health Sciences* (ACHS) is the first school in the USA to offer this government approved certificate, although there are other excellent courses available, endorsed by the AHNA.

Academic programmes range from study at university (usually in phytotherapy) to distance learning, including those endorsed by accrediting bodies such as the American Holistic Nurses Association (AHNA) and approved providers offering Continuing Education Units (CEUs) to health-care professionals. The ACHS and the *Institute of Integrative Aromatherapy* in Colorado (IIAC) and Washington are now offering registered nurses continuing educational units in aromatherapy by distance learning. *The Institute of Aromatic Studies* (IAS) in San Francisco offers the same to registered nurses in California. The Aromatherapy Registration Council (ARC) provides an aromatherapy curriculum and offers a national exam – the Registration Examination in Aromatherapy – twice per calendar year in 30 states, open to anyone who has completed a minimum of the Level 2 aromatherapy programme (200 hours) instigated by the National Association of Holistic Aromatherapy (NAHA – see below). This programme can be completed at any college or school following the NAHA Educational Guidelines. The ARC exam is also open to anyone who can provide evidence of equivalent training. Successful candidates qualify for insurance (see Associations below)

Use of essential oils use in medical establishments

Clinical aromatherapy is recognized and respected among nurses, with successfully conducted studies in pain control, cardiology, psychiatry, obstetrics and gynecology, paediatrics, dermatology, oncology, senior care and immunology, etc. Aromatherapy is also gaining acceptance in the care of the chronically and terminally ill and patients are now rarely given hypnotics to regulate sleep patterns. Several hospitals use aromatherapy to aid sore muscles, bruises and vein relief, etc, as well as stress and insomnia. Where essential oils are used on the elderly, the need for antipsychotic drugs has been noticeably reduced.

The main methods of use are inhalation, baths, compresses and massage.

Associations

The National Association of Holistic Aromatherapy (NAHA)

This was founded in 1990 and is the largest aromatherapy organization in the USA, with nearly 1000 members. It is an educational, non-profit organization, dedicated to enhancing public awareness of the benefits of true aromatherapy. It hosts bi-annual international conferences and trade shows and offers a quarterly Aromatherapy Journal.

NAHA promotes and raises academic standards in aromatherapy education and practice and has established a code of ethics for teachers, practitioners and students. It is also active in furthering public perception and knowledge of true aromatherapy, its safety and effectiveness in everyday life. It provides a listing of schools, colleges and educators offering their accredited Level 1 and Level 2 syllabi, which include practical tuition, essential oil studies and anatomy and physiology.

In 2001 NAHA created a True Aromatherapy Product (TAP) registered certification mark approved by the Federal government, demonstrating dedication to purity and high standards. Currently 25 schools carry and can use this mark of approval (not yet to be used on product), showing that they fulfil the National Education criteria set out by NAHA's Council of Aromatherapy Schools and Educators. Strict guidelines for use of the seal allow schools and educators to use it on their websites and brochures.

NAHA offers professional, product and general liability insurance to its professional members.

The Aromatherapy Registration Council (ARC)

This council was established in 1999 as a public

benefit, non-profit making corporation, independent from any paid membership organization or educational facility, ensuring an impartial and unbiased body.

The ARC provides an aromatherapy curriculum and sponsors a national examination (see Education above). Successful candidates may use the trade marked RA (Registered Aromatherapist) after their name. The ARC verifies an individual's registration status on request by employers, governmental agencies and the public, for whom they provide a register of aromatherapists (147 in 2004).

The Associated Bodywork and Massage Professionals (ABMP)

The ABMP offers membership to aromatherapists who have completed 100 hours or more of training with an institution or educator registered by the state in which they operate. Membership includes professional liability insurance for aromatherapists, aestheticians, massage therapists and body workers.

Research

Dr Tim Culbert is currently doing a project at the Children's Hospital in Minneapolis on aromatherapy and palliative care for children with cancer, focusing on pain management, sleep disorders, nausea and fatigue. Results will not be available until 2005.

In Illinois a study of the effectiveness of aromatherapy care in the psychiatric unit is to be carried out. The National Library of Medicine (PubMed) has many essential oil research papers (see websites), although not all are related to complementary alternative medicine.

SUMMARY

It can be seen that aromatherapy in most countries seems to have developed from contact with aromatherapy as practised in the UK. Some countries are not yet allowed to practise in hospitals, others can work with the express permission of the nurse or doctor in charge – and others have advanced still further than the UK in their freedom to work in these establishments.

ACKNOWLEDGEMENTS

Thanks to those who responded to the author's request for an update – and those who sent in information for the new countries. Their names appear beside their country.

Appendices, Glossary and Useful addresses

CONTENTS

Appendix A

Botanical name [common name]

Abies alba fol. [European silver fir, white fir]

Abies balsamea [Canada balsam]

Abies sibirica fol. [Siberian pine]

Achillea millefolium herb. [yarrow]

Acorus calamus [sweet flag, calamus]

Aloysia triphylla [lemon verbena]

Anethum graveolens [dill]

Angelica archangelica [angelica]

Aniba rosaeodora fol. [rosewood, bois de rose]

Boswellia carteri res. dest. [frankincense, olibanum]

Cananga odorata flos [ylang ylang]

Carum carvi fruct. [caraway]

Cedrus atlantica lig. [Atlas cedarwood, satinwood]

Chamaemelum nobile (= *Anthemis nobilis*) flos [Roman chamomile]

Cinnamomum verum cort. [cinnamon bark]

Cinnamomum verum fol. [cinnamon leaf]

Cistus ladaniferus ram., fol. [labdanum]

Citrus aurantifolia (*C. medica* var. *acida*) per. [lime]

Citrus aurantium var. *amara* flos [neroli bigarade]

Citrus aurantium var. *amara* fol. [petitgrain bigarade]

Citrus aurantium var. *amara* per. [orange bigarade]

Citrus bergamia per. [bergamot]

Citrus limon per. [lemon]

Citrus paradisi per. [grapefruit]

Citrus reticulata per. [mandarin]

Citrus sinensis per. [sweet orange]

Commiphora myrrha var. *molmol* (= *C. molmol*, *Balsamodendron myrrha*) res. dist. [myrrh]

Coriandrum sativum fruct. [coriander]

Cuminum cyminum fruct. [cumin]

Cupressus sempervirens fol., strob. [cypress]

Cymbopogon citratus, *C. flexuosus* [lemongrass]

Cymbopogon nardus and *Cymbopogon winterianus* [citronella]

Elettaria cardamomum fruct. [cardamom]

Eucalyptus citriodora fol. [lemon scented gum]

Eucalyptus dives ct. piperitenone fol. [broad-leaved peppermint]

Eucalyptus globulus fol. [Tasmanian blue gum]

Eucalyptus radiata subsp. *radiata* (= *E. numerosa*, *E. lindleyana*) fol. [black peppermint, narrow-leaved peppermint]

Eucalyptus smithii fol. [gully gum]

Eucalyptus staigeriana [lemon scented ironbark]

Foeniculum vulgare var. *dulce* fruct. [sweet fennel]

Helichrysum angustifolium (= *H. italicum*) flos [everlasting, immortelle]

Hyssopus officinalis flos, fol. [hyssop]

Illicium verum [star anise]

Inula graveolens flos, fol. [elecampane]

Juniperus communis fruct. [juniper berry]

Juniperus communis ram. [juniper twig]

Kunzea ericoides [kanuka, burgan]

Laurus nobilis [bay]

Lavandula angustifolia (= *L. officinalis*, *L. vera*) flos [lavender]

Lavandula x *intermedia* 'Super' flos [lavandin]

Leptospermum citratum

Leptospermum scoparium [manuka]

Litsea cubeba fruct. [may chang]

Matricaria recutita (= *M. chamomilla, Chamomilla recutita*) flos [German chamomile]

Melaleuca alternifolia fol. [tea tree]

Melaleuca leucadendron (= *M. cajuputi*) fol. [cajuput]

Melaleuca viridiflora (= *M. quinquenervia*) fol. [niaouli]

Melissa officinalis fol. [melissa]

Mentha arvensis [cornmint]

Mentha spicata [spearmint]

Mentha x *piperita* fol. [peppermint]

Myristica fragrans sem. [nutmeg]

Myrtus communis [myrtle, red and orange]

Nardostachys jatamansi (= *N. grandiflora*) rad. [spikenard]

Nepeta cataria var. *citriodora* flos, fol. [catnep]

Ocimum basilicum fol. [European basil]

Origanum majorana flos, fol. [sweet marjoram]

Origanum vulgare subsp. *viride* (= *O. heracleoticum*), [Greek oregano, green oregano]

Ormenis multicaulis, Ormenis mixta flos [Moroccan chamomile]

Pelargonium graveolens fol. [geranium]

Picea nigra, P. mariana [black spruce]

Pimenta dioica fruct. [allspice]

Pimenta racemosa fruct. fol. [West Indian bay]

Pimpinella anisum fruct. [aniseed]

Pinus mugo var. *pumilio* [dwarf pine]

Pinus sylvestris fol. [Scots pine]

Piper nigrum fruct. [black pepper]

Pogostemon patchouli, Pogostemon cablin fol. [patchouli]

Ravensara aromatica fol. [aromatic ravensara]

Rosa damascena, R. centifolia flos (dist.) [rose otto]

Rosmarinus officinalis (ct. cineole, ct. camphor) fol. [rosemary]

Rosmarinus officinalis (ct. verbenone) fol. [rosemary]

Ruta graveolens [rue]

Salvia officinalis fol. [sage, Dalmatian sage]

Salvia sclarea flos, fol. [clary]

Santalum album lig. [sandalwood]

Satureia hortensis fol. [summer or garden savory]

Satureia montana fol. [winter or mountain savory]

Syzygium aromaticum flos [clove bud]

Tagetes minuta (= *T. glandulifera, T. patula, T. erecta*) flos [taget, French marigold]

Thymus mastichina flos, fol. [Spanish marjoram]

Thymus satureioides [Moroccan thyme, borneol thyme]

Thymus vulgaris (population) herb. [thyme]

Thymus vulgaris (ct. geraniol, ct. linalool) herb. [sweet thyme]

Thymus vulgaris (ct. thujanol-4) herb. [sweet thyme]

Thymus vulgaris (ct. thymol, ct. carvacrol) herb. [thyme]

Valeriana officinalis rad. [valerian]

Valeriana wallichii rad. [Indian valerian]

Vetiveria zizanioides rad. [vetiver]

Zingiber cassumunar [phrai, plai]

Zingiber officinale rhiz. [ginger]

PART I
ESSENTIAL OILS FOR GENERAL USE IN HEALTH-CARE SETTINGS

This appendix is not intended to be a comprehensive list of essential oils and their properties. It is designed with health-care situations in mind, and includes enough information to cover most eventualities where treatment with essential oils is appropriate. Several essential oils mentioned in the text of this book that do not appear here are shown in the chart in Appendix B9.

It is not possible in a general list such as this to give precise figures for the presence of a component in a given essential oil, particularly when the essential oils used in aromatherapy are not standardized but are taken directly from the still and used without any further treatment. The percentages shown for the constituents are aggregated and show the highs and lows for given compounds, hence the variation, sometimes remarkably wide, in these. A common misinterpretation of aggregated data is that a species might appear to be high in two closely related compounds, e.g. thymol and carvacrol. It must be borne in mind that there is often compensation between the two compounds so that when the quantity of one is raised another is lowered (Beckstrom-Sternberg & Duke 1996). The factors that affect the variability of components have been discussed in Section 1, Essential oil science. Different authors do give widely varying information – and sometimes fail to identify accurately the plant being discussed. It cannot be ruled out that some sources may be referring to standardized or adulterated oils.

Asterisks (*) are used to indicate where the authors have found essential oils to be particularly effective.

The tables listed below summarize various properties of essential oils and are to used in conjunction with this Appendix A(I):

Table B1 General properties
Table 4.4 Antibacterial properties
Table 4.5 Antifungal properties
Table 4.6 Antiinflammatory properties
Table 4.7 Antiviral properties
Table 4.8 Digestive properties
Table 4.9 Hormonal properties

Table 4.10 Insect repellent and insecticidal properties

ABIES ALBA FOL.
(*European silver fir, white fir*)
ABIETACEAE

Representative constituents

Hydrocarbons
monoterpenes (90–95%) fenchene 0.2%, bornylene 0.05%, santene 1.8%, tricyclene 1.8%, (–)-α-pinene 23.6%, β-fenchene 0.2%, α-fenchene 2.0%, camphene 21.1%, β-pinene 8.7%, sabinene 0.2%, δ-3-carene 0.1%, α-phellandrene 0.2%, α-terpinene 0.7%, (–)-limonene 34.2%, β-phellandrene 1.3%, γ-terpinene 0.3%, α-terpinolene 1.1%, α-thujene *trace*, β-myrcene 1.0%
aromatic p-cymene 1.0%

Esters *(5–10%)*
monoterpenyl (–)-bornyl acetate

Properties	Indications
analgesic	rheumatism, arthritis
anticatarrhal	bronchitis
antiseptic, pulmonary	respiratory tract infections
expectorant	
rubefacient	arthritis
stimulant, uplifting	sadness, withdrawal

Observations

- no contraindications known at normal aromatherapeutic dose.
- caution advised with oral use (Franchomme & Pénoël 2001 p. 347)
- conifers are rich in terpenes, and so are good decongestants (also indicated for fluid retention), respiratory system cleansers
- *in vitro* tests showed Turkish *Abies alba* oil to have moderate activity against 10 bacteria and

Candida albicans but none against *E. coli* (Bagci & Digrak 1996a)

- *in vitro* testing of 9 Turkish *Abies* sp essential oils against 6 bacteria and *Candida albicans* showed the least active to be *Abies alba* which also had little activity towards yeast (Bagci & Digrak 1996)

ABIES BALSAMEA FOL., RAM. [BALSAM FIR NEEDLE, CANADA FIR NEEDLE] ABIETACEAE

Representative constituents

Hydrocarbons
monoterpenes (75-90%) tricyclene 0.4–2.2%, santene 1.2–4.0%, α-pinene 4.7–10.6%, (–)-camphene 3.9–16%, β-pinene 21.4–54%, δ-3-carene 7.3–35.6%, (–)-limonene 2.7–19.7%, α-terpinolene 0.3–2.2%, β-phellandrene 2.7–5.8%, β-myrcene 1.0–2.5%

Alcohols
monoterpenols borneol 0.1–2.2%, terpinen-4-ol <0.2%, α-terpineol 0.1–0.8%

Phenols
thymol 0–*trace*

Methyl ethers *0–trace*

Esters *(10–25%)*
monoterpenyl bornyl acetate 8.3–27.6%

Ketones
monoterpenones camphor 0.2%, piperitone 1.6%
sesquiterpenone-ester juvabione *trace*

Properties	Indications
antiarthritic	arthritis
antibacterial	*Staphylococcus, E. coli,* see Table 4.4
antiparasitic	ascaridiosis (thread worms)
antiseptic, pulmonary	asthma, catarrh, rhinitis, bronchitis, sinusitis
antiseptic urinary	cystitis
antispasmodic	muscular tension
antitussive	
stimulant, neurotonic	depression, stress
cicatrizant	burns, wounds, cuts

Observations

- none known at normal aromatherapeutic dose
- caution advised with oral use (Franchomme & Pénoël 2001 p. 347)
- very balancing oil to the energy (avoid evening use)
- for the respiratory system use blended with an essential oil having a high 1,8-cineole content
- balsam fir needle oil is not to be confused with *Canada balsam*, which is the oleoresin collected by tapping the trunk of the same species (Bruneton 1995 p. 473)
- an oil distilled from the oleoresin is used in pharmacy in the formulation of haemorrhoid creams
- an essential oil obtained from the twigs contains santene 0.1–1.2%, α-pinene 7.6–20.5%, camphene 1.7–7.4%, β-pinene 12.1–40.8%, δ-3-carene 0.8–29.6%, limonene 6.0–20.9%, β-phellandrene 2.0–8.8%, bornyl acetate 3.6–12.2%
- the twig oil has no oxygenated compounds
- Lawless (1992 p. 49) gives this oil as being purgative and diuretic

ABIES SIBIRICA FOL. [SIBERIAN FIR NEEDLE] ABIETACEAE

Representative constituents

Hydrocarbons
monoterpenes (–)-camphene 10–26%, (–)-α-pinene 10–22%, δ-3-carene 10–15%, limonene, β-pinene, α-phellandrene, santene
sesquiterpene bisabolene

Alcohols
monoterpenols borneol, α-terpineol
diterpenols isoabienol *trace*

Esters
monoterpenyl (–)-bornyl acetate 25–42%, terpenyl acetate

Properties	Indications
antiinflammatory	pyorrhoea, see Table 4.6
antispasmodic	spasmodic colitis, bronchial asthma

Observations

- no contraindications known at normal aromatherapeutic dose

■ Siberian fir needle oil is not to be confused with the essential oil derived from the cones (templin oil) (Bruneton 1995 p. 473)

ACHILLEA MILLEFOLIUM HERB. [*YARROW*] ASTERACEAE

Representative constituents

Hydrocarbons
monoterpenes α-pinene 1.5–3.5%, β-pinene 6–12.3%, camphene < 2.5%, sabinene 7.5–41.5%, β-myrcene 0.6–2%, α-terpinene 0.5–1.1%, limonene 0.4–1%, γ-terpinene 1.3–3.6%, α-terpinolene 0.2–0.6%
sesquiterpenes chamazulene 5–33.2%, dihydroazulenes, caryophyllene 2.7–4.9%, germacrene D 9.3–13.6%
aromatic p-cymene 0.1–1.2%

Alcohols
monoterpenols terpinen-4-ol 2.1–5.6%, borneol 0.2–9.5%
sesquiterpenols cadinols 0.4–1.1%

Oxides
monoterpenoid 1,8-cineole 1.9–11%
sesquiterpenoid caryophyllene oxide 0.4–1.7%

Ketones
monoterpenones isoartemisia ketone 9%, camphor <2.9%, thujone

Esters
monoterpenyl bornyl acetate <2.2%

Lactones
sesquiterpenyl achilline

Phenols
eugenol

Properties	Indications
analgesic	neuralgia, sprained ankle, sprains
anticatarrhal*	colds, catarrh
antiinflammatory*	prostatitis, neuritis, rheumatism, see Table 4.6
antiseptic	urinary infections
choleretic*	hepatobiliary deficiency, poor digestion
cicatrizant*	
decongestant	dysmenorrhoea
digestive stimulant	see Table 4.8
diuretic	
emmenagogic*	oligomenorrhoea, amenorrhoea
expectorant	
febrifuge	fevers
hypotensor	hypertension
litholytic	kidney stones
vulnerary	varicose ulcers

Observations

■ not normally used for babies, children and pregnant women
■ neurotoxic and abortive (Franchomme & Pénoël 2001 p. 348)
■ yarrow contains little or no thujone (Leung 1980)
■ some individuals show positive patch test reactions to yarrow
■ cross-sensitivity between other Asteraceae members and yarrow has been demonstrated (Duke 1985)
■ yarrow oil is obtained from the *A. millefolium* complex, a group of hardly separable species or subspecies of Asteraceae found throughout the temperate and boreal zones of the northern and southern hemispheres; the taxonomic problem is extensive and confusing (Lawrence 1984) and what is known as yarrow oil may come from one of several species
■ at least 14 different chemical races have been identified in Europe (Mills 1991)
■ yarrow has been universally used for the treatment of rheumatism, colds, catarrh, fevers, hypertension and amenorrhoea (Wren 1988)
■ yarrow is diaphoretic, a peripheral vasodilator (Mills 1991)
■ persons known to be allergic to ragweeds should be cautious about drinking chamomile or yarrow teas (Tyler 1982)
■ isoartemisia ketone 9% is listed by Franchomme & Penoël (2001 p. 348) for this oil, but not by Lawrence; according to Guenther (1948–1952) it is found in *Artemisia annua*

- camphor chemotype should be used with caution; when taken orally camphor causes convulsions if sufficient quantity is taken (Craig 1953)
- antiinflammatory properties are associated with azulenes (Chandler, Hooper & Harvey 1982)
- CNS-depressant activity in mice has been documented (Kudrzycka-Bieloszabska & Glowniak 1966)

ACORUS CALAMUS RHIZ.
[*SWEET FLAG*, *CALAMUS*] ARACEAE

Representative constituents

Hydrocarbons
monoterpenes camphene 0.9%, α-pinene 0.6%, β-pinene *trace*–0.3%, limonene 0.1–2.8%
sesquiterpenes β-gurjunene 0.2–3.4%, calamenene 0.1–3.8%, calacolene *trace*–0.2%, β-elemene 0.6–1.5%, α-selinene, δ-cadinene 0.5–2.1%, α-ylangene
aromatic p-cymene *trace*–0.1%

Phenols
eugenol 0–0.1%, *cis*-isoeugenol 2.5–25%, *trans*-isoeugenol 0.5–2%

Methyl ethers
methyl eugenol *trace*–1.8%, *cis*-methyl isoeugenol 2.4–49%, *trans*-methyl isoeugenol 1.1–7.9%, α-asarone 1–16%, β-asarone 20.5–75.6%

Aldehydes
monoterpenals geranial
aromatic asaronal 0.2–6%

Alcohols
monoterpenols geraniol, linalool 0.3–12%, terpinen-4-ol 0.1–1%, α-terpineol
sesquiterpenols α-cadinol, calamol
diols calamendiol, isocalamendiol

Oxides
monoterpenoid 1,8-cineole *trace*–0.2%

Ketones
monoterpenones camphor
sesquiterpenones shyobunone *trace*–3.7%, epi-shyobunone 0.1–4.8%, isoshyobunone

0.6–9.4%, acolamone, isoacolamone, acoragermacrone, acorenone, acorone, sekishone *trace*–1.3%

Ethers
trimethyl elemicin 0.1–1.3%, *cis*-isoelemicin *trace*–0.1%

Properties	Indications
antiinflammatory	gout, gastritis, bronchitis, cystitis, see Table 4.6
antispasmodic, spasmolytic	dysentery, diarrhoea, enterocolitis
carminative	flatulence
digestive	poor appetite, sluggish digestion, see Table 4.8
diuretic	uric acid elimination
hypnotic	
sudorific	fever
sedative	

Observations

- short-term use only (Franchomme & Pénoël 2001 p. 348)
- neurotoxic and abortive (Franchomme & Pénoël p. 349)
- oral use best avoided altogether (Tisserand & Balacs 1995a p. 204)
- the USA Food and Drug Administration bans the use of oil of calamus for food use because β-asarone was found to be a hepatocarcinogen in rats (Lawrence 1981 p. 47)
- long-term administration of Indian calamus oil to rats induces duodenal tumours (Bruneton 1995 p. 463, Taylor et al 1967)
- Baxter et al (1962) showed that β-asarone has a *cis* configuration and asarone has a *trans*-configuration; both isomers were found to have hypnotic potentiating activity.
- β-asarone was found to possess sedative activity (Baxter, Fan & Kardel 1962)
- reported to have hypotensive activity in cats and rabbits (Leung & Foster 1996 p. 112)
- β-asarone (Z-isoasarone) is absent from the essential oil of the American variety but is dominant in the oil of the Indian variety and also the Chinese variety (up to 85%)

- β-asarone is banned in the USA as a pharmaceutical ingredient; the alpha isomer is permitted (Harborne & Baxter 1993)
- it is possible that β-asarone is the most active carcinogenic compound to be found in essential oils (Tisserand & Balacs 1995b p. 95)
- calamus oil has been found to induce sterility in male houseflies and insects (Mathur & Saxena 1975, Saxena et al 1977)
- Indian calamus root oil repels houseflies (Adler & Jacobson 1982)
- used to flavour gin and beers (Grieve 1998)
- *Acorus calamus* var. *americanus,* diploid form, contains a mixture of shyobunones 13–45% and virtually no β-asarone (Keller & Stahl 1983); the triploid forms (*Acorus calamus* var. *calamus*) contain a mixture of shyobunones (23–32%) and β-asarone (8–19%); tetraploid forms (*Acorus calamus* var. *angustatus*) contain *cis*-methyl isoeugenol (0.4%), a mixture of shyobunones (1–53%) and β-asarone (12–96%) (Röst & Bos 1979)
- shyobunone chemotype contraindicated for use on babies, young children and in pregnancy (Franchomme & Pénoël 2001 p. 349)
- shyobunone chemotype given as anticatarrhal and mucolytic (Franchomme & Pénoël 2001 p. 348)

ALOYSIA TRIPHYLLA (= *LIPPIA CITRIODORA*) [*VERBENA*] VERBENACEAE

Representative constituents

Hydrocarbons

monoterpenes α-pinene 0.1–1%, β-pinene 0.5%, β-myrcene 0.1%, limonene 4.2–15%, *cis*-β-ocimene, *trans*-β-ocimene 0.8–2.5%, camphene *trace*, sabinene *trace*–2.5%, α-terpinene *trace*, α-terpinolene *trace*

sesquiterpenes α-cedrene 0.3%, β-elemene 0.1%, isocaryophyllene, β-caryophyllene 3–3.8%, thujopsene 0.2%, alloaromadendrene 0.4%, germacrene D 1.8%, α-farnesene and bicyclogermacrene 4.8%, δ–cadinene 0.5%, γ-cadinene 0.2%, β-curcumene 2%, β-cubebene 0.3%, β-maaliene 2%, copaene 0.3%

aromatic p-cymene 0.1%, ar-curcumene 3–4.5%

Alcohols

monoterpenols geraniol 0.5–6%, nerol 0.5–5.2%, linalool 0.5%, isopulegol 0.1%, terpinen-4-ol 0.3%, α-terpineol 1.5–2.5%, citronellol 1% , *cis*-thujanol-4-ol 0.2%

sesquiterpenols (+)-nerolidol 1.3–2% cedrol 0.1%, spathulenol 2–3%, cadinol 0.7%, farnesol 0.1%, caryophylla-1-(12), 8(15)-dien-9-α-ol, caryophylla-1(12),7-dien-9-α-ol, caryophylla-1(12)7-dien-9-β-ol, muurolol

other hexenol, 3-octanol 0.2%, 1-octen-3-ol 1%

Aldehydes

monoterpenals neral 12%, geranial 15–26%, citronellal 1%

other decanal *trace*, octanal *trace*, 2,5-dimethyl-2-vinyl-4-hexenal

Ketones

other 3-octanone 0.1%, β-ionone 0.2%, methyl heptenone 1.7–4%, 2-isopropyliden-5-methylcyclopentanone, kubosone

Oxides

monoterpenyl 1,8-cineole 3–6%, *cis*- and *trans*-limonene epoxide *trace*, nerol oxide

sesquiterpenyl caryophyllene oxide 2%, 2,6-epoxy-caryophyllene *trace*

Esters

monoterpenyl citronellyl acetate 0.2%, neryl acetate 4%, geranyl acetate 1.5–1.8%

other cis-3-hexanyl acetate *trace*

Coumarins *(trace)*

Properties	Indications
antiinfectious	amoebiasis
antiinflammatory	rheumatism, cystitis, see Table 4.6
antipyretic	malaria
calming	tachycardia, hypertension, stress, asthma
digestive	indigestion, flatulence, see Table 4.8
hormonelike	see Table 4.9
litholytic	kidney stones (gravel)
sedative	depression, insomnia, stress

| stimulant (gall bladder, pancreas) | diabetes |
| stimulant (skin) | psoriasis, pallid skin |

Observations

- no known contraindications at normal aromatherapeutic dose, but avoid use on the skin because of the presence of furanocoumarins (Franchomme & Pénoël 2001 p. 395)
- no contraindications with physiological dosage; contains *trace*s of furocoumarin; can have sensitizing effects on the skin (Schnaubelt 1998 p. 77)
- genuine *Aloysia triphylla* does not irritate the skin, unlike other oils with similar concentrations of citral (Schnaubelt 1998 p. 117)
- should not be used in therapy, either internally or externally (Tisserand & Balacs 1995b p. 177); this is based on tests carried out at 12% of fragrance quality oils (Opdyke 1992 p. 30); concentrations used in aromatherapy are very much less than 12%, probably only in the region of 1%
- the true oil can be difficult to source; most lemon verbena oils are blends made of lemon, citronella, lemongrass, etc: the genuine oil is expensive
- IFRA recommendation is that lemon verbena oil should not be used in fragrance formulations because of its possible phototoxicity and sensitization
- infusions of lemon verbena are used to treat various digestive ailments and sleeplessness (Bruneton 1995 p. 462)
- *in vitro* tests showed Italian oil to have poor antifungal activity (Guarrera et al 1995)

ANETHUM GRAVEOLENS SEM.
[DILLSEED] APIACEAE

Representative constituents

Hydrocarbons
monoterpenes (25–50%) (+)-limonene 25–40%, α-phellandrene 1–25%, β-phellandrene 0.2%, α-pinene 0.1%, β-myrcene 0.2%
sesquiterpenes β-caryophyllene
aromatic p-cymene 0.2–0.3%, α-p-dimethyl styrene 0.1%

Aldehydes
other anisic aldehyde *trace*

Phenols
carveol 2%, eugenol

Methyl ethers
anethole, dillapiole

Benzodioxoles
myristicin

Ketones *(40–60%)*
monoterpene (+)-carvone (28–60%), cis-dihydrocarvone 3.7%, trans-dihydrocarvone 1.8%

Coumarins *(<4%)*
umbelliferone, umbelliprenine dill furan 0.4%

Properties	Indications
anticatarrhal	respiratory catarrh
anticoagulant	infarction, *hemogliase*
bactericidal	
carminative	flatulence
cholagogic, choleretic	low bile production
digestive	dyspepsia, gastric upsets, constipation, see Table 4.8
hypotensor	hypertension
mucolytic	bronchitis
sedative	sleep-inducing
spasmolytic	smooth muscle spasm, colic, hiccups

Observations

- non-toxic, non-irritant and not phototoxic at normal dose levels (Tisserand & Balacs 1995b p. 204)
- undiluted oil was not irritating when applied to the backs of hairless mice and pigs
- moderately irritating when applied full strength to both intact and abraded rabbit skin for 24 hours under occlusion
- 4% in petrolatum did not produce irritation after a 48-hour closed-patch test on humans
- no sensitization was obtained with 4% of oil in petrolatum

- no phototoxicity was reported when undiluted oil was applied to hairless mice and pigs
- dill seed essential oil is neurotoxic and abortive (Franchomme & Pénoël 2001 p. 351)
- contraindicated for babies, young children and in pregnancy (Franchomme & Pénoël 2001 p. 351)
- used in soaps and in the preparation of dill water for flatulence in infants
- chemically very similar to caraway oil; both oils consist largely of carvone and limonene
- East Indian dill seed oil *Anethum sowa* [SOYAH] may be substituted but can be distinguished by a higher specific gravity (0.945 to 0.972) and a lower optical rotation (+48 to +57); dillapiole is present (about 20%), making this oil abortifacient and toxic to liver and kidneys; there is a lower content of carvone
- Indian dill seed oil shows antifungal activity (Ramadan et al 1972a)
- anethofuran, carvone and limonene were tested on mice; all acted as inducers of the detoxifying enzyme glutathione S-transferase in the liver; carvone was the most potent inducer (Zheng et al 1992)

ANGELICA ARCHANGELICA RAD. [*ANGELICA*] APIACEAE ANGELICA ROOT OIL CONSTITUENTS

Representative constituents

Hydrocarbons
monoterpenes (73%) α-pinene 24–27%, β-pinene 4.4–8.7%, limonene 13%, camphene 0.9–1.2%, β-myrcene 4–11.5%, α-thujene 0.7%, γ-terpinene 2.7–4.2%, α-phellandrene, 12.4–14.7%, sabinene 0.6%, (+)-α-phellandrene
sesquiterpenes β-caryophyllene <0.2%
aromatic p-cymene 5%

Alcohols
monoterpenols linalool, borneol

Aldehydes
other acetaldehyde

Esters *(1.5–2%)*
monoterpenyl bornyl acetate 0.75%, *trans*-verbenyl acetate 0.45%

Oxides
monoterpenoid 1,8-cineole 14%

Coumarins *(2%)*
umbelliferone, archangelicin, angelicin, bergapten, osthol, osthenol, imperatorin, xanthotoxol, xanthotoxin, and others

Lactones
pentadecanolide <1%, ambrettolide <1%, heptadecanolide, tridecanolide

Properties	Indications
antibacterial	see Table 4.4
anticoagulant	
antifungal	see Table 4.5
antiseptic	urinary infections, respiratory tract infections
antispasmodic	spasmodic enterocolitis, painful periods
carminative	flatulence
diuretic	
digestive	see Table 4.8
emmenagogic	
digestive	dyspepsia, indigestion, griping, colic, anorexia, dyspepsia, stomach ulcers, see Table 4.8
expectorant	asthma, bronchitis
febrifuge	
neurotonic	
sedative	anxiety, nervous fatigue, insomnia
soothing	irritated skin, arthritis, rheumatism

ANGELICA ARCHANGELICA FRUCT. [*ANGELICA*] APIACEAE

Representative constituents

Hydrocarbons
monoterpenes: β-phellandrene 16–35%, α-phellandrene 2.7–20%, α-pinene 9.2%, camphene 0.4%, β-pinene 0.7%, sabinene 0.3%, β-myrcene 1.5%, α-terpinene *trace*, limonene 38.7%, *cis*-β-ocimene 0.15%, γ-terpinene *trace*, *trans*-β-ocimene 0.3%, α-terpinolene *trace*

sesquiterpenes β-caryophyllene 3.3%, α-copaene
0.3%, α-humulene 0.7%
aromatic p-cymene 0.7%

Oxides
sesquiterpenoid caryophyllene oxide 0.13%

Coumarins *(1–3%)*
imperatorin 0.5%, xanthotoxin, bergapten 0.1%,
isoimperatorin, xanthotoxol, 8-hydroxy-5-
methoxypsoralen, 4-methoxy-7-
hydroxypsoralen and others

Properties	Indications
carminative	flatulence, dyspepsia, colitis
sedative (high dose)	anxiety
tonic, uplifting (low dose)	

Observations, root and seed oils

- root oil is photosensitizing when used on the skin due to the presence of coumarins (Franchomme & Pénoël 2001 p. 351)
- root oil phototoxicity is due to the presence of the coumarins bergapten, xanthotoxin; IFRA (1992) recommends a maximum of 0.8% presence of the root oil in product applied to skin which is to be exposed to UV rays
- both angelica root and seed oil are non-irritant on the skin
- angelica root oil should not be used during pregnancy or by diabetics (Lawless 1992 p. 44)
- angelica seed oil is cheaper than the root oil and is often added to the root oil
- umbelliferone is a proven antifungal agent (Mabey 1988 p. 117)
- pinene is antimicrobial and expectorant (Opdyke 1975b p. 713)
- angelica root oil is antispasmodic (Wagner et al 1979)
- root oil is antibacterial and antifungal (Saksena & Tripathi 1985)
- bergapten, xanthotoxin and other coumarins which have been shown to be effective in the treatment of psoriasis and vitiligo
- both root and seed oils are used at a maximum of 0.1% in perfumes (Leung & Foster 1996 p. 33)
- seed oil is photosensitizing when used on the skin due to the presence of furocoumarins (Franchomme & Pénoël 2001 p. 351)
- Opdyke (1974c p. 12) gives angelica seed oil as being not phototoxic

ANIBA ROSAEODORA FOL. *[ROSEWOOD]* LAURACEAE

Representative constituents

Hydrocarbons
monoterpenes α-pinene 0.15%, camphene 0.03%,
β-pinene 0.5%, β-myrcene 0.04%, limonene
0.6%, β-phellandrene
sesquiterpenes caryophyllene 0.03%, α-selinene,
β-elemene, γ-cadinene
aromatic p-cymene

Alcohols
monoterpenols linalool 82–95%, geraniol, terpinen-
4-ol 0.4%, α-terpineol 3.5%
other (C8) methyl heptenol

Aldehydes
monoterpenals neral, geranial
aromatic benzaldehyde

Esters
monoterpenyl geranyl acetate 0.14%

Ketones
other methyl heptenone

Oxides
monoterpenoid cis-linalool oxide 1.5%, *trans-*
linalool oxide 1.3%, 1,8-cineole 0.2–2.3%

Properties	Indications
antifungal*	*Candida*, see Table 4.5
antiinfectious	respiratory infections*, coughs
antiparasitic	
antiseptic	skin problems
antiviral*	colds, influenza, see Table 4.7
astringent	
bactericidal*	
cicatrizant	
stimulating*	general debility, overwork, sexual debility
tonic	nervous depression, stress-related headaches

Observations

- no known contraindications to aromatherapy use
- potent antibacterial agent (Lis-Balchin, Deans & Hart 1994)
- non-toxic when applied externally (Opdyke 1978a)
- linalool was found to have weak tumour-promoting properties in mice (Homburger & Boger 1968, Opdyke 1975c)
- anticonvulsant activity in mice and rats; spasmolytic activity on isolated guinea pig ileum and antimicrobial properties have been reported (Opdyke 1975)
- maximum level allowed in perfumes is 1.0% (Opdyke 1975a)

BOSWELLIA CARTERI RES. DIST.
[FRANKINCENSE, OLIBANUM] BURSERACEAE

Representative constituents

Hydrocarbons

monoterpenes (40%) α-pinene 21%, α-thujene 24%, limonene 8%, sabinene 6%, camphene, β-myrcene, α-terpinene 3.5%, β-pinene, γ-terpinene, α-terpinolene, α- and β-phellandrene
sesquiterpenes α-gurjunene, α-guaiene, copaene, caryophyllene
aromatic *p*-cymene 6%

Alcohols

other octanol 12%
monoterpenols borneol, terpinen-4-ol, *trans*-pinocarveol, linalool 2%
sesquiterpenols farnesol

Ketones

monoterpenone verbenone

Esters

other octyl acetate 60%

Oxides

diterpenoid incensole 3%

Properties	Indications
analgesic	rheumatism, sports injuries
antibacterial	see Table 4.4
anticatarrhal*	asthma, bronchitis*
antidepressive*	nervous depression*
antiinfectious	respiratory tract
antiinflammatory	rheumatism, see Table 4.6
antioxidant	combats ageing process
cicatrizant	scars, ulcers, wounds
energizing	
expectorant	
immunostimulant*	immunodeficiency*

Observations

- no contraindications yet known for this gentle, effective, distilled oil
- olibanum absolute produces no skin irritation or sensitization reactions at 8% dilution when tested on humans, no phototoxic effects when undiluted (Opdyke 1978b)
- antibacterial action including *Listeria monocytogenes* (Lis-Balchin, Deans & Hart 1994)
- mild antifungal activity (Maruzzella 1960)
- olibanum distilled oils were tested at 10% and 100% concentrations against *Staphylococcus aureus, Sarcina lutea, Mycobacterium phlei, Bacillus subtilis, Escherichia coli* and *Neisseria catarrhalis* and all were found to be inhibited to some extent by the undiluted oil: an n-hexane extract of the oleogum resin had markedly less antimicrobial activity (Abdel Waheb et al 1987)
- the leaf oil of *Boswellia serrata* has antifungal effects (Garg 1974)

CANANGA ODORATA FOL. [YLANG YLANG] ANNONACEAE

Representative constituents

(Percentage composition figures are given as a guide – ylang ylang is an oil of variable make-up.)

Hydrocarbons

monoterpenes α-pinene, β-pinene
sesquiterpenes α-farnesene and γ-cadinene 6.5–17.4%, β-caryophyllene 15–22%, germacrene D 15–25%, δ-cadinene 2–4.7%, α-humulene 0.9–2.5%

Alcohols

monoterpenols linalool 11.6–30%, geraniol, nerol
sesquiterpenols farnesol
aromatic benzyl alcohol

Phenols

eugenol, isoeugenol

Methyl ethers

p-cresyl methyl ether 15%, methyl eugenol

Benzodioxoles

safrole, isosafrole

Esters *(15%)*

monoterpenyl geranyl acetate 5–10%
sesquiterpenyl farnesyl acetate 1–7%
aromatic methyl anthranilate, methyl salicylate
    1–10%, benzyl benzoate 5–12%, benzyl acetate
    3–8%, benzyl salicylate, methyl benzoate
    1–5.5%, *p*-cresyl acetate

Properties	Indications
antidiabetic	diabetes
antiseptic	intestinal infections
antispasmodic*	cramp, colic
balancing*	
calming	tachycardia*, hyperpnoea, insomnia
hypotensor*	hypertension
tonic	scalp, hair growth
reproductive stimulant	frigidity, impotence
sedative	

Observations

- no contraindications known to normal aromatherapy use
- ylang ylang oil has been recognized as an allergen and removed from certain cosmetics (Mitchell & Rook 1979)
- no sensitization reactions at 10% dilution (Draize 1959)
- no irritation when tested at 10% dilution on humans (Opdyke 1974d)
- no phototoxic effects reported (Opdyke 1974d)
- can produce dermatitis in sensitized individuals (Duke 1985)
- the oil has been suggested as a possible substitute for quinine in malaria (Burkhill 1966)

- an essential oil is also prepared from the leaves
- stimulant when applied as a mask or by spraying (Rovesti & Colombo 1973)
- a folk remedy for asthma, boils, diarrhoea, headache, malaria, ophthalmia, rheumatism, stomach ailments (Duke & Wain 1981)

CARUM CARVI FRUCT. *[CARAWAY]* APIACEAE

Representative constituents

Hydrocarbons

monoterpenes (38–45%) limonene 10–45%, carvene
    30%, caryophyllene 0.1%, α-terpinolene 0.2%,
    β-myrcene
aromatic p-cymene

Alcohols

monoterpenols (2–6%) *cis*-carveol 5.5%, *cis*-perillyl
    alcohol 0.1%, dihydrocarveol
aromatic cuminyl alcohol

Ketones

monoterpenones (50–60%) carvone 45–80%,
    dihydrocarvones 0.7%

Aldehydes

aromatic cuminaldehyde 0.1%

Coumarins

herniarin *trace*

Properties	Indications
antibacterial	see Table 4.4
antihistaminic	hay fever
antispasmodic*	gastric spasm*, large intestine spasm, intestinal problems
aperitive	loss of appetite
calming	anger, vertigo
carminative*	flatulence*, aerophagy*
cholagogic, choleretic	insufficient bile, indigestion
diuretic	
emmenagogic	
larvicidal	
mucolytic*	bronchitis*
stimulant	scalp problems

Observations

- although caraway oil contains a substantial proportion of carvone, tests have proved that the whole oil is safe in normal use; however, it is best not used on infants under 3 years or expectant mothers
- in excessive dose it is neurotoxic and abortive
- no irritation or sensitization when tested at 4% dilution on humans (Opdyke 1973b)
- has a low level of phototoxicity (Opdyke 1973b)
- carvone and limonene have been shown to have an experimental cancer chemopreventative effect; overall carvone was the most potent, attributed to its α,β-unsaturated ketone system (Zheng, Kenney & Lam 1992d)
- the seeds are chewed to relieve toothache and for carminative effect (Foster 1993b p. 59)
- it is a well-known digestive stimulant and this property is made use of in drinks such as Benedictine, Grand Chartreuse and Izarra
- caraway seeds have been found in 3000-year-old Egyptian tombs
- caraway and peppermint oils combined in enteric coated capsules (Enteroplant®) were found to improve non-ulcer dyspepsia (May et al 1996): those with and without irritable bowel syndrome profited equally from the treatment
- the effect of peppermint (90 mg) – caraway (50 mg) combination was investigated on the gastromobility of six healthy volunteers; the subjects were given either enteric coated (Enteroplant®) or non-enteric coated capsules; both coated and non-coated preparations were concluded to be safe and acted locally to cause smooth muscle relaxation; the effect of the non-enteric coated capsules was not as pronounced due to dilution of the oils by gastric juices (Micklefield, Greving & May 2000)
- the oil exhibits antibacterial and larvicidal activities (Oishi et al 1974, Ramadan et al 1972a)
- has antispasmodic and antihistaminic activities (Debelmas & Rochat 1967)
- carvone induces the detoxifying enzyme glutathione S-transferase (GST) in mouse tissue. Compounds that induce increased GST detoxification are considered potential inhibitors of carcinogenesis (Zheng, Kenney & Lam 1992d)
- Enteroplant®, containing a hydrophobic phase galenic auxiliary material with *Mentha* x *piperita* and *Carum carvi* essential oils in an enteric coated capsule, was examined; peppermint oil caused significant reduction in contractions in the duodenum and gastric corpus; caraway oil induced significant reduction in the duodenum, gastric corpus and antrum; the effect of both of the oils exceeded that of either the carrier or hydrophobic phase in producing smooth muscle relaxation (Micklefield et al 2003)

CEDRUS ATLANTICA LIG. [ATLAS CEDARWOOD, SATINWOOD] ABIETACEAE

Representative constituents

Hydrocarbons
sesquiterpenes (50%) cedrene

Alcohols
sesquiterpenols (30%) atlantol, α-caryophyllene alcohol, epi-β-cubenol

Ketones
sesquiterpenones (20%) α-atlantone, γ-atlantone
other α-ionone

Other
epoxy-β-himachalene and its epimer deodarone

Properties	Indications
antiseptic	skin problems, scalp (with cade oil), urinary tract, eczema, pruritus (with bergamot oil)
arterial regenerator*	arteriosclerosis*
cicatrizant	skin problems, wounds
lipolytic*	cellulite*
lymph tonic*	cellulite*, lymph circulation problems, water retention
mucolytic	bronchitis*
stimulant	scalp problems

Observations

- it is important to specify this oil accurately: the term cedarwood oil has little meaning, because many oils are sold under this name, many of them from the Cupressaceae family
- considered in France to be neurotoxic and abortive, and not normally used there for pregnant women and infants
- Duraffourd (1982) recommends leaving internal use of this oil to a doctor
- the Moroccan oil *C. atlantica* showed no irritation or sensitization at 8% dilution when tested on humans (Opdyke 1976g)
- has no phototoxic effects reported, although the use of toilet preparations containing unspecified cedarwood oils followed by exposure to various wavelengths sometimes causes dermatitis (Winter 1984)

CHAMAEMELUM NOBILE
(= *MATRICARIA CHAMOMILLA, ANTHEMIS NOBILIS*) [ROMAN CHAMOMILE] ASTERACEAE

Representative constituents

Hydrocarbons
monoterpenes α-terpinene 0–10%, α-pinene 0–10%, β-pinene 0–10%, sabinene 0–10%, camphene, β-myrcene, γ-terpinene
sesquiterpenes caryophyllene 0–10%, chamazulene, copaene, β-copaene, δ-cadinene
aromatic p-cymene

Alcohols
monoterpenols trans-pinocarveol 5%
sesquiterpenols (5–6%) farnesol, nerolidol

Aldehydes
monoterpenal myrtenal 0–10%

Ketones
monoterpenones pinocarvone 13%

Esters *(75–80%)*
other 2-methylbutyl 2-methyl propionate 0.5–25%, 2-methylpropyl butanoate 0.5–10%, 2-methylbutyl 2-methylbutanoate 0.5–25%, 2-methylpropyl 3-methylbutanoate 0–10%, propyl angelate 0.5–10%, 2-methylpropyl angelate 0.5–25%, butyl angelate 0.5–10%, 3-methylpentyl angelate 0–10% (Nano, Sacco & Frattini 1974), isobutyl angelate 36–40%, isobutyl isobutanoate 4%, 2-methylbutyl methyl-2-butanoate 3%, isoamyl methyl-2-butanoate 3%, propyl angelate 1%, hexyl acetate 0.5–10%, isobutyl tiglate, isoamyl tiglate, hexyl tiglate, crotanoates, methacrylates

Oxides
monoterpenoid 1,8-cineole 0–25%

Lactones
sesquiterpenyl 3-deshydronobiline

Properties	Indications
antianaemic	anaemia
antiinflammatory*	eczema, gout, inflamed skin, rheumatic pain, urticaria, skin irritation after shaving, cracked nipples, inflamed gums, neuritis, see Table 4.6
antineuralgic	
antiparasitic*	
antispasmodic*	migraines, headaches, (relaxes neuromuscular tension), infantile diarrhoea
calming, sedative	insomnia*, irritability, migraine, nervous depression*, nervous shock*
carminative	gas, intestinal colic
digestive	indigestion, loss of appetite, see Table 4.8
emmenagogic	nervous menstrual problems
menstrual	menopause, amenorrhoea, dysmenorrhoea
ophthalmic	conjunctivitis, sore tired eyes
stimulant	
sudorific	
vulnerary	boils, burns, wounds

Observations

- no contraindications known
- no irritation or sensitization at 4% dilution when tested on humans (Opdyke 1974e)
- no phototoxic effects reported (Opdyke 1974e)
- chamomile tea may cause anaphylaxis, contact dermatitis or other hypersensitivity reactions in allergic individuals; persons known to be allergic to ragweeds should be cautious about drinking chamomile or yarrow teas (Tyler 1982)
- the oil mixed with flour is a folk remedy for indurations of the liver, stomach and spleen (Duke 1985)
- oil is used in 'Kamillosan' ointment at 0.5% to treat nappy rash and cracked nipples; two women developed severe bilateral eczema using Kamillosan with 10.5% oil (McGeorge & Steele 1991)
- included in shampoos and for rinsing blond hair (Reynolds 1972)
- the oil is considered antispasmodic, carminative, cordial and sudorific (Duke 1985 p. 111)
- generally non-toxic when applied externally (Food and Drug Administration 1978)
- oil is active against *Staphylococcus aureus* and *Candida albicans* and is used as an inhalant (Bartram 1995 p. 106)
- in animals large dose produced sedation with drop in body temperature (Rossi et al 1988)
- the oil has antiinflammatory activity, antidiuretic and sedative effects following intraperitoneal administration in rats (Melegari et al 1988)

CINNAMOMUM VERUM FOL. [*CINNAMON LEAF*] LAURACEAE

Representative constituents

Hydrocarbons

monoterpenes β-phellandrene
sesquiterpenes (8%) α-ylangene 0.25–1%, β-caryophyllene 1.9–5.7%, humulene, *iso*-caryophyllene, α-copaene *trace*

Alcohols

monoterpenols α-terpineol 0.2–0.4%, linalool 2–5%
aromatic cinnamic alcohol 0.5–7%, benzyl alcohol *trace*

Esters *(9%)*

aromatic methyl cinnamate *trace*–0.3%, ethyl cinnamate *trace*–0.02%, benzyl benzoate *trace*–4.1%, 2-phenyl ethyl benzoate *trace*–2%, cinnamyl acetate, 3-phenyl propyl acetate 1%, decinnamyl acetate 0.8–1.6%, *trans*-cinnamyl acetate 0.8–4.6%, eugenol acetate 1–8.1%

Phenols *(80%)*

eugenol 68–87%, isoeugenol 0.15%, phenol 0.2%, 2-vinyl phenol *trace*

Aldehydes

aromatic cis-cinnamaldehyde 0.2–2%, hydroxycinnamaldehyde 0.15%, benzaldehyde *trace*–0.2%, coniferaldehyde, phenyl propanal *trace*

Ketones

monoterpenones camphor *trace*

Oxides

monoterpenoid 1,8-cineole

Properties	Indications
analgesic	toothache, rheumatism, gout pain
antiinfectious	oropharyngitis, cystitis, acute bronchitis, rhino-pharyngitis
antiinflammatory	stomatitis, salpingitis, enterocolitis, see Table 4.6
antifungal	see Table 4.5
antiparasitic	
antiviral	see Table 4.7
immunostimulant	increase IgA
neurotonic	
stimulating	

Observations

- cinnamon leaf oil has a different composition from the bark oil; the leaf oil consists chiefly of a phenol, is a powerful antiseptic but must be used sparingly because of the risk of skin irritation

- eugenol (present in cinnamon leaf oil) is reported to have weak tumour promoting action on mouse skin and weak cytotoxic activity against HeLa cells
- cinnamon leaf oil is dermocaustic on mucous surfaces and should not be used on babies and young children
- undiluted cinnamon leaf oil was moderately irritating when applied to the backs of hairless mice and strongly irritating when applied under occlusion to both intact and abraded rabbit skin
- 10% cinnamon leaf oil in petrolatum did not produce irritation or sensitization in humans
- leaf oil is used in soaps, creams, perfumes at a maximum level of 0.8% (Leung & Foster 1996 p. 168)
- eugenol, eugenol acetate and methyl eugenol are reported to enhance trypsin activity *in vitro* (Leung & Foster 1996 p. 168)

CINNAMOMUM VERUM CORT.
[CINNAMON BARK] LAURACEAE

Hydrocarbons
monoterpenes pinene, β-phellandrene 1–2%
sesquiterpenes β-caryophyllene 1.3–3.3%, α-copaene 0.5%
aromatic p-cymene

Aldehydes
aromatic cis-cinnamaldehyde (60–76%), benzaldehyde *trace*–2.2%, cuminaldehyde <1%, hydroxycinnamaldehyde 0.4%, phenyl propanal 0.6–1%
other furfurole

Phenols
phenol *trace*, 2-vinyl phenol 0.03%, eugenol 2–13%, iso-eugenol 0.02%

Methyl ethers
methyl eugenol

Benzodioxoles
safrole

Esters
aromatic benzyl benzoate <1%, 2-phenyl ethyl ester *trace*, menthyl cinnamate *trace*, eugenol acetate, *trans*-cinnamyl acetate 0.3–10.6%

Alcohols
monoterpenols linalool 0.2–3.1%, benzyl alcohol *trace*, terpinen-4-ol 0.6–1.1%, α-terpineol 0.4–1.4%
aromatic 2-phenyl ethyl alcohol 0.4%, cinnamyl alcohol 0.2%

Coumarins *(<1%)*

Ketones
monoterpenone camphor *trace*–1.4%

Oxides
monoterpenoid 1,8-cineole

Properties	Indications
alexipharmic	snake bites
analgesic	rheumatism
antibacterial	see Table 4.4
anticoagulant	
antifungal	see Table 4.5
antiinfectious	influenza, coughs, colds, diarrhoea, typhoid fever, tropical fevers, haemoptysis
antiparasitic	scabies, pediculosis
antiputrescent	
antiseptic	sprays to purify foul atmospheres, urinary infections
antispasmodic	colic, spasm due to infected enterocolitis
antiviral	warts, viral infections, see Table 4.7
astringent	tooth socket pyorrhoea, diarrhoea
bactericidal	dysentery, enterocolitis, diarrhoea, cystitis (bacterial), urinary infection, vaginitis, leucorrhoea
carminative	flatulence
emmenagogic	oligomenorrhoea

digestive	see Table 4.8
haemostatic	
larvicidal	
respiratory	bronchitis, pleurisy, sinus
tonic	impotence
uplifting, stimulating	fatigue, depression, asthenia, depression, tiredness
vermifuge	oxyures, amoebiasis

Observations

- cinnamon bark oil may be adulterated with cinnamon leaf oil and oil of cassia
- following ingestion of cinnamon, contact dermatitis may flare up as pompholyx (Mitchell & Rook 1979 p. 787)
- neither the bark nor leaf oil should be used on young children (Franchomme & Pénoël 2001 p. 362) or old people
- undiluted cinnamon bark oil was mildly irritating when applied to the backs of hairless mice and strongly irritating under occlusion to both intact and abraded rabbit skin
- 8% in petrolatum did not cause irritation but gave sensitization reactions in humans (Opdyke 1975a p. 13)
- cases of contact sensitivity to a dentifrice containing the oil have been reported
- low level phototoxicity is reported
- cinnamon bark oil must be regarded as a potential sensitizer on the skin and therefore used with great caution
- IFRA recommends that cinnamic bark oil should be used on the skin at a maximum presence of less than 1% in a mix to reduce the risk of sensitization reactions (IFRA 1992)
- IFRA make no recommendation regarding the leaf oil but there is a distinct risk of skin irritation particularly in people with sensitive skins, and both of these oils – as with any of the essential oils used in aromatherapy – should be employed only with great care, technical knowledge and respect
- some practitioners use the essential oil *per os* in case of urinary infections, since a urinary bacteriostatic activity has been demonstrated clinically (Bruneton 1995 p. 452)
- cinnamaldehyde has been shown experimentally to be CNS sedative in the mouse, and respiratory and myocardial stimulant in the dog (Bruneton 1995 p. 452)
- cinnamaldehyde is used mainly for flavouring cola-type drinks
- studies on cinnamon essential oil (unspecified) vapour showed complete inhibition of *Aspergillus niger* and *A. flavus* and a broad range of activity against a further 35 fungal species (Tiwari, Dixit & Dixit 1994)
- the wood and leaf oils of *Cinnamomum zeylanicum* were tested against *Candida albicans, C. glabrata, Microsporum canis, Trichophyton rubris* and *T. mentagrophytes* and found to be moderately active (Mastura et al 1999)
- essential oils of *Cinnamomum zeylanicum, Syzygium aromaticum* and their components cinnamal and eugenol respectively were studied for their effect on growth and aflatoxin production of *Aspergillus parasiticus*; the essential oils (above 250 ppm) and the two components (above 200 ppm) completely inhibited fungal growth and toxin production was not started (Bullerman, Lieu & Seier 1977)
- cinnamon bark oil and cinnamal were used in vapour toxicity tests against a range of fungi involved in respiratory tract mycoses; they were considered promising chemotherapeutic agents for respiratory tract mycoses as they could be inhaled and were lipolytic (Singh et al 1995)
- cinnamon oil and cinnamaldehyde were shown to have strong antibacterial properties against *Staphylococcus aureus, Streptococcus faecalis* and *Pseudomonas aeruginosa* (Lens-Lisbonne et al 1987)
- cinnamon bark oil *per os* might be best avoided in liver conditions, alcoholism, when taking paracetamol (Tisserand & Balacs 1995b p. 130) because of glutathione depleting action of cinnamaldehyde (Swales & Caldwell 1992)

CISTUS LADANIFERUS [LABDANUM] CISTACEAE

Representative constituents

Hydrocarbons

monoterpenes camphene 3–10.3%, α-pinene 3.5–50%, *p*-menthatriene 3.5%, limonene 2.3%, γ-terpinene 1.6%, α-terpinene 0.7%, β-pinene 0.5%, β-phellandrene 0.5%, α-phellandrene 0.2%

sesquiterpenes alloaromadendrene 1.2%, α-cubebene 0.2%, α-amorphene 1.0%, α-copaene 0.6%, γ-muurolene 0.4%, δ-cadinene 0.3%, calacorene 0.3%

aromatic p-cymene 4.0%, α-o-dimethyl styrene 0.1%, α-p-dimethyl styrene 1.6%

Alcohols

monoterpenols pinocarveol 3.4%, borneol 2%, linalool 0.5–1.9%, terpinen-4-ol, geraniol 0.8%, nerol

others cis-3-hexen-1-ol, *trans*-2-hexen-1-ol

Oxides

monoterpenoid 1,8-cineole 0.2%, *cis*-rose oxide 0.5%

Ketones

monoterpenones isopinocamphone 3.5%, verbenone 2.0%, fenchone 1%, pinocamphone, pinocarvone 0.6%, α-thujone, isomenthone

other 2,2,6-trimethylcyclohexanone 2–5.7%, acetophenone 1.5%, 2,2,6-trimethylcyclohex-2-enone 0.3%, 3-nonen-2-one 0.6%

Esters

monoterpenyl bornyl acetate 3–4%, linalyl acetate, *cis*-carvyl acetate, geranyl acetate

aromatic methyl benzoate, benzyl benzoate, thymol benzoate

Aldehydes

monoterpenals α-campholenic aldehyde 0.8%, γ-campholenic aldehyde

aromatic benzaldehyde

other dodecanal 1.1%, 2-methyl decanal 0.2%

Lactones

bicyclobutyrolactone, tuberolactone, 12-nor-ambeinolide

Phenols

eugenol 1%, thymol

Acids

α-campholytic acid, γ-campholytic acid

Properties	Indications
antibacterial	urinary tract infections, scarlet fever, see Table 4.4
antihaemorraghic	menorrhagia, haemorrhage
antiinfectious	childhood ailments (chicken pox, measles, whooping cough)
antiinflammatory	arteritis, rheumatoid arthritis, inflamed, sensitive skin, see Table 4.6
antiviral	childhood viral infections, see Table 4.7
cicatrizant	wounds, ulcers
diuretic	
neurotonic	regulates the parasympathetic system (sedative), chronic fatigue syndrome, anxiety, insomnia, multiple sclerosis

Observations

- no contraindications known at normal aromatherapeutic dose (Franchomme & Pénoël 2001 p. 363)
- labdanum oil is reported to be non-irritant, non-sensitizing and non-phototoxic to human skin (Opdyke 1974a, Opdyke 1976f)
- labdanum oil is obtained by distilling the oleo resin, labdanum gum, which is derived from boiling the plant material in water (Leung & Foster 1996 p. 337) or by distilling the leaves and twigs directly (Lawless 1992 p. 115)
- the myrrh of the Bible is now recognized to be correctly translated as labdanum (Tucker 1986) – but see also observation under *Commiphora myrrha*
- labdanum oil is used in perfumes at a maximum of 0.8%
- labdanum essential oil is active against *Staphylococcus aureus, Escherichia coli, Candida albicans* and other microbes (Leung & Foster 1996 p. 337); α-pinene, eugenol, 1,8-cineole and benzaldehyde were the most active components

CITRUS AURANTIFOLIA (C. MEDICA VAR. ACIDA) PER. [LIME] RUTACEAE
Expressed essence

Representative constituents

Hydrocarbons
monoterpenes (+)-limonene 36–60%, γ-terpinene 6–17.6%, α-pinene 0.2–1.9%, β-pinene 4.9–11.6%, camphene 0.4%, sabinene, α-terpinolene 1.2%, α-phellandrene 0.3–2.5%, β-myrcene 1–2.6%
sesquiterpenes β-caryophyllene 1.3–3.4%, α-bisabolene 2.3%, α-bergamotene, germacrene B 0.35%
aromatic p-cymene 0.1–6.8%

Alcohols
monoterpenols (–)-linalool 1.4–16.9%, borneol 0–0.9%, geraniol 0–0.5%, nerol, (–)-α-terpineol 13–23%, α-fenchyl alcohol 0.9%, β-terpineol 0–3%
other 3-methyl-3-buten-2-ol 0.2%, 3-methyl-2-butanol 0.4% , ethyl alcohol, *cis*-3-hexanol, isoamyl alcohol, *cis-p*-menth-2-en1-ol, methyl alcohol, 2-methyl-2-butanol, 2-methyl-3-buten-2-ol, 3-methyl-2-buten-1-ol

Aldehydes
monoterpenals perillaldehyde, geranial, neral, citronellal 0–5.3%
other hexanal, 2-hexanal, decanal 1.3%, octanol 0–6.5%, nonanal 0–0.9%, acetaldehyde

Esters *(10%)*
monoterpenyl linalyl acetate 26–27%, neryl acetate, *trans*-carvyl acetate 0.2%, *cis*-carvyl acetate
other ethyl acetate

Ketones
monoterpenone piperitone

Oxides
monoterpenoid 1,8-cineole 1.8%, *cis*-linalool oxide, *trans*-linalool oxide, 1,4-cineole

Coumarins *(7%)*
auropten, bergamottin, byakangelicin, 5-geranoxy-7-methoxycoumarin 2–2.5%, isopimpinellin, limettin, sesilin, bergapten, imperatorin, isoimperatorin, 8-geranoxypsoralen, 6,7-dimethoxycoumarin, bergaptol

Properties	Indications
antirheumatic	rheumatism
antiscorbutic	scurvy
antiseptic	sick rooms
antiviral	colds, influenza, warts, verrucas, see Table 4.7
aperitive, digestive	loss of appetite, nausea, see Table 4.8
bactericidal	unspecified
diuretic	
febrifuge	fever
tonic	

Observations

- expressed lime essence contains more coumarins than other citrus oils and has been reported to be phototoxic to humans (Opdyke 1974s p. 731)
- cold pressed lime essence contains similar compounds to the distilled oil but with fewer degradation products
- distilled lime oil is reported to be non-irritating, non-sensitizing and non-phototoxic to human skin (Opdyke 1974t p. 729)
- the total annual yield of lime essential oil is 400 metric tons, of which distilled oil forms the greatest part: distilled oil is much cheaper than the expressed essence which is preferred for aromatherapy
- the distilled oil is won from crushed whole fruit which is a by-product of the juice industry and contains few or no coumarins
- cymene results from the unavoidable decomposition of citral, especially during distillation
- maximum level of use in perfumery is 1.5%
- the lime grown in Italy is known as *Citrus limetta;* the peel is cold pressed to give limette essence; this is given as antispasmodic by Franchomme & Pénoël (2001 p. 367) who recommend it for enterocolitis spasm
- Roulier (1990 p. 297) groups under one heading the properties of lime and limette essences
- Lawless (1992) says that the home uses of lime essence are the same as for lemon essence

CITRUS AURANTIUM VAR. AMARA
FLOS [NEROLI BIGARADE] RUTACEAE

Representative constituents

Hydrocarbons
monoterpenes (35%) α-pinene 0.84%, β-pinene 13–14.3%, limonene 12–18%, sabinene 0.73%, β-myrcene 1.62%, *trans*-β-ocimene 3.65%

Alcohols
monoterpenols (40%) linalool 30–36.4%, α-terpineol 2–5%, geraniol 2–3%, nerol 1–3%
sesquiterpenols (6%) *trans*-nerolidol 3–6%, farnesol 1.7%
aromatic phenyl ethyl alcohol, benzyl alcohol

Esters *(7–21%)*
monoterpenyl linalyl acetate 4–8.9%, neryl acetate 0.8–3%, geranyl acetate 1–1.8%
aromatic methyl anthranilate B

Aldehydes *(2.5%)*
2.5-dimethyl-2-vinyl-hex-4-enal (Corbier & Teisseire 1974) and others (unspecified)

Ketones
monoterpenone jasmone

Oxides
monoterpenoid cis-linalool oxide

Properties	Indications
antibacterial	see Table 4.4
antidepressive*	nervous depression, neurasthenia
antiinfectious	colitis
antiparasitic*	
antitumoral	
digestive	liver and pancreas (diabetes), see Table 4.8
hypotensor	hypertension
neurotonic*	fatigue, aids sleep, sympathetic nervous system imbalance, spasms, cardiovascular erethism, sustains uterus tone
phlebotonic	haemorrhoids, varicose veins

tranquillizing (light)	anxiety
unspecified	bronchitis
unspecified	tuberculosis

Observations

- no known contraindications
- no irritation or sensitization at 4% dilution when tested on humans (Opdyke 1976h); devoid of irritating properties (Peterson & Hall 1946)
- it is essential to use the genuine version of this much adulterated and simulated oil. Neroli Portugal, the oil distilled from the flowers of the sweet orange tree, is of a lesser quality
- the vapour of neroli showed strong antibacterial activity *in vitro* against one of five bacteria (Maruzella & Sicurella 1960)
- a 1:50 dilution of neroli oil exhibited antifungal activity against all of a group of eight phytopathogenic fungi (Rao & Joseph 1971)
- no phototoxic effects reported (Opdyke 1976h)
- Huang et al (1981) showed that myrcenol and nerol possessed antiasthmatic activity
- bactericidal action five times greater than that of phenol (Reynolds 1972)
- some antifungal action (Maruzzella 1960)
- tests (on mice) demonstrated that neroli oil, citronellal and phenylethyl acetate all had sedative properties (Jäger et al 1992)

CITRUS AURANTIUM VAR. AMARA
FOL. [PETITGRAIN BIGARADE] RUTACEAE

Representative constituents

Hydrocarbons
monoterpenes (10%) β-myrcene 1–6%, β-pinene 0.7–1.7%, sabinene <0.4%, α-phellandrene *trace*–0.2%, limonene 0.7–1.1%, *cis*-β-ocimene *trace*–1.1%, γ-terpinene 0.5–1.1%, *trans*-β-ocimene *trace*–3.3%, α-terpinolene *trace*–0.1%, α-pinene *trace*, α-terpinene *trace*
aromatic p-cymene 1–3%

Alcohols
monoterpenols (30–40%) linalool 20–27.9%, α-terpineol 4.6–7.6%, nerol 1–2%, geraniol 2–4%, terpinen-4-ol 0.5–0.8%, citronellol *trace*–0.2%

Esters (50–70%)

monoterpenyl linalyl acetate 44–55%, neryl acetate 0.55–2.6%, geranyl acetate 2–3%, α-terpinyl acetate 0.2–2.2%

Aldehydes

monoterpenals neral *trace*, geranial *trace*
other decanal *trace*

Phenols

thymol *trace*

Coumarins

citropten, bergapten

Properties	Indications
antibacterial	see Table 4.4
antiinfectious	boils, infected acne*, respiratory infections
antiinflammatory	acne, see Table 4.6
antispasmodic*	
balancing*	sympathetic nervous system
calming	

Observations

- no known contraindications
- no irritation at 5% dilution when tested on humans (Fujii, Furukawa & Suzuki 1972)
- no irritation at 8% dilution when tested on humans (Ford, Api & Letizia 1992a)
- no phototoxic effects when tested on mice (Forbes, Urbach & Davies 1977)
- strong antibacterial and antifungal action (Lis-Balchin, Deans & Hart 1994, Maruzzella 1960, Maruzzella & Liguori 1958, Maruzzella & Sicurella 1960)
- the common name 'petitgrain' is used as a general term for oils distilled from the leaves of citrus trees, and so should be qualified to indicate from which tree the oil was obtained – orange (bitter or sweet), lemon, mandarin, etc.

CITRUS AURANTIUM VAR. AMARA
PER. [ORANGE BIGARADE] RUTACEAE
Expressed essence

Representative constituents

Hydrocarbons

monoterpenes (90–92%) limonene 90%, β-myrcene 1–2%, α-terpinolene, α-pinene 0.1–1%, camphene
sesquiterpenes caryophyllene, copaenes, farnesene, α-humulene

Alcohols (0.3–0.5%)

monoterpenols citronellol, α-terpineol, nerol, linalool, nerol

Aldehydes (0.9–3%)

monoterpenals geranial, neral
sesquiterpenals α-sinensal, β-sinensal
other undecanal

Esters (2%)

monoterpenyl linalyl acetate 1%, geranyl acetate, neryl acetate, citronellyl acetate

Coumarins (<1%)

osthol (7-methoxy-8-isopentenoxycoumarin), auraptenol (7-methoxy-8-(2-hydroxy-3-methyl-3-butenyl) coumarin), bergapten (5-methoxypsoralen), 7-geranoxycoumarin, 7-hydroxycoumarin, 5-isopentenoxypsoralen

Non-volatiles

β-carotene, flavonoids, fatty acids, triterpenoids

Properties	Indications
antiinflammatory	see Table 4.6
anticoagulant	poor circulation
calming*	gastric spasm, nervousness, sympathetic nervous system, vertigo, palpitations
cholagogic	
digestive	constipation*, liver stimulant, indigestion*, see Table 4.8
sedative*	anxiety

tonic*

tonic for the gums,
mouth ulcers

Observations (see also sweet orange oil)

- no irritation or sensitization at 10% dilution when tested on humans (Opdyke 1974g); cutaneous irritation has been reported (Schwarz, Tulipan & Peck 1947)
- a case of dermatitis has been reported in a girl employed to peel bitter orange (Murray 1921)
- phototoxic effects have been reported (Opdyke 1974g)
- it is lightly hypnotic (P Collin personal communication)
- the majority of the compounds in this oil are present at less than 1%
- orange oil spray had an antidepressant effect on patients (Rovesti & Colombo 1973)
- dried orange peel is used commonly by Puerto Ricans to treat sleep disorders, gastrointestinal disorders, respiratory ailments and raised blood pressure (Reynolds 1972)
- mouse skin tumours have been shown to be promoted by orange peel oil, assumed to be due to (+)-limonene; the oil is a very weak promoter of skin papillomas and carcinomas; neither the oil nor (+)-limonene had promotional activity when given orally (Elegbede et al 1986)
- fractions of orange and lime oils (terpinyl formate, terpinyl acetate and limonene oxide) were found to possess antifungal properties and activity against *Aspergillus*, *Fusarium* and *Rhizopus* species (Appaiah et al 1983)
- essential oils of German chamomile, orange and mandarin were tested in aqueous gels at 5% concentration; all three gels produced an immediate hydrating effect on the skin, with German chamomile producing a more intense and longer lasting hydration (Monges et al 1994)
- exposure to ambient odour of *C. sinensis* oil had a relaxant and anxiety reducing effect on female patients in dental premises, masking the smell of eugenol (Lehrner et al 2000)

CITRUS AURANTIUM VAR. *SINENSIS* PER. [SWEET ORANGE] RUTACEAE
Expressed essence

Representative constituents

Hydrocarbons
monoterpenes (95%) (+)-limonene >90%, β-myrcene 2.3%, camphene, α-pinene 0.9%, β-pinene 0.3%, *cis*- and *trans*-β-ocimenes, α-terpinolene *trace*, β-phellandrene 1.5%, sabinene 0.6%, γ-terpinene
sesquiterpenes β-caryophyllene *trace*, valencene, α-ylangene (Ramaswami et al 1988 p. 951)
aromatic p-cymene 0.2%

Alcohols
monoterpenols (+)-linalool 1.8%, (+)-α-terpineol 0.1–0.7%, nerol, geraniol 0.4%, *cis*-carveol, *trans*-carveol
sesquiterpenols farnesol, nerolidol
other octanol 0.2%

Aldehydes *(1.2–2.5%)*
monoterpenal citronellal 0.5%, neral
other decanal, *n*-octanal, nonanal, *n*-decanal, dodecanal, *trans*-2-hexenal, acetaldehyde, formaldehyde

Ketones
monoterpenone carvone 1.8%
other jasmone, α-ionone 0.7%

Esters *(0.2–0.4%)*
monoterpenyl linalyl acetate, geranyl acetate 0.1%
other ethyl butanoate, decyl pelargonate, octyl acetate

Coumarins
bergapten, aurapten, isoimperatorin, auraptenol

Free acids *(0.1–0.3%)*
octadecadienoic acid

Oxides
monoterpenoid trans-linalool oxide *trace*

Properties	Indications
antibacterial	unspecified
antidepressant	
antifungal	see Table 4.5
antiseptic	sore throat
antispasmodic	stomach cramp, spasm, diarrhoea, constipation
calming, mildly	anxiety, nervousness,
sedative	insomnia
carminative	dyspepsia
hypnotic, mildly	palpitations
stomachic	chronic diarrhoea, constipation (normalizing effect on peristalsis)

Observations (see also bitter orange oil)

- the expressed oils of bitter orange, sweet orange and neroli are reported to be non-irritating and non-sensitizing to humans but no phototoxicity is reported for expressed sweet orange oil despite the presence of coumarins (Opdyke 1974b p. 735, Opdyke 1974c p. 733, Opdyke 1976e p. 813)
- said by Franchomme & Pénoël (2001 p. 369) to be photosensitizing when used on the skin
- (+)-limonene (the major constituent of the oil) may cause contact dermatitis in humans
- orange oils, both bitter and sweet, are cold expressed from the fresh peel for aromatherapy use; alternatively the fresh or already pressed peel may be distilled to yield oils of a different quality; yet a third method is the distillation of the essences resulting from the production of orange juice
- orange oil is a source of (+)-limonene used for the synthesis of carvone
- (+)-limonene is reported to have anticarcinogenic activity (Opdyke 1974c p. 733)
- its normalizing effect on peristalsis makes it helpful in the treatment of constipation and diarrhoea
- sweet orange is recommended for those suffering from a deficiency of magnesium and calcium pectate (Rouvière & Meyer 1983 p. 30)
- sweet orange is used widely for care of skin problems (Rouvière & Meyer 1983 p. 30)
- sweet orange oil has been reported to promote tumour formation on mouse skin treated with a primary carcinogen (Nacino et al 1975)

- both bitter and sweet orange oils and neroli oil have been reported to exhibit antifungal and antibacterial activities *in vitro* (Murdock & Allen 1960, Opdyke 1976h p. 813, Rao & Joseph 1971)
- reported maximum level of use of sweet orange oil is 0.75% in sauces
- 21 essential oils were tested against seven bacteria and orange oil was found to be one of the most active (Kivanc & Akgul 1986)
- antimicrobial action of lemon and orange oils was investigated against seven bacteria, three yeasts and three *Aspergillus* species; orange oil was more effective than lemon oil and only orange oil inhibited the *Aspergillus* species (Subba et al 1967)
- sweet orange oil exhibited strong fungitoxicity against several fungal pathogens including *Aspergillus niger, A. flavus, A. parasiticus* and was shown to be more effective than commercial synthetic fungicides (Singh et al 1993)
- aurapten has been indicated as a chemopreventative of skin tumorigenesis (Murakami et al 1997)

CITRUS BERGAMIA PER. [BERGAMOT] RUTACEAE *Expressed essence*

Representative constituents

Hydrocarbons
monoterpenes α-pinene 0.5–1%, camphene trace–0.03%, limonene 26.7–42.5%, β-pinene 2.9–5.1%, sabinene 0.6–0.7%, β-myrcene 0.4–1.4%, δ-3-carene 0–2%, γ-terpinene 1.2–4.8%
sesquiterpenes β-bisabolene 0.02–0.9%
aromatic p-cymene 0.1–3.6%

Alcohols
monoterpenols (45–65%) linalool 11–22%, nerol, geraniol 0–5.6%, α-terpineol, dihydrocumin alcohol

Esters
monoterpenyl linalyl acetate 30–60%, geranyl acetate 0.6–1.3%, neryl acetate 0.5–0.9%

Aldehydes
monoterpenals geranial 0.1–0.5%, neral 0.04–0.4%

Coumarins, furanocoumarins
bergamottin 5% (5-methoxyfurano-2, 3, 6,
    7-coumarin)

Properties	Indications
antibacterial	see Table 4.4
antiinfectious	wounds
antiseptic*	intestinal, gas, colic, gargles for mouth and throat
antispasmodic*	colic, indigestion
antiviral	*Herpes simplex* I, see Table 4.7
calming*	insomnia
cicatrizant	burns
photosensitizers	vitiligo
sedative	agitation
stomachic*	loss of appetite
tonic	digestive system, central nervous system
unspecified	psoriasis

Observations

- not normally used prior to exposure to ultraviolet (UV) light because it is phototoxic to human skin on account of the bergamottin and bergapten compounds, which accelerate sun tanning (Musajo, Rodighiero & Caporale 1953, 1954, Pathak & Fitzpatrick 1959, Zaynoun, Johnson & Frain-Bell 1977)
- for the same reason some perfumes (e.g. eau de Cologne) should be used with care
- there is a melanoma risk associated with sun creams containing bergamot oil, but thought to be so because people who use these creams are more likely to spend more time in the sun
- in 1995 the EU limited furanocoumarins to 1 ppm in sun products
- a rectified oil did not exhibit any phototoxic effects; berloque dermatitis is due to bergapten (5–methoxypsoralen) and this must be reduced to 0.001% to obviate bergapten dermatitis (Marzulli & Maibach 1970)
- no sensitization at 30% dilution when tested on humans (Opdyke 1973c)
- undiluted oil is slightly irritating to skin

- distilled oil is obtained from the residue of cold extraction and small, unripe fruits which cannot be cold extracted
- bergamot oil is used in most perfumes as a natural fixative
- there are three cultivars of bergamot, namely Castagnaro, Feminello, Fantastico (by far the most popular (80%))
- natural bergamot is 60% of consumption, but reconstituted oils are often found
- there are approximately 350 constituents in bergamot essential oil
- in the presence of UVA, 5-methoxypsoralen is mutagenic *in vitro* (Averbeck et al 1990) and was carcinogenic when tested on mice (Young et al 1990, Zajdela & Bisagni 1981), but Mezzadra et al (1981) found no increase in cutaneous carcinogenesis in Calabrian workers in contact with bergamot oil and fruits
- berloque dermatitis, or bergapten dermatitis, is caused by exposure to UV light following bergapten application (Young et al 1990)
- the non-volatile residue of the cold-pressed oil has a CNS depressant action in rats (Occhiuto et al 1995)
- bergamottin has antiarrhythmic and antianginal effects on guinea pigs; the activity of bergamottin was equivalent to that of verapamil (Occhutio & Circosta 1996)
- tests showed that bergamottin (5-geranyloxypsoralen) possessed the characteristics of an antiarrhythmic drug with calcium antagonistic properties (class 4) (Occhutio & Circosta 1997)
- it has sedative action (Manley 1993)
- accidental bullous phototoxic reactions to bergamot oil have been reported: first, a woman used a bergamot 'aromatherapy' oil and then spent several hours outdoors on a sunny day; second, a woman took a sauna where bergamot oil was vaporized, then went directly to a tanning salon: both were treated with topical steroids and there was no residual hyper-pigmentation (Kaddu, Helmut & Wolf 2001). [Author's note: this could easily have been avoided by simply not exposing the skin to sunlight (or UV) for 2 hours. The sun tanning clinic was irresponsible.]

CITRUS LIMON PER. [LEMON]
RUTACEAE *Expressed essence*

Representative constituents

Hydrocarbons
monoterpenes (90–95%) limonene 55–80%,
α-pinene 1.9–2.4%, β-pinene 10–17%,
γ-terpinene 3–10%, sabinene 2%, α-thujene
0.01–0.4%, β-myrcene, α-phellandrene,
α-terpinene 0.2–0.4%
sesquiterpenes β-bisabolene 0.5–4%,
α-bergamotene 0.4%, β-caryophyllene 0.2%
aromatic p-cymene 1%

Alcohols
monoterpenols linalool 0.1%, terpinen-4-ol 0.05%,
α-terpineol 0.1–0.2%
other hexanol, N-heptanol, octanol, nonanol,
decanol

Aldehydes
monoterpenals geranial 0.9–1.6%, neral 0.5–1%,
citronellal 0.1%
other nonanal, octanal, decanal 0.05%

Esters
monoterpenyl neryl acetate 0.5%, geranyl acetate
0.5%, α-terpinyl acetate 0–0.7%

Coumarins, furanocoumarins
bergamottin 0.2%, citroptene, bergaptol *trace*,
phellopterin, bergapten 0.6%, oxypeucedanin,
imperatorin, isoimperatorin

Properties	Indications
antianaemic	anaemia
antibacterial*	see Table 4.4
anticoagulant	hypertension, phlebitis, poor circulation, thrombosis, varicose veins
antifungal	thrush, see Table 4.5
antiinfectious	respiratory system
antiinflammatory	boils, gout, insect bites, rheumatism, see Table 4.6
antimelanistic	brown skin spots, freckles
antisclerotic	combats ageing process
antiseptic* (air)	crèches, burns units, hospital wards
antispasmodic	diarrhoea
antiviral	colds, *Herpes simplex* I, verrucas, warts, see Table 4.7
astringent	diarrhoea, seborrhoea (scalp and face), oily skin, broken capillaries
calming	headache, insomnia, nightmares
carminative	flatulence, aerophagy
digestive	nausea, painful digestion, loss of appetite, see Table 4.8
diuretic	obesity, oedema
expectorant	respiratory system
immunostimulant	white cell deficiency
litholytic*	gall stones, urinary stones
pancreatic stimulant*	diabetes
phlebotonic	
stomachic	gastritis, stomach ulcers

Observations

- no irritation or sensitization at 10% dilution when tested on humans (Opdyke 1974h)
- no phototoxic effects reported for distilled lemon oil (Opdyke 1974i)
- the expressed oil is phototoxic (Opdyke 1974h), therefore exposure to sunlight is to be avoided for 1 hour after skin application
- in the case of expressed oils it is very important to ensure that the fruits have not been sprayed with chemicals
- non-volatile constituents make up about 2% of expressed lemon oil
- weak antibacterial and antifungal activity (Deans & Ritchie 1987)
- (+)-limonene preparation used to dissolve gall stones (Reynolds 1972)
- lemon oil spray relieved depression of patients (Rovesti & Colombo 1973)
- oil of lemon was found to have expectorant activity in guinea pigs (Boyd & Pearson 1946)
- lemon oil exhibits antimicrobial activity (Poretta & Casolari 1966, Subba et al 1967)
- patch tests showed a barman, who complained of chronic eczematous lesions on the hands

and occasional lip swelling and axillary itching, to be sensitive to lemon, lemongrass and neroli essential oils and the component geraniol; sensitivity was attributed to (+)-limonene (structurally similar to geraniol) (Audicana & Bernaola 1994)

- the phototoxic substances in lemon oil were found to be oxypeucedanin and bergapten; bergapten is four times more potent than oxypeucedanin (Naganuma et al 1985)

CITRUS PARADISI PER. [GRAPEFRUIT] RUTACEAE *Expressed essence*

Representative constituents

Hydrocarbons
monoterpenes (+)-limonene 93–98%, α-thujene *trace*, camphene *trace*, α-pinene 0.6%, β-pinene 0.1–0.2%, sabinene 0.5%, β-myrcene 1.9%, β-phellandrene 1.3%, γ-terpinene 0.1–0.3%, α-terpinolene *trace*, α-phellandrene *trace*, δ-3-carene *trace*, α-terpinene *trace*, *trans*-β-ocimene 0.15%
sesquiterpenes β-caryophyllene 0.3%, δ-cadinene <0.1%
aromatic p-cymene

Aldehydes *(1.5%)*
monoterpenals citronellal, neral, geranial, perillaldehyde
sesquiterpenals sinensals *trace*
other nonanal *trace*, decanal 0.26%, octanal 0.3%

Alcohols
monoterpenols geraniol *trace*, terpinen-4-ol, citronellol *trace*, linalool *trace*, α-terpineol *trace*, nerol *trace*

Ketones
sesquiterpenones nootkatone 0.1–0.3%

Esters
monoterpenyl neryl acetate *trace*–0.1%, geranyl acetate <0.1%, α-terpinyl acetate *trace*, citronellyl acetate *trace*, *trans*-carvyl acetate

Coumarins, furocoumarins
aesculetine, auraptene, limettin, bergaptol, 7-geranoxycoumarin, marmesin, osthol, bergapten, bergamottin
flavonoids, carotenoids

Properties	Indications
antiinfectious	colds, flu
antiseptic (air)	room disinfection
aperitive	
cleansing	to liver, kidneys, blood
digestive	see Table 4.8
haemostatic?	
slimming	cellulite
uplifting, refreshing	depression, headaches, exhaustion

Observations

- grapefruit oil is non-irritating, non-sensitizing and non-phototoxic to humans (Opdyke 1974v p. 723)
- care should be taken with external use of expressed grapefruit oil because of possible photosensitization (Franchomme & Pénoël 2001 p. 368)
- during storage, and on chilling, a yellowish brown flocculent precipitates which disappears again when warmed. This sediment may collect in cold storage for up to 2 years (95% of it after only 2 months)
- grapefruit oil can also be recovered by distillation of the crushed peel but has different properties, lower yield and is usually of a poorer quality
- distilled grapefruit oil has a higher aldehyde content than expressed oil, which may indicate that during expression aldehydes are lost by oxidation and reduction through the action of enzymes
- grapefruit oil has been reported to promote tumour formation on mouse skin (Rose & Field 1965)
- the aldehydes present make grapefruit essence prone to oxidation; it deteriorates upon exposure to moisture, air and light; the addition of antioxidants is not uncommon as this prolongs the shelf-life; they are effective in concentrations as low as 0.002%, which is far below the odour perception threshold
- used at a maximum level of 1% in perfumes
- grapefruit oil is not infrequently partially deterpenized; this is to be avoided for aromatherapy

CITRUS RETICULATA PER. [MANDARIN] RUTACEAE

Representative constituents

Hydrocarbons
monoterpenes limonene 65–77%, α-pinene 1.5–3%, β-pinene 1.3–2.5%, β-myrcene 1.6–2.2%, γ-terpinene 13.7–20.9%, α-terpinolene 0.6–1%, α-phellandrene 0.05–0.1%
aromatic p-cymene 1.2–3.6%

Alcohols
monoterpenols citronellol, linalool 1–5%, α-terpineol 0.1–0.25%
other nonanol, octanol 1%

Aldehydes *(1%)*
monoterpenal perillaldehyde <0.1%
sesquiterpenal α-sinensal 0.15–0.3%
other decanal 0.05–0.17%, octanal 0.1%

Phenols
thymol <0.1%

Esters
aromatic methyl N-methyl anthranilate 0.1–0.7%, benzyl acetate

Properties	Indications
antiepileptic	
antifungal	see Table 4.5
antispasmodic	hiccoughs, stomach cramp, spasm
calming*	insomnia, nervous tension, cardiovascular erethism, excitability
cholagogic	
digestive	indigestion, constipation, see Table 4.8
hepatic	
sedative	
stomachic	stomach pains

Observations

- because mandarin oil may be phototoxic, exposure to sunlight should be avoided for 2 hours after skin application
- no irritation or sensitization at 8% dilution when tested on humans (Ford, Api & Letizia 1992b)
- no coumarins were detected in mandarin oil by Shu, Waradt & Taylor (1975) but Franchomme & Pénoël (2001 p. 368) identify a presence
- an aqueous gel containing 5% mandarin produced an immediate hydrating effect on skin (Monges et al 1994)

COMMIPHORA MYRRHA VAR. MOLMOL (= C. MOLMOL, BALSAMODENDRON MYRRHA) RES. DIST. [MYRRH] BURSERACEAE

Representative constituents

Hydrocarbons
monoterpenes cis-β-ocimene 1.9%, *trans*-β-ocimene 1.27%, α-thujene 0.76%, β-myrcene 0.45%, limonene 0.42%, α-pinene
sesquiterpenes δ-elemene 28.79%, α-copaene 10.02–11.9%, β-elemene 6.19%, bourbonene 4.9%, α-bergamotene 4.9%, α-muurolene 0.14%, γ-cadinene 0.12%, curzerene (iso-furanogermacrene) 0.09–11.9%, α-caryophyllene 0.08%, heerabolene, β-elemene, lindestrene 3.5%, furanoeudesm-1,3-diene 12.5%
aromatic p-cymene 1.51%, xylene 2.84%

Ketones
sesquiterpenones curzerenone 11.7%
other methyl isobutyl ketone 5.68%, 3-methoxy-10 (15)-dihydrofuranodien-6-one 1.5%, 1, 10 (15)-furanodien-6-one 1.2%, dihydropyrocurzerenone (dihydrofuranoeudesmadiene) 1.1%, 3-methoxy-10-methylenefuranogermacr-1-en-6-one 0.9%, furanodien-6-one 0.4%, 6-methyl-5-hepten-2-one 0.23%, 3 methoxy-4,5-dihydrofuranodien-6-one 0.2%, 3-methoxyfuranoguai-9-en-8-one 0.1%

Aldehydes
aromatic benzaldehyde 0.53%, cuminaldehyde, cinnamaldehyde
other 5-methylfurfural 1.66%, furfural 1.44%

Phenols
m-cresol, eugenol

Methyl ethers
methyl anisole 0.14%

Alcohols
aromatic cuminyl alcohol

Acids
other acetic acid, formic acid, palmitic acid

Other
2-methyl-5-isopropenylfuran 4.63%,
   2-methylfuran 1.93%, 2-methyl-5-
   isopropylfuran 1.18%, 4,4-dimethyl-2-
   butenolide 1.04%, 2-phenyl-2-methylbutane
   0.14%, rosefuran 0.09%, tridecane 0.09%

Properties	Indications
antiinflammatory	see Table 4.6
antiseptic	urinary tract, cleansing sores, wounds, ulcers
antispasmodic	
astringent	
cardiac tonic	
carminative	flatulence, aerophagy
cicatrizant	wounds, skin diseases, mouth ulcers
emmenagogic?	
expectorant	bronchitis, laryngitis, influenza
sedative	
stomachic	
tonic	

Observations

- the oil was not irritating when applied to the backs of hairless mice and pigs (Urbach & Forbes 1973); 5% in petrolatum was not irritating and 8% in petrolatum was non-sensitizing (Epstein 1973)
- no phototoxicity on mice and swine has been noted (Urbach & Forbes 1973)
- acute oral toxicity LD_{50} 1.65 g/kg in rats (Moreno 1973)
- a flavour component of foods; a fragrance component or fixative in soaps, detergents, creams and lotions; used in perfumes (0.8% max.) (Opdyke 1976i)

- a leukocytogenic agent (increases number of white cells in blood) bacteriostatic against *Staphylococcus aureus* and other Gram-positive bacteria; perhaps the most widely used herbal antiseptic (Bartram 1995 p. 304)
- myrrh was always present in the coffins and as salve on the bodies in ancient Egypt
- Dioscorides mentioned myrrh as warming, astringent and 'numbing'; it was to some extent used as an anaesthetic in operations
- the condemned Christ was offered wine spiced with myrrh to diminish his suffering on the cross (Mark 15: 23). This use of wine containing myrrh or incense at the Flagellation and Crucifixion seems to have been customary in ancient times in order to diminish to some extent the sufferings of martyrdom (Storp 1996)
- bisabol myrrh is believed by some to be the myrrh of the Bible (Holmes 1916) – but see observation under *Cistus ladaniferus*

CORIANDRUM SATIVUM FRUCT.
[*CORIANDER*] APIACEAE

Representative constituents

Hydrocarbons
monoterpenes (10–20%) γ-terpinene 1–8%,
   limonene 0.5–4%, α-pinene 0.2–8.5%,
   camphene *trace*–1.4%, β-myrcene 0.2–2%
aromatic p-cymene *trace*–3.5%

Alcohols
monoterpenols (60–80%) linalool 60–87%, geraniol
   1.2–3.3%, terpinen-4-ol *trace*–3%, α-terpineol
   <0.5%

Ketones *(7–9%)*
monoterpenone camphor 0.9–4%

Esters
monoterpenyl geranyl acetate 0.1–4.7%, linalyl
   acetate 0–2.7%

Coumarins, furanocoumarins
umbelliferone *trace*, bergapten *trace*

Properties	Indications
analgesic	osteoarthritis, rheumatic pain
antibacterial*	see Table 4.4
antiinfectious*	cystitis, influenza
antiinflammatory	gastroenteritis, see Table 4.6
antispasmodic	digestive, uterine
carminative*	flatulence, aerophagy
euphoric*	sadness
larvicidal	
neurotonic*	anorexia, debility, general fatigue, mental fatigue
stomachic	indigestion, sluggish digestion

Observations

■ no irritation or sensitization at 6% dilution when tested on humans (Opdyke 1973d)

■ weakly cytotoxic

■ the linalool content depends upon the ripeness of the fruits and the geographical source, as do the proportions of the constituents

■ coriandrol is a synonym for (+)-linalool (Foster 1993b)

■ the leaf oil has the fragrance of decylaldehyde and other fatty aldehydes (Prakash 1990)

■ experimentally coriander is antiinflammatory and hypoglycaemic (Foster 1993b)

■ a Chinese remedy for measles, of value in diabetes (hypoglycaemic), gastroenteritis, also used for schistosomiasis (Bartram 1995 p. 128)

■ coriander oil is larvicidal, bactericidal and cytotoxic (Abdullin 1962, Silyanovska et al 1969)

■ coriander, laurel and sage oils, tested *in vitro* against 25 bacteria, demonstrated significant activity against seven species including *S. aureus* and exhibited antioxidant activity (Baratta, Dorman & Deans 1998)

CUMINUM CYMINUM FRUCT. [CUMIN] APIACEAE

Representative constituents

Hydrocarbons

monoterpenes (30–50%) β-pinene 14.4–18.7%, α-terpinene 12–28%, β-phellandrene 0.1–0.4%, α-terpinolene 0.04%, limonene 0.2–0.3%, α-pinene 0.3–0.9%, camphene 0.02%, β-myrcene 0.6–1%, δ-3-carene 0.5–0.8%, γ-terpinene 3.8–15.7%

sesquiterpenes β-caryophyllene, isocaryophyllene 0.2–0.3%, *cis*-β-farnesene 0.01–0.5%, cadinene, α-cubebene, β-cubebene, copaene, *trans*-α-bergamotene 0.01–0.1%

aromatic p-cymene 3–23%

Alcohols

monoterpenols linalool 0.03–0.1%, terpinen-4-ol 0.1–0.2%, α-terpineol 0.05–0.08%, *cis*-sabinene hydrate 0.1–0.2%

sesquiterpenol   cadinol

aromatic cuminol 0.1–0.8%

Aldehydes *(30–40%)*

aromatic cuminal 19.6–27.7%

monoterpenals p-menth α-1,3-dien-7-al 4.3–12.2%, *p*-menth-1,4-dien-7-al 24.5–49%

Phenols

thymol 0.02%, carvacrol 0–0.03%, *p*-isopropyl phenol 0.1–0.2%

Esters

monoterpenyl bornyl acetate 0.02%

Coumarins

scopoletin *trace*

Properties	Indications
analgesic	
antifungal	see Table 4.5
antiinflammatory	enterocolitis, arthritis, rheumatism, hepatitis, orchitis, see Table 4.6
antiseptic (urinary)	
antispasmodic	enterocolitis
aperitive	
calming*	insomnia, hyperthyroidism
carminative	aerophagy, flatulence
digestive	dyspepsia, colic, dyspeptic headache, see Table 4.8

Observations

- phototoxic effects have been reported for cumin oil but not for cuminal (Opdyke 1975 p. 12)
- cumin oil does not cause sensitization and may be mildly irritant on the skin (Tisserand & Balacs 1995b p. 205)
- weak antiviral activities in rats and antibacterial activity *in vitro* (Leung & Foster 1996 p. 200)
- cumin oil is used in veterinary digestive and carminative preparations
- the fruit essential oils of *Apium graveolens* and *Cuminum cyminum* were mixed in equal proportions and shown to have antifungal activity against *Aspergillus flavus* and *A. parasiticus*; individually the oils were not as effective (Mishra, Samuel & Tripathi 1993)
- *in vivo* studies in animals showed cumin oil increased significantly glutathione S-transferase activity in the liver (Aruna & Sivaramakrishnan 1996)
- cumaldehyde isolated from cumin essential oil produced 100% inhibition of *Aspergillus niger* and *A. flavus*; the residual oil had no activity (Singh & Upadhyay 1991)

CUPRESSUS SEMPERVIRENS FOL., STROB. [CYPRESS] CUPRESSACEAE

Representative constituents

Hydrocarbons
monoterpenes α-pinene 35–55%, β-pinene 3%, δ-3-carene 15–25%, limonene 2.5–5%, α-terpinolene 2.4–6%, sabinene 0.1–3%, γ-terpinene 0.3%, *cis-* and *trans-*β-ocimenes 0.4%
sesquiterpenes α-cedrene 0.4%, δ-cadinene 1.5–3%, β-cedrene 0.3%
aromatic p-cymene 0.2–1.5%

Alcohols
monoterpenols terpinen-4-ol, α-terpineol 1–2%, borneol 1–8.7%, linalool 0.8%, sabinol
sesquiterpenols cedrol 5.3–21%
diterpenols (*trace*) manool, abienols, pimarinols, totarol

Oxides
monoterpenoid 1,8-cineole 0.3%
manoyl oxide 0.5%

Esters
monoterpenyl α-terpenyl acetate 4–5%, terpinen-4-yl acetate 1–2%

Other
sandaracopimar-8(14),15-diene 1.3%

Properties	Indications
antibacterial	see Table 4.4
antiinfectious	bronchitis, influenza
antispasmodic	cramp
antisudorific	excessive perspiration
antitussive	whooping cough, bronchitis
astringent	broken capillaries
calming	regulates sympathetic nervous system, irritability
deodorant	sweaty feet
diuretic	oedema, rheumatic swelling
hormonelike	ovary problems, see Table 4.9
neurotonic*	debility
phlebotonic*	varicose veins, haemorrhoids, poor venous circulation, protects capillary circulation

Observations

- no contraindications known
- has a very remarkable astringent action, much superior to that of witch hazel (Duraffourd 1982)
- oil of cypress is a homologue of the ovarian hormone (Valnet 1980)
- no irritation or sensitization at 5% dilution when tested on humans (Opdyke 1978c)
- no phototoxic effects reported (Opdyke 1978c)
- found to be active against *Staphylococcus aureus*; antibacterial due to a synergy between citronellal and citronellol (90:7.5) producing a four-fold increase in activity (Low et al 1974)

CYMBOPOGON CITRATUS, C. FLEXUOSUS [LEMONGRASS] POACEAE

Representative constituents

Hydrocarbons

monoterpenes α-pinene 0.1–0.24%, β-pinene 0.2–1.65%, α-thujene 0.03%, β-myrcene 2.34–21%, limonene 2.4–2.6%, α-terpinolene <0.1%, δ-3-carene 0.2%, β-phellandrene <1%, camphene <0.1, *cis*-β-ocimene <0.1%, *trans*-β-ocimene <0.1%

sesquiterpenes β-elemene 1.3%, α- and β-caryophyllene

aromatic p-cymene 0.1–0.2%

Ketones

monoterpenone α-thujone 0.1%

other methyl heptenone 1.4–2.6%, 2-nonanone <0.1%, 6-methyl-5-hepten-2-one 0.5–2.3%, 2-undecanone 0.4–0.6%, 2-tridecanone 0.3%

Alcohols

monoterpenols α-terpineol 0.2–2.3%, borneol 0.1–1.9%, geraniol 0.1–4.4%, nerol 0.3–0.4%, linalool 0.8–1.5%, citronellol 0.1–8%, *trans-p*-menth-2-en-1-ol *trace*–0.1%

sesquiterpenols farnesol 12.8%

Aldehydes

monoterpenals (60–85%) neral 25–41.8%, geranial 4.5–58%, citronellal 0.1–9%

sesquiterpenals farnesal 3%

other nonanal <1%

Oxides

monoterpenoid 1,8-cineole 1.2%, β-caryophyllene oxide 0.6%

Esters

monoterpenyl linalyl acetate, geranyl acetate 1–3%, citronellyl acetate 1%, lavandulyl acetate 0.6%

Properties	Indications
analgesic	
antibacterial	Gram +ve organisms (Gyane 1976, Kokate & Varma 1971, Ramadan et al 1972), *Bacillus subtilis, Staphylococcus aureus, Escherichia coli* (Onawunmi & Oguniara 1981), see Table 4.4
antifungal	see Table 4.5
antiinflammatory	cellulite, inflamed arteries, see Table 4.6
antioxidant	
antipyretic	
digestive	digestion problems, see Table 4.8
insectifuge	see Table 4.10
sedative	CNS depressant effects
vasodilator	

Observations

- mildly irritating when applied to the backs of hairless mice and pigs
- moderately irritating under 24-hour occlusion on both intact and abraded rabbit skin
- 4% in petrolatum is non-irritant and non-sensitizing on human skin (Opdyke 1976b p. 457)
- no phototoxicity has been recorded
- source of citral (used for the synthesis of ionones and Vitamin A)
- used in perfumery, soap, laundry products and widely in food flavourings
- when taken internally caused damage to the intestines and death (Winter 1999 p. 276)
- citral has been reported to produce sensitization in humans when applied alone but to produce no such reactions when applied as a mixture with other compounds (Opdyke 1976a p. 197)
- a mild hormonelike (oestrogenic) action may be assumed from the citral content (Tisserand & Balacs 1995a p. 146)
- oral use of citral may cause a rise in ocular tension
- lemongrass oil is used in perfumes at a maximum of 0.7%
- the oil possesses biological activity against storage pests and has been used as a post harvest pesticide (Monograph 1990c p. 22)
- a geraniol chemotype exists with 35–50% geraniol, citral 10–20% and methyl eugenol (Atal & Bradu 1976)
- a borneol chemotype exists which has borneol 30% and citral 0% (List & Hörhammer 1969–1979)

- lemongrass oil was found to have a marked depressive effect on the central nervous system when tested on rats (Seth, Kokate & Varma 1976)
- *Cymbopogon martinii* and *C. citratus* were tested in vitro against *Aspergillus, Candida* and *Mucor* species, *Trichophyton rubrum* and *T. viollacellium*; both oils were fungicidal to all species tested (Singatwadia & Katewa 2001)
- citral possesses strong antiseptic and antibacterial activity (Onawunmi & Oguniana 1981)

CYMBOPOGON NARDUS [Sri Lanka citronella] and CYMBOPOGON WINTERIANUS [Java citronella] POACEAE

Representative constituents

Hydrocarbons

monoterpenes (15%) α-pinene 0.5–2.2%, camphene 2–7.6%, β-pinene *trace*, limonene 2.6–11.3%, sabinene 0.1–0.3%, α-terpinene, β-myrcene 0.2–0.8%, α-terpinolene 0.3–0.6%, δ-3-carene *trace*, α-phellandrene 0.1%, β-phellandrene 0.2–0.4%, tricyclene 1.2%, *cis*-β-ocimene 2.1%, *trans*-β-ocimene 1.1%

sesquiterpenes β-elemene 0.7%, δ-cadinene 0.6%, α-caryophyllene 1%, β-caryophyllene 0.1%, α-bergamotene *trace*–1%

aromatic p-cymene 0.1%

Alcohols

monoterpenols linalool 0.5%, nerol 0.6%, geraniol 17%, α-terpineol, citronellol 6.5%, terpinen-4-ol 0.4%, isopulegol 0.4%, α-terpineol 0.5–1%, borneol 5%

sesquiterpenols elemol 0.7%

Aldehydes

monoterpenals citral, citronellal 13–14%, geranial 0.6%, neral 0.4%

Ketones

methylheptenone 0.2%

Methyl ethers

methyl eugenol, *cis*-methyl isoeugenol 0.4%, *trans*-methyl isoeugenol 10%

Esters

monoterpenyl citronellyl acetate 1.1–2.3%, geranyl acetate 0.06–2.1%, bornyl acetate 0.5%, geranyl formate *trace*, β-terpinyl acetate 0.4%, geranyl butanoate 0.5%

Oxides

monoterpenoid 1,8-cineole
sesquiterpenoid caryophyllene oxide 0.1%

Properties	Indications
antibacterial	see Table 4.4
antifungal	see Table 4.5
antiinfectious	enterocolitis
antiinflammatory	arthritis, muscular rheumatism, see Table 4.6
antiseptic	(air) sickrooms
antispasmodic	colitis
deodorant	
diaphoretic	excessive perspiration
febrifuge	
insectifuge	mosquitoes, vermin, see Table 4.10
tonic, stimulant	fatigue
vermifuge	

Observations

- citronella oil reported to cause contact dermatitis in humans (Opdyke 1973a p. 1067)
- should not be used in case of pregnancy (Abrissart 1997 p. 166)
- citronella oil caused irritation on both intact and abraded rabbit skin
- some cases of an eczematous, contact-type of hypersensitivity to the oil have been reported
- citronella oil is a primary irritant in perfumes
- dilute preparations are non-irritating and non-sensitizing
- solubility decreased in 80% alcohol, relative density increased
- storage leads to polymerization, and polymers are not revealed by normal GC fingerprint (quantitative gas chromatography necessary with internal standards to detect the presence of polymeric material)
- the essential oils come from many sources (Sri Lanka, Java, Taiwan, Malaysia, Madagascar,

Central and South America, India, China) all differing slightly in composition

■ Ceylon citronella and Java citronella have similar compositions and many properties in common, although the Java oil is considered to be superior because it has a higher content of aldehydes (up to 50% citronellal) and the anti-infectious property is enhanced

■ the Java citronella oil (*C. winterianus*) has up to 45% geraniol

■ the fragrance of citronella oil is similar to that of melissa oil and according to Weiss (1988a p. 33) the two oils have similar actions

■ spirit of melissa compound listed in the German Pharmacopoeia does not contain melissa but citronella oil instead (Weiss 1988a p. 33)

■ citronella oil may cause allergic reactions such as stuffy nose, hay fever, asthma and skin rash when used in cosmetics (Winter 1999 p. 130)

■ a slow release citronella formulation was shown in a double blind randomized study to be effective in significantly lowering the incidence of head lice reinfestation in children (Kosta et al 2004)

ELETTARIA CARDAMOMUM
[CARDAMOM] ZINGIBERACEAE

Representative constituents

Hydrocarbons
monoterpenes (5–17%) limonene 1.7–14%, sabinene 2.5–5%, α-pinene 0.6–1.6%, camphene *trace*, β-pinene 0.2–0.4%, β-myrcene 0.2–2.2%, α-phellandrene *trace*, α-terpinene 0.1%, γ-terpinene 0.3%, α-terpinolene 0.3%, *cis*-β-ocimene *trace*, *trans*-β-ocimene *trace*
sesquiterpenes (<1%) β-caryophyllene *trace*, δ-cadinene *trace*
aromatic p-cymene 0.2%

Alcohols
monoterpenols linalool 0.4–6.9%, borneol <0.3%, terpinen-4-ol 0.1–3.2%, α-terpineol 0.8–4.3%, citronellol *trace*, nerol 0.1–0.7, geraniol 0.2–1.6%
sesquiterpenols farnesol *trace*, *trans*-nerolidol 0.1–2.7%, *cis*-nerolidol 0.2–1.6%
other octanol 0.7%

Aldehydes
monoterpenals neral 0.1–0.2%, geranial 0.3%

Phenols
p-cresol *trace*

Methyl ethers
methyl eugenol *trace*

Esters
monoterpenyl α-terpinyl acetate 29–52%, linalyl acetate 0.2–7.7%, neryl acetate *trace*, geranyl acetate *trace*, α-terpinyl propionate *trace*

Ketones
methyl heptenone *trace*

Oxides
monoterpenoid 1,8-cineole 23–50%, 1,4-cineole

Acids
acetic acid, butanoic acid, decanoic acid, dodecanoic acid, citronellic acid, geranic acid, hexanoic acid, heptanoic acid, nerylic acid, perillic acid

Properties	Indications
analgesic	
antiinflammatory	see Table 4.6
antiseptic	pulmonary disorders, coughs, halitosis
antispasmodic	griping caused by purgatives, colic
carminative	flatulent dyspepsia
cephalic	
digestive	sluggish digestion, nausea, digestive headaches, see Table 4.8
diuretic	
stimulant	

Observations

■ essences of cardamom (or cardamum) come from the distillation of either the fruit (shells and seeds) of *Elettaria cardamomum* or the white almonds of *Amomum afzelii* (grains of paradise)

■ non-toxic, non-irritating and non-sensitizing and no phototoxic effects reported

■ antispasmodic on excised mouse intestine

- an ingredient in Compound Cardamom Spirit to flavour pharmaceuticals (Leung & Foster 1996 p. 122)
- seed pods from other members of the ginger family are frequently offered as cardamom but are inferior (Stuart 1982 p. 57)
- used as a flavouring agent in curries, pickles and mixed spices; also used in mulled wine and Persian coffee (Stuart 1982 p. 57)
- three drops of cardamum oil in honey after meals promotes digestion, removes odour of garlic, onions, etc (Bartram 1995 p. 98)
- in tests on animals the oil was confirmed to be antiinflammatory, analgesic and antispasmodic (Al-Zuhair et al 1996, El Tahir, Shoeb & Al-Shora 1997)
- when tested cardamom essential oil had considerable effect against seven pathogenic moulds – *Aspergillus flavus, A. parasiticus, A. ochraceous* and four *Penicillium* species – and had a strong inhibitory effect against the formation of aflotoxins (Badei 1992a,b)

EUCALYPTUS CITRIODORA FOL. [*LEMON SCENTED GUM*] MYRTACEAE

Representative constituents

Hydrocarbons

monoterpenes (1–12%) α-pinene 0.2–1.9%, camphene *trace*, β-pinene 0.4–1.5%, α-phellandrene, limonene <7.1%, γ-terpinene <0.9%, p-menth-3,8-diene 0.2%, α-terpinolene 0.1–0.8%, β-myrcene <0.6%
sesquiterpenes caryophyllene 0.3–3.9%, α-humulene 0.1%, β-cubebene 0.1%, α-elemene 0.1%, aromadendrene
aromatic p-cymene 0.1–0.9%
other isopropyl hexane 0.3%, *trans-p*-menthane, (1-methyl-4-isopropyl-cyclohexane) *trace*

Alcohols

monoterpenols citronellol 4.6–14.4%, geraniol <5%, α-terpineol 0.1%, nerol *trace*, linalool 0.3–1.5%, *trans*-pinocarveol, isopulegol 0.3–29.8%, 1,8-terpin hydrate 0.8%
sesquiterpenols (2–4%) spathulenol 0.1%
diols trans- and *cis-p*-menthan-3,8-diols

Phenols
eugenol

Aldehydes
monoterpenals citronellal 26.7–90.1%, geranial, citronellal *trace*, hydroxycitronellal
other 2,6-dimethyl-5-heptenal 0.2%

Esters
monoterpenyl citronellyl acetate 0.4–3.1%, citronellyl butanoate, citronellyl citronellate, methyl-*cis*-9-octadecenoate *trace*

Ketones
monoterpenones carvone, menthone *trace*

Oxides
monoterpenoid 1,8-cineole 0.4–17.9%, *cis*-rose oxide 0.4%, linalool oxide 0.4%

Properties	Indications
analgesic*	
antidiabetic	diabetes (some)
antifungal	see Table 4.5
antiinfectious	shingles
antiinflammatory	arthritis, cystitis, vaginitis, pericarditis, coronaritis, see Table 4.6
antirheumatic*	rheumatoid arthritis
antispasmodic	
bactericidal	*Staphylococcus aureus*
calming, sedative	hypertension

Observations

- no known contraindications
- makes a synergistic mix with copaiba balsam, wintergreen and *Helichrysum italicum* (Roulier 1990)
- the tree is grown in many tropical areas for its wood and as a source of citronellal
- four forms have been identified (Penfold & Willis 1961):
  1. citronellal 65–85%, citronellol 15–20%, esters
  2. citronellal 1–14%, citronellol, esters
  3. citronellal 10–50%, guaiol
  4. hydrocarbons

- bacteriostatic properties are due to natural synergism between citronellal and citronellol. The oil is active against *S. aureus* and has a minimal inhibitory concentration of 1:32. Tests on the individual components of this oil showed them to be relatively inactive but a combination of the three major components in the ratio found in the natural oil produced a fourfold increase in antimicrobial activity (Low, Rawal & Griffin 1974)
- inhibits *Trichophyton mentagrophytes* and *Microsporum audonii* (Yadav & Dubey 1994); active antibacterial agent (Asre 1994)
- effective against *Candida* and other fungi (Asre 1994)
- *E. citriodora* was found to be effective against *Escherichia coli, Bacillus megaterium, Staphylococcus aureus, Candida albicans, Saccharomyces cereviciae, Aspergillus niger* and *Zygorrhynchus* species; activity was due to synergy between citronellal and its derivative alcohol, acid and ester and was not necessarily due to the amount of 1,8-cineole as previously thought (Hmamouch et al 1990)
- of 21 Moroccan eucalyptus oils tested against *E. coli, Staphylococcus aureus, Bacillus megaterium, Aspergillus niger* and *Candida albicans* the volatile constituents of *E. citriodora* were the most effective (Hajji & Fkih-Tetouani 1993)
- *trans-* and *cis-p*-menthan-3,8-diols are allelopathic substances

EUCALYPTUS DIVES CT. PIPERITENONE *FOL. [BROAD-LEAVED PEPPERMINT]* MYRTACEAE

Representative constituents

Hydrocarbons
monoterpenes α-phellandrene 30%
sesquiterpenes α-cubebene, β-caryophyllene, longifolene, γ-elemene, δ-cadinene

Alcohols
monoterpenols α-terpineol, linalool, terpinen-1-ol-4, piperitol

Ketones
monoterpenones piperitone 40–50%

Properties	Indications
antibacterial	see Table 4.4
anticatarrhal	
antifungal	see Table 4.5
antiinfectious	sinusitis, otitis, bronchitis, nephritis, vaginitis (leucorrhoea)
antiviral	see Table 4.7
cicatrizant	wound healing
diuretic	
lipolytic	
mucolytic	

Observations

- contraindicated for babies and pregnant women (Franchomme & Pénoël 2001 p. 379)
- generally regarded as safe in normal aromatherapy use
- this species is not generally cultivated therefore the oil comes from wild plants (Weiss 1997 p. 279)
- there are at least four distinct chemotypes of *E. dives* (Boland, Brophy & House 1991) including a cineole type (up to 75%) closely related to *E. radiata* and a phellandrene type (up to 80%) used in industrial perfumery and insecticides
- piperitone is antiasthmatic and insectifuge (Beckstrom-Sternberg & Duke 1996 p. 411)

EUCALYPTUS GLOBULUS FOL. [*TASMANIAN BLUE GUM*] MYRTACEAE

Representative constituents

Hydrocarbons
monoterpenes α-pinene 3–27%, limonene 1.8–9%, camphene 0.2–0.4%, α-phellandrene 0.2%
sesquiterpenes aromadendrene 0.1–6%
aromatic p-cymene 1.2–3.5%

Alcohols
monoterpenols α-fenchyl alcohol 1–2%, α-terpineol 0.1–0.6%, myrtenol 1.3%, *trans*-pinocarveol 0.8–4.5%
sesquiterpenols globulol 0–6%, ledol 1–2%, viridiflorol, epi-globulol

Aldehydes

monoterpenals myrtenal, geranial
other valeraldehyde, butyraldehyde,
    caproaldehyde

Ketones

monoterpenones pinocarvone 1–2%, carvone 0.1%,
    fenchone 0.4%

Oxides

monoterpenoid 1,8-cineole 60–85%, α-pinene
    epoxide 0.2%

Esters

monoterpenyl α-terpenyl acetate 0.1–2%

Properties	Indications
antibacterial	see Table 4.4
anticatarrhal	coughs, sinusitis
antifungal	*Candida*, see Table 4.5
antiinfectious	acute bronchitis, coughs, influenza, pneumonia, respiratory tract infections, sinusitis, laryngitis
antiinflammatory	pleurisy, bronchitis, sinusitis, laryngitis, cystitis, see Table 4.6
antimigraine	migraine
antiseptic*	cystitis, urinary tract infection
antiviral	colds, influenza, see Table 4.7
balsamic	combats fever and acts like a balm
decongestant	asthma, headaches, migraine
expectorant*	bronchitis, cough, catarrh, cold
insectifuge	gnats, mosquitoes, see Table 4.10
mucolytic	cough, sinusitis
rubefacient	subcutaneous infection, arthritis

Observations

- contraindicated for very young children and babies because of the high cineole content: several cases of poisoning in children have been reported (Craig 1953, Foggie 1911, Kirkness 1910, McPherson 1925, Neale 1893, Patel & Wiggins 1980, Sewell 1925)
- as with many essential oils in excessive dose, eucalyptus oil has caused fatalities from intestinal irritation (Morton 1981); death is reported from ingestion of widely differing quantities of 4–24 ml essential oil, but recoveries are also reported for the same amounts (Reynolds 1972)
- eliminated from the body via the respiratory tract
- it may be necessary to rid certain eucalyptus oils of some short chain aldehydes (e.g. valerian aldehyde, butyraldehyde, capronaldehyde), which are irritant and tussigenic (Belaiche 1979, Wagner, Bladt & Zgainski 1984)
- no irritation or sensitization at 10% dilution when tested on humans (Opdyke 1975d)
- hypersensitivity has been reported (Goodman & Gilman 1942, Löwenfeld 1932, Schwartz & Peck 1946, Schwartz, Tulipan & Peck 1947)
- no phototoxic effects reported (Opdyke 1975d)
- there is a difference between the oils from the young leaves and those from the old leaves
- *E. globulus* oil is used in catarrhal conditions, given orally on a lump of sugar or as an emulsion with olive oil (Reynolds 1972)
- found to increase output of respiratory tract fluid in guinea pigs (Boyd & Pearson 1946)
- the oil is used in cough drops as antiseptic, rubefacient and stimulant (Morton 1981)
- used in Cuba for bronchitis, bladder and liver infections, lung ailments, malaria and stomach trouble (Morton 1981)
- the oil has antibacterial and expectorant properties (Maruzella & Henry 1958, Pizsolitto 1975, Prakash et al 1972)
- strongly antibacterial against several *Streptococcus* strains (Benouda, Hasser & Benjilali 1988)
- oil is used as an antiseptic, febrifuge and expectorant (Bisset 1994, Wren 1988)
- the oil is taken orally for catarrh and applied as a rubefacient (Reynolds 1989)
- eucalyptole (1,8-cineole) and α-pinene were found not to be responsible for antimicrobial activity of 21 Moroccan eucalyptus oils (Zakarya, Fkih-Tetouani & Hajji 1993)

- different eucalyptus oils were investigated for antibacterial activity against 15 pathogenic and non-pathogenic bacteria; Gram-positive organisms were found to be more sensitive than Gram-negative (Kumar et al 1988)
- a commercial repellent (Mosi-guard Natural®) containing principally *p*-menthane-3,8-diol with isopulegol and citronellol tested on humans gave 6–8 hours' protection against mosquitoes *Anopheles gambiae* and *Anopheles funestus* (Trigg 1996)
- a component of eucalyptus oil, *p*-menthane-3,8-diol, had good insect repellency against *Anopheles gambiae* lasting 5 hours, comparing favourably with DEET and was better than citronella; also afforded protection against the biting midge *Culicoides variipennis* for 6 hours (Trigg & Hill 1996)
- Tovey & McDonald (1997) showed that a low concentration of eucalyptus oil used in a washing cycle killed live house dust mites (*Dermatophagoides pteronyssinus*)
- it was shown *in vitro* that the oils of *Melaleuca alternifolia* and *Eucalyptus globulus* had a concentration dependent antiviral effect when in contact with *Herpes simplex* prior to or during adsorption (Schnitzler, Schon & Reichling 2001)
- a blend of phytochemicals (*Eucalyptus globulus*, *Melaleuca alternifolia*, *Thymus species*, *Syzygium aromaticum*, citrus extracts and bioethanol) was successfully used in two cases to treat methicillin resistant *Staphylococcus aureus*; there was no recurrence of the infection (Sherry, Boeck & Warnke 2001)
- *E. citriodora* (60% citronellal), *Eucalyptus tereticornis* and *E. globulus* (both 60–90% 1,8-cineole) showed antiinflammatory, peripheral and central analgesic effects on animals (Silva et al 2003)

EUCALYPTUS RADIATA SUBSP. *RADIATA* (= *E. NUMEROSA*, *E. LINDLEYANA*) FOL. [BLACK PEPPERMINT, NARROW LEAVED PEPPERMINT] MYRTACEAE

Representative constituents

Hydrocarbons
monoterpenes α-pinene 3.7%, β-pinene 1.0%, β-myrcene 2.0%

Alcohols
monoterpenols linalool 0.4%, geraniol 2.6%, (–)-α-terpineol 14.0%, isoterpineol 4 2.0%, borneol

Aldehydes
monoterpenals geranial, neral, citronellal, myrtenal

Oxides
monoterpenoid 1,8-cineole 62–72%, caryophyllene oxide

Properties	Indications
anticatarrhal	
antiinfectious	acute and chronic respiratory infections, influenza*
antiinflammatory	rhinitis, rhinopharyngitis, otitis, bronchitis, conjunctivitis, vaginitis, acne, see Table 4.6
antiseptic	strong antiseptic
antiviral	influenza, see Table 4.7
energizing*	chronic fatigue, immune deficiency
expectorant	
mucolytic	coughs, powerful expectorant and fluidification properties (especially when blended with *Eucalyptus smithii*)

Observations

- long-lasting action, quick penetration
- particularly indicated for children (Roulier 1990)
- no contraindications known
- it is important to blend with a terpene rich oil for best results
- Weiss (1997 p. 294) gives phellandrene as a major constituent at up to 40%

EUCALYPTUS SMITHII FOL. [*GULLY GUM*] MYRTACEAE

Representative constituents

Hydrocarbons
monoterpenes (20%) limonene 9–10%, α-pinene 7%
aromatic p-cymene

Alcohols
monoterpenols terpineol, terpineol-4, geraniol,
   linalool
sesquiterpenols eudesmol

Oxides
monoterpenoid 1,8-cineole 70–80%

Esters
small quantities

Aldehydes
isovaleraldehyde

Properties	Indications
analgesic	painful joints and muscles
anticatarrhal	bronchitis, coughs
antiinfectious	respiratory system
antiviral	colds, influenza, see Table 4.7
balancing	calming and stimulating
decongestant	asthma, headaches
digestive	stimulant, sluggish digestion, see Table 4.8
expectorant	bronchitis, coughs
prophylactic	colds, influenza

Observations

- no contraindications known
- the oil has great synergistic and quenching properties (Pénoël 1993)
- an effective chest rub; may be used undiluted

EUCALYPTUS STAIGERIANA [*LEMON SCENTED IRONBARK*] MYRTACEAE

Representative constituents

Hydrocarbons
monoterpenes limonene 1–14%, β-phellandrene
   12–34%
aromatic p-cymene 2%

Alcohols
monoterpenols nerol 3%, geraniol 9–18%

Aldehydes
monoterpenals neral 8–12%, geranial 13%

Oxides
monoterpenoid 1,8-cineole 6%

Esters
monoterpenyl methyl geranate 11–18%, geranyl
   acetate 4–14%

Properties	Indications
antiinfectious	
antiinflammatory	see Table 4.6
antispasmodic	
calming	anxiety

Observations

- no known contraindications

FOENICULUM VULGARE VAR. *DULCE* FRUCT. [*SWEET FENNEL*] APIACEAE

Representative constituents

Hydrocarbons
monoterpenes α-pinene 1.4–10%, limonene 1.4–17%,
   α-phellandrene 0.2–4%, α-thujene 0.2%,
   camphene 0.2%, β-pinene 0.3–1%, sabinene 2%,
   β-myrcene 0.5–3%, α-terpinene 0.5–1%, β-
   phellandrene 0.4–2.6%, γ-terpinene 10.5%, *cis*-β-
   ocimene 12%, α-terpinolene *trace*–3.3%
aromatic p-cymene 0.4–4.7%

Alcohols
monoterpenols fenchol 3–4%

Ketones
monoterpenones fenchone *trace–22%*

Methyl ethers
methyl chavicol 2–12%, *cis*-anethole *trace–1.7%*,
trans-anethole 50–90%

Aldehydes
anisaldehyde *trace–0.5%*

Oxides
monoterpenoid 1,8-cineole 1–6%

Coumarins, furanocoumarins
bergapten, umbelliferone

Properties	Indications
analgesic	backache, gout, painful menstruation
antibacterial	see Table 4.4
antifungal	see Table 4.5
antiinflammatory	cystitis, gout, see Table 4.6
antiseptic	urinary tract infections
antispasmodic	gastroenteritis
cardiotonic	heart palpitations
carminative*	flatulence
cholagogic	
circulatory stimulant	
decongestant	breast engorgement, bruises
digestive	indigestion, loss of appetite, see Table 4.8
diuretic	cellulite, oedema
emmenagogic	lack of, irregular or scanty menstruation*
hormonelike	see Table 4.9
lactogenic*	lack of milk in breastfeeding mothers*
laxative	constipation
litholytic	urinary stones
oestrogen-like*	ovary problems, PMS, menopause
respiratory tonic	hyperpnoea

Observations

- must be well-diluted for young children and is best avoided in pregnancy until last 2 months
- if the oil is given in excessively high dose it may cause disturbance of the nervous system, but is safe when used in the amounts normally employed in aromatherapy
- no irritation or sensitization at 4% dilution when tested on humans (Opdyke 1974j)
- no phototoxic effects reported (Opdyke 1974j)
- large doses of oil reduced the body weight of mice
- has an epileptic action at high dose (Roulier 1990)
- special consideration must be given to the amount used when treating young children (note: it is an ingredient of gripe water); fennel oil is used as a carminative for children (Reynolds 1972)
- has caused pulmonary oedema, respiratory problems, and seizures in quantities of 1–5 ml; for this reason, self-medication with fennel should be restricted to moderate use of the fruits (seeds), and the volatile oil should not be used (Tyler 1982)
- anethole is reported to have allergenic and toxic properties; its structural similarity to catecholemines (adrenalin, noradrenalin, dopamine) may help to explain its ephedrine-like bronchodilator action and amphetamine-like facilitation of weight loss; similarity of anethole to the psychoactive compounds mescaline, asarone and myristicin has been noted (Mills 1991); fennel oil is oestrogen-like (Albert-Puleo 1980, Zondek et al 1938)
- therapeutic doses of the distilled oil of fennel occasionally induced epileptiform madness and hallucinations; dill, anise and parsley (plants) all have similar oils, and it has been demonstrated that *in vivo* amination of these ring-substituted oils can result in a series of three hallucinogenic amphetamines (Emboden 1972)
- due to anethole content it is best avoided in liver disease and when taking paracetamol
- the oil is recommended for hookworm (Council of Scientific and Industrial Research 1948–1976)
- best avoided in alcoholism, liver disease, and if taking paracetamol owing to anethole content
- exhibits antibacterial activities (Ramadan et al 1972b)
- potentially carcinogenic depending on dosage, assumed owing to estragole content, oral dose

not recommended (Drinkwater et al 1976, Swanson et al 1981, Zangouras et al 1981)

- the essential oil of fennel is used as a lactogenic in cases of deficiency of milk in nursing mothers, but puerperal lactation may be suppressed by the use of the flowers and inhalation of *Jasminum sambac* (Abraham et al 1979, Shrivastav et al 1988)
- *in vitro* investigation of the antimicrobial activity showed synergistic blends of essential oil of *Foeniculum vulgare* and paraben effective against *Escherichia coli, Staphylococcus aureus* and *Candida albicans* (Hodgson, Stewart & Fyfe 1998)
- essential oils of fennel bulb, leaf and flowering umbels were found *in vitro* to be antispasmodic on rat ileum and urinary bladder (Saleh, Hashem & Grace 1996)
- studies on isolated rat uterus showed significant reduction in intensity of oxytocin and prostaglandin induced muscle contractions, with a reduction in frequency of contractions by prostaglandin but not by oxytocin (Ostad et al 2001)
- 0.1% fennel seed oil emulsion was effective in decreasing the intensity of infantile colic with no side-effects (Alexandrovitch et al 2003)
- fennel oil showed strong fungitoxic activity against *Aspergillus flavus* and *Penicillium italicum* and showed a broad spectrum of activity against 31 other fungi including nine *Aspergillus* species (Shukla & Tripathi 1987b)

HELICHRYSUM ANGUSTIFOLIUM (= H. ITALICUM) FLOS [EVERLASTING, IMMORTELLE] ASTERACEAE

Representative constituents

Hydrocarbons
monoterpenes α-pinene, camphene, β-pinene, β-myrcene, limonene, *cis*-β-ocimene, *trans*-β-ocimene

Alcohols
monoterpenols linalool, terpinen-4-ol, nerol, geraniol

Phenols
eugenol

Ketones
diones italidiones 15–20%, beta-diketones, 2,5,7-trimethyldec-2-en-6,8-dione, 2,5,7,9-tetramethyldec-2-en-6,8-dione, 2,5,7,9-tetramethylundec-2-en-6,8-dione, 3,5-dimethyloctan-4,6-dione, 2,4-dimethylheptan-3,5-dione
other 4,7-dimethyloct-6-en-3-one

Esters
monoterpenyl neryl acetate 75%

Oxides
monoterpenoid 1,8-cineole

Properties	Indications
antiallergic	asthma, hay fever, eczema
anticoagulant	
antidiabetic	
antifungal	*Candida albicans*, see Table 4.5
antiinfectious	
antiinflammatory	arthritis, polyarthritis (with wintergreen or sweet birch), dermatitis, salivary gland inflammation, rhinitis, sinusitis, whooping cough, gastritis, colitis, see Table 4.6
antispasmodic	coughs
antiviral	colds, influenza, see Table 4.7
cicatrizant	bruises, skin regeneration, acne, burns, scars, ulcers, open wounds
digestive	aerophagy, see Table 4.8
hepatic	stimulates liver function
lipolytic	
mucolytic	bronchitis, pulmonary cleanser
neurotonic	solar plexus, nervous depression
phlebotonic	red veins (couperose), haematoma (even old), thromboses, prevention of bruises

Observations

- the oil from Corsica was found to contain 64% esters (Zola & LeVanda 1975)
- everlasting oil is used as a source of nerol, which is found in its free state and esterified (Guenther 1949)
- sometimes called the super arnica of aromatherapy (Pénoël 1991)
- isovaleric aldehyde, furfurol have also been mentioned as compounds sometimes present in *H. angustifolium*
- RIFM monograph (1979 p. 821) refers to immortelle absolute
- in case of trauma can be applied to the skin neat or diluted 10–50% in a carrier oil (Roulier 1990 p. 272)
- the essential oil and main components were tested against *Staphylococcus aureus, Staphylococcus epidermidis, Pseudomonas aeruginosa, Escherichia coli, Klebsiella pneumoniae* and *Enterobacter cloaceae*; geraniol was the most active component, the *Staphylococcus* species the most sensitive and *E. coli* the most resistant (Chinou et al 1996)
- helichrysum oil of Spanish origin showed significant activity towards *Staphylococcus aureus, Staphylococcus epidermidis, Klebsiella pneumoniae* and *Pseudomonas aeruginosa*; there was variable activity towards Gram-negative species (Tsoukatou et al 1999)

HYSSOPUS OFFICINALIS FLOS, FOL. [HYSSOP] LAMIACEAE

Representative constituents

Hydrocarbons

monoterpenes (25–30%) β-pinene 8.8–22.9%, limonene 0.7–1%, α-pinene 0.7–1.4%, camphene 0.1–0.4%, α-phellandrene 0.03–0.3%, sabinene 1.5–2%, β-myrcene 0.7–2%, *cis*-β-ocimene 0.1–3.6%, *trans*-β-ocimene 0.3–0.5%

sesquiterpenes (12%) β-caryophyllene 0.4–3.2%, germacrene D 0.4–2.8%, alloaromadendrene 0.5–0.8%, δ-cadinene 0.1%, calamenene *trace*, α-caryophyllene

aromatic p-cymene 0.1–0.9%

Alcohols

monoterpenols (5–10%) borneol, geraniol, terpinen-4-ol 0.1%, α-terpineol 1–1.8%, myrtenol 0.4–2.2%, linalool

sesquiterpenols elemol 0.4–1.7%, nerolidol 0.1–1%, spathulenol 0.7–2.2%

other 1-octen-3-ol 0.1%

Esters

monoterpenyl bornyl acetate

methyl myrtenate 2%

Ketones

monoterpenones (45–58%) α-thujone *trace*-0.08%, β-thujone 0.1–0.3%, camphor, pinocamphone 12–58%, isopinocamphone 25–32.6%, 2-hydroxyisopinocamphone 0.3–0.7%

Phenols

carvacrol *trace*

Methyl ethers (4%)

myrtenyl methyl ether 0.8–3.9%, methyl chavicol 0.1–1.3%, methyl eugenol 0.1–0.5%

Oxides

monoterpenoid 1,8-cineole 0.6%, caryophyllene oxide 0.2%

Properties	Indications
antibacterial	see Table 4.4
anticatarrhal	bronchitis, coughs
antiinfectious	colds, coughs, influenza
antiinflammatory	bronchitis, rhinopharyngitis, sinusitis, emphysema, cystitis, rheumatism, see Table 4.6
antitussive	coughs, influenza
astringent, styptic	
cicatrizant	wounds, bruises*, scars, eczema
decongestant	
digestive	loss of appetite, dyspepsia, sluggish digestion, see Table 4.8
diuretic	
emmenagogic	scanty periods, irregular periods

expectorant	
hypertensor	hypotension
lipolytic	
litholytic	urinary stones
mucolytic*	bronchitis, coughs, sinusitis, pneumonia, asthma*, hay fever, dyspnoea
sudorific	
tonic	asthenia (general debility)
vermifuge	intestinal parasites
unspecified	multiple sclerosis
unspecified	leucorrhoea

Observations

- hyssop essential oil can be neurotoxic and abortive in overdose
- not normally used on babies, children, pregnant women and the elderly
- no irritation or sensitization at 4% dilution on humans (Opdyke 1978d)
- no phototoxic effects reported (Opdyke 1978d)
- makes a synergistic mix together with *Eucalyptus globulus*, *Ravensara aromatica* and *Melaleuca viridiflora* for respiratory problems (Roulier 1990)
- maximum dose is four drops per day for a 70 kg adult
- may cause epileptic attack in those so predisposed (Valnet 1980)
- high dose of hyssop essential oil can cause muscular spasm (Bunny 1984); hyssop is a convulsant, owing to pinocamphone and iso-pinocamphone (Millet 1979, Millet et al 1981)
- eliminated via the lungs
- the essence neutralizes the tuberculosis bacillus at 0.2 parts per 1000 (Valnet 1980)
- extracts of hyssop have had antiviral effects against herpes virus (unspecified) (Foster 1993b)
- also mentioned for leprosy and scrofula (Gattefossé 1937)
- plant extracts and the essential oil, used in minute amounts as commercial flavourings in foods, are generally recognized as safe
- the essential oil is used to flavour Benedictine and Grand Chartreuse
- hyssop oil had a dose dependent fungistatic effect on *Aspergillus fumigatus* (Ghfir, Fonvieille & Dargent 1977, Ghfir et al 1994)

- in tests *Hyssopus officinalis* var. *decumbens*, consisting mainly of linalool, has a much broader and stronger antimicrobial action than *Hyssopus officinalis* (Mazzanti et al 1998)

ILLICIUM VERUM [STAR ANISE] MAGNOLIACEAE, ILLICIACEAE

Representative constituents

Hydrocarbons
monoterpenes (3–16%) (+)-α-pinene *trace*–2.1%, α-phellandrene 0.1–0.5%, limonene 0.7–5%, α-terpinene, γ-terpinene 0.3%, camphene, sabinene, β-pinene, β-myrcene 0.4%, δ-3-carene 0.6%, β-phellandrene
sesquiterpenes (0.5–2.5%) β-bisabolene 0.2%, *trans*-β-farnesene 0.4%, α-copaene 0.1%, *cis*-bergamotene, *trans*-bergamotene, β-caryophyllene 0.3–2,% cadinene, isocaryophyllene 0.3%, alloaromadendrene 0.2%, elemene
aromatic p-cymene 0.3%

Alcohols
monoterpenols α-terpineol, linalool 0.4–2.3%, isoborneol 0.05%, borneol
sesquiterpenols farnesol, elemol, nerolidol 0.1%

Aldehydes
anisaldehyde 0.3–0.9%

Methyl ethers
trans-anethole 72–91%, *cis*-anethole *trace*–0.4%, *trans*-isoeugenol methyl ether 0.1%, methyl chavicol 0.3–6.7%

Benzodioxoles
safrole

Ketones
monoterpenone camphor 0.02%

Oxides
monoterpenoid 1,4-cineole, 1,8-cineole 0.2%

Esters
methylanisoate

Other
foeniculin 0.5–14.6%

Properties	Indications
antibacterial	see Table 4.4
antifungal	see Table 4.5
antispasmodic	indigestion, spasmodic colitis, coughs
carminative	aerophagy, eructations, flatulence
expectorant	bronchitis, catarrh
hormonelike (mildly oestrogenic)	oligomenorrhoea, menopause, see Table 4.9
spasmolytic (mild)	
stimulant	

Observations

- used in aperitifs
- not to be recommended in home aromatherapy because of the risk of harming the nervous system if used without knowledge
- avoid during pregnancy and breast feeding
- several cases of sensitization have been reported; this is attributed to the presence of anethole
- star anise oil was not irritating or phototoxic when applied to the backs of hairless mice
- no irritation or sensitization was reported from a 4% mixture in petrolatum (Opdyke 1974u)
- star anise oil is used to mask undesirable odours in drug and cosmetic products (Leung & Foster 1996 p. 37)
- anethole has been reported to cause dermatitis (erythema, scaling and vesiculation) in some individuals; cis-anethole is reported to be 15–38 times more toxic than the trans-isomer (Opdyke 1975a)
- research suggests that polymers of anethole, such as dianethole and photoanethole, are active oestrogenic compounds (Albert-Puleo 1980 p. 337)
- anise flavoured oils increase the basal tone and the contractions of smooth intestinal muscle (Brandt 1988)
- the antimicrobial activity of star anise oil was tested in vitro against 18 bacteria and 12 fungal species; the essential oil inhibited the majority of the bacterial species and all the fungi were completely inhibited (Sharma et al 1985)

INULA HELENIUM (= INULA GRAVEOLENS) FLOS, FOL. [ELECAMPANE] ASTERACEAE

Representative constituents

Hydrocarbons
monoterpenes camphene, α-pinene 27%
sesquiterpenes trans-β-farnesene
other azulene

Alcohols
monoterpenols borneol

Esters
monoterpenyl bornyl acetate

Lactones (very active)
alantolactone 4.4%, isolactone, dihydroisolantolactone, dihydralantolactone, isoalantolactone, 1-β-hydroxyalantolactone

Acids
alantic acid

Ketones (12%)
monoterpenones elecampane camphor, alant camphor

Properties	Indications
antiinfectious	pulmonary infections
antiinflammatory	dermatitis, tracheitis, laryngitis, cystitis, vaginitis, chronic bronchitis, see Table 4.6
antiseptic	tubercle bacillus, food poisoning
antispasmodic	all cramps, coughs
antitussive	chronic bronchitis, chronic coughs
antiviral	viral enteritis, see Table 4.7
aperitive	weak digestion, gall bladder malfunction
calming	hypertension
cardiotonic	arrhythmia*, tired heart
expectorant	bronchitis, whooping cough, croup, silicosis, chronic catarrh

heart regulator   hypertension, tachycardia

mucolytic*   catarrh

vermifuge

Observations

- no known contraindications at normal aromatherapeutic dose
- some individuals are very sensitive to elecampane oil when applied to the skin (Opdyke 1976c)
- contains the sesquiterpenic lactone alantolactone (also known as helenin) which is mucolytic
- the strongest mucolytic found in aromatherapy (Schnaubelt 1998 p. 73)
- the presence of alantolactone gives anthelmintic properties (Guenther 1949 p. 453)
- alantolactone has been reported as immunostimulant (Wagner & Proksh 1985)
- recommended by Mills (1993 p. 585) during post pneumonia convalescence
- research on 105 plant lactones found that alantolactone and isoalantolactone in elecampane are powerful antibacterial and antifungal agents (Vichkanova et al 1977) and they inhibit the growth of *Microsporum cookei, Trichophyton mentagrophytes, Trichothecium roseum* and others (*Trichophyton, Epidermophyton*) (Bruneton 1995 p. 503)
- helenin inhibits the growth of the tubercle bacillus; also is reported to have strong inhibitory effects on seed germination and growth (Rodriguez et al 1976)
- the root oil is reported to consist of 88% lactones: alantolactone 54%, isoalantolactone 33%, dihydroalantolactone 0.4% (Bourrel, Vilarem & Perineau 1993)

JUNIPERUS COMMUNIS FRUCT. [JUNIPER BERRY] CUPRESSACEAE

Representative constituents

Hydrocarbons

monoterpenes (60–80%) α-pinene 26.5–70%, β-pinene 1.7–13.6%, limonene 2.5–40%, camphene 0.3–0.8%, α-thujene 1.2–3%, sabinene 0.3–8.8%, β-myrcene 2.6–9.5%, γ-terpinene 0.3–4%, α-terpinene 0.1–2.2%, δ-3-carene 0.03%, α-terpinolene 0.3–1.8%, α-phellandrene 0.3%, β-phellandrene 0.7%
sesquiterpenes β-caryophyllene *trace*–2%, α-copaene 0.1–0.4%, δ-cadinene 0.2–2.9%, α-humulene 1.9%, germacrene D 2.7%, α-cubebene 0.4%
aromatic p-cymene 1.3–2.4%, p-2-methylstyrene 0.3%, α-p-dimethyl styrene 0.2%

Alcohols

monoterpenols terpinen-4-ol 2.1–9.5%, α-terpineol 0.5%, geraniol 0.1%
sesquiterpenols elemol, α-eudesmol, α-cadinol 0.7%

Oxides

monoterpenoid caryophyllene oxide 0.1%

Esters

monoterpenyl bornyl acetate, terpinyl acetate

Coumarins

umbelliferone

Properties	Indications
analgesic	articular pain
antidiabetic	diabetes, pancreatic stimulant
antiseptic	cystitis
depurative	skin affections
digestive*	cirrhosis, loss of appetite, see Table 4.8
diuretic*	cellulite, oedema
litholytic	bladder and kidney stones
soporific	insomnia

Observations

- not to be used where there is inflammation of the kidneys; α-terpineol and terpinen-4-ol are diuretic principals, and excessive doses may produce kidney irritation
- the diuretic action is due to a direct irritation of the urinary tubule wall by terpineol (Mills 1991)
- this oil has a general augmenting action on mucous secretions; elimination by all natural paths; aids active elimination of unwanted

material, which then cannot be deposited in the joints
- juniper and extracts should not be used by expectant mothers
- symptoms of external poisoning caused by the essential oil on the skin include burning, redness, inflammation with blisters and swelling; internal overdoses cause pain in or near the kidney, strong diuresis, albuminuria, hematuria, accelerated heartbeat and blood pressure elevation (Duke 1985, List & Horhammer 1969–1979)
- undiluted oil when patch tested on 20 subjects showed two irritant reactions (Opdyke 1976j)
- no irritation or sensitization at 8% dilution when tested on humans (Opdyke 1976j)
- no phototoxic effects reported (Opdyke 1976j)
- makes a synergistic mix with rosemary
- juniper berry oil imparts to the urine a smell of violets (Mabey 1988)
- juniper berry oil is commonly adulterated; care in procurement is necessary
- terpinen-4-ol increases glomerular filtration rate, responsible for the diuretic activity (Tyler 1993) and may produce kidney irritation (Tyler 1982)
- the oil is carminative, cephalic, deobstruent, depurative, diaphoretic, digestive, diuretic, emmenagogic, stimulant and sudorific (Duke & Wain 1981, Tierra 1980, Watt & Breyer-Brandwijk 1962)
- uterine-stimulating activity has been reported (Farnsworth 1975)
- oil is used in folk remedies for cancer, indurations, polyps, swellings, tumours and warts (Hartwell 1967–1971)
- in an investigation of nephrotoxicity, two juniper berry oils of slightly differing composition and terpinene-4-ol were orally administered to rats; neither the oils nor terpinene-4-ol induced changes in the morphology and function of the kidneys: they were considered non-toxic (Schilcher & Leuschner 1997)

JUNIPERUS COMMUNIS RAM. [JUNIPER TWIG] CUPRESSACEAE

Representative constituents

Hydrocarbons
monoterpenes α-pinene 35%, β-pinene, limonene 3–40%, camphene 0.3%, α-thujene 3%, sabinene 5%, β-myrcene 9%, γ-terpinene 4%
sesquiterpenes β-caryophyllene 2%

Alcohols
monoterpenols terpinen-1-ol–4

Properties	Indications
analgesic	
anticatarrhal*	bronchitis, rhinitis
antiinflammatory	see Table 4.6
antiseborrhoeic	greasy scalp
antiseptic*	acne, cystitis, weeping eczema
depurative	kidneys, digestive system, urinary stones
diuretic*	gout, rheumatism* (uric acid excretion)
expectorant	
neurotonic	debility, fatigue
unspecified	arteriosclerosis

Observations
- no known contraindications
- see also notes under *J. communis* fruct. [juniper berry]

KUNZEA ERICOIDES [KANUKA, BURGAN] MYRTACEAE

Representative constituents

Hydrocarbons
monoterpenes α-pinene 60–68%
aromatic p-cymene 5.8–12.6%

Alcohols
sesquiterpenols viridiflorol 7.2%

Oxides
monoterpenoid 1,8-cineole 4.3–6.2%

Observations

- Kunzea oils had no antibacterial activity against the bacteria tested and had only weak antifungal activity to *Trichophyton rubrum* (Perry et al 1997a)
- spasmolytic when tested on isolated guinea pig ileum (Lis-Balchin & Hart 1998)

LAURUS NOBILIS FOL. [BAY LEAF]
LAURACEAE

Representative constituents

Hydrocarbons
monoterpenes (−)-α-pinene 2.7–7.6%, β-pinene 2–5%, (−)-sabinene 6.2–8.3%, α-terpinolene 1.9–2.2%, β-myrcene <0.1%, α-phellandrene 0.2–0.55%, δ-3-carene 0.15–0.3%, α-thujene 0.3%, camphene <0.1%, γ-terpinene 0.5–0.7%
sesquiterpenes β-elemene, β-caryophyllene *trace*–0.3, α-humulene
aromatic p-cymene 0.7–1%

Alcohols
monoterpenols (−)-linalool 3–16%, (−)-α-terpineol 1.5–4.5%, terpinen-1-ol-4 2.5–3.75%, borneol, geraniol *trace*–0.2%, *cis*-thujan-4-ol, α-fenchyl alcohol 0.1%, dihydro-α-terpineol 0.2–0.3%

Aldehydes
monoterpenals citral 0.2–0.35%

Esters
monoterpenyl linalyl acetate <0.1%, α-terpinyl acetate <0.1%

Phenols
eugenol 15–16.7%

Methyl ethers
methyl eugenol 2.4%, acetoeugenol 0.2–0.4%

Ketones
monoterpenones α-thujone 0.3–0.5%, β-thujone 0.2–0.4%, camphor 0.15%

Oxides
monoterpenoid 1,8-cineole 35–48.5%, dehydro-1,8-cineole

Lactones
costunolide 1.8%, artemorin 0.5%, deacetyllaurenobiolide

Properties	Indications
analgesic	arthritis, rheumatism, rheumatism (bone and muscle)
anticatarrhal	
anticoagulant	
antifungal	see Table 4.5
antiinfectious	influenza, ENT infections, mouth ulcers, boils, skin infections, malaria, adenitis, stomatitis
antiparasitic	phthiriasis (pediculosus)
antispasmodic	muscle cramp
antiviral	viral neuritis, see Table 4.7
bactericidal	infected acne
digestive	slow digestion, impaired digestion, epigastric bloating, eructations, see Table 4.8
hypotensor	
expectorant	
emmenagogic	scanty periods
mucolytic	
skin	greasy skin, millium, boils, ulcers

Observations

- no contraindications known at normal aromatherapeutic dose; use sparingly in external application to avoid potential sensitization (because of the presence of sesquiterpenic lactones) (Schnaubelt 1998 p. 74)
- do not use in pregnancy (Abrissart 1997 p. 193)
- do not use on children younger than 2 years
- three different samples of laurel leaf oil produced no sensitization reactions when tested on 25, 25 and 49 volunteers (Opdyke 1976d)
- bay laurel or sweet bay is not to be confused with the cherry laurel or common laurel (*Prunus laurocerasus*) which is highly poisonous (Mabey 1988 p. 76)
- bay laurel or sweet bay is not to be confused with the West Indies bay oil *Pimenta racemosa*

- sweet bay leaves can be used safely both fresh or dried as long as you have the correct plant (Herbalism: newsletter of The Herb Society March 1994, No 17)
- there is a volatile oil from the berries which contains 1,8-cineole, geraniol, and linalool; the volatile oil from the leaves is richer in 1,8-cineole (up to 50%)
- bay leaf oil is extensively used in processed foods
- maximum use level of the oil in perfumes is 0.2% in perfumes (Opdyke 1976d)
- bay leaf oil depressed the heart rate and lowered blood pressure in animals (Leung & Foster 1996 p. 70)
- formulations containing bay leaf and the volatile oil have been claimed to have antidandruff activities
- some of the volatile compounds in bay leaf have been shown to repel cockroaches (Verma 1981)
- bay oil (alcohol extracted) was found to be much more effective than the bay leaf against *Salmonella typhimurium, Staphylococcus aureus* and *Vibrio parahaemolyticus* (Aktug & Karapinar 1986)
- laurel oil will produce a relieving effect on swollen lymph nodes (Schnaubelt 1998 p. 75)

LAVANDULA ANGUSTIFOLIA (= L. OFFICIANALIS, L. VERA) *FLOS [LAVENDER]* LAMIACEAE

Representative constituents

Hydrocarbons
monoterpenes (4–5%) α-pinene 0.02–1.1%, *cis*-β-ocimene 1.3–10.9%, *trans*-β-ocimene 0.8–5.8%, limonene 0.2–7%, β-pinene 0.1–0.2%, camphene 0.1–0.3%, δ-3-carene 0.5%, allo-ocimene <1%
sesquiterpenes β-caryophyllene 2.6–7.6%, β-farnesene 1%

Alcohols
monoterpenols linalool 26–49%, terpinen-4-ol 0.03–6.4%, α-terpineol 0.1–1.4%, borneol 0.8–1.4%, geraniol 1%, lavandulol 0.5–1.5%
other cis-3-hexen-1-ol *trace*

Aldehydes *(2%)*
monoterpenals myrtenal 0.1%, neral and geranial 0.4%
aromatic cuminal 0.4%, benzaldehyde 0.2%
other trans-2-hexenal 0.4%

Esters *(40–55%)*
monoterpenyl linalyl acetate 36–53%, lavandulyl acetate 0.2–5.9%, terpenyl acetate 0.5%, geranyl acetate 0.5%
2,6-dimethyl-3, 7-octadiene–2-ol-6-yl acetate

Oxides *(2%)*
monoterpenoid 1,8-cineole 0.5–2.5%, linalool oxide
sesquiterpenoid caryophyllene oxide

Ketones *(4%)*
monoterpenones camphor <1%
other octanone-3 0.5–3%, *p*-methyl-acetophenone

Lactones, coumarins *(0.3%)*
herniarin *trace*, butanolides *trace*, coumarin 0.04%, umbelliferone, santonine

Properties	Indications
analgesic*	arthritis, muscular aches and pains, rheumatism
antibacterial	see Table 4.4
antifungal	*Candida, Tinea pedis* (including infection of the nails) see Table 4.5
antiinflammatory	eczema (dry), insect bites, phlebitis, sinusitis, otitis, cystitis, bruises, sprains, acne, pruritus, see Table 4.6
antiseptic	acne, bronchial secretions, cystitis, otitis, infectious skin complaints, influenza, sinusitis, tuberculosis, pityriasis
antispasmodic	cramp, spasmodic coughing
balancing	nervous system regulator
calming, sedative	headaches*, migraines, anxiety, insomnia and sleep problems

	(opposite effect at high dose),
cardiotonic	tachycardia
carminative	flatulence, colic
cicatrizant*	burns, scars, varicose ulcers, wounds
emmenagogic	scanty periods
hypotensor*	hypertension
tonic	debility, melancholy
unspecified	leucorrhoea, psoriasis

Observations

- no known contraindications
- a remarkable balancing effect on the CNS (Duraffourd 1982)
- no irritation or sensitization at 16% dilution when tested on humans (Opdyke 1976k)
- the oil can cause dermatitis (Duke 1985)
- no phototoxic effects reported (Opdyke 1976k)
- fine lavender oils have ketones belonging to the amyl group, while in the hybrids and lavender species other than *L. angustifolia* the ketones take on the form of camphor (Foster 1993b)
- there are more than 30 different types of lavender oils traded on commercial markets; buying a high quality one is an art known only to a few experienced specialists (Foster 1993b)
- Prager & Miskiewicz (1979) came to the conclusion that two oils imported as lavender oils were in fact blends of lavender oils and lavandin oils, while one further sample was found to be a blend of spike lavender oil and lavender oil
- Bulgarian lavender oils have 35.2–37.6% linalyl acetate (Ognyanov 1984)
- used as an insect repellent (Hartwell 1967–1971, Reynolds 1972)
- maximum acceptable daily intake of the components linalool and linalyl acetate is 500 mg/kg body weight per day (Reynolds 1972)
- found to be sedative in mice (Buchbauer et al 1991) and humans (Buchbauer et al 1993)
- sedative influence of lavender oil and the excitatory effects of jasmine oil on human behaviour was clearly shown (Karamat et al 1992)
- oil has antimicrobial activities (Uzdenikov 1970)

- percutaneous absorption of *Lavandula angustifolia* essential oil via massage was proved by Jäger et al (1992); main components were detected 5 minutes afterwards and 90 minutes later most were eliminated from the blood
- lavender, sage, winter savory and thyme oils showed good antibacterial activity against the majority of 25 species tested: lavender was most effective against *Cl. sporogenes* and *Staphylococcus aureus*: all were active against *Moraxella* species (Piccaglia et al 1993)
- lavender, geranium and Bulgarian rose sprayed in the room were shown to stimulate neuro-psychic activity in humans, with an increase in concentration, attention span, work rhythms and shortening of reflex times (Tasev, Toleva & Balabanova 1969)
- lavender ambient aroma adversely affected arithmetic reasoning (Ludvigson & Rottman 1989).
- lavender was found to be more sedative than jasmin in human tests (Yagyu 1994)
- it was shown that lavender oil had a depressive effect on the central nervous system (Atanasova-Shopova & Rousinov 1970)
- lavender oil was shown to have an anticonvulsive effect in mice (Yamada, Mimaki & Sashida 1994)
- lavender was found to be sedative and to potentiate the effects of barbiturate (Guillemain, Rousseau & Delaveau 1989)
- *in vitro* tests proved *L. angustifolia* to be spasmolytic on smooth muscle; mode of action of linalool reflected that of the whole oil (Lis-Balchin & Hart 1999)
- animal test results indicated that mast cell mediated immediate type allergic reactions were inhibited by lavender essential oil (Kim & Cho 1999)
- local anaesthetic activity of *L. angustifolia* was demonstrated *in vitro* and thought to be due to blockage of sodium or calcium channels (Ghelardini et al 1999)
- acaricidal activity against *Psoroptes cuniculi* by inhalation was shown; whole oil was more effective than linalool (Perucci et al 1996)

LAVANDULA × INTERMEDIA 'SUPER' FLOS [LAVANDIN] LAMIACEAE

Representative constituents

Hydrocarbons
monoterpenes α-pinene 0.05–0.5%, β-pinene
0.05–0.4%, β-myrcene 0.4–2.5%, limonene
0.2–1.6%, camphene 0.2%, sabinene 0.06%,
δ-3-carene 0.02%, *cis*-β-ocimene 1.3%,
γ-terpinene 0.02%, α-terpinolene 0.1%
sesquiterpenes caryophyllene 0.6–1.7%
aromatic p-cymene 0.7%

Alcohols
monoterpenols linalool 23–48%, lavandulol 0.2–1%,
α-terpineol 0.5–6.3%, nerol 0.05–0.6%, geraniol
0.2–1.3%, terpinen-4-ol 0.4%, borneol 2.27%
other 1-octen-3-ol 0.2%

Esters *(25%)*
monoterpenyl linalyl acetate 32–52%, neryl acetate
0.1–0.5%, geranyl acetate 0.4–2%, lavandulyl
acetate 1.5%
other hexyl isobutanoate 0.1%, 1-octen-3-yl
acetate 0.5%, hexyl butanoate 0.6%

Oxides
monoterpenoid 1,8-cineole 1.8–10.8%, *trans*-linalool
oxide 0.2%, *cis*-linalool oxide 0.08%

Ketones
monoterpenones camphor 5–14.8%

Coumarins
coumarin, dihydrocoumarin, 70-
methoxycoumarin and others

Properties	Indications
anticatarrhal	bronchitis, rhinopharyngitis
antifungal	athlete's foot, *Candida albicans,* see Table 4.5
antimigraine	chronic migraine
antiviral*	viral enteritis, see Table 4.7
expectorant	bronchitis, coughs
neurotonic	nervous debility, listlessness
sedative	post cardiac surgery (Buckle 1993)

Observations

- no known contraindications
- no irritation or sensitization at 5% dilution when tested on humans (Opdyke 1976l)
- no phototoxic effects reported (Opdyke 1976l)
- see notes on *Lavandula angustifolia*: *L. × intermedia* 'Super' is a lavandin clone which is close to *L. angustifolia* in its constituents, and therefore in its properties and effects
- *L. x intermedia* 'Grosso' was found to be highly effective against *Mycobacterium, M. fortuitum, M. kansasii, M. marinum* and *M. scrofulaceum* (Gabrielli et al 1988)

LEPTOSPERMUM CITRATUM

Representative constituents

Aldehydes
monoterpenals citrals 40–50%, citronellal 35%

Alcohols
monoterpenols geraniol, citronellol

Esters
formates, acetates

Properties	Indications
antiinflammatory	indigestion, see Table 4.6
digestive	enterocolitis, see Table 4.8
sedative	anxiety, stress, depression

LEPTOSPERMUM SCOPARIUM
[MANUKA, MANEX] MYRTACEAE

Representative constituents

Hydrocarbons
monoterpenes α-pinene 1.1–1.5%, β-pinene 0.1%,
β-myrcene 0.2–0.3%, limonene <0.4%,
γ-terpinene 0.1–0.2%, α-thujene *trace*,
γ-terpinene *trace*, α-terpinolene *trace*

sesquiterpenes (12–17%) α-cubebene 3.9–4%,
α-ylangene 0.3%, α-copaene 5.6–6%,
β-elemene 0.6%, α-gurjunene 0.9–1.1%,
β-caryophyllene 2.4–2.6%, aromadendrene
1.9–2.3%, α-humulene 0.3–0.4%, alloaromadendrene 0.8%, β-selinene 3.6–3.8%,
α-selinene 4.2–4.5%, α-farnesene 0.6–1.0%,
calamanene 11.8–17%, α-cadinene 5.9–6.1%,
cadin-1,4-diene 4.7–5.4, selinene, arnorphene,
muurolene and cadinene isomers
aromatic p-cymene 0.15%

Alcohols

monoterpenols terpinen-4-ol *trace*, α-terpineol *trace*
sesquiterpenols (4%) nerolidol, viridiflorol, ledol,
spathulenol 0.40–0.63%, cubenol 0.86–1.12%

Ketones

triketones flavesone 4.65–5.18%, isoleptospermone
4.47–4.76%, leptospermone 15.1–15.9%

Esters *(0.55–50%)*

(mainly C10. MWt 168–172)

Oxides

monoterpenoid 1,8-cineole 0.2%
sesquiterpenoid β-caryophyllene oxide 0.23–0.26%

Properties	Indications
analgesic	muscular tension and sprains, joint stiffness and aches, rheumatism
antibacterial	*Staphylococcus aureus*, colitis, see Table 4.4
antifungal	*Tinea pedis*, ringworm, *Candida albicans*, see Table 4.5
antimicrobial astringent digestive respiratory skin uplifting	dyspepsia, see Table 4.8 bronchitis (inhalation) skin infections, psoriasis anxiety, depression, stress

Observations

- no known contraindications at normal aromatherapeutic dose
- extracts of this plant have been consumed

traditionally in infusions, perhaps low toxicity
may be inferred
- found to be effective against *Staphylococcus aureus* and ringworm; manuka oil was found to be much stronger against Gram-positive organisms (about 20 times stronger than tea tree) (Cooke & Cooke 1994, Perry et al 1997b)
- manuka and kanuka oils grow in the same regions and are difficult to differentiate morphologically, also there are manuka chemotypes, hence there are available manuka essential oils of variable antimicrobial activity (Porter & Wilkins 1998)

LITSEA CUBEBA FRUCT. [MAY CHANG] LAURACEAE

Representative constituents

Hydrocarbons

monoterpenes limonene 0.2–8%, β-myrcene 3%,
β-pinene, α-pinene, camphene
sesquiterpenes β-caryophyllene
aromatic p-cymene

Alcohols

other 6-methyl-5-hepten-2-ol, β-methyl heptanol
monoterpenols (5%) linalool 2.8%, α-terpineol,
citronellol, nerol, geraniol 51%

Aldehydes *(66–76%)*

monoterpenals neral 34–41%, geranial 40–51%,
citronellal 0.6%
other 2,6-dimethyl-5-heptenal

Ketones

methyl ionone, methyl heptanone 1.5–4%,
acetone, methyl heptenone 1.5%

Esters

monoterpenyl linalyl acetate, neryl acetate, geranyl
acetate, terpenyl acetate

Properties	Indications
antibacterial	see Table 4.4
antifungal	see Table 4.5
antiinfectious	
antiinflammatory	dermatitis, see Table 4.6
antiviral	viral neuritis, see Table 4.7

calming, sedative	anxiety, hysteria, vertigo, insomnia, nervous depression, memory loss, stress
digestive	gastric/duodenal ulcers, poor digestion, see Table 4.8
insecticidal	*Pediculosus capitis*, nits, see Table 4.10

Observations

- used in various medicines for headache, dizziness, hysteria, paralysis and loss of memory
- the distilled oil recalling citral odour is widely used in flavouring industries
- reported to be active against *Fusarium moniliforme, F. solani, Alternaria alternata* and *Aspergillus niger*; antifungal activity increased with concentration (Gogoi, Baruah & Nath 1997)

MATRICARIA RECUTITA (= M. CHAMOMILLA, CHAMOMILLA RECUTITA) FLOS [GERMAN CHAMOMILE] ASTERACEAE

Representative constituents

Hydrocarbons

monoterpenes α-terpinene *trace*, limonene, β-ocimene 1.7%
sesquiterpenes chamazulene 1–35%, bisabolenes, trans-β-farnesene 2–13%, trans-α-farnesene 27%, δ-cadinene 5.2%, α-copaene 0.2%, caryophyllene 0.5%, γ-muurolene 1.3%, α-muurolene 3.4%
aromatic p-cymene

Alcohols

sesquiterpenols α-bisabolol 2–67%, spathulenol, farnesol

Oxides

monoterpenoid 1,8-cineole
sesquiterpenoid α-bisabol oxide A 0–55%, α-bisabolol oxide B 4.3–19%, epoxybisabolol, bisabolone oxide A 0–64%

Coumarins

herniarin (7-methoxycoumarin), umbelliferone (7-hydroxycoumarin)

Ethers

en-yn-dicycloether 0.7%

Properties	Indications
antiallergic	
antifungal	see Table 4.5
antiinflammatory*	eczema, gastritis, skin problems, rheumatism, see Table 4.6
antispasmodic	gastric spasm
cicatrizant	infected wounds, ulcers
decongestant	dysmenorrhoea
digestive	duodenal ulcers, gastric ulcers, indigestion, morning sickness, nausea, see Table 4.8
hormonelike	amenorrhoea, PMS, see Table 4.9

Observations

- no known contraindications
- there are several chemotypes of this plant, hence the wide limits for the constituents quoted
- no irritation or sensitization at 4% dilution when tested on humans (Opdyke 1974f)
- no phototoxic effects reported (Opdyke 1974f)
- bisabolol type chamomile extracts have low sensitizing activity but there are reports of allergenic properties perhaps due to a linear sesquiterpene lactone (anthecotulide) (Hausen, Busker & Carle 1984)
- the azulenes and bisabolol are anti-inflammatory and antispasmodic, reducing histamine induced reactions such as anaphylaxis and hay fever, allergic asthma and eczema (Mills 1991): the oil has anti-inflammatory activity (Reynolds 1972)
- (–)-α-bisabolol possesses low acute toxicity after oral administration in mice, rats, dogs and rhesus monkeys (Habersang et al 1979)
- the sesquiterpenol (–)-α-bisabolol has been found to possess ulcer protective (Szelenyi & Thiemer 1979), spasmolytic (Achterrath-Tuckermann et al 1980), antiphlogistic

(Jakovlev et al 1979) and antiinflammatory (Tubaro et al 1984) properties

- Foster (1991, 1993a) says that it is now generally believed that the chief pharmacological benefits are primarily due to α-bisabolol

- bisabolol has been shown to reduce the amount of proteolytic enzyme pepsin secreted by the stomach without any change occurring in the amount of stomach acid (Szelenyi & Thiemer 1979); it has also shown anti-inflammatory action on granulomas, and shortens the healing time of cutaneous burns (Isaac 1979)

- chamazulene is anodyne, antispasmodic, anti-inflammatory and antiallergenic (Foster 1993b)

- chamazulene is active against *Staphylococcus aureus* (Bartram 1995)

- azulenes reduce histamine-induced tissue reactions, calm the nervous system both peripherally as in visceral tension and centrally as in anxiety, nervous tension and headaches; their activity also extends to reducing the anaphylaxis due to the allergic response and so are indicated for hay fever, allergic asthma and eczema (Mills 1991)

- included in the pharmacopoeia of 26 countries (Salamon 1992)

- it has been shown that the use of the herbicide propyzamide caused an increase in essential oil content; it has also been stated that the use of herbicides over extended periods could readily affect the plant's metabolism and it is recommended that all medicinal and essential oil plants be screened against a number of herbicides to see if there is any long-term effect on secondary product metabolism; it is noteworthy that the effects under discussion were found in plants in which residual amounts of the herbicide were absent (Reichling, Becker & Drager 1978, Vömel et al 1977)

- the tea induced deep sleep (Reynolds 1972)

- antioxidant action and weak antibacterial, antifungal action (Lis-Balchin, Deans & Hart 1994)

- used externally for neuralgia (Bartram 1995)

- azulene components of the oil are thought to inhibit histamine release and prevent allergic seizures in guinea pigs (Mann & Staba 1986)

- azulenes have the ability to regenerate liver tissue in partially hepatectomized rats (Mann & Staba 1986)

- the oil reduced serum urea concentration in rabbits with induced uraemic conditions (Grochulski & Borkowski 1972)

- essential oils of German chamomile, orange and mandarin were tested in aqueous gels at 5% concentration; all three gels produced an immediate hydrating effect on the skin, with German chamomile producing a more intense and longer lasting hydration (Monges et al 1994)

MELALEUCA ALTERNIFOLIA FOL. *[TEA TREE]* MYRTACEAE

Representative constituents

Hydrocarbons
monoterpenes (25–40%) α-pinene 0.8–3.6%, β-pinene 0.1–1.6%, α-terpinene 4.6–12.8%, γ-terpinene 9.5–28.3%, limonene 0.4–2.77%, α-terpinolene 1.6–5.4%, α-thujene 0.1–2.1%, sabinene 0–3.2%, β-myrcene 0.1–1.8%, α-phellandrene 0.1–1.9%, β-phellandrene 0.4–1.6%
sesquiterpenes β-caryophyllene 1%, aromadendrene 0.1–6.6%, viridiflorene 0.3–6.1%, δ-cadinene 0.1–7.5% alloaromadendrene 0.3%, α-muurolene 0.1%, α-gurjunene 0.2%, calamenene 0.1%
aromatic p-cymene 0.4–12.4%

Alcohols
monoterpenols terpenen-4-ol 28.6–57.9%, α-terpineol 1.5–7.6%
sesquiterpenols globulol 0.1–3.0%, viridiflorol 0.1–1.4%, cubenol 0.1%

Oxides
monoterpenoid 1,8-cineole 0.5–17.7%, 1,4-cineole *trace*

Properties	Indications
analgesic	
antibacterial	see Table 4.4
antifungal	*Candida** see Table 4.5
antiinfectious*	abscesses, skin infections, intestinal infections, bronchitis, genital infections

antiinflammatory	abscesses (including dental), pyorrhoea, vaginitis, sinusitis, otitis, see Table 4.6
antiparasitic	lamblias, ascaris, ankylostoma
antiviral	viral enteritis, see Table 4.7
immunostimulant	low immunoglobulin A and immunoglobulin M
neurotonic	debility, depression, PMS, anxiety
phlebotonic	haemorrhoids, varicose veins, aneurysm

Observations

- no known contraindications
- no irritation or sensitization at 1% dilution when tested on humans (Ford, Letizia & Api 1988)
- no phototoxic effects reported (Ford, Api & Letizia 1988)
- said to prevent postoperative shock due to anaesthetic (Franchomme & Penoël 1990)
- tea tree oil has a low cineole content and is non-irritant to the skin or the mucous surfaces
- in a single-blind randomized study on 124 patients with mild to moderate acne, tea tree oil was compared with benzoyl peroxide: both treatments produced a significant improvement, while fewer patients using the tea tree oil reported unwanted effects (Bassett, Pannowitz & Barnetson 1990)
- tea tree was active against *Staph. aureus, Staph. epidermidis* and *Propionibacterium acnes*, supporting its use in treatment of acne (Rama, Weir & Bloomfield 1995)
- see observation under *Melaleuca viridiflora* concerning possible radio protective property
- tea tree oil may be useful in removing transient skin flora owing to its ability to penetrate the outer layers of the skin giving a residual effect, while suppressing but maintaining resident flora. *Staphylococcus aureus* and Gram-negative bacteria were susceptible to tea tree oil (Hammer, Carson & Riley 1996)
- excellent antimicrobial and antifungal action including *Listeria monocytogenes, Candida albicans, Pityrosporum ovale* and *Trichophyton* (Asre 1994, Lis-Balchin, Deans & Hart 1994, Maruzzella 1960, Millet et al 1981); this is probably due to *p*-cymene content
- *in vitro* tests on *S. aureus* suggest tea tree oil may be useful in the treatment of MRSA carriage (Carson, Hammer & Riley 1995, Carson et al 1995); of 66 isolates tested, 64 were methicillin resistant and 33 were mupirocin resistant; all were susceptible to *M. alternifolia* essential oil
- tea tree has been used to treat skin conditions such as acne and furunculosis (boils); vaginal thrush; foot problems; coughs and colds (Mayo 1992)
- tea tree oil cream reduced symptomatology of *Tinea pedis* as effectively as tolnaftate but was not more effective than placebo in achieving a mycological cure (Tong, Attman & Barnetson 1992). Satchell et al (2002) suggest using a 25% tea tree oil solution for *Tinea pedis* but emphasize that this is less effective than standard topical treatments
- tea tree oil is as effective as clotrimazole as an antifungal agent (Anon 1994a, Buck, Nidorf & Addino 1994). Was effective *in vitro* against a range of isolated fungi but was less effective than micanozole (Nenoff, Haustein & Brandt 1996)
- tea tree oils inhibited *Candida albicans, Escherichia coli, Staphylococcus aureus, Bacteroides fragilis, Mycobacterium smegmatis* and *Clostridium perfringens* but *Pseudomonas aeruginosa* was resistant (Carson & Riley 1994). Anticandidal activity demonstrated *in vitro* (Hammer, Carson & Riley 1998, D'Auria et al 2001)
- tea tree is not recommended for treatment of burns as it could decrease healing and increase scarring (Faoagali, George & Leditschke 1997)
- Koh et al (2002) showed that *Melaleuca alternifolia* oil reduced experimentally induced skin inflammation in humans
- *Melaleuca alternifolia* used in the antiseptic treatment of furuncles encouraged more rapid healing without scarring than conventional treatment (Feinblatt 1960)
- several cases are reported of non-fatal poisoning where relatively large amounts of the oil have been ingested (Carson & Riley 1993, Jacobs & Hornfeldt 1994, Morris et al 2003)

- the EU Scientific Committee on Consumer Products (SCCP) concluded that the sparse data available suggest that the use of undiluted tea tree oil as a commercial product is not safe (SCCP 2004)

MELALEUCA LEUCADENDRON (= M. CAJUPUTI) FOL. [CAJUPUT] MYRTACEAE

Representative constituents

Hydrocarbons
monoterpenes α-pinene 4%, β-pinene 35%, limonene 7%
sesquiterpenes β-caryophyllene 5.9%

Alcohols
monoterpenols (–)-α-terpineol 6.4%
sesquiterpenols (+)-viridiflorol, nerolidol

Oxides
monoterpenoid 1,8-cineole 50–75%

Aldehydes
valeraldehyde, butanal, benzaldehyde

Esters
monoterpenyl terpineol acetate

Properties	Indications
analgesic	earache, gout, painful periods, rheumatism, toothache, painful joints, neuralgia, arthritis
antibacterial	see Table 4.4
antifungal	see Table 4.5
antiinfectious	bronchitis, colds, coughs, enteritis
antiseptic	intestines, urinary tract, cystitis, respiratory tract, cholera, pityriasis, psoriasis
antispasmodic	gastroenteritis, colic
decongestant	haemorrhoids, varicose veins
expectorant	bronchitis, coughs, lungs
insectifuge	mosquitoes, lice, fleas, see Table 4.10
phlebotonic	varicose veins, haemorrhoids
sudorific	helps influenza

Observations

- no known contraindications, but care is advisable with pregnancy
- no irritation or sensitization at 4% dilution when tested on humans (Opdyke 1976m)
- no phototoxic effects reported (Opdyke 1976m)
- see observation under *Melaleuca viridiflora* concerning possible radio protective property
- widely used in the East; Indochina–arthritis, rheumatism, colds, rhinitis; Indonesia–burns, cramp, colic, earache, headache, skin disease, toothache; New Guinea–malaria; Malaysia–pain relief, stomachic, cholera, colic (Perry 1980)
- very good antimicrobial action (Cuong et al 1994, Jedlickova, Motl & Sery 1992, Maruzzella & Sicurella 1960)
- used internally as a carminative and externally as a rubefacient (Reynolds 1972)
- *Melaleuca leucadendron* essential oil was shown to possess a broad range of antifungal activity against 24 fungal species (Dubey , Kishore & Singh 1983)

MELALEUCA VIRIDIFLORA (= M. QUINQUENERVIA) FOL. [NIAOULI] MYRTACEAE

Representative constituents

Hydrocarbons
monoterpenes α-pinene 7.5%, β-pinene 3%, 1-limonene 4–8%
sesquiterpenes β-caryophyllene 2%, aromadendrene, alloaromadendrene, viridiflorene, α-humulene, α-cadinene

Alcohols
monoterpenols linalool, α-terpineol 9–14%, terpinen-1-ol-4 2%
sesquiterpenols viridiflorol 6–15%, globulol, nerolidol 1–7%

Aldehydes
isovaleraldehyde, benzaldehyde <1%

Oxides
monoterpenoid 1,8-cineole 38–65%,
sesquiterpenoid epoxycaryophyllene II

Other
sulphur constituents

Properties	Indications
analgesic	labour
antibacterial	see Table 4.4
anticatarrhal	chronic catarrh
antiinfectious	respiratory infections, skin fungal infections, insect bites, boils
antiinflammatory	sinusitis*, rhinopharyngitis, bronchitis*, blepharitis, vulvovaginitis, urethritis, prostatitis, inflammation of coronary arteries, see Table 4.6
antiparasitic	
antipruritic	insect bites
antirheumatic	rheumatoid arthritis
antiseptic	infected wounds, respiratory
antitumoral	breast cancer (non-hormonal), rectal cancer, fibroma (some)*
antiviral*	viral hepatitis*, viral enteritis, genital herpes*, see Table 4.7
digestive	aerophagy, gastritis, gastric and duodenal ulcers, diarrhoea, see Table 4.8
expectorant*	bronchitis*, coughs, colds
febrifuge	fevers
hepatic stimulant	
hormonelike	amenorrhoea, oligomenorrhoea, irregular menses, see Table 4.9
hypotensor	atherosclerosis, hypertension
immunostimulant	activates defences and augments leukocytes and antibodies in infected areas
litholytic	gall stones
phlebotonic	varicose veins*, haemorrhoids*
skin tonic	psoriasis, boils, wrinkles, fungal infections
tonic	post-viral nervous depression
unspecified	leucorrhoea

Observations

- no known contraindications but care is advised for pregnant women and children
- used in New Caledonia to purify air (Duraffourd 1982)
- procuring the genuine natural oil is not easy
- the French pharmacopoeia lists natural niaouli and purified niaouli; only the latter can be used in anticatarrhal preparations or for applications for use on burns or on wounds (Belaiche 1979)
- niaouli is thought by some to act as a radio protective, i.e. as a preventative for radiotherapy burns by attenuating the effects of burning of the epidermis. The neat essential oil may be applied before irradiation sessions, and afterwards may be applied as a mixture consisting of 50% niaouli oil and 50% of either *Rosa mosquetta* [rose hip oil] or *Hypericum perforatum* [St John's wort] macerated oil (Roulier 1990 p. 230). This same characteristic has been attributed also to *Melaleuca alternifolia* and *M. leucadendron* (Franchomme & Pénoël 1990 pp. 369–370)

MELISSA OFFICINALIS FOL. [MELISSA] LAMIACEAE

Representative constituents

Hydrocarbons
monoterpenes trans-β-ocimene 0.2%, limonene 0.2%
sesquiterpenes β-caryophyllene 8–10%, δ-cadinene 1%, γ-cadinene 1%, α-humulene <1%, α-copaene 4–5%, β-elemene <1%, β-bourbonene 0.3%

Alcohols

monoterpenols linalool 0.4–1.3%, nerol <1%,
  geraniol <1%, citronellol <1%, isopulegol <1%
sesquiterpenols α–cadinol 0.3%, elemol <1%,
other cis-3-hexenol 0.1%, 1-octen-3-ol 1.3%

Ketones

6-methyl-5-hepten-2-one 4.5%,
  hexahydrofarnesyl-acetone 0.2%, 3-octanone
  0.6%, methyl heptanone 0.6%

Esters

monoterpenyl geranyl acetate <0.5%, neryl acetate,
  citronellyl acetate

Oxides

monoterpenoid 1,8-cineole
sesquiterpenoid caryophyllene oxide 2.5–3.6%

Aldehydes

monoterpenals neral 22–24%, geranial 32–37%,
  citronellal 0.7–2.2%

Coumarins

aesculetine

Properties	Indications
antiinflammatory	see Table 4.6
antispasmodic	stomach cramp
antiviral	*Herpes simplex* I, see Table 4.7
calming	hysteria, palpitations, headaches, vertigo*, erethism
choleretic	regularizes secretions (bile, stomach)
digestive	indigestion*, nausea, morning sickness*, sluggish liver, see Table 4.8
hypotensor*	hypertension
sedative	insomnia, calming to CNS, depression, grief
vasodilator (capillaries)	palpitations, angina

Observations

- no known contraindications, but care may be necessary in sunlight

- often adulterated or reconstructed: caution is advised when procuring it, because the properties given above relate only to the true oil; melissa is frequently adulterated by mixing with lemongrass or citronella to increase its bulk, but is more usually totally simulated; these reconstructed oils have a similar 'lemony' aroma and contain some of the compounds found in natural melissa oil, e.g. citral, citronellal
- citronellal is the terpene to which sedative action is primarily attributed (Foster 1993b)
- skin allergies and respiratory problems are often made worse if not treated with a suitably low concentration of melissa oil (usually less than 1%)
- a powerful choleretic which triples the volume of bile in 30 minutes (Duraffourd 1982)
- the hydrosol is useful for regulating fever in children (Roulier 1990)
- studies have indicated that a cream with lemon balm (available in Germany) reduces the healing time of *Herpes simplex* type I lesions and lengthens the time before recurrence (Tyler 1992)
- two chemotypes of melissa are known to exist: citral (as above) and citronellal (Lawrence 1989b)
- melissa oil was found to be a strong antioxidant (Lis-Balchin, Deans & Hart 1994) and a relaxant (Torii et al 1988)
- citral can cause an increase in ocular tension (Leach & Lloyd 1956)
- the oil has antibacterial (Wagner & Sprinkmeyer 1973) and antifungal (Mulkens et al 1985) activity
- essential oils of lemon balm containing up to 80% citral had a pseudo-narcotic effect on the central nervous system (Masakova et al 1979)

MENTHA ARVENSIS [CORNMINT] LAMIACEAE

Representative constituents

Hydrocarbons

monoterpenes (–)-limonene 0.48–9.8%, α-pinene
  0.1–1.54%, β-pinene 0.06–2.9%
sesquiterpenes β-caryophyllene

Alcohols
monoterpenols (–)-menthol 56.7–80.2%,
(+)–neomenthol + neoisomenthol 2.41–12.32%,
cis-thujan-4-ol 0–0.8%
diols (–)-2,5-*trans-p*-menthane diol

Esters
monoterpenyl menthyl acetate 0.22–4%
other β-hexanyl phenyl acetate, γ-hexanyl phenyl
acetate

Ketones *(34%)*
monoterpenones (–)-menthone 15–30%, isomenthone
0.1–6%, piperitone 0.1–5.9%, pulegone 0.3–4%

Oxides
monoterpenoid 1,8-cineole *trace*–2.6%

Methyl ethers *(5%)*

Properties	Indications
analgesic	neuralgia, toothache, sciatica, migraine, headaches, periarticular pain
antibacterial	*Bacillus brevis*, *Staphylococcus*, *Bacillus subtilis*, meningococcus, see Table 4.4
antifungal	*Aspergillus* species and others, see Table 4.5
antiinfectious	rhinitis, rhinopharyngitis, laryngitis, sinusitis
antiparasitic	parasites, lice, fleas, bugs
calming (high dose)	headaches
cooling	eczema, pruritus, urticaria
digestive, aperitive, eupeptic	constipation, dyspepsia, ulcers, nausea (indigestion, pregnancy) see Table 4.8
tonic (low dose)	

Observations

- contraindicated for nursing mothers and children under 3: danger of respiratory arrest due to laryngeal or nasal reflex

- the essential oil from *Mentha arvensis* (cornmint) is similar to peppermint oil, but the former contains a much higher level of menthol: 70 to 80%
- menthol is probably the main analgesic component; the properties of this essential oil are due almost entirely to the menthol content.
- Japanese *Mentha arvensis* may contain 20–30% of the ketone pulegone (Guenther 1949 vol 3 p. 663): therefore not to be used at all during pregnancy
- menthol is removed from this oil for use in perfumery, pharmacy, thus artificially raising the level of menthone perhaps up to 26%
- cornmint oil is much adulterated and should be used with great care: not at all on children under 3 years old
- a dementholized oil was tested against 23 fungi and found to have a wide range of fungicidal activity, inhibiting 22 species (Singh, Dikshit & Dixit 1983)
- a gel containing 30% *Mentha arvensis* oil was tested on patients suffering periarticular pain; it was concluded that mint oil therapy was safe and effective in treating subacute and acute periarticular complaints (Krall & Kraus 1993)
- in tests the oil was found to have antibacterial and antifungal activities, but *Sarcina* species and *E coli* were resistant to the oil (Singh et al 1992)

MENTHA × PIPERITA FOL. [PEPPERMINT] LAMIACEAE

Representative constituents

Hydrocarbons
monoterpenes (3–18%) α-pinene 0.2–2%, β-pinene
0.3–4%, limonene 0.6–6%, menthene, α- and
β-phellandrene, sabinene <1%, β-myrcene
<1%, *cis*-β-ocimene *trace*–1.5%, α-terpinolene
trace–0.2%, α-terpinene <1%, γ-terpinene <1%
sesquiterpenes β-caryophyllene <1%, *trans*-β-
farnesene *trace*–0.5%, α-muurolene *trace*–0.5%,
germacrene D 2.1–4.3%, γ-cadinene
trace–0.7%, β-bourbonene <1%
aromatic p-cymene *trace*–0.5%

Alcohols
monoterpenols (50%) menthol 28–46%, isomenthol, neomenthol 2–7.7%, piperitol, piperitenol, isopiperitenol, α-terpineol 0.1–1.9%, linalool <1%, terpinen-4-ol 0–2.4%, *cis*-thujan-4-ol 0.2–1.4%, *trans*-thujan-4-ol *trace*–0.8%
sesquiterpenols viridiflorol 0.5–1.3%, 10-α-cadinol *trace*–0.3%
other 3-octanol <1%

Ketones
monoterpenones menthone 16–36%, isomenthone 4–10.4%, neomenthone 2–3%, piperitone 0.5–1.2%, isopiperitone, pulegone <1%, piperitenone *trace*–0.7%

Oxides
monoterpenoid 1,8-cineole 3–7.4%, *trans*-piperitonoxide 0.5–3.1%
sesquiterpenoid caryophyllene oxide *trace*–0.5%

Esters
monoterpenyl menthyl acetate 1.6–10%, neomenthyl acetate, isomenthyl acetate, menthyl butanoate, menthyl isovalerate

Coumarins
aesculetine

Benzofurans
menthofuran 0.1–5.7%

Properties	Indications
analgesic	migraine, neuralgia, sciatica
antibacterial	see Table 4.4
antifungal	ringworm, skin infections see Table 4.5
antiinfectious	
antiinflammatory	bronchitis, colitis, cystitis, eczema*, enteritis, gastritis, hepatitis, laryngitis, sinusitis, urticaria*, see Table 4.6
antilactogenic	prevents milk forming
antimigraine	headache, migraine
antipyretic	fever
antispasmodic	colic, gastric spasm
antiviral	zoster, viral hepatitis, viral neuritis, see Table 4.7
carminative	flatulence
decongestant	cirrhosis
digestive	indigestion, nausea, painful digestion, digestive problems, irritable bowel syndrome, see Table 4.8
expectorant	bronchial asthma, bronchitis
hepatic stimulant	cirrhosis, jaundice
hormonelike	irregular periods (ovarian stimulant), hot flushes, see Table 4.9
hypertensor	hypotension
insectifuge	gnats, mosquitoes, see Table 4.10
mucolytic	bronchial asthma, bronchitis
neurotonic	apathy, nervous vomiting, travel sickness, palpitations, vertigo, (excites the motor nerves but damps the excitation of sensor nerves)
reproductive stimulant	impotence
soothing	skin irritation, rashes, redness
uterotonic	facilitates delivery

Observations

- contraindicated for babies and young children, where it can produce reflex apnoea or laryngospasm; an ointment containing menthol applied to the nostrils of infants for the treatment of cold symptoms has been reported to cause instantaneous collapse (Tester-Dalderup 1980)
- may cause allergic reactions such as contact dermatitis, flushing and headache in some individuals
- skin irritations may be made worse unless used in suitably low concentration
- should not be used externally in high concentration (i.e. low dilution) as in certain adults it may result in sleep disturbance

- peppermint oil is reported to be effective as an analgesic when used in conjunction with *Ravensara aromatica* (Roulier 1990)
- helps local circulation in the head
- there is a consensus of opinion that peppermint should not be used concurrently with homoeopathic treatment, although the reasons given vary
- menthol is cooling and anaesthetic when applied to the skin, increasing blood flow to the area to which it is applied (Mabey 1988)
- whole peppermint has more antispasmodic effect than menthol alone (Trease & Evans 1983)
- oil of peppermint is antispasmodic (Leung 1980); studies have shown peppermint oil to inhibit gastrointestinal smooth muscle spasms and reduce colonic motility (Duthie 1981, Leicester & Hunt 1982, Sigmund & McNally 1969, Taylor, Luscombe & Duthie 1983)
- *M.* x *piperita* is a hybrid of *Mentha spicata* [spearmint] and *Mentha aquatica* [watermint]
- local anaesthetic and counterirritant for muscular aches and pains (Dew, Evans & Rhodes 1984, Rees 1979, Reynolds 1972)
- peppermint and caraway oils combined in enteric-coated capsules (Enteroplant®) were found to improve non-ulcer dyspepsia (May et al 1996, Micklefield, Greving & May 2000, Micklefield et al 2003)
- Colpermin enteric coated capsules with 187 mg of peppermint essential oil proved to reduce pain associated with IBS and could be used in children (Dew, Evans & Rhodes 1984, Kline et al 2001, Rees, Evans & Rhodes 1979)
- the oil is reported to have antimicrobial (Abdullin 1962, Pizsolitto 1975, Ramadan et al 1972c, Sanyal & Varma 1969) and antiviral (Hermann & Kucera 1967) activity
- reported to have cytotoxic properties (Silyanovska et al 1969)
- 18 different peppermint oils showed a significant variability in antiseptic qualities, but spasmolytic activity was consistent for all samples (Lis-Balchin, Deans & Hart 1997)
- mosquito larvicidal and with repellent activity to mosquitoes comparable to commercial preparations containing dimethyl and dibutyl phthalates (Ansari et al 2000)
- the inclusion of peppermint oil during barium enema is a safe method of reducing colonic spasm during examination (Sparks et al 1995)
- a significant analgesic effect with reduction in sensitivity to headache was produced by peppermint applied to temples and foreheads (Gobel, Schmidt & Soyka 1994)
- Kiel University in 1996 compared the analgesic effects of *Mentha* x *piperita* versus paracetamol on people with tension headaches and found that 10% of the peppermint oil in ethanol had the same effect as 1000 mg of paracetamol, leading to the development of Euminz®

MENTHA SPICATA [SPEARMINT] LAMIACEAE

Representative constituents

Hydrocarbons
monoterpenes (–)-α-pinene 0.2–0.9%, β-pinene 0.3–2.3%, β-myrcene 1.2–5.5, (–)-limonene 2–25%, α-thujene 0.03–0.7, sabinene 0.3–0.9, *cis*-β-ocimene 0.3–1, γ-terpinene *trace*, camphene, α-terpinolene
sesquiterpenes β-caryophyllene 0.3–2.6%, α-elemene, farnesene, β-bourbonene *trace*–2%, germacrene D 0–2%
aromatic p-cymene 0.2–0.47

Alcohols
monoterpenols dihydrocarveol 1.3%, linalool 0–1.1%, (–)-menthol 0.5–2%, terpinen-4-ol *trace*–6.1%, α-terpineol 0–2.7%, neodihydrocarveol, *cis*-carveol 0–0.6%, *trans*-carveol 0–0.2%
sesquiterpenols viridiflorol 0–0.6%
other 3-octanol 0–1.26%, 1-octen-3-ol 0.3–1.5%

Esters
monoterpenyl dihydrocarvyl acetate 1.2–24.8%, *cis*-carvyl acetate 0.2–5.5%, *trans*-carvyl acetate 0.7–5.9%, neoisodihydrocarveol acetate 0–21%, menthyl acetate 2%
other 3-octyl acetate 0–0.3%, 1-octen-3-yl acetate <0.1%

Ketones
monoterpenones (–)-carvone 39–67%, menthone *trace*–5.2%, isomenthone *trace*–0.5%, *cis*-dihydrocarvone 3.1–21.6%, *trans*-

dihydrocarvone 0–21%, (+)-pulegone <0.5%, 6-hydroxycarvone, piperitenone *trace*

Oxides
monoterpenoid 1,8-cineole 0.5–3.2%

Benzofurans
menthofuran 2%

Properties	Indications
anticatarrhal	respiratory infections, bronchitis, influenza
antifungal	see Table 4.5
antiinflammatory	cystitis, see Table 4.6
antiseptic	
antispasmodic	colic
calming	
carminative	flatulence
cicatrizant	wounds, scars
choleretic	poor digestion
diaphoretic, sudorific	feverish condition
digestive	nausea, constipation, diarrhoea, flatulence, dyspepsia, travel sickness, poor appetite, poor digestion, vomiting due to pregnancy, see Table 4.8
insecticide	see Table 4.10
mucolytic	common cold
stimulant, uplifting	depression, mental fatigue

Observations

- spearmint is reported to be non-toxic, very mildly irritant (mucous membrane irritant) and non-sensitizing (Tisserand & Balacs 1995b)
- spearmint has GRAS (Generally Recognized as Safe) status (§182.10 and §182.20)
- despite this, spearmint oil is given by Franchomme & Pénoël (2001 p. 403) as contra-indicated in pregnancy, babies and children, due to the high carvone content
- carvone is said to be neurotoxic and abortive by Franchomme & Pénoël (2001 p. 403); however, this is not the general view (Price 1993, Tisserand & Balacs 1995b) and (–)-carvone is listed by Winter (1999 p. 113) as having no known toxicity; as with most essential oils, if

the correct doses are used under the supervision of a qualified aromatherapist, spearmint oil is safe to use
- Adam et al (1998) found spearmint oil, among others, to be active against *Malassezia furfur, Trichophyton rubrum* and *T. beigelii* which cause human skin infections

MYRISTICA FRAGRANS SEM. [NUTMEG] MYRISTICACEAE

Representative constituents

Hydrocarbons
monoterpenes (70–75%) α-pinene 14–25%, β-pinene 10–15%, β-myrcene 2%, sabinene 14–35%, α-terpinene 2–4%, γ-terpinene 1.9–7.7%, limonene 3.7–4%, β-phellandrene, camphene < 1%, α-phellandrene 0.7–1%, α-terpinolene 0.9–1.7%
sesquiterpenes β-caryophyllene 0–1%
aromatic p-cymene 1.1–3.1%

Alcohols
monoterpenols terpinen-4-ol 4–8.2%, α-terpineol 0.4–1.2%, *cis*-thujan-4-ol <1%, *trans*-thujan-4-ol <1%

Phenols
eugenol 0.2%

Methyl ethers
elemicin 0.4–2.1%, methyl eugenol 0.6%

Benzodioxoles
safrole 0.7–1.7%, myristicin 2.9–10.4%

Oxides
monoterpenoid 1,8-cineole 2–3%

Properties	Indications
analgesic	aches and pains, rheumatism, sprains, toothache, neuralgia
antibacterial	see Table 4.4
antiseptic	chronic diarrhoea
carminative	flatulence
circulatory stimulant	

digestive — loss of appetite, sluggish digestion, difficulty with starches and heavy meals, speeds up intestinal transit, see Table 4.8

emmenagogic — scanty periods
neurotonic — debility
psychoactive
reproductive stimulant — impotence, frigidity
uterotonic — facilitates delivery

Observations

- requires great care in use on account of the myristicin content (a hallucinogen); ingestion of an overdose may produce epileptiform convulsions, coma and death (Åkesson & Wålinder 1965, Dale 1909)
- doses exceeding 5 ml take effect within 2–5 hours, producing time–space distortions and sometimes visual hallucinations accompanied by dizziness, headache, illness and rapid heartbeat (Duke 1985)
- it has been hypothesized that myristicin and elemicin can readily be modified in the body to amphetamines (Duke 1985)
- no irritation or sensitization at 2% dilution when tested on humans (Opdyke 1976n)
- Valnet (1980) lists the *monoterpenols* linalool, geraniol and borneol as constituents of this oil
- inhibits prostaglandin synthesis (Reynolds 1972) and platelet aggregation (Shafran, Maurer & Thomas 1977)
- used to treat diarrhoea owing to eugenol content (Bennett et al 1988)
- myristicin has been shown to cross the placenta causing an increase in the foetal heartbeat (Lavy 1987)
- oral doses of the oil together with pethidine is not advisable as myristicin has been shown to inhibit monoamine synthesis (Reynolds 1993)
- oil is recommended for inflammation of the bladder and urinary tract
- nutmeg oil has larvicidal activity (Oishi et al 1974)
- expectorant action of inhaled nutmeg oil (by animals) was shown (Boyd & Sheppard 1970)
- myristicin (from parsley leaf oil) considered to be a chemopreventative agent (Zheng, McKenney & Lam 1992c, Zheng et al 1992)

MYRTUS COMMUNIS FOL. [*MYRTLE, RED AND ORANGE*] MYRTACEAE

Representative constituents

Hydrocarbons
monoterpenes α-pinene 8.1–56.7%, camphene 0.01–0.2%, β-pinene 0.1–0.8%, β-myrcene 0.1–0.3%, α-terpinolene 0.03–0.6%, sabinene 0.03–0.2%, α-terpinene *trace*–0.6%, α-thujene 0.1–1.5%, limonene 4.1–19%, γ-terpinene *trace*–0.6%, α-phellandrene 0.03–0.4%, δ-3-carene *trace*–0.6%, *cis*-β-ocimene 0.04–0.6%, *trans*-β-ocimene 0.04–0.3%
sesquiterpenes α-copaene 0.1%, β-caryophyllene 0.2–0.8%, α-caryophyllene 0.1–1.4%, δ-cadinene 0.03–2.5%, dihydroazulenes
aromatic p-cymene 0.2–1.8%

Alcohols
monoterpenols (+)-myrtenol 0.3–1.6%, (–)-myrtenol, α-terpineol *trace*–4.2%, terpinen-1-ol-4 0.2–0.3%, nerol *trace*–0.4%, linalool 0.5–13.7%, geraniol 0.1–0.9%, borneol <0.1%
other propanol *trace*–0.8%

Aldehydes
monoterpenal myrtenal 0.1–0.4%
other trans-2-hexanal, n-decanal, furfural, 2-methyl butanal

Esters
monoterpenyl linalyl acetate 0.02–2%, bornyl acetate *trace*–2.1%, α-terpenyl acetate 0.15–4.4%, myrtenyl acetate 0.1–36%, *cis*-myrtenyl acetate, *trans*-carvyl acetate, geranyl acetate 1–3.9%, neryl acetate 0.02–0.2%, methyl myrtenate, citronellyl acetate 0.05–0.2%
other (0.5%) myrtenyl 2-methylpropionate, geranyl 2-methylpropionate, isobutyl isobutanoate 0.2–2.2%, isobutyl 2-methyl butanoate 0.03–0.4%

Oxides
monoterpenoid 1,8-cineole 8–37%, limonene oxide
sesquiterpenoid caryophyllene oxide *trace*–0.9%
other 2-methyl furane

Phenols
carvacrol 0.2–0.6%, eugenol 0.03–0.3%

Methyl ethers
methyl eugenol 0.08–2.3%

Lactones
myrtucommulones A and B

Properties (variation with country of origin)	Indications
anticatarrhal	bronchitis, sinusitis, catarrhal conditions
antiinfectious	throat infections, colds, flu, infectious disease, head lice, nits
antiinflammatory antiseptic (air)	prostatitis, see Table 4.6
antiseptic (urinary, pulmonary, respiratory)	urinary infection, hay fever, asthma
astringent, skin	wrinkles , acne, oily skin, open pores
expectorant	chronic coughs
hormonelike (thyroid, ovary)	hypothyroid, amenorrhoea, dysmenorrhoea, see Table 4.9
sedative (slight), calming	insomnia, relaxing by inhalation
tonic	hepatobiliary deficiency

Myrtus communis ct. myrtenyl acetate

decongestant	varicose veins, lymph congestion, haemorrhoids, prostate congestion

Observations

- no known contraindications at normal aromatherapeutic dose (Franchomme & Pénoël 2001 p. 406)
- well-tolerated on the skin, no phototoxicity, no sensitization, not irritant to the skin
- no oral toxicity, safe to use (Tisserand & Balacs 1995b p. 208)
- very effective in inhalations and aerosols (Roulier 1990 p. 287)
- Dioscorides recommended a maceration of the leaves in wine for bladder infections and for the lungs
- the leaves and flowers were major ingredients in the sixteenth century skin care lotion Angel's Water
- the essential oil of myrtle is seldom used in pharmacy (Bruneton 1995 p. 462)
- the leaves are used in alcoholic beverages (Winter 1999 p. 307)
- North African myrtle essential oil has a reddish colour and contains about 20% of the ester myrtenyl acetate and approximately 45% of 1,8-cineole
- green myrtle is produced in Corsica for aromatherapy purposes; it also contains about 45% 1,8-cineole but little myrtenyl acetate
- oils of differing composition due to different stages of growth and methods of extraction were tested against the human head louse and its eggs; the study confirmed that essential oils of *Myrtus communis* were effective pediculocides but that the method of use depended upon their chemical composition (Gauthier, Agoumi & Gourai 1989)
- the acute oral toxicity of the leaf oil was determined as 3.7 ml/kg; after repeated daily oral administration of essential oil of 0.5–2 ml/kg the toxicity decreased considerably and after 10 days was 6.6 ml/kg; after cessation of oil administration liver weight slowly returned to normal, due to adaptive liver stimulation (Uehleke & Brinkschulte-Freitas 1979): it is very unlikely that humans receiving the much smaller normal aromatherapeutic dose would experience adaptive liver stimulation
- the undiluted essential oil of *Myrtus communis* var. *microphylla* was tested against 13 fungi and caused strong inhibition of *Trichoderma viride, Candida albicans, Aspergillus niger* and others; all fungi tested were inhibited to some extent by a 1:200 dilution of the essential oil (Garg & Dengre 1988)

NARDOSTACHYS JATAMANSI (= N. GRANDIFLORA) RAD. [SPIKENARD] VALERIANACEAE

Representative constituents

Hydrocarbons
monoterpenes α-pinene 0.1%, β-pinene 0.1%, limonene 0.1%

sesquiterpenes aristolene 5%, dihydroazulenes, α-gurjunene 0.6%, β-gurjunene 29%, α-patchoulene 29%
β-patchoulene 0.7%, seychellene 1.7%, β-maaliene

Alcohols
sesquiterpenols calarenol, nardol, valeranol, patchouli alcohol 6%, maaliol

Aldehydes
sesquiterpenals valeranal

Ketones
sesquiterpenones valeranone, β-ionone 1.4%, 3,4-dihydro-β-ionone *trace*, 1-hydroxyaristolenone 6%, aristolenone 0.7%

Oxides
monoterpenoid 1,8-cineole 0.2%

Coumarins
coumarin

Properties	Indications
antiepileptic	
antifungal	see Table 4.5
antispasmodic	convulsions, intestinal colic
calming	tachycardia, epilepsy, hysteria
cardiotonic	arrhythmia
phlebotonic	varicose veins, haemorrhoids
skin	psoriasis*
unspecified	anaemia, ovarian insufficiency

Observations

■ no known contraindications
■ it is sometimes used in place of valerian
■ a history of religious use; used in meditation
■ in tests *N. jatamansi* inhibited the growth of *Aspergillus flavus*, *A. niger* and *Fusarium oxysporum*; it was also active against a wide range of other fungi (Mishra et al 1995)

NEPETA CATARIA VAR. *CITRIODORA* FLOS, FOL. [CATNEP] LAMIACEAE

Representative constituents

Hydrocarbons
monoterpenes β-myrcene *trace*–1.5%, limonene *trace*–0.4%, β-ocimenes *trace*–0.7%
sesquiterpenes β-caryophyllene 1.1–6.8%, α-caryophyllene *trace*–4.3%

Alcohols
monoterpenols geraniol 13.7%, citronellol 48.3%

Esters
hexanyl benzoate and other acetates, valeronates and butanoates

Aldehydes
monoterpenals neral 4.9%, geranial 5.6%

Lactones *(>15%)*
nepetalactone 9.4%, epinepetalactone 1.6%, dihydro nepetalactone 1.2%

Ketones
monoterpenone piperitone

Methyl ethers
thymol methyl ether

Oxide
humulene oxide

Properties	Indications
antiinfectious	urinary infections
antiinflammatory*	irritable bowel syndrome, rheumatism*, arthritis, see Table 4.6
antiviral*	*Herpes*, see Table 4.7
calming*, sedative	anxiety
litholytic	gall stones
neurotonic*	nervous depression

Observations

■ no known contraindications
■ the nepetalactone chemotype is described as diaphoretic and expectorant (Secondini 1990)

- the chemical structure of nepetalactone is similar to the valepotriates, the sedative principle in valerian
- the lactone content is highest at the time of flowering (up to 60%) (Bourrel et al 1993)
- fungistatic activity was observed against *Candida albicans* and *Aspergillus niger* (Bourrel et al 1993)
- nepetalactone (from *Nepeta caesarea*) possesses significant analgesic and strong sedative action (Aydin et al 1998)

OCIMUM BASILICUM
FOL. [EUROPEAN BASIL] LAMIACEAE

Representative constituents

Hydrocarbons
monoterpenes (2%) α-pinene, β-pinene, camphene, limonene, *cis*-β-ocimene, γ-terpinene
sesquiterpenes isocaryophyllene, β-caryophyllene 2–3%, β-elemene
aromatic p-cymene
other cis-3-hexanol

Alcohols
monoterpenols linalool 40–55%, α-fenchyl alcohol 3–12%, terpinen-4-ol 1.6%, α-terpineol 2%, citronellol 1.5%, geraniol 1.2%

Esters
monoterpenyl linalyl acetate, α-fenchyl acetate <1%, α-terpinyl acetate *trace*
other methyl cinnamate 0.1–7%

Phenols
eugenol 1–19%, iso-eugenol 2%

Methyl ethers
methyl chavicol 3–31%, methyl eugenol 1–9%

Oxides
monoterpenoid 1,8-cineole 2–8%

Ketones
monoterpenone camphor 0.1%

Properties	Indications
analgesic	gout, migraine, rheumatoid arthritis
anthelmintic	threadworms
antibacterial	coliform cystitis, see Table 4.4
antifungal*	see Table 4.5
antiinflammatory*	gout, wasp stings, see Table 4.6
antiseptic	intestinal infections, gastritis
antispasmodic	gastric spasm, muscle cramp
antiviral	viral hepatitis, see Table 4.7
cardiotonic	arrhythmia, arteriosclerosis, tachycardia
carminative, eupeptic	flatulence, sluggish digestion, see Table 4.8
digestive	stimulates digestive secretions, ulcers, see Table 4.8
hypertensor	hypotension
insecticidal	housefly, mosquito, see Table 4.10
liver stimulant	hepatobiliary deficiency
nervous system	anxiety*, epilepsy, insomnia, nervousness, travel sickness, vertigo
neurotonic	debility, mental strain, convalescence, depression
reproductive	uterine and prostatic congestion
unspecified	dry eczema

Observations

- no known contraindications
- no irritation or sensitization at 4% dilution when tested on humans (Opdyke 1973e)
- no phototoxic effects reported (Opdyke 1973e)
- this oil may be used with safety when the methyl chavicol content is low; methyl chavicol causes liver cancer when fed to mice; no tests have been carried out on the application to the skin of humans and subsequent metabolization. There are no reports of cancer ever having been caused in

humans owing to the use of essential oils
(Tisserand & Balacs 1995b)

- a prolonged daily intake of five drops would
be ill advised (Caldwell 1991)
- the fact that it is a uterine decongestant does
not mean that it is emmenagogic
- there is a natural variation in the chemical
constituents of this essential oil both between
plants and according to where the plant is grown
- oil has insecticidal and insect repellent
properties, effective against house flies and
mosquitoes (Deshpande & Ripnis 1977); out of
250 insects of *Allocophora foveicollis* tested, basil
oil repelled 134, attracted 59 and 57 were non-
reactive (Dube, Upadhyay & Tripathi 1988);
also bactericidal against *Salmonella typhi*
- insecticidal against mosquito species *Anopheles
stephensi, Aedes aegypti, Culex quinquefasciatus*
(Bhatnagae et al 1993)
- estragole is metabolized to 1-hydroxyestragole
in humans (Sangster et al 1987) but small
amounts are detoxified easily (Anthony et al
1987, Zangouras et al 1981)
- *O. basilicum* essential oil inhibited the mycelial
growth of 22 species of fungi (Dube,
Upadhyay & Tripathi 1988)
- the oil is a stimulant (Manley 1993)

ORIGANUM MAJORANA FLOS, FOL. [SWEET MARJORAM] LAMIACEAE

Representative constituents

Hydrocarbons
monoterpenes (40%) sabinene 2–10%, β-myrcene
1–9%, α-terpinolene 1–7%, α-pinene 1–5%,
β-pinene 0.2–2.5%, *cis-* and *trans-*β-ocimenes
6.4%, 3-carene 6.2%, α-terpinene 6–8%,
γ-terpinene 14–20%, α-phellandrene,
β-phellandrene 0.9%, limonene 0.6%
sesquiterpenes β-caryophyllene 2–4.6%,
α-caryophyllene 0.1%, δ-cadinene 4.2%
aromatic p-cymene 1–6%

Alcohols
monoterpenols (50%) terpinen-1-ol-4 14–20%, *cis-*
thujan-4-ol 4–13%, *trans-*thujan-4-ol 1–5%,
linalool 2–9.5%, α-terpineol 7–27%, *cis-*p-
menth-2-en-1-ol 2%, *trans-*p-menth-2-en-ol
2%, *cis-*piperitol 0.5%

Esters
monoterpenyl terpenyl acetate 0–3%, geranyl
acetate 1–7.8%, linalyl acetate 0.1%

Aldehydes
monoterpenal citral 5.4%

Properties	Indications
analgesic*	arthritis*, migraine, muscular pain*, rheumatism*, toothache, headaches,
antibacterial antiinfectious	see Table 4.4 whooping cough, bronchitis, respiratory infections, rhinitis, sinusitis
antispasmodic	colic, muscles, respiratory spasm, nervous spasm
calming	ether addiction, psychoses, agitation, anxiety, epilepsy, insomnia, migraine, sexual obsessions, vertigo
carminative	flatulence
digestive	gastroduodenal ulcers, indigestion, see Table 4.8
diuretic expectorant	catarrh, coughs, bronchitis
hormonelike	hyperthyroidism, see Table 4.9
hypotensor	hypertension, tachycardia, palpitations, fainting
neurotonic	debility*, mental instability, nervous spasm (by balancing the parasympathetic nervous system), anguish, agitation, nervous depression
respiratory tonic stomachic vasodilator	nervous breathing diarrhoea, enteritis

Observations

- no known contraindications at normal dose
- marjoram oil stimulates the vagus (parasympathetic) nerve and does not act on the sympathetic nerve, therefore its action is tranquillizing and lightly narcotic, a nervous sedative (Duraffourd 1982)
- no irritation or sensitization at 6% dilution when tested on humans (Opdyke 1976o)
- used in Vermouth
- the naming and correct identification of this group of herbs presents difficulties even to the expert: there are some 30 species of marjoram with the generic name *Origanum*
- has antiviral activities against *Herpes simplex* (Herrmann & Kucera 1967)
- *O. majorana* achieved total inhibition of a range of yeasts, moulds and lactic acid bacteria (except *Pediococcus damnosus*) (Charai, Mosaddak & Faid 1996)
- when tested *in vitro O. majorana* inhibited the growth of five fungal and 25 bacterial species (Deans & Svoboda 1990)

ORIGANUM VULGARE SUBSP. VIRIDE (= O. HERACLEOTICUM)
[GREEK OREGANO, GREEN OREGANO]
LAMIACEAE

Representative constituents

Hydrocarbons
monoterpenes α-terpinene 0.8–1%, γ-terpinene 3.6%, α-thujene and α-pinene 0.95%, camphene 0.14%, β-pinene 0.1%, β-myrcene 0.93%, limonene 0.1%
sesquiterpenes caryophyllene 1.05%, β-bisabolene
aromatic p-cymene 7–10%

Alcohols
monoterpenols linalool 0.2%, terpinen-4-ol 0.85%, borneol 0.74%, *trans*-thujan-4-ol 0.1%
other pentyl alcohol *trace*

Phenols
carvacrol 50–75%, thymol *trace*–7%

Esters
monoterpenyl linalyl acetate 3.5%

Oxides
monoterpenoid 1,8-cineole 0.2%
other 4,5-epoxy-*p*-menth-l-ene

Ketones
monoterpenone carvone *trace*

Properties	Indications
antiinfectious***	wide range of action, infections of the respiratory tract, digestive tract, genitourinary system
antiparasitic***	
immunostimulant	
tonic**	asthenia

Observations

- no known contraindications at normal aromatherapeutic dose
- prudence should be exercised in dermal application because of the high phenol content
- *Origanum vulgare* essential oil was effective against three strains of *Candida albicans*; the main component carvacrol had the same effect (Stiles et al 1995)
- *Origanum vulgare* subsp. *hirtum* was found to have strong antifungal activity against *Malassezia furfur, Trichophyton rubrum T. beigelii* (Adam et al 1998); also strong activity against *Escherichia coli, Pseudomonas aeruginosa, Staphylococcus aureus, Salmonella typhimurium* and *Bacillus subtilis* (Sivropoulou et al 1996)
- possessed strong action against 19 bacteria and the fungus *Aspergillus niger* (Baratta, Dorman & Deans 1998)
- emulsified oregano oil was used successfully by oral administration to treat patients having enteric parasites (Force, Sparks & Ronzio 2000)
- *in vitro* the oil was a potent antifungal agent against *Candida albicans* and *in vivo* was comparable to amphotericin B for systemic candidiasis; activity of the whole oil was superior to the major component carvacrol (Manohar et al 2001)

ORMENIS MIXTA FLOS [MOROCCAN CHAMOMILE] ASTERACEAE

Representative constituents

Hydrocarbons

monoterpenes α-pinene 15%, camphene 0.4%, limonene 8%, γ-terpinene 0.1%, α-terpinolene 0.25%

sesquiterpenes germacrene 5%, β-caryophyllene 1.5%, bisabolene 2.5%, δ-elemene 0.7%

Alcohols

monoterpenols α-terpineol, linalool 0.3%, borneol 1%, ormenol, *trans*-pinocarveol 3%, santolina alcohol 32%, yomogi alcohol 2.4%, artemisia alcohol 2.3%

Ketones

monoterpenones camphor, pinocarvone 0.5%

Oxides

monoterpenoid 1,8-cineole

Esters

monoterpenyl bornyl acetate 2.2%, bornyl butanoate 1.3%

Properties	Indications
antibacterial*	colibacillosus, see Table 4.4
antiinfectious	acne, cysts
antiinflammatory	rheumatism, colitis, cystitis, see Table 4.6
antiinflammatory (skin)	dermatitis, eczema, inflamed skin, sunburn
antiirritant	pruritus
hepatobiliary tonic	gall bladder and pancreas, sluggish liver
neurotonic*	nervous depression*
parasiticide	*Oxyures, Amibes* intestinal parasites, *Kystes amibiens*
tonic general	gall bladder and pancreas, sluggish liver
other	atherosclerosis, allergic reactions

Observations

- no known contraindications at normal aromatherapeutic dose
- Moroccan chamomile essential oil is unlikely to present any hazard in aromatherapy (Tisserand & Balacs 1995b p. 215)
- at a presentation to the Royal Society of Medicine it was stated that *Ormenis mixta* essential oil, in common with several other oils, was effective against MRSA (cited in Buckle 1997 p. 125)

PELARGONIUM GRAVEOLENS FOL. [GERANIUM] GERANIACEAE

Representative constituents

Hydrocarbons

monoterpenes (1–2%) α-phellandrene *trace*, β-phellandrene, α-pinene 1%, β-pinene 0.2%, β-myrcene 0.2%, limonene 0.2%, *cis*-β-ocimene 0.2%

sesquiterpenes (1–2%) guai-6,9-diene 3.9–5.3%, guaiazulene, α-copaene, δ-cadinene, γ-cadinene, α-bourbonene, β-bourbonene, caryophyllene 0.7%

Alcohols

monoterpenols (55–65%) citronellol 21–45%, geraniol 17–25%, linalool 1–13%, nerol 1.2%, α-terpineol 0.7%

sesquiterpenols 10-epi-γ-eudesmol 1%

aromatic phenyl ethyl alcohol <1%

Esters *(15%)*

monoterpenyl citronellyl formate 8–18%, geranyl formate 1–6%, citronellyl propionate 1–3%, geranyl propionate 0–1%, geranyl angelate 1–2%, geranyl acetate 0.4%, citronellyl butanoate 1.3%, geranyl butanoate 1.3%,

other phenyl ethyl isobutanoate, phenyl ethyl angelate

Aldehydes *(Bourbon variety) (0–10%)*

monoterpenals neral, geranial 0–9%, citronellal 0–1%

Ketones *(1–8%)*

monoterpenones menthone 0.6–3%, isomenthone 4–8.4%, piperitone *other* methyl heptanone, furopelargone 0.4%

Oxides *(only in Chinese variety) (2–3%)*
monoterpenoid cis-rose oxide 2–25%, *trans*-rose
oxide 1%, *cis*-linalool oxide 0.6%, *trans*-
linalool oxide 0.2%

Properties	Indications
analgesic	facial neuralgia, osteoarthritis, rheumatism
antibacterial*	see Table 4.4
antidiabetic	sluggish pancreas, diabetes
antifungal*	athlete's foot and other skin and nail fungi, *Candida*, see Table 4.5
antiinfectious	infectious colitis, acne, wounds, impetigo, infectious skin diseases
antiinflammatory	arthritis, colitis, pruritus, rheumatism, tonsillitis, see Table 4.6
antiseptic	
antispasmodic	colic, cramp, gastroenteritis, painful menstruation
astringent	diarrhoea, haemorrhoids, varicose veins
cicatrizant	burns, cuts, ulcers, uterine haemorrhage, stretch marks, wounds
decongestant	breast congestion, lymph congestion
digestive	jaundice, sluggish liver, see Table 4.8
haemostatic, styptic	burns, cuts, ulcers, uterine haemorrhage, wounds
insectifuge	gnats, mosquitoes, see Table 4.10
phlebotonic* (lymph*)	haemorrhoids, varicose ulcers, varicose veins
relaxant*	agitation, anxiety, debility, nervous fatigue

Observations

■ no known contraindications

■ to be used with care on the skin of hypersensitive individuals (Winter 1984)
■ no irritation or sensitization at 10% dilution when tested on humans (Opdyke 1974k)
■ no phototoxic effects reported (Opdyke 1974k)
■ contact with the leaves of the plant has been reported to cause vesicular dermatitis (Anderson 1923)
■ maximum acceptable daily intake of 500 mg/kg body weight of citral, geranyl acetate, citronellol and linalool is recommended (Reynolds 1972)
■ 32 scented leaf *Pelargonium* essential oils were tested *in vitro* and found to be spasmolytic (Lis-Balchin, Hart & Roth 1997)
■ the primary alcohols in *P. graveolens* were shown to be chiefly responsible for the fungitoxic activity of the oil against *Colletotrichum gloeosporioides* (Nidiry 1998)

PICEA MARIANA, PICEA NIGRA
[BLACK SPRUCE] PINACEAE

Representative constituents

Hydrocarbons
monoterpenes (+)-camphene 10–15%, tricyclene 1–3%, (–)-α-pinene 13–16%, (+)-δ-3-carene 5–15%
sesquiterpenes longifolene, longicyclene, cadinene

Alcohols *(2.5%)*
monoterpenols (+)-borneol 1%
sesquiterpenols longiborneol

Esters *(30–45%)*
monoterpenyl bornyl acetate 35–45%

Properties	Indications
antifungal	intestinal *Candida*, see Table 4.5
antiinfectious	air antiseptic
antiinflammatory	prostatitis, rheumatism, see Table 4.6
antiparasitic	lamblia, ankylostoma
antispasmodic	abdominal spasm
hormonelike	cortisone like, hyperthyroidism, see Table 4.9

immunostimulant**	lowered immune system
neurotonic	asthenia, tired out
skin	acne, dry eczema

Observations

- no contraindications known at normal aromatherapeutic dose (Franchomme & Pénoël 2001 p. 415)
- Schnaubelt (1998 p. 90) advises only the external use of black spruce oil

PIMENTA DIOICA FRUCT. [ALLSPICE, PIMENTO, JAMAICAN PEPPER, CLOVE PEPPER] MYRTACEAE

Representative constituents

Hydrocarbons
monoterpenes limonene 0.1–0.4%, α-pinene 0.2%, α-thujene 0.2%, β-pinene 0.1%, β-myrcene 0.2–0.8%, α-phellandrene 0.5–1.2%, α-terpinene 0.1–0.3%, *trans*-β-ocimene + γ-terpinene 0.3–0.7%, α-terpinolene 0.5–1.5%, β-phellandrene 0.1%, camphene 0.2%
sesquiterpenes β-caryophyllene 2.5–5.4%, + iso-caryophyllene, calamenene 0.1%, α-humulene 1.1–2.7%, α- and β-selinene 0.7–1.0%, δ-cadinene 0.4–0.9%, β-elemene 0.2–0.3%, alloaromadendrene 0.1%, β-caryophyllene 0.5%, α-copaene 0.1%, γ-muurolene 0.1%, γ-cadinene *trace*
aromatic p-cymene 0.2–0.7%, ar-curcumene 0.1–0.2%

Phenols
eugenol 69–87%, chavicol 0.2–0.5%

Methyl ethers
methyl eugenol 2.9–13.1%

Oxides
monoterpenoid 1,8-cineole 0.2–3.3%
sesquiterpenoid humulene oxide *trace*, caryophyllene oxide 0.2%

Alcohols
monoterpenols α-terpineol 0.2–0.5%, linalool 0.15%, terpinen-4-ol 0.3–0.5%
sesquiterpenols β-caryophyllene alcohol 0.4–0.6%

Aldehydes
sesquiterpenal caryophyllene aldehyde 0.2%

PIMENTA DIOICA FOL. [LEAF OIL]

Representative constituents

Hydrocarbons
monoterpenes β-myrcene 0.1–0.2%, α-pinene *trace*, α-phellandrene *trace*, limonene 0.2–0.4%, γ-terpinene *trace*, trans-β-ocimene 0–0.7%, α-terpinolene *trace*
sesquiterpenes β-caryophyllene 0.1–8%, α-humulene 1–2.1%,, α-gurjunene <0.5%, β-elemene 0.1–0.4%, aromadendrene <0.05%, alloaromadendrene 0–0.9%, β-selinene 0.4–0.9%, α-selinene 0.6–1%, δ-cadinene 0–0.6%
other undecane, dodecane, octane
aromatic p-cymene <0.1%

Alcohols
monoterpenols α-terpineol 0–0.3%
sesquiterpenols viridiflorol 0–0.8%, palustrol 0–0.6%, ledol 0–0.2%, β-eudesmol 0–0.5%

Oxides
monoterpenoid 1,8-cineole 1.1–2.5%
sesquiterpenoid caryophyllene oxide 0.2–1.8%

Phenols
eugenol 65–95%, isoeugenol 6%, chavicol <1%

Methyl ethers
methyl eugenol 1–4%

Properties	Indications
anaesthetic	toothache
antibacterial	infected acne, dysentery, cystitis, salpingitis, urethritis, see Table 4.4
antifungal	see Table 4.5
antiinfectious	dental infections, cholera, influenza, colds
antiseptic	
antiviral	hepatitis, neuritis, *Herpes zoster*, MS, poliomyelitis, enterocolitis, see Table 4.7

carminative	flatulence, indigestion
hypertensor	hypotension
neurotonic	
parasiticide	skin parasites
stimulant	general fatigue, asthenia, depression
uterotonic	

Observations

- N.B. The situation regarding the properties and indications for *Pimenta dioica* oil is somewhat confused because writers do not always make clear whether leaf, fruit or leaf and fruit oil is being discussed; also there are chemotypes of this plant and this is not usually specified. Those listed above must be viewed in the light of this. Other uses that have been mentioned are cramp, intestinal problems, rheumatism, muscular strains, as a tonic and also as a tranquillizer

- when the oil and eugenol were applied to intact shaved abdominal skin of mice no percutaneous absorption was observed within 2 hours

- the oil was not irritant when applied to the backs of hairless mice and pigs

- 8% in petrolatum was not irritant or sensitizing

- no phototoxicity was reported

- both the oil and eugenol enhance trypsin activity and have larvicidal properties

- eugenol is a local anaesthetic and antiseptic

- compared to the Jamaican oil, Honduran and Mexican oils contain a lower eugenol content (52–62% and 49% respectively) and increased methyl eugenol (up to 28%) and β-myrcene (6–9%)

- oil from Grenada has a similar eugenol content to Jamaican oil and a decreased methyl eugenol (0.5%) and an increased cineole (3.2%) content

- Guatamalan oil has a similar range of values to Jamaican oil

- the leaf oil contains a higher proportion of eugenol (up to 96%)

- used medicinally as an aromatic carminative and stomachic, also used in cosmetics as an ingredient in fragrance formulations and extensively used in food products

PIMENTA RACEMOSA (= PIMENTA ACRIS) FRUCT., FOL. [WEST INDIAN BAY] MYRTACEAE

Representative constituents

Hydrocarbons

monoterpenes α-pinene 0.1–0.3%, sabinene 0.3%, β-pinene 0.1%, β-myrcene 13.9–31.6%, α-phellandrene 0.4%, limonene 1.4%, β-phellandrene 0.1%, *trans*-β-ocimene 0.4–2.1%, α-terpinolene 0.1–0.3%
sesquiterpenes β-caryophyllene 0.9%, copaene 0.2%, α-amorphene 0.1%
aromatic p-cymene 0.1–0.5%

Aldehydes

monoterpenals neral 0.5%

Alcohols

monoterpenols linalool 1.7–3%, terpinen-4-ol 0.3%, α-terpineol 0.1–0.8%
other 3-octanol 0.5–0.6%, 1-octen-3-ol 1–1.3%

Phenols

eugenol 38–75%, chavicol 11–22%, isoeugenol

Methyl ethers

methyl chavicol 0.3%

Oxides

monoterpenoid 1,8-cineole 0.2–2%

Ketones

3-octanone 1–1.1%, methyl heptenone 0.7%

Esters

monoterpenyl geranyl acetate 0.8%

Properties	Indications
analgesic	muscular and joint pains, sprains, strains
antiseptic	respiratory tract infections, bronchitis, tonsillitis
antiviral	influenza, viral infections
aperitive	loss of appetite, anorexia
astringent	

carminative

emmenagogic

digestive

sudorific

tonic (scalp)

flatulence

scanty periods

dyspepsia, see Table 4.8

fevers

falling hair, poor circulation

Observations

- N.B. The situation regarding the properties and indications for *Pimenta racemosa* (=*Pimenta acris*) oil is somewhat confused because writers do not always make clear whether the leaf, fruit or leaf and fruit oil is being discussed; also there are chemotypes of this plant and these are not usually specified. Those listed above must be viewed in the light of this. Other uses that have been mentioned are sinusitis, bronchitis, tuberculosis, malaria, thyroid malfunction, and rheumatoid arthritis
- non-irritant on human skin at 10% (Opdyke 1973a p. 869)
- oral toxicity classed as mild by Tisserand & Balacs (1995a p. 203)
- it is sometimes falsified with clove or turpentine essential oils
- although this oil also has the common name of bay it must not be confused with *Laurus nobilis*
- used in hair lotions, aftershave lotions and men's line fragrances
- Duraffourd (1982 p. 37) writes that the properties are very similar to that of clove in that it has very strong antiseptic properties especially on the respiratory tract
- once important as the source for bay rum but this is now synthesized
- there exist 2 chemotypes, one with anise scented essential oil (with methyl chavicol 32% and methyl eugenol 43%) and the other lemon scented (containing mostly citral >80%) (Leung & Foster 1996 pp. 71–72)
- an additional third chemotype was identified by Aurore et al (1998) having chavicol 17% and eugenol 56%; all three chemotypes were tested for antibacterial and antifungal activity; the citral chemotype possessed the most potent antimicrobial action
- eugenol is an inhibitor of platelet activity (Janssens et al 1990) and it may be assumed that the oil inhibits blood clotting (Tisserand &

Balacs 1995b p. 121); caution is recommended for anyone taking anticoagulants

PIMPINELLA ANISUM FRUCT. [ANISEED] APIACEAE

Representative constituents

Hydrocarbons

sesquiterpenes γ-himachalene *trace*, β-caryophyllene

Alcohols *(0.5–4%)*

monoterpenols anisol 0.5–4%, linalool <1.5%, α-terpineol <1.5%

Phenols *(0.5%)*

Methyl ethers *(90–95%)*

cis-anethole 0–1%, *trans*-anethole 90–93%, methyl chavicol 0–2%

other isochavibetol 0.5%

Benzodioxoles

myristicin *trace*

Aldehydes

anisaldehyde 1–2%

Ketones

p-methoxyphenylacetone

Coumarins, furanocoumarins

umbelliferone, scopoletin

Properties	Indications
analgesic	arthritis, backache, nauseous migraine, period pains, rheumatism, sciatica, vertigo
antispasmodic	bronchial spasm, colic, enteritis, flatulence, indigestion, infantile colic, vomiting (of nervous origin), painful periods
aperitive	stimulates digestive juices

cardiotonic	cardiovascular erethism, palpitations, tired heart
carminative*	flatulence, indigestion
diuretic	oliguria
emmenagogic	amenorrhoea, oligomenorrhoea*
expectorant*	catarrh
lactogenic	lack of milk
narcotic (gentle)	
oestrogen-like*	menopause, PMS
psychoactive*	
respiratory tonic	asthma, bronchitis, congestion in lungs, nervous breathing
sexual tonic	frigidity, impotence
uterotonic	facilitates delivery

Observations

- not normally used on babies, young children and pregnant women
- like fennel oil, anise oil contains compounds that can be aminated *in vivo* resulting in a series of three dangerous hallucinogenic amphetamines (Emboden 1972)
- the major component of aniseed oil, anethole, can cause dermatitis (erythema, scaling and vesiculation) in some individuals
- anethole has two isomers, the *cis* isomer being 15 to 38 times more toxic than the *trans* isomer (Leung 1980)
- several cases of sensitization have been reported (Loveman 1938, Schwarz 1934, Tulipan 1938), and attributed to the presence of anethole (Schwarz, Tulipan & Peck 1947)
- no irritation or sensitization at 4% dilution when tested on humans (Opdyke 1973f); not a primary irritant to normal skin (Harry 1948)
- *trans*-anethole and its derivatives are oestrogen-like; avoid oral intake during pregnancy and breastfeeding (Albert-Puleo 1980, Zondek et al 1938)
- found to be a most effective expectorant in guinea pigs (Boyd & Pearson 1946)
- anethole, anisaldehyde, (+)-carvone and myristicin have mild insecticidal properties (Carter 1976); anethole inhibits also the growth of toxin-producing *Aspergillus* species (Hitokoto et al 1980)
- anethole is considered to be an oestrogenic

agent; however, research suggests that dianethole and photoanethole (polymers of anethole) are the active oestrogenic compounds (Albert-Puleo 1980)
- anethole is structurally related to the hallucinogenic compound myristicin (Reynolds 1989)
- anethole is responsible for contact dermatitis reactions (Chandler & Hawkes 1984, Mitchell & Rook 1979)
- ingestion of 1–5 ml of the oil can cause nausea, vomiting, seizures and pulmonary oedema (Chandler & Hawkes 1984)
- essential oil *Pimpinella anisum* was found to be fungistatic due to anethole content (Shukla & Tripathi 1987a)

PINUS MUGO VAR. *PUMILIO*
[*DWARF PINE*] PINACEAE

Representative constituents

Hydrocarbons
monoterpenes (70%) (+)-limonene 42.1%, δ-3-carene 11.5%, (−)-α-pinene 18.4%, β-pinene 8.1%, α-phellandrene; β-phellandrene; camphene 4.3%, α-terpinolene, α-terpinene, γ-terpinene, β-myrcene 3.6%
sesquiterpenes α-humulene, β-bisabolene, α-curcumene, caryophyllene, longifolene, α-muurolene, γ-muurolene, *trans*-muurolene, δ-cadinene
aromatic p-cymene
other chamazulene, elemazulene

Alcohols
monoterpenols borneol 1%

Esters
monoterpenyl bornyl acetate 4–10%, bornyl propionate, bornyl caproate

Oxides
monoterpenyl 1,8-cineole

Aldehydes
monoterpenals geranial, neral
aromatic cuminaldehyde, anisaldehyde
other hexenal

Ketones
monoterpenone camphor, (+)-cryptone

Properties	Indications
antiinflammatory (mild)	see Table 4.6
antimicrobial	sore throat, respiratory problems and chest infections, colds,
antiseptic (pulmonary)	catarrh, bronchitis, asthma, sinusitis, pleurisy
diuretic	bladder and kidney disorders
energizing	
litholytic	gall stones
rubefacient	muscular aches and pains, massage for circulatory problems, rheumatism

Observations

- the oil was non-irritant when applied to the backs of hairless mice and pigs and when applied under 24-hour occlusion to both intact and abraded rabbit skin (Opdyke 1976 p. 483)
- 12% in petrolatum was tested on 22 humans and three irritant responses were obtained (Opdyke 1976 p. 483)
- in patch tests on 21 patients with essential oil dermatoses positive reactions to full-strength or diluted oils were attributed to δ-3-carene and α-phellandrene
- dwarf pine oil may be irritant if oxidized (Tisserand & Balacs 1995b p. 164)
- no phototoxicity has been reported
- limonene, dipentene and bornyl acetate have been reported as being responsible for the antiviral and antibacterial activity (Joubert & Gattefossé 1968, Opdyke 1976)
- much used in Italy for chest [respiratory] problems; balsamic (Cesare Giordano personal communication)
- bornyl acetate has a strong pine odour and can cause nausea, vomiting if ingested (Winter 1999 p. 347)
- for cough remedies volatile oils are used for inhalation, above all oil of dwarf pine needles (Weiss 1988 p. 216)

- dwarf pine was included in a study of various essential oils and was found to have a mild antiinflammatory effect (Wagner, Wierer & Bauer 1986)

PINUS SYLVESTRIS FOL. [PINE] PINACEAE

Representative constituents

Hydrocarbons
monoterpenes (60–70%) α-pinene 22–43%, β-pinene 3–33%, limonene 0.7–4.1%, δ-3-carene 0.4–31%, β-caryophyllene 0.7–5.5%, camphene 1.6–3.3%, sabinene 0.2–0.6%, γ-terpinene 0.1–0.5%, *trans*-β-ocimene 0.7–1.4%, α-terpinolene 0.3–3%
sesquiterpenes longifolene, γ-cadinene 0.5–5.4%, α-copaene 0–0.2%, δ-elemene *trace*, α-ylangene *trace*, longifolene 0–0.2%, β-guaiene 0.2–0.7%, β-farnesene *trace*, γ-muurolene *trace*–0.4%, α-humulene *trace*–0.5%, γ-patchoulene 0–0.2%, γ-cadinene *trace*–0.3%, α-muurolene *trace*–1%, cubenene *trace*, calamenene *trace*, β-phellandrene 1–2.7%
aromatic p-cymene 0–0.2%

Alcohols
monoterpenols borneol 2%, terpinen-4-ol 1%
sesquiterpenols epi-α-cadinol <1%, epi-α-muurolol <1%, α-cadinol 0–0.2%

Aldehydes
monoterpenals citronellal 0–0.2%

Esters *(1–10%)*
monoterpenyl bornyl acetate 0–3%

Properties	Indications
analgesic	gastralgia, intestinal pains, arthritis, rheumatism
antibacterial	see Table 4.4
antifungal	see Table 4.5
antiinfectious*	antiseptic (air), respiratory infections, asthma*, bronchitis*, colds, influenza,

	pneumonia, sinusitis*, tracheitis, tuberculosis, urinary infections (cystitis, prostatitis, pyelitis)
antiinflammatory	inflammatory and allergic conditions, arthritis, gall bladder inflammation, gout, rheumatism, see Table 4.6
antisudorific balsamic	hyperidrosis of the feet
cortisone-like	stimulates suprarenal cortex
decongestant	congested lymph, uterine or ovarian congestion, breaks down bronchial secretions
expectorant	respiratory tract
hypertensor*	hypotension*
insulin-like	pancreatic diabetes
litholytic	gall stones
neurotonic*	debility*, fatigue, insufficient semen (nervous origin), multiple sclerosis
rubefacient	arthritis, rheumatism
testosterone-like	impotence

Observations

- no known contraindications
- in patch tests on 21 patients with essential oil dermatoses, positive reactions to full-strength or diluted oils including *P. sylvestris* oil were attributed to δ-3-carene (a major component of pine oil), α-phellandrene and eugenol (Woeber & Krombach 1969)
- no irritation or sensitization at 12% dilution when tested on humans (Opdyke 1976p)
- no phototoxic effects reported (Opdyke 1976p)
- limonene, dipentene and bornyl acetate are responsible for antiviral and antibacterial activity (Joubert & Gattefossé 1968)

PIPER NIGRUM FRUCT. [BLACK PEPPER]
PIPERACEAE

Representative constituents

Hydrocarbons

monoterpenes α-pinene 2–9%, β-pinene 5–14%, α-thujene 0.5–3.5%, sabinene 9–19%, α-terpinene 0.4–2.8%, δ-3-carene 1–15%, β-myrcene 1.6–2.5%,(–)-limonene 17%, α-phellandrene 5–9%, δ-elemene 2.6%, γ-terpinene 0.5–3.9%, α-terpinolene 0.5–1.5%, camphene

sesquiterpenes β-caryophyllene 9–29%, α-caryophyllene 1–2%, α-guaiene, α- and β-cubebene 0.2–1.6%, α– and β-selinene 0.5–7.7%, α- and β-elemene 0.3–2.4%, β-bisabolene 2–5%, calamenene, α-copaene 0.5–1.5%, β-farnesene 1–3%, zingiberene *trace*, bergamotene 0.5%

aromatic p-cymene 1–2.8%, ar-curcumene 0.5%

Alcohols

monoterpenols terpinen-4-ol <1%, α-terpineol 0.1%, linalool <1%, *trans*-pinocarveol, *trans*-carveol

sesquiterpenols α-bisabolol 0.1%, elemol 0.5%

Methyl ethers

p-cymene methyl ether, carvacrol methyl ether *trace*

Benzodioxoles

myristicin *trace*, safrole *trace*

Ketones *(1–8%)*

monoterpenones dihydrocarvone 0.05%, piperitone <1%

Aldehydes

monoterpenals piperonal

Oxides

sesquiterpenyl caryophyllene oxide 0.6%

Properties	Indications
analgesic*	rheumatic pain, toothache*
antibacterial	see Table 4.4

anticatarrhal	chronic bronchitis, laryngitis, colds
antiseptic	urinary system
digestive	sluggish liver, pancreas and digestion, see Table 4.8
expectorant	bronchitis, coughs
febrifuge	fevers
sexual tonic	frigidity, general

Observations

- no known contraindications to *P. nigrum*
- no irritation or sensitization at 4% dilution when tested on humans (Opdyke 1978e)
- low level (insignificant) phototoxic effects (Opdyke 1978e)
- myristicin and elemicin can be readily modified in the body to amphetamines (Buchanan 1978, Duke 1985)
- it is mutagenic with *Leptospira*; in large doses it has a bactericidal effect and has an inhibiting effect on *Lactobacillus plantarum*, *Escherichia coli* and *Streptococcus faecalis* (Duke & Ayensu 1985)
- smoking withdrawal symptoms are lessened by the inhalation of the vapour from an extract of black pepper (Rose & Behm 1994)

POGOSTEMON PATCHOULI, P. CABLIN FOL. [PATCHOULI] LAMIACEAE

Representative constituents

Hydrocarbons

monoterpenes α-pinene <1%, β-pinene <1%, limonene *trace*, α-thujene

sesquiterpenes (40–50%) α-bulnesene 10–19.6%, β-bulnesene 14–16%, α-guaiene 6–15.6%, β-guaiene, α-patchoulene 3–5.3%, β-patchoulene 1.9–6.6%, γ-patchoulene, seychellene 5–12%, cycloseychellene <1%, β-caryophyllene 2–4.2%, δ-cadinene 1–2.8%, aromadendrene 10.8–20.9%, α-humulene, β-gurjunene <0.1%, α-gurjunene 0–2.8%, β-elemene <1%, α-copaene 2%

Alcohols

monoterpenols borneol

sesquiterpenols (35–45%) patchouli alcohol 23.6–45.9%, pogostol 1–3%, bulnesol 1%, guaiol, norpatchoulenol <1%

Aldehydes

aromatic benzaldehyde, cinnamaldehyde

Ketones

monoterpenones camphor

sesquiterpenones patchoulenone *trace*–2.2%, isopatchoulenone 1%

Oxides

monoterpenoid α-guaiene oxide 1%, α-bulnesene oxide 4%

sesquiterpenoid caryophyllene oxide 0.5–1%, 1,5-epoxy-α-guaiene 0.1–0.4%, 1,10-epoxy-α-bulnesene 0.2–0.6%, epoxy-1α,5α-V-α-guaiene *trace*, epoxy-1β, 5β-α-guaiene *trace*, epoxycaryophyllene *trace*, epoxy-1,10α-bulnesene <1%

Lactones

pogostone

Properties	Indications
antibacterial	see Table 4.4
antiinfectious	enteritis
antiinflammatory	acne*, allergies, inflamed skin, seborrhoeic eczema,
antiseptic	
cicatrizant	cracked skin, scar tissue, abnormal epidermis
decongestant	
digestive	infected enterocolitis, see Table 4.8
febrifuge	
immunostimulant	low natural defences
insectifuge	see Table 4.10
phlebotonic*	haemorrhoids*, varicose veins*
sedative	

Observations

- no known contraindications (Franchomme & Pénoël 2001 p. 419)
- no irritation was produced by the oil on humans at 20% in petroleum jelly or in an ointment, or at 0.1% in a non-irritant cream base in subjects with dermatoses (Fujii, Furukawa & Suzuki 1972)
- no irritation or sensitization at 10% dilution when tested on humans (Opdyke & Letizia 1982a)

- no phototoxic effects reported (Opdyke & Letizia 1982a)
- slightly irritating when applied at full strength to either intact or abraded rabbit skin for 24 hours under occlusion
- no phototoxicity for undiluted oil on hairless mice and pigs
- mild phototoxic reaction when hairless mice were irradiated with UV light after treatment with patchouli oil
- bactericidal property is attributed to the presence of pogostone (Terhune et al 1974)
- short-term feeding study indicates patchouli oil to be non-toxic to rats (Oser et al 1965)
- eugenol, cinnamaldehyde and benzaldehyde, isolated from the oil, are reported to be insecticidal against insects in stored grain (Deshpande et al 1974)
- patchouli oil is extensively adulterated
- *Trichophyton rubrum, T. mentagrophytes, T. interdigitale, T. violaceum, T. souclanense, Microsporum canis, M. gypseum, Epidermophyton floccosum* and bacteria responsible for foot odour were all found to be susceptible to a Chinese patchouli oil high in patchoulol (41%) (Yang et al 1996)
- *Pogostemon patchouli* oil from China proved superior *in vitro* in antifungal and bacterial properties compared with Indonesian and Indian oils (Yang et al 1996)

RAVENSARA AROMATICA FOL.
[AROMATIC RAVENSARA] LAURACEAE

Representative constituents

Hydrocarbons
monoterpenes α-pinene, β-pinene, sabinene 13.5–15%
sesquiterpenes β-caryophyllene

Alcohols
monoterpenols α-terpineol 6–7%, terpinen-4-ol 2%

Esters
monoterpenyl terpenyl acetate

Oxides
monoterpenoid 1,8-cineole 61%

Properties	Indications
antibacterial	see Table 4.4
antifungal	see Table 4.5
antiinfectious*	glandular fever, bronchitis, influenza*, sinusitis, whooping cough
antiinflammatory	rhinopharyngitis, see Table 4.6
antiviral*	chicken pox, dendritis*, herpes zoster*, viral enteritis, viral hepatitis*, see Table 4.7
detoxicant	
expectorant*	bronchitis, coughs
neurotonic	insomnia*, muscle fatigue, neuromuscular problems

Observations

- no contraindications known
- well-tolerated on the skin
- relaxing when massaged over the vertebral column

ROSA DAMASCENA, R. CENTIFOLIA
FLOS (DIST.) [ROSE OTTO] ROSACEAE

Representative constituents

Hydrocarbons *(25%)*
monoterpenes α-pinene, β-pinene, α-terpinene, limonene, β-myrcene, *cis-* and *trans-*β-ocimene, camphene
sesquiterpenes β-caryophyllene 0.3%
other octadecane 0.2%, nonadecane and nonadecene 2–15%, eicosane 1%, heneicosane, docosane 0.1–0.4%, tricosane 0.04–0.9%, tetracosane 0.2%, pentacosane 0.4%, stearoptene 16–22%
aromatic p-cymene <1%

Alcohols
monoterpenols geraniol 15.8–22.2%, citronellol 22.5–60?%, nerol 8.5%, linalool 1.5–2.7%, iso-borneol 0.4%, α-terpineol <1%
sesquiterpenols farnesol 0.2–2%
aromatic phenyl ethyl alcohol 0.9–3%

Aldehydes
monoterpenal neral 0.5%

Esters *(2–6%)*
monoterpenyl citronellyl acetate 0.5%, geranyl and
    neryl acetate 1.2%

Methyl ethers
methyl eugenol 1.4%

Oxides
monoterpenoid rose oxide 0.3%

Ketones
sesquiterpenone damascenone 0.2–1.6%

Properties	Indications
antibacterial	see Table 4.4
antiinfectious	acute and chronic bronchitis, asthma, mouth ulcers
antiinflammatory	blotchy skin, gingivitis, conjunctivitis, see Table 4.6
astringent	
cicatrizant	mouth ulcers, skin problems, sprains, wounds
general tonic	chronic bronchitis
neurotonic*	debility, depression
sexual tonic	frigidity, sexual debility
styptic	wounds

Observations

- no known contraindications
- no irritation or sensitization at 2% dilution when tested on humans (Opdyke 1974l, 1975e)
- no phototoxic effects reported (Opdyke 1974l, 1975e)
- rose absolute is produced in a different way from rose otto and has a different chemical composition
- French rose absolute produced one sensitization reaction in a test on 25 individuals (Opdyke 1975f)
- Bulgarian rose, lavender and geranium (all unspecified) sprayed into the atmosphere increased attention spans, concentration capacity and work rhythms, and shortened reflex times in 48 medical students (Tasev, Toleva & Balabanova 1969)
- rose oil was shown to have hepatoprotective action in rats against the toxic action of ethanol (Kirov et al 1988)
- rose oil was shown to have inhibitory effect *in vitro* on *Helicobacter pylori* and to be antiulcerous (Boyanova & Neshev 1999)
- rose oil had a strong choleretic effect in humans and a strong antiulcer effect in animals (Kirov & Vankov 1988)
- rose oil (unspecified) tested *in vivo* showed an anxiolytic effect similar to benzodiazepine (Umezu 1999); the effect was not antagonized by flumazenil, a benzodiazepine antagonist

ROSMARINUS OFFICINALIS CT. CINEOLE, CT. CAMPHOR *FOL.* [ROSEMARY] LAMIACEAE

N.B. The cineole and camphor chemotypes have almost the same constituents, properties and indications. They are therefore considered together here.

Representative constituents

Hydrocarbons
monoterpenes (30–37%) α-pinene 1.4–12%,
    β-pinene 3–9%, camphene 3–22%, β-myrcene
    1–2%, α-phellandrene, β-phellandrene,
    α-terpinene, γ-terpinene, limonene 1.9–2.4%
sesquiterpenes β-caryophyllene 0.9–3%,
    α-humulene 0.6–1.2%
aromatic p-cymene 1.1–2%

Alcohols
monoterpenols linalool 0.6–2%, α–terpineol
    1–4.5%, borneol 3.4–12%, isoborneol,
    terpenen-4-ol 0.6–1.5%, *cis-* and *trans*-thujan-
    4-ol, verbenol
aromatic p-cymene-8-ol

Esters
monoterpenyl isobornyl acetate *trace*–1.2,
    α-fenchyl acetate

Oxides
monoterpenoid 1,8-cineole 30–55%
sesquiterpenoid caryophyllene oxide, humulene
    oxides

Ketones

monoterpenones α-thujone, β-thujone, camphor
    6.4–30%, verbenone *trace*, carvone 1%
other 3-hexanone, methyl heptanone

Properties	Indications
analgesic	migraine, painful digestion
antibacterial	see Table 4.4
antifungal	see Table 4.5
antiinfectious	chills, diarrhoea, enteritis, influenza
antiinflammatory	cystitis, gout, muscular pains, otitis, rheumatism, inflamed gall bladder, see Table 4.6
antispasmodic	muscle cramp
antitussive	coughing, whooping cough
antiviral	see Table 4.7
cardiotonic	palpitations, weak heart
carminative	flatulence
choleretic*	insufficient bile
cicatrizant	burns, wounds
decongestant (venous)	migraine, headache, poor circulation, arteriosclerosis, bruises
detoxicant	hepatitis, jaundice, cirrhosis, enlarged liver, gall bladder malfunction
digestive	indigestion, sluggish digestion, colitis, constipation, painful digestion, see Table 4.8
diuretic	liver*, gall bladder*
emmenagogic	amenorrhoea, oligomenorrhoea
hyperglycaemic	
hypertensor (high dose)	hypotension
hypotensor (low dose)	hypertension
litholytic	gall stones
lowers cholesterol	high cholesterol
mucolytic*	chronic bronchitis, sinusitis
neuromuscular action*	multiple sclerosis, painful muscles,
	epilepsy, neuralgia, rheumatism
neurotonic	fainting, general debility, general fatigue, hysteria, loss of memory, vertigo
sexual tonic	impotence
stimulant	adrenal cortex
unspecified	enuresis (bedwetting)

Observations

■ usually regarded as having no contraindications
■ there are conflicting opinions regarding the use of rosemary oils in pregnancy and epilepsy:
  – some cite it as an oil to avoid in the first 4 months of pregnancy
  – Roulier (1990) warns against its use in pregnancy but does not give this warning for the verbenone chemotype
  – Franchomme & Penoël (1990) warn against using the verbenone chemotype on pregnant women, but do not mention the cineole and camphor chemotypes
  – some contraindicate its use on people prone to epilepsy
  – Valnet (1980) recommends its use on epileptics
  – thought to induce epileptic fits in epileptic patients receiving massage with the oil (Betts 1994)
■ bath preparations containing the oil can cause erythema (Duke 1985)
■ toiletries containing the oil can cause dermatitis in hypersensitive individuals (Mitchell & Rook 1979)
■ the essential oil in wine is said to help cancers (Hartwell 1967–1971)
■ no irritation or sensitization at 10% dilution when tested on humans (Opdyke 1974n)
■ stimulating action in humans and mice (Buchbauer et al 1991); in mice (Kovar et al 1987)
■ neurotoxic due to camphor content, which can cause convulsions in oral use (Craig 1953); some oils have low camphor level
■ tests suggest that the volatile oil of *R. officinalis* has hyperglycaemic and insulin release

inhibitory effects in the rabbit (Al-Hader, Hasan & Aqel 1994)

- carminative and a mild irritant (Reynolds 1972)
- potent antibacterial action (Aureli, Constantini & Zolea 1992, Deans & Ritchie 1987, Lis-Balchin, Deans & Hart 1994, Maruzzella 1960, Maruzzella & Sicurella 1960), poor antifungal action (Lis-Balchin, Deans & Hart 1994, Maruzzella 1960, Maruzzella & Liguori 1958)
- active against *Staphylococcus aureus*, *S. albus*, *Vibrio cholerae*, *Escherichia coli* and *Corynebacterium* (Opdyke 1974n)
- *Rosmarinus officinalis* diffused into the air significantly enhanced overall quality of memory in healthy participants but impaired speed of memory (Moss et al 2003)
- rosemary, sage, laurel, oregano and coriander essential oils all showed antioxidant activity (Baratta, Dorman & Deans 1998)
- rosemary oil at 3% in ointment (optimal antimicrobial concentration) was found to be effective *in vivo* against *Trichophyton rubrum* (Suleimanova et al 1995)
- essential oil of R. officinalis was listeriostatic (*Listeria monocytogenes*) at concentrations of 10–30 µl/100 ml (Pandit & Shelef 1994)
- peppermint, sage and rosemary essential oils were tested on guinea pig ileum and all were similar in inhibiting muscle contraction (Taddei et al 1988)
- examination of 10 commercial samples of rosemary oil and 39 samples of sage oil showed that most bore no resemblance to oils obtained from laboratory distilled plants (Svoboda & Deans 1990)

ROSMARINUS OFFICINALIS CT. VERBENONE *FOL.* [*ROSEMARY*] LAMIACEAE

Representative constituents

Hydrocarbons

monoterpenes α-pinene 15–34%, β-pinene, camphene, β-myrcene, limonene, α-terpinene, α-terpinolene
sesquiterpenes β-caryophyllene

Alcohols

monoterpenols borneol *trace–7%*

Esters

monoterpenyl bornyl acetate

Ketones

monoterpenones verbenone 15–37%, camphor 1–15%

Oxides

monoterpenoid 1,8-cineole *trace–20%*

Properties	Indications
antibacterial	see Table 4.4
antiinfectious	leucorrhoea, vaginitis
anticatarrhal	bronchitis, sinusitis
antifungal	*Candida*, see Table 4.5
antispasmodic	digestive tract, cardiovascular
antiviral*	viral colic*, viral hepatitis, see Table 4.7
cardiotonic	angina pectoris, arrhythmia, tachycardia
cicatrizant	
detoxicant	liver and bilious affections [but see Observations]
expectorant	bronchitis, coughs
hormone regulator	ovaries, testicles, sexual problems
mucolytic	bronchitis, coughs, sinusitis
nervous system regulator	fatigue, nervous depression, nervous indigestion*

Observations

- not normally used on those inclined to liver problems, children and in pregnancy (except where necessary)
- the oil is neurotoxic and abortive (Franchomme & Pénoël 1990); not to be used in pregnancy (Roulier 1990)
- tests showed verbenone rosemary (Hungarian origin) to inhibit Gram-positive bacteria (three *Staphylococcus* species, six *Streptococcus* species, *Mycobacterium fortuitum*) and *Candida albicans* (Domokos et al 1997)

RUTA GRAVEOLENS [*RUE*] RUTACEAE

Representative constituents

Hydrocarbons
monoterpenes α-pinene, β-pinene, limonene
sesquiterpenes β-caryophyllene *trace*,
   α-caryophyllene *trace*
other heptadecane 0.3%, pentadecane 0.24%,
   geijerene 0.8%, naphthalene *trace*

Ketones
2-nonanone 18–35%, 2-undecanone (methyl-
   nonyl ketone) 2.5–30.7% (90% in Algerian oil),
   2-heptanone, 2-octanone, 9-methyl-2-
   decanone 0.15%, 2-decanone 1, isooctyl
   methyl ketone *trace*

Alcohols
2-nonanol 0.6%, 2-undecanol *trace*, tetradecanol
   0.2%, eicosanol 0.2%

Aldehydes
nonanal 0.15%, decanal 0.2%, dodecanal 0.8%

Esters
undecyl-2-acetate, 2-octyl acetate 0.25%,
   2-nonyl acetate 11%, 2-decyl acetate 0.2%,
   2-undecyl acetate 1.2%, isoundecyl acetate 0.1%

Acids
anisic acid

Phenols
phenol, guaiacol

Ketones
2-undecanone (up to 90%), 2-tridecanone 0.9%,
   4-(3,4-methylenedioxyphenoyl)-2-butanone
   3.1%, 2-nonanone 18%, 2-decanone 1%,
   2-heptanone, 2-octanone, 9-methyl-2-
   decanone 0.15%

Coumarins
bergapten 7.2%, herniarin, xanthotoxin, psoralen
   1.3%, xanthotoxin, isoimperatorin, rutamarin

Oxides
monoterpenoid 1,8-cineole

Properties	Indications
anthelmintic	worm, leech, nematode
antiparasitic	skin parasites
antispasmodic	

Observations

- the oil may produce a burning sensation, erythema and blisters when applied to human skin
- undiluted oil was not irritating when applied to the backs of hairless mice but was slightly irritating when applied under occlusion on abraded rabbit skin
- 1% in petrolatum did not cause sensitization in humans
- taken internally causes severe stomach pain, vomiting, exhaustion, confusion and convulsion
- toxic when ingested due to the presence of methyl-nonyl ketone
- large doses may be fatal; a single oral dose (400 mg/kg) in guinea pigs reported fatal due to internal haemorrhages (Leung & Foster 1996 p. 452)
- reported to cause abortion in humans and in guinea pigs (Anon 1974)
- reported to cause phototoxicity
- neurotoxic and strong abortifacient; not to be used on babies, young children or during pregnancy (Franchomme & Pénoël 2001 p. 422)
- rue should never be used for perfumes, food flavouring (Arctander 1960 p. 563)
- said to be harmful to the mucous membranes (Arctander 1960 p. 563) but Tisserand & Balacs (1995b p. 60) give it as non-irritant to the mucous membranes with the caution that it may cause irritation if used undiluted
- bergapten, xanthotoxin and psoralen all have phototumorigenic properties and all are found in rue oil (Grube 1977)
- the toxicity of rue oil in humans remains unclear, but there seems no reason to restrict its use except during pregnancy and the normal cautions for phototoxicity (Tisserand & Balacs 1995b p. 166)
- 2-undecanone (methyl-*n*-nonyl ketone) was a major component (90%) in an Algerian rue oil

- coumarin derivatives present contribute to the spasmolytic properties (List & Hörhammer 1979 pp. 204–208)

SALVIA OFFICINALIS FOL. [*SAGE, DALMATIAN SAGE*] LAMIACEAE

Representative constituents

Hydrocarbons
monoterpenes (3–15%) α-pinene 3.2–6.4%, β-pinene 1.9%, camphene 1–5.4%, β-myrcene 0.4–1.1%, limonene 0.9–4%, α-terpinolene, salvene, α-phellandrene 0.1%, β-phellandrene 0.1%, α-thujene *trace*, sabinene 0.2%, α-terpinene 0.2%, γ-terpinene 0.3%, tricyclene 0.3%
sesquiterpenes β-caryophyllene 1–7%, aromadendrene, α-humulene 4–5%, α-cadinene, β-cadinene, β-copaene
other cis-2-methyl-3-methylene-5-heptene 0.7%, trans-2-methyl-3-methylene-5-heptene 0.1%
aromatic p-cymene 1–2%

Alcohols
monoterpenols (3–38%) linalool 0.4–12%, terpinen-4-ol 0.2–4%, α-terpineol *trace*–9%, borneol 1.5–14%, salviol, *trans*-sabinol *trace*, *cis*-thujan-4-ol 0.2%, *trans*-thujan-4-ol
sesquiterpenols viridiflorol 0–10%

Esters
terpenyl bornyl acetate 0.1–3%, linalyl acetate 1–2%, sabinyl acetate
other linalyl isovalerate, methyl isovalerate

Phenols
thymol *trace*

Oxides
monoterpenoid 1,8-cineole 5–14%
sesquiterpenoid caryophyllene oxide 0.4–2.1%

Ketones
monoterpenones (20–70%), α-thujone 12–35.7%, β-thujone 2–33%, camphor 4.1–26%, fenchone 0.2%

Aldehydes
3-hexanal *trace*

Coumarins
aesculetine *trace*

Methyl ethers
methyl chavicol 0.4%

Properties	Indications
analgesic	angina, rheumatism, toothache
antibacterial	see Table 4.4
anticancer	malignant conditions
anticatarrhal	asthma, bronchitis, coughs
antifungal*	*Candida albicans**, see Table 4.5
antiinfectious	influenza, gingivitis, insect bites, intermittent fevers, leucorrhoea, sore throat
antilactogenic	see Observations
antipyretic	hot flushes
antispasmodic	
antisudorific	excessive hand and armpit hyperidrosis, night sweating
antiviral	genital herpes, thrush, viral enteritis, viral meningitis, viral neuritis, see Table 4.7
choleretic	insufficient bile*
cicatrizant	
circulatory regulator	poor circulation, rheumatism, congestion
digestive (low dose)	indigestion, loss of appetite, sluggish digestion, see Table 4.8
diuretic	oliguria, urinary disorders
drains biliary canal	
emmenagogic	amenorrhoea, irregular periods, scanty periods, dysmenorrhoea
expectorant	bronchitis, coughs
hormonelike	conducive to conception, facilitates delivery, sterility, menopause, premenopause*, see Table 4.9

hypertensor	hypotension
hypoglycaemiant	prediabetes
insecticidal	see Table 4.10
lipolytic*	cellulite
mucolytic	coughs, sinusitis
neurotonic	alopecia, general debility, nervous debility, tremors, vertigo

Observations

- not normally used for breastfeeding mothers and young children
- antilactogenic: halts lactation in nursing mothers (Roulier 1990, Valnet 1980)
- neurotoxic and abortive; may cause malformed heart in babies if used throughout pregnancy (Franchomme & Pénoël 1990)
- because of its potential toxicity, sage oil, like all essential oils, should be used only in very small quantities (Foster 1993b)
- no irritation or sensitization at 8% dilution when tested on humans (Opdyke 1974o)
- German authorities recommend an internal dosage level of one drop of the essential oil per cup of water in infusion, perhaps taken up to three times per day
- although sage has more thujone than wormwood it seems a far safer plant: but the tea should only be taken for a week or two at a time because of the potentially toxic effects of thujone (Mabey 1988)
- cheilitis and stomatitis follow some cases of sage tea ingestion (Duke 1985)
- the distilled oil is said to be a violent epileptiform convulsant, resembling the essential oils of absinth, nutmeg and wormwood (Duke 1985)
- the Flavourings and Food Regulations 1992 allow 0.5 mg/kg food of α- and β-thujone
- salvin and salvin monomethyl ether (phenolic acids) have antimicrobial activities especially against *Staphylococcus aureus* (Alimkhodzhaeva & Khazanovich 1972, Dobrynin et al 1976)
- thujone is responsible for the antimicrobial activity (Jalsenjak, Peljnjak & Kustrak 1987)
- antimicrobial activity of the oil was demonstrated against *Escherichia coli, Shigella sonnei, Salmonella* species, *Klebsiella ozanae*, *Bacillus subtilis, Candida albicans* and *Cryptococcus neoformans* (Recio et al 1989)
- reported to show anticonvulsive activity in animals (Atanasov-Shopova & Rusinov 1970)
- is a relaxant (Kubota et al 1992)
- has antifungal activities (Dikshit & Husain 1984)
- antibacterial activity of the encapsulated oil was the same as the pure oil but antifungal activity was much lower (Jalsenjak, Peljnjak & Kustrak 1987)
- sage (unspecified) was found to be very effective against *Acinetobacter calcoacetica, Clostridium sporogenes* and *Moraxella* species (Piccaglia et al 1993)
- a detergent with sage and thyme essential oils applied to feet removed *Pseudomonas aeruginosa, Staphylococcus aureus, Proteus* and *Streptococcus* species and skin pH was reduced (Sparavigna, Viscardi & Galbiati 1993)

SALVIA SCLAREA FLOS, FOL. [CLARY] LAMIACEAE

Representative constituents

Hydrocarbons
monoterpenes (2–3%) α-pinene 0.1–0.25%, β-pinene 0.3%, sabinene *trace*, camphene, β-myrcene 0.1–1.7%, α-terpinolene 0.1–0.4%, α-terpinene *trace*, limonene 0.1–0.8%, *trans-*β-ocimene 0.4–1%
sesquiterpenes (5%) β-caryophyllene 0.8–3%, germacrene D 1.6–4%, *trans-*calamenene, α-cubebene *trace*, α-copaene 0.1–0.5%, β-bourbonene 0.1%
aromatic ar-curcumene, *p*-cymene *trace*

Alcohols
monoterpenols (15%) linalool 5–26%, α-terpineol 1%, citronellol, nerol *trace*–1%, geraniol 0.1–3.2%, borneol, isoborneol, thujol, terpinen-4-ol *trace*–0.1%
sesquiterpenols α-bisabol, junerol, spathulenol *trace*
diterpenols (5–7%) sclareol 1–7%
other cis-3-hexanol *trace*–0.3%, trans-2-hexanol 0.2%, 1-octen-3-ol *trace*

Aldehydes
sesquiterpenals caryophyllenals
other trans-2-hexanal *trace*–0.1%

Esters
monoterpenyl linalyl acetate 49–75%, citronellyl
    acetate, geranyl acetate 0.3–3.2%, neryl acetate
    0.2–1.7%, bornyl acetate 0.2%, α-terpinyl
    acetate *trace*–0.1%
other butanoates, valeronates

Oxides
monoterpenoid 1,8-cineole, *trans*-linalool oxide
    trace, *cis*-linalool oxide *trace*
sesquiterpenoid caryophyllene oxide 0.2–0.5%
diterpenoid sclareol oxide

Ketones
monoterpenones α-thujone, β-thujone

Coumarins
coumarin

Properties	Indications
antifungal	dermal fungal conditions, see Table 4.5
antiinfectious	genital infections (connected with hormone deficiency)
antispasmodic	
antisudorific	hyperidrosis
decongestant	dysmenorrhoea
detoxicant	
hormone (oestrogen-like)	amenorrhoea*, oligomenorrhoea, premenopause
neurotonic	epilepsy, nervous fatigue, calming to parasympathetic nervous system, alopecia
phlebotonic	circulatory problems, haemorrhoids, varicose veins, venous aneurysm, cholesterol
regenerative	cellular ageing, poor hair growth, alopecia

Observations

- no known contraindications, but is not normally used on people with cancers or tumours
- no irritation or sensitization at 8% dilution when tested on humans (Opdyke & Letizia 1982b)
- there are in excess of 250 constituents in clary oil
- contains a diterpenol (sclareol) which is rare in distilled oils

SANTALUM ALBUM LIG. [SANDALWOOD] SANTALACEAE

Representative constituents

Hydrocarbons
sesquiterpenes α- and β-santalene 10%, epi-β-
    santalene 6%, α- and β-curcumene, farnesene

Alcohols
sesquiterpenols α-santalol 46–60%, β-santalol
    20–30%, epi-β-santalol 4–5%, *trans*-β-santalol
    1–2%, *cis*-lanceol 1.5%, *cis*-nuciferol 1%, a
    monocyclic sesquiterpenol 5%, a tricyclic
    sesquiterpenol 1%

Aldehydes
sesquiterpenals teresantalal

Properties	Indications
antiinfectious	pulmonary: chronic bronchitis, colibacillosus; urinary: cystitis, gonorrhoea, urinary tract infections
astringent	diarrhoea
cardiotonic*	tired heart, haemorrhoids, varicose veins
decongestant*	pelvic congestion*, acne, skin problems
dilator (bronchial)	restricted bronchioles
diuretic	
moisturizer	dry skin
nerve relaxant	lumbago, neuralgia, sciatica, meditation

sedative
sexual tonic   impotence
tonic

Observations

- no known contraindications
- regarded as a general and sexual tonic
- does not irritate the mucous linings of the stomach or intestine
- no irritation or sensitization at 10% dilution when tested on humans (Opdyke 1974o)
- no phototoxic effects reported (Opdyke 1974o)
- approved for food use (Duke 1985)
- isolated santalol can cause dermatitis in sensitive individuals (Claus 1961, Leung 1980, Lewis & Elvin-Lewis 1977, Reynolds 1972)
- the oil has diuretic and urinary antiseptic properties (Leung 1980)
- two major components α-santalol and β-santalol were found to have sedative effect *in vivo* in mice and were considered neuroleptic (Okugawa et al 1995)
- sandalwood essential oil could be a chemoprentative against skin cancer (Dwivedi & Abu-Ghazaleh 1997)

SATUREIA HORTENSIS FOL.
[SUMMER OR GARDEN SAVORY] LAMIACEAE

Representative constituents

Hydrocarbons

monoterpenes (34%) α-thujene <1%, α-pinene <1%, β-pinene *trace*, β-myrcene 1–2.8%, α-terpinene 1–3.1%, γ-terpinene 20–24%, camphene *trace*, δ-3-carene, δ-4-carene, α-phellandrene, β-phellandrene *trace*, limonene *trace*, sabinene *trace*

sesquiterpenes (3–4%) β-caryophyllene 2–4%, β-bisabolene 1%, δ-cadinene 3%, calacorene and γ-cadinene 3.6%

aromatic p-cymene 3.7–20%

Alcohols

monoterpenols linalool, terpinen-4-ol, borneol, α-terpineol, nerol *trace*, geraniol *trace*

Phenols *(39–40%)*

thymol, carvacrol 35–40%, eugenol

Ketones

monoterpenone camphor *trace*
sesquiterpenone damascenone 1%

Aldehydes

monoterpenal piperonal

Oxides

monoterpenoid 1,8-cineole

Properties	Indications
antibacterial	see Table 4.4
antifungal	see Table 4.5
antiinfectious*	wide range of action
antioxidant	
antiparasitic	
antiseptic	respiratory tract infections
antiviral	see Table 4.7
cardiotonic	
carminative	flatulence
choleretic	
digestive	indigestion, facilitates elimination, sluggish bile, see Table 4.8
expectorant	
general tonic/ stimulant	debility*
nervous system balancer	
revitalizing	

Observations

- no irritation or sensitization at 6% dilution when tested on humans (Opdyke 1976q)
- no phototoxic effects reported (Opdyke 1976q)
- two species of *Satureia* – *S. hortensis* and *S. montana* – have a pronounced thyme-like odour and flavour, and the oils of the two plants are closely related in chemical composition (Guenther 1949)
- carvacrol has antidiuretic properties

SATUREIA MONTANA FOL. [WINTER OR MOUNTAIN SAVORY] LAMIACEAE

Representative constituents

Hydrocarbons
monoterpenes (40–50%) α- and γ-terpinenes 2–20%,
    α-pinene, β-pinene, camphene, sabinene,
    β-myrcene, limonene, α-phellandrene
sesquiterpenes β-caryophyllene, α-caryophyllene,
    aromadendrene, β-bisabolene, α-cadinene,
    γ-cadinene, calacorene
aromatic p-cymene 10–25%

Alcohols
monoterpenols linalool 9–54%, *cis*-thujan-4-ol,
    trans-thujan-4-ol, terpinen-4-ol *trace*–7%,
    α-terpineol 6–9%, geraniol, borneol

Esters
monoterpenyl linalyl acetate, terpinen-4-yl acetate,
    geranyl acetate, α-terpinyl acetate

Phenols *(25–50%)*
carvacrol 25–50%, thymol 1–5%, eugenol

Methyl ethers
carvacrol methyl ether

Oxides
monoterpenyl 1,8-cineole 1%
sesquiterpenyl caryophyllene oxide

Ketones
monoterpenones camphor
sesquiterpenone damascenone

Properties	Indications
analgesic*	rheumatoid arthritis*
antibacterial	see Table 4.4
anticatarrhal	bronchitis, coughs
antifungal	*Candida albicans*, fungal infections of the mouth, see Table 4.5
antiinfectious*	wide range of action, colitis, enteritis, tonsillitis, sore throat, tuberculosis, diarrhoea, cystitis, malaria*, skin infections, abscesses, impetigo, lichen
antiparasitic*	oxyurids, ascaris, taenia, amoebiasis*
antispasmodic	intestinal spasm, colic, muscle spasms
antiviral	see Table 4.7
carminative	flatulence
cicatrizant	insect bites, sores
digestive	painful digestion, see Table 4.8
expectorant	asthma, bronchitis, catarrh
general tonic*	general debility
hypertensor	hypotension*
immunostimulant	repetitive infections
mental stimulant	mental debility
neurotonic	lymph ganglion inflammation*, debility, nervous fatigue*, depression

Observations

- possible skin irritant and therefore to be used in low concentration
- savory oil is an efficient antidiuretic because of the carvacrol present (Duke 1985 p. 432)
- winter savory is used for catarrh, colic, otitis, sclerosis and spasms (Duke 1985 p. 432)
- winter savory has diuretic activity in rats (Stanic & Samarzija 1993)
- *Satureia montana* was particularly effective towards *Streptococcus faecalis* (Melegari et al 1985)
- antimicrobial activity of *S. montana* was 2 to 20 more than lavender or rosemary and 2 to 8 times more potent than thyme (Pellecuer et al 1975)
- diuretic activity of *S. montana* was shown (Stanic & Samarzija 1993)

SYZYGIUM AROMATICUM FLOS [CLOVE BUD] MYRTACEAE

Representative constituents

Hydrocarbons
monoterpenes pinene

sesquiterpenes α- and β-caryophyllene 5–13%, β-humulene 0.5–1.5%, α-cubebene 0.01–0.3%, α-copaene 0.01–0.2%, calamenene 0.2–0.5%

Phenols *(60–90%)*
eugenol 36–85%, isoeugenol 0.1–0.25%

Esters *(20–25%)*
monoterpenyl α-terpinyl acetate 0.1–0.2%, benzyl acetate *trace*, methyl benzoate 0.04–0.13%
other eugenyl acetate 0.5–12%, 2-nonanyl acetate *trace*, acetoeugenol 11–21.8%

Oxides
sesquiterpenoid caryophyllene oxide *trace*–1.8%, humulene epoxide *trace*

Properties	Indications
analgesic	rheumatoid arthritis, toothache, neuralgia*
antibacterial	see Table 4.4, tuberculosis*
antifungal	see Table 4.5
antiinfectious	abscesses, gum infections, infected acne, ulcers, wounds
antiinflammatory	bronchitis, salpingitis, sinusitis, arthritis, bursitis, see Table 4.6
antiseptic	prevention of disease, cystitis, diarrhoea, sinusitis
antispasmodic	diarrhoea, intestinal spasm
antiviral*	enteritis*, influenza, hepatitis, *Herpes simplex*, see Table 4.7
carminative	flatulence
cicatrizant	infected acne, ulcers, wounds
hormonelike	thyroid imbalance, see Table 4.9
hypertensor	hypotension
immunostimulant	low immunity
insectifuge	mosquitoes, clothes moths, see Table 4.10
mental stimulant*	memory loss, mental fatigue
neurotonic*	debility, fatigue*
sexual tonic	impotence
unspecified	stimulates secretion of saliva
uterotonic*	difficult labour, long labour

Observations

- should not be applied undiluted to skin because clove oils may cause irritation at high dosage levels
- considered non-toxic at normal usage levels
- 20% dilution of clove bud oil on humans produced erythema in two of the 25 tested; no irritation or sensitization occurred at 2%, or at 0.2% on subjects with dermatoses (Fujii, Furukawa & Suzuki 1972)
- no irritation or sensitization at 5% dilution when tested on humans (Opdyke 1975g)
- no phototoxic effects reported for any of the clove oils (Opdyke 1975g)
- is used as an antiseptic mouthwash
- eugenol sensitizes some people causing contact dermatitis (Duke 1985)
- clove bud oil and savory oil create a synergistic mix (Duraffourd 1982)
- used externally in patented treatments of bone degeneration, joint inflammation, bursitis and treatment of sinuses
- antiviral due to eugeniin, present in buds; eugeniin has strong antiviral activity against herpes simplex virus (Takechi & Tanaka 1981)
- oil is used widely for toothache
- the oil is an irritant and stimulates peristalsis; used as an expectorant in bronchitis and phthisis (Duke 1985)
- eugenol is responsible for the anodyne and mild antiseptic properties; exhibits broad antimicrobial activities against Gram-positive, Gram-negative and acid fast bacteria as well as fungi (Anon 1977, Martinez Nadal et al 1973, Ramadan et al 1972b)
- also has larvicidal and anthelmintic properties (Oishi et al 1974)
- essential oil demonstrated antithrombotic effect comparable to 50 mg/K of aspirin (Saeed & Gilani 1994)
- five *sesquiterpenes* isolated from the essential oil were considered to be potential chemopreventative agents (Zheng, Kenney & Lam 1992b)

- *Cinnamomum verum* and *Syzygium aromaticum* and their principal constituents cinnamic aldehyde and eugenol inhibited fungal growth and toxin production of *Aspergillus parasiticus* (Bullerman, Lieu & Seier 1977)
- essential oil has antioxidant properties (Deans et al 1995, Lee & Shibamoto 2001)
- leaf, bud and stem oils had significant antimicrobial activity against 23 of 25 bacteria especially *Clostridium perfringens*; antimycotic properties were more pronounced than antibacterial activity – notably *Aspergillus niger* and *Aspergillus ochraceous* (Deans et al 1995)

TAGETES GLANDULIFERA, TAGETES PATULA, TAGETES MINUTA [TAGET, FRENCH MARIGOLD] ASTERACEAE

Representative constituents

Hydrocarbons

monoterpenes (+)-limonene 0.03–7.3%, β-myrcene 0.3%, α-phellandrene 0.4%, β-phellandrene 0.1%, γ-terpinene *trace*, α-terpinolene *trace*, cis-β-ocimene 27.9–54.5%, *trans*-β-ocimene 0.5%
sesquiterpenes trans-β-farnesene 0.05%, γ-elemene 0.8%, β-caryophyllene 0.5%, aromadendrene 16%
aromatic p-cymene 0.1%

Alcohols

monoterpenols linalool 0.4%, menthol 0.3%, geraniol 0.1%
other phenyl ethanol 14%,

Ketones

monoterpenones tagetone 20–60%, *trans*-ocimenone + *cis*-ocimenone 26%, *trans*-tagetone 1%, dihydrotagetone 5.1–28%, *cis*-tagetone 2–10%, *cis*-tagetenone 0.3–7.6%, *trans*-tagetenone 0.5–5.3%, α-thujone *trace*, β-thujone 0.5%, piperitenone
other 2,6-dimethyl-7-octen-4-one

Phenols

thymol 0.2%, carvacrol *trace*, eugenol *trace*

Methyl ethers

methyl eugenol 0.03%, thymolhydroquinone dimethyl ether 0.9%

Esters

monoterpenyl linalyl acetate 0.3%

Coumarins

coumarin

Properties	Indications
anthelmintic	parasitic enteritis
anticatarrhal	catarrhal infections
antifungal	*Candida, Tinea pedis*, ungueal infections, see Table 4.5
antiinfectious	catarrhal infections
antiinflammatory	see Table 4.6
bronchodilator	
cicatrizant	scratches, burns, chronic skin lesions, bruises, slow healing wounds
emmenagogic	amenorrhoea
hypotensor	
mucolytic	bronchitis, coughs
phototoxic	
spasmolytic	
tranquillizing	

Observations

- avoid use on babies, children and in pregnancy because of ketone content; tagetone may be harmful (Arctander 1960)
- phototoxic when used inappropriately; IFRA recommends not more than 0.05% in preparations for use on skin exposed to sunlight (IFRA 1992)
- given as photosensitizing by Franchomme & Pénoël (1990)
- stated to be non-toxic, not phototoxic, non-irritant, not a sensitizer (Opdyke 1982b)
- hypotensive in rats (Chandhoke & Ghatak 1969)
- has tranquillizing, hypotensive, bronchodilatory, tranquillizing, spasmolytic and antiinflammatory properties in experimental animals (rats) (Bye 1986, Chandhoke & Ghatak 1969)
- stated to be non-toxic, not phototoxic, non-irritant, not a sensitizer (Opdyke 1982b)
- Hethelyi et al (1986) demonstrated that oil of *Tagetes minuta* inhibited (95–100%) growth of Gram-positive and Gram-negative bacteria in

agar diffusion tests; in atmospheric diffusion bacterial inhibition was 23–30% while inhibition of fungal growth was 100%

- the oil was tested for antibacterial activity and found to be effective against *Staphylococcus albus, Bacillus subtilis, B. pumilis* and *B. mycoides* and also against some Gram-negative organisms (Garg & Dengre 1986)
- tested *in vitro* the oil demonstrated antimicrobial activity against *Bacillus subtilis, Escherichia coli, Salmonella typhi, Staphylococcus aureus, Aspergillus niger* and *Trichoderma viride* (Razdan, Wanchoo & Dhar 1986)
- the essential oil, paste and tincture of *Tagetes erecta* was used in the treatment of hyperkeratotic plantar lesions and found effective for the reduction of corn and callus width, length and pain levels (Khan et al 1996)
- tests on the oil of *Tagetes minuta* suggest that the essential oil possessed antidepressant-like and anxiogenic-like properties (Martijena et al 1998)
- (Z,E)-ocimenone has larvicidal activity against mosquito larvae (Maradufu et al 1978)

THYMUS MASTICHINA FLOS, FOL. [*SPANISH MARJORAM*] LAMIACEAE

Representative constituents

Hydrocarbons
monoterpenes α-terpinolene 4%, limonene 2–2.8%, α-pinene 2.6%, β-pinene 2–3%, sabinene 0.8–1.1%, α-thujene 0.2–0.5%, β-myrcene 0.2–1%, camphene 0.2–1.4%, γ-terpinene <1%
sesquiterpenes β-caryophyllene 0.1%, β-gurjunene 0.3%, alloaromadendrene 0.2–1%, γ- and δ-cadinene 0.1%, β-bourbonene 0.1%, caryophyllene 1–1.5%
aromatic p-cymene 1.3–3.4%

Alcohols
monoterpenols borneol *trace*–3.5%, linalool 8.5–43%, α-terpineol 8%, geraniol 0.2%, *cis-* and *trans-*thujanol-4 0.2%, *trans-*pinocarveol 1%, 3-terpinen-l-ol 0.2%, terpinen-4-ol 0.1–0.7%, *cis-*thujan-4-ol 0.2%

Phenols
thymol 0–5%

Ketones
monoterpenone camphor *trace*–4%

Oxides
monoterpenyl 1,8-cineole 41–75%
sesquiterpenyl caryophyllene oxide *trace*

Esters
monoterpenoid linalyl acetate 1–1.5%, 3-terpinen-l-yl acetate 0.2%, bornyl acetate 0.2%, *trans-*pinocarveol acetate 1.5%, α-terpinyl acetate 3%, geranyl acetate 0.1%

Properties	Indications
antibacterial	see Table 4.4
antifungal	see Table 4.5
antiinfectious	sinusitis, catarrhal bronchitis*, viral and bacterial infections

Observations

- no contraindications known at normal dose
- no irritation or sensitization at 6% dilution when tested on humans (Opdyke 1976r)
- no phototoxic effects reported (Opdyke 1976r)

THYMUS SATUREIOIDES [*MOROCCAN THYME, BORNEOL THYME*] LAMIACEAE

Representative constituents

Hydrocarbons
monoterpenes α-pinene 0.1–17%, γ-terpinene 0–4.2%, camphene 0.1–20%, α-thujene 0–0.8%, sabinene 0–0.2%, β-pinene 0–1.3%, β-myrcene 0–1%, α-phellandrene 0–0.1%, α-terpinene 0–0.7%, limonene 0.1–1.1%, α-terpinolene 0–0.3%, tricyclene 0–0.5%
sesquiterpenes β-caryophyllene 1.8–7.0%, δ-cadinene 0.1–1.3%, α-copaene 0–0.6%, β-bourbonene 0–0.1%, aromadendrene 0–0.3%, α-caryophyllene 0–0.5%, alloaromadendrene 0–0.2%, γ-muurolene 0–0.2%, α-muurolene 0–0.3%, β-guaiene 0–1%
aromatic p-cymene 0–10%

Alcohols

monoterpenols borneol 13.0–77.6%, α-terpineol 4.7–21%, terpinen-4-ol 0.7–4.8%, linalool 0.4–12.3%, *trans*-pinocarveol 0–0.4%, *trans*-thujan-4-ol 0–0.5%, *p*-menth-1(7), 2-dien-8-ol 0–0.1%

aromatic p-cymen-8-ol 0.1–0.7%

other 3-octanol 0–0.8%

Aldehydes

monoterpenal campholenic aldehyde 0–0.4%

Phenols

thymol 0–21.3%, carvacrol 0.5–49.5%

Methyl ethers

carvacrol methyl ether 0–7.1%, thymol methyl ether 0–0.1%

Ketones

monoterpenones dihydrocarvones 0.2–3%, verbenone 0–0.1%, camphor 0.1–2.6%

other α-irone 0–0.5%

Esters

monoterpenyl bornyl acetate 0.1–5.4%, linalyl acetate 0–0.2%

Oxides

monoterpenoid 1,8-cineole 0–0.16%, *cis*-linalool oxide 0–0.1%

sesquiterpenoid caryophyllene oxide 0.4–3.7%

Properties	Indications
antibacterial	tuberculosis*, see Table 4.4
antiinfectious	acne, chronic sinusitis, cystitis, infections (viral and bacterial)
antiinflammatory	tonsillitis, arthritis*, cystitis, see Table 4.6
immunostimulant*	autoimmune deficiency
neurotonic*	debility*, general fatigue*
tonic sexual*	sexual apathy*
tonic general	gall bladder malfunction, gall stones, hepatic deficiency
uterotonic	lack of uterine muscle tone

Observations

- no known contraindications at normal dose
- possible skin irritant

THYMUS VULGARIS (POPULATION)
HERB. [*THYME*] LAMIACEAE

Representative constituents

Hydrocarbons

monoterpenes γ-terpinene 0.3–12.4%, α-pinene 0.9–3.7%, camphene 0.5–2.4%, β-myrcene *trace*–2.6%, α-terpinene 0.8–1.5%, limonene 0.4–2.1%, α-terpinolene *trace*–2%, α-thujene 0.5%, δ-3-carene 0.1%, sabinene 0.6%, α-phellandrene 0.1–0.2%, β-pinene *trace*

sesquiterpenes β-caryophyllene 0.2–2.9%

aromatic p-cymene 2.2–42.8%

Phenols

thymol 30–48.2%, carvacrol 0.5–5.5%

Alcohols

monoterpenols borneol *trace*–1.8%, linalool 1.3–12.4%, terpinen-4-ol 0.3–9.5%, α-terpineol 0.4–9.4%, geraniol 0.1–0.2%, β–terpineol 0.6–0.9%

sesquiterpenols nerolidol 0–0.8%

Ketones

monoterpenones camphor 2.3–16.3%, α-thujone 0.2%

Esters

monoterpenyl linalyl acetate 0.9%, α-terpinyl acetate 0.7–1.4%, geranyl acetate 0–0.5%

Oxides

monoterpenoid 1,8-cineole 0.4–7.4%, *trans*-linalool oxide 0.5%, *cis*-linalool oxide 1%

Properties	Indications
antibacterial	see Table 4.4
antifungal	see Table 4.5
antioxidant	
antiseptic	acne, boils, skin problems, etc.
antispasmodic	
capillary stimulant	anaemia, circulatory

carminative	disorders, hair loss flatulence
cicatrizant	
digestive	sluggish digestion, see Table 4.8
diuretic	
expectorant	bronchial secretions, bronchitis, sinusitis, asthma
hypertensor	hypotension
mental stimulant	depression, exam nerves
neurotonic	anxiety, debility
parasiticide	
stomachic	
sudorific	
tonic general	general fatigue
vermifuge	intestinal parasites
warming	rheumatism, stiff joints
unspecified	leucorrhoea

Observations

- irritant to the skin
- the volatile oil is toxic in any quantity and internal use should be restricted to professionals (Mabey 1988)
- oil of thyme is largely eliminated through the alveoli of the lung (Weiss 1988a)
- the German Bundes Gesundsheitamt (BGA) publishes monographs on acceptable labelling for herb products and permits thyme to be designated for symptoms of bronchitis, whooping cough and catarrh of the upper airways (Foster 1993b)
- carvacrol stimulates mucosal secretory activity (Mills 1991)
- thyme oil has been shown to be antispasmodic owing to its phenols
- thyme plants grown from seed (known as population thyme) yield an essential oil with a rich variety of components
- there is wide variation of constituents in oils from *T. vulgaris*, hence the broad limits given above
- like many of the herbaceous members of the Lamiaceae family that have achieved economic importance, there are nomenclatural and botanical authenticity problems associated with thyme (Lawrence 1979); there are about 400 species, or 100 species with 400 names

(Foster 1993b). Phillips (1989, 1991) has attempted to sort out the confusion of species occurring in the USA

- at least nine naturally occurring chemotypes are known
- *T. vulgaris* ct. thymol and *T. vulgaris* ct. carvacrol have thymol and carvacrol respectively as major components
- *T. vulgaris* ct. geraniol has geraniol 60–80%; *T. vulgaris* ct. linalool has linalool 60–80%
- see Observations under other types of *T. vulgaris*
- has antispasmodic, expectorant and carminative properties as well as antimicrobial activities, owing to thymol and carvacrol (Patakova & Chladek 1974, Pizsolitto 1975, Simeon de Bouchberg et al 1976, Van Den Broucke & Lernli 1981, Vincenzi & Dessi 1991)
- reported to be lethal to mosquito larvae (Novak 1968)

THYMUS VULGARIS CT. GERANIOL HERB. *[SWEET THYME]* LAMIACEAE

Representative constituents

Hydrocarbons
monoterpenes very low

Alcohols
monoterpenols geraniol 60–80%

Esters
monoterpenyl geranyl acetate

Properties	Indications
antibacterial	acne (*S. alba*), see Table 4.4
antifungal*	see Table 4.5
antiinfectious	bronchitis, sinusitis, tuberculosis, rhinopharyngitis, urethritis, cystitis, vaginitis, psoriasis, weeping eczema
antiseptic	sore throat, tonsillitis, colitis, infected acne
antiviral*	verrucas, viral enteritis*, people prone to

	repeated viral attacks*, see Table 4.7
cardiotonic	tired heart
choleretic	
neurotonic*	fatigue, insomnia
uterotonic*	

THYMUS VULGARIS CT. LINALOOL HERB. [*SWEET THYME*] LAMIACEAE

Representative constituents

Hydrocarbons
monoterpenes very low

Alcohols
monoterpenols linalool 60–80%

Esters
monoterpenyl linalyl acetate

Properties	Indications
antibacterial	*Staphylococcus** nephritis, see Table 4.4
antispasmodic	bronchiole spasm
antiinfectious	
antiinflammatory	bronchitis, cystitis, muscular rheumatism, otitis, urethritis, prostatitis, dry eczema, see Table 4.6
antiviral	verrucas, viral enteritis*, people prone to repeated viral attacks*, see Table 4.7
diuretic	
fungicidal	*Candida albicans*, vaginitis
immunostimulant	diabetes
neurotonic*	nervous fatigue, insomnia, psoriasis
parasiticide	colitis
uterotonic*	
vermifuge	ascariasis, taeniasis, enterobiasis (oxyuriasis)

Observations on geraniol and linalool chemotypes

- no known contraindications

- sweet thyme oils do not contain the aggressive elements of the red thymes
- preferred for general use, children and the elderly (Price 2000)

THYMUS VULGARIS CT. THUJANOL-4 HERB. [*SWEET THYME*] LAMIACEAE

Representative constituents

Hydrocarbons
monoterpenes β-myrcene, γ-terpinene

Alcohols
monoterpenols (+)-*trans*-thujan-4-ol, (+)-terpinen-4-ol, *cis*-myrcenol-8, (–)-linalool

Properties	Indications
antiinfectious	influenza, bronchitis, sinusitis, rhinopharyngitis, otitis, urethritis, cystitis
antiinflammatory	dermatitis, arthritis, tendonitis, see Table 4.6
antiviral	see Table 4.7
bactericide	*Chlamydia**
hepatic	inadequate liver function
hormonelike	diabetes
immunostimulant*	increase IgA
neurotonic	balancing to CNS, asthenia*

Observations

- no contraindications known at normal aromatherapeutic dose
- this clone does not survive well under cultivation and therefore the oil is rare today, making caution necessary when procuring it; strenuous efforts are being made to overcome this problem and it is hoped to be resolved in the near future (Lamy 1997 personal communication)
- due to this fact, reliable information on ct. thujanol-4 is hard to find
- said to be useful for warming by improving the circulation (Franchomme & Pénoël 1990 p. 403)

THYMUS VULGARIS CT. THYMOL, CT. CARVACROL HERB. *[THYME]* LAMIACEAE

Properties	Indications
anthelmintic*	
antibacterial*	tuberculosis, see Table 4.4
antidiuretic (ct. carvacrol)	enuresis
antifungal	see Table 4.5
antiinfectious	influenza, general infections*, head colds, infectious diseases, sinusitis
antioxidant	
antiparasitic	
antiseptic	
mental stimulant	mental strain, depression
mucolytic*	asthma, emphysema, pulmonary diseases
warming*	rheumatism of joints and muscles, sciatica, lumbago

Observations

■ red thymes are powerful antiseptic and antibacterial agents

■ to be used with care because of the high phenol content

■ no irritation or sensitization at 8% dilution when tested on humans; can be irritating at full strength (Opdyke 1974p)

■ thymol is a dermal and mucous membrane irritant (Anon 1994b, Tisserand & Balacs 1995)

■ no phototoxic effects reported (Opdyke 1974p)

■ it is to be avoided in pregnancy as the carvacrol content stimulates the mucosal secretory systems (Mills 1991)

■ thymol is an antiseptic 20 times stronger than phenol, yet, unlike phenol, does not irritate or corrode the skin or mucosa

■ thymol can be highly toxic; it is strongly fungicidal, antibacterial, antioxidant (Simpson 1993) and toxic to the hookworm (Foster 1993b)

■ thymol is a starting material for synthetic menthone and is used in embalming fluids

■ thymol is an effective antifungal agent and anthelmintic: it is poorly absorbed into body fluids, so finds its main use within the gut or on the surface of the body; it is ideal for toothpastes and mouthwashes (Mills 1991)

■ thymol has caused dermatitis in dentists, and (in toothpaste) has caused glossitis (Duke 1985)

■ the oil of thyme used in bath preparations has caused hyperaemia and inflammation (Rook 1979)

■ effective *in vitro* against *Salmonella typhimurium* and *Staphylococcus aureus* (Juven et al 1993)

VALERIANA OFFICINALIS RAD. *[VALERIAN]* VALERIANACEAE

Representative constituents

Hydrocarbons
monoterpenes α-pinene, camphene 8–14%, α-fenchene, β-pinene, β-myrcene, limonene, β-phellandrene, α-terpinene, α-terpinolene
sesquiterpenes β-caryophyllene, azulene, β-elemene, alloaromadendrene, β-bisabolene, α-cadinene, eremophilene, valene
aromatic ar-curcumene

Alcohols
monoterpenols α-terpineol, geraniol, borneol
sesquiterpenols valeranol

Esters
monoterpenyl isobornyl acetate 15–31%, bornyl isovaleronate, bornyl formiate, bornyl butanoate, bornyl acetate 1–17%

Aldehydes
sesquiterpenals valeranal 3–16%

Acids
isovaleric acid, valerianic acid, acetoxyvaleric acid

Ketones
sesquiterpenones valeranone 0–32%
other methyl-2-pyrrole ketone

Properties	Indications
antiinflammatory	see Table 4.6
antispasmodic	spasm
sedative	agitation, anxiety, tachycardia, insomnia
temperature reducing	fever
tranquillizing	long standing depression
vermifuge	

Observations

- no contraindications known to this essential oil at normal aromatherapeutic dose (Von Skramlik 1959)
- the drug should not be taken in large doses or for an extended period of time (Stuart 1987 p. 278)
- essential oil from the root of *Valeriana officinalis* var. *latifolia* was used in a clinical study on coronary heart disease patients with angina pectoris which found a remission of symptoms, decreased frequency with shorter duration of angina attacks; no toxic effects were noted (Gui-Yuan & Wei 1994)
- valerian essential oil and its components valerenal, valeranic acid, valeranone and isoeugenyl isovalerate were found to be sedative and/or muscle relaxant (Hendricks et al 1981, 1985)
- essential oil has a powerful action on the nervous system and the use of this oil undiluted should be restricted to therapists who have received appropriate training
- approved for food use by the FDA 172.510; extracts and the essential oil are added as flavouring in many processed foods (0.01% max)
- essential oil and absolute are used in perfumery and flavouring of tobacco, beer and fruit juices
- valerian has always been a mainstay ingredient of countless love potions, philtres and aphrodisiacs
- the result of a study on rats showed that although valerian depressed the central nervous system, neither the tested valepotriates, nor the sesquiterpenoids valerenic acid or valeranone, nor the volatile oil itself displayed any activity (Kriegelstein & Grusla 1988)

VALERIANA WALLICHII RAD.
[*INDIAN VALERIAN*] VALERIANACEAE

Representative constituents

Hydrocarbons
sesquiterpenes α-patchoulene, β-patchoulene, γ-patchoulene

Alcohols
sesquiterpenols patchoulol, maaliol

Ketones
sesquiterpenones valeranone

Esters
amyl α-hydroxy-isovaleronate

Oxides
maalioloxide

Acids
isovaleranic acid

Properties	Indications
neurotonic	asthenia
phlebotonic	haemorrhoids, varicose veins

Absolute

Properties	Indications
antispasmodic	
carminative	
stimulant	depression
sedative	epilepsy, hysteria, cholera, neurosis, anxiety
vermifuge	

Observations

- essential oil has a powerful action on the nervous system
- use of this oil undiluted should be restricted to therapists who have received appropriate training

VETIVERIA ZIZANIOIDES
RAD. [VETIVER] POACEAE

Representative constituents

Hydrocarbons
sesquiterpenes vetivene <1%, vetivazulene <1%, tricyclovetivene <1%

Alcohols
sesquiterpenols vetiverol <1%, bicyclovetiverol 10–12%, tricyclovetiverol 3–4%

Esters
sesquiterpenyl vetiverol acetate 1–2%

Ketones
sesquiterpenones α-vetivone 3–6%, β-vetivone 3–6%

Acids
sesquiterpenyl vetivenic acid <1%
other palmitic acid <1%, benzoic acid <1%

Properties	Indications
antiinfectious	general infections, skin infections, acne
circulatory tonic*	inflamed coronary artery
emmenagogic	amenorrhoea, oligomenorrhoea
glandular tonic	insufficient pancreatic secretion, liver congestion
immunostimulant	low immunity
unspecified	arthritis
unspecified	urticaria

Observations

- no known contraindications
- no irritation or sensitization at 8% dilution when tested on humans (Opdyke 1974q)
- no phototoxic effects reported (Opdyke 1974q)

ZINGIBER CASSUMUNAR RHIZ.
[PLAI, PHRAI] ZINGIBERACEAE

Representative constituents

Hydrocarbons
monoterpenes sabinene 25–45%, α-pinene 1.3%, β-pinene 3%, camphene, α-thujene 1%, β-myrcene 1.5%, α-terpinene 2–5%, β-phellandrene 1%, γ-terpinene 5–10%, terpinolene 1%
sesquiterpenes zingiberene, cassumunene, β-bisabolene, *cis*-β-farnesene, β-sesquiphellandrene 0.5%
aromatic ar-curcumene, *p*-cymene 1.5%

Alcohols
monoterpenols terpinen-1-ol-4 25–45%, nerol, *cis*-thujan-4-ol 0.8%, *trans*-thujan-4-ol 0.7%, α-terpineol 0.7%, *trans*-piperitol 0.2%, *cis*-piperitol 0.3%
sesquiterpenols zingiberol, β-eudesmol

Aldehydes
monoterpenals geranial

Oxides
1,8-cineole 0.4%
cis-*p*-menth-2-en-1-ol 0.9%
trans-*p*-menth-2-en-1-ol 0.7%
trans-1-(3,4-dimethoxyphenyl)butadiene 1–10%

Properties	Indications
antiinflammatory* antipyretic	colitis, arthritis, rheumatism, sports injuries, bursitis, tendonitis, inflamed joints, muscles, see Table 4.6
antioxidant	
bronchodilator	asthma
carminative	digestion problems
uterorelaxant	dysmenorrhoea

Observations

- several studies have found cassumunarins A, B and C to be antiinflammatory antioxidants (Jitoe et al 1994, Masuda & Jitoe 1994, Masuda et al 1995)

- has been suggested for use in ME
- Piromrat et al (1986) investigated the antihistaminic of plai on histamine skin test in asthmatic children
- to allay hip pain plai has been used in a 10% dilution together with *Laurus nobilis* [bay] and *Pimenta racemosa* [West Indian bay] (Louise Krijgsman)
- plai, nutmeg and lemon were used in a post operative blend to reduce joint pain more than a year following a knee operation and after removal of the screws (Marianne Debock)
- *Zingiber cassumunar* essential oil exhibited topical antiinflammatory effect in rats (Pongprayoon et al 1996)
- a test on antiinflammatory activity showed the component *trans*-1-(3,4-dimethoxyphenyl) butadiene to be twice as potent as the reference drug Diclofenac (Voltarol) which is used for rheumatoid arthritis, osteoarthritis and ankylosing sponolytis and other conditions (Thailand Institute)
- antiinflammatory activity was shown on carrageenan induced oedema in rats; results pointed to the antiinflammatory and analgesic action of (*E*)-1-(3,4-dimethoxyphenyl) but-1-ene (Ozaki, Kawahara & Harada 1991)

ZINGIBER OFFICINALE RHIZ. [GINGER]
ZINGIBERACEAE

Representative constituents

Hydrocarbons

monoterpenes (20%) α-pinene 0.4–4.2%, β-pinene 0.1–2.3%, camphene 1.1–8%, β-myrcene 0.1–1%, limonene 1.2–3% β-phellandrene 1.3–4%

sesquiterpenes (55%) zingiberene 11.3–50.9%, β-sesquiphellandrene 1.6–9%, *cis*-γ-bisabolene 7%, copaene, sesquithujene, β-ylangene, β-elemene, β-farnesene 19.8%, β-caryophyllene, calamenene, β-bisabolene 0.2%, α-selinene 1.4%

aromatic p-cymene 0.2–10.8%, ar-curcumene 0.1–32.9%

Alcohols

monoterpenols citronellol 6%, linalool 1–5.5%

sesquiterpenols nerolidol *trace*–8.9%, elemol 0.2%, β-bisabol, zingiberenol 0.5%, *trans*-β-sesquiphellandrol 0.4%, *cis*-sesquisabinene hydrate 0.2%, β-eudesmol 0.6%

aromatic cuminic alcohol

other 2-butanol, 2-nonanol 2.1–7.8%, 2-heptanol *trace*

Aldehydes

monoterpenals citronellal 0.4%, myrtenal, phellandral, neral 0.5%, geranial 1%

other butanal, 2-methyl,3-methyl-butanal, pentenal

Ketones

monoterpenones cryptone, carvotanacetone

other acetone, 2-hexanone, 2-heptanone, methyl-heptanone, 2-nonanone, gingerone

Oxides

monoterpenoid 1,8-cineole 1%

Properties	Indications
analgesic*	angina, painful indigestion, rheumatism, toothache
anticatarrhal	chronic bronchitis
carminative*	flatulence
digestive	constipation, loss of appetite, sluggish digestion, nausea, see Table 4.8
expectorant	chronic bronchitis
general tonic	fatigue
sexual tonic	impotence
stomachic	diarrhoea

Observations

- no known contraindications at normal dose
- gingerols and shogaols do not appear in the distilled essential oil
- no irritation or sensitization at 4% dilution when tested on humans (Opdyke 1974r)
- low level insignificant phototoxic effects reported (Opdyke 1974r)
- both eugenol and ginger (unspecified) essential oil proved potent antiinflammatory agents related to kallikrein levels (Sharma et al 1997)

PART II
INDICATIONS FOR USES OF ESSENTIAL OILS

Condition	Essential oils	Condition	Essential oils
abscesses	*Melaleuca alternifolia; Satureia montana*	anxiety, agitation	*Angelica archangelica* rad.; *Cistus ladaniferus; Citrus aurantium* var. *amara* fol.; *Citrus aurantium* var. *amara* per.; *Citrus bergamia; Citrus aurantium* var. *sinensis* per.; *Eucalyptus staigeriana; Leptospermum scoparium; Lavandula angustifolia; Litsea cubeba; Melaleuca alternifolia; Nepeta cataria* var. *citriodora; Ocimum basilicum; Origanum majorana; Pelargonium graveolens; Pogostemon patchouli; Thymus vulgaris* [population]; *Valeriana officinalis*
acne	*Citrus aurantium* var. *amara* fol.; *Eucalyptus radiata; Helichrysum angustifolium; Juniperus communis* ram.; *Lavandula angustifolia; Laurus nobilis* (infected); *Myrtus communis; Ormenis mixta; Pelargonium graveolens; Picea nigra; Pimenta dioica* (infected); *Pogostemon patchouli; Santalum album; Syzygium aromaticum* (infected); *Thymus satureioides; Thymus vulgaris* [population]; *Thymus vulgaris* ct. geraniol, (infected); *Vetiveria zizanioides*		
		apathy	*Mentha x piperita; Salvia officinalis*
		appetite (poor, loss of)	*Acorus calamus; Carum carvi; Chamaemelum nobile; Citrus aurantifolia; Citrus bergamia Citrus limon; Foeniculum vulgare; Hyssopus officinalis; Juniperus communis* fruct.; *Mentha spicata; Myristica fragrans; Pimenta racemosa; Salvia officinalis; Zingiber officinale*
aerophagy	*Carum carvi; Citrus limon; Coriandrum sativum; Cuminum cyminum; Helichrysum angustifolium; Illicium verum; Melaleuca viridiflora;*		
ageing	*Salvia sclarea* (cellular)		
allergies	*Ormenis mixta; Pogostemon patchouli*		
alopecia	*Salvia officinalis; Salvia sclarea; Thymus vulgaris* [population]		
amenorrhoea	*Achillea millefolium; Chamaemelum nobile; Matricaria recutita; Melaleuca viridiflora; Myrtus communis; Pimpinella anisum; Rosmarinus officinalis* ct. cineole, ct. camphor; *Salvia officinalis; Salvia sclarea; Tagetes minuta; Vetiveria zizanioides*	arrhythmia	*Inula graveolens; Nardostachys jatamansi; Ocimum basilicum; Rosmarinus officinalis* ct. verbenone
		arteriosclerosis	*Juniperus communis* ram.; *Ocimum basilicum; Rosmarinus officinalis* ct. cineole, ct. camphor, *Cedrus atlantica*
anaemia	*Chamaemelum nobile; Citrus limon; Nardostachys jatamansi; Thymus vulgaris* [population]	arteritis	*Cistus ladaniferus; Cymbopogon citratus*
		arteritis, coronary	*Melaleuca viridiflora; Vetiveria zizanioides*
aneurysm	*Melaleuca alternifolia; Salvia sclarea* (venous)	arthritis	*Abies alba* fol.; *Abies balsamea; Angelica archangelica* rad.; *Cuminum cyminum; Cymbopogon nardus; Eucalyptus citriodora; Eucalyptus globulus; Helichrysum angustifolium;*
angina	*Melissa officinalis; Rosmarinus officinalis* ct. verbenone; *Salvia officinalis; Zingiber officinale*		
anorexia nervosa	*Angelica archangelica* rad.; *Coriandrum sativum; Pimenta racemosa*		

Condition	Essential oils	Condition	Essential oils
	Lavandula angustifolia; Laurus nobilis; Melaleuca leucadendron; Nepeta cataria var. *citriodora; Origanum majorana; Pelargonium graveolens; Pimpinella anisum; Pinus mugo* var. *pumilio; Pinus sylvestris; Thymus satureioides; Thymus vulgaris* ct. thujanol-4; *Vetiveria zizanioides; Zingiber cassumunar*	breast, engorgement	*Foeniculum vulgare*
arthritis, rheumatoid	*Abies alba* fol.; *Cistus ladaniferus; Eucalyptus citriodora; Melaleuca viridiflora; Ocimum basilicum; Satureia montana; Syzygium aromaticum*	bronchitis	*Abies alba* fol.; *Abies balsamea; Acorus calamus; Anethum graveolens* sem.; *Angelica archangelica* rad.; *Boswellia carteri; Carum carvi; Cedrus atlantica; Cinnamomum verum* fol.; *Cinnamomum verum* cort.; *Citrus aurantium* var. *amara* flos; *Cupressus sempervirens; Eucalyptus dives; Eucalyptus globulus* (acute); *Eucalyptus radiata; Eucalyptus smithii; Helichrysum angustifolium; Hyssopus officinalis; Illicium verum; Inula graveolens* (chronic); *Juniperus communis* ram.; *Lavandula* x *intermedia; Leptospermum scoparium* (inhalation); *Melaleuca alternifolia; Melaleuca leucadendron; Melaleuca viridiflora; Mentha* x *piperita; Mentha spicata; Myrtus communis; Origanum majorana; Pimenta racemosa; Pimpinella anisum; Pinus mugo* var. *pumilio; Pinus sylvestris; Piper nigrum* (chronic); *Ravensara aromatica; Rosa damascena, R. centifolia; Rosmarinus officinalis* ct. cineole, ct. camphor (chronic); *Rosmarinus officinalis* ct. verbenone; *Salvia officinalis; Santalum album* (chronic); *Satureia montana; Syzygium aromaticum; Tagetes minuta; Thymus mastichina* (catarrhal); *Thymus vulgaris* [population]; *Thymus vulgaris* ct. geraniol, ct. linalool; *Thymus vulgaris* ct. thujanol-4; *Zingiber officinale* (chronic)
asthenia	*Cinnamomum verum* cort.; *Hyssopus officinalis; Origanum vulgare; Picea nigra; Pimenta dioica; Thymus vulgaris* ct. thujanol-4		
asthma	*Abies balsamea; Aloysia triphylla; Angelica archangelica* rad.; *Boswellia carteri; Eucalyptus globulus; Eucalyptus smithii; Helichrysum angustifolium; Hyssopus officinalis; Myrtus communis; Pimpinella anisum; Pinus mugo* var. *pumilio; Pinus sylvestris; Rosa damascena, R. centifolia; Salvia officinalis; Satureia montana; Thymus vulgaris* [population]; *Thymus vulgaris* ct. thymol, ct. carvacrol; *Zingiber cassumunar*		
asthma, bronchial	*Abies sibirica; Mentha* x *piperita; Salvia officinalis*		
atherosclerosis	*Melaleuca viridiflora; Ormenis mixta*		
backache	*Foeniculum vulgare; Pimpinella anisum*		
bite, insect	*Citrus limon; Lavandula angustifolia; Melaleuca viridiflora; Salvia officinalis*		
boils	*Chamaemelum nobile; Citrus aurantium* var. *amara* fol.; *Citrus limon; Laurus nobilis; Melaleuca viridiflora; Melaleuca viridiflora; Thymus vulgaris* [population]	bruises	*Foeniculum vulgare; Helichrysum angustifolium; Hyssopus officinalis; Lavandula angustifolia; Rosmarinus officinalis* ct. cineole, ct. camphor; *Tagetes minuta*

Condition	Essential oils
burns	*Abies balsamea; Chamaemelum nobile; Citrus bergamia; Helichrysum angustifolium; Lavandula angustifolia; Pelargonium graveolens; Rosmarinus officinalis* ct. cineole, ct. camphor; *Tagetes minuta*
bursitis	*Syzygium aromaticum*
Candida albicans	*Aniba rosaeodora; Citrus limon, Eucalyptus globulus; Helichrysum angustifolium; Lavandula angustifolia; Lavandula x intermedia; Leptospermum scoparium; Melaleuca alternifolia; Pelargonium graveolens; Picea nigra* (intestinal); *Rosmarinus officinalis* ct. verbenone; *Salvia officinalis; Satureia montana; Tagetes minuta*
capillaries, broken	*Citrus limon; Cupressus sempervirens; Helichrysum angustifolium*
catarrh	*Abies balsamea; Achillea millefolium; Anethum graveolens* sem.; *Commiphora myrrha; Eucalyptus dives; Illicium verum; Inula graveolens* (chronic); *Lavandula x intermedia; Melaleuca viridiflora* (chronic); *Myrtus communis; Origanum majorana; Pimpinella anisum; Pinus mugo* var. *pumilio; Satureia montana; Tagetes minuta* (infection)
cellulite	*Citrus paradisi; Foeniculum vulgare; Salvia officinalis, Cedrus atlantica; Cymbopogon citratus;*
chickenpox	*Ravensara aromatica*
cholera	*Melaleuca leucadendron; Pimenta dioica*
circulation, poor	*Citrus aurantium* var. *amara* per.; *Citrus limon; Cupressus sempervirens; Foeniculum vulgare; Pimenta racemosa; Rosmarinus officinalis* ct. cineole, ct. camphor; *Salvia officinalis*

Condition	Essential oils
cirrhosis	*Juniperus communis* fruct.; *Mentha x piperita; Rosmarinus officinalis* ct. cineole, ct. camphor; *Salvia officinalis*
colds	*Achillea millefolium; Aniba rosaeodora; Cinnamomum verum* cort.; *Citrus aurantifolia; Citrus limon; Citrus paradisi; Eucalyptus globulus; Eucalyptus smithii; Helichrysum angustifolium; Hyssopus officinalis; Melaleuca leucadendron; Melaleuca viridiflora; Mentha spicata; Myrtus communis; Pimenta dioica; Pinus sylvestris; Piper nigrum; Rosmarinus officinalis* ct. cineole, ct. camphor (chills); *Thymus vulgaris* ct. thymol, ct. carvacrol (head)
colic	*Anethum graveolens* sem.; *Angelica archangelica* rad.; *Cananga odorata; Chamaemelum nobile* (intestinal); *Cinnamomum verum* cort.; *Citrus bergamia; Cuminum cyminum; Elettaria cardamomum; Lavandula angustifolia; Melaleuca leucadendron; Mentha x piperita; Mentha spicata; Nardostachys jatamansi* (intestinal); *Origanum majorana; Pelargonium graveolens; Pimpinella anisum; Rosmarinus officinalis* ct. verbenone (viral); *Satureia montana*
colitis	*Abies sibirica* (spasmodic); *Acorus calamus; Angelica archangelica* rad. (spasmodic); *Cinnamomum verum* fol.; *Cinnamomum verum* cort.; *Citrus aurantifolia* (spasmodic); *Citrus aurantium* var. *amara* flos; *Cuminum cyminum; Cymbopogon nardus; Helichrysum angustifolium; Illicium verum* (spasmodic); *Leptospermum scoparium; Mentha x piperita; Ormenis*

Condition	Essential oils	Condition	Essential oils
	mixta; Pelargonium graveolens (infectious); *Pimenta dioica; Pogostemon patchouli; Rosmarinus officinalis* ct. cineole, ct. camphor; *Satureia montana; Thymus vulgaris* ct. geraniol, ct. linalool; *Zingiber cassumunar*	cramp (spasm)	*Abies balsamea; Citrus reticulata; Cupressus sempervirens; Ocimum basilicum; Origanum majorana; Rosmarinus officinalis* ct. cineole, ct. camphor; *Satureia montana*
conception, difficult	*Salvia officinalis*	cramp	*Anethum graveolens* sem. (smooth muscle); *Cananga odorata; Inula graveolens; Laurus nobilis; Lavandula angustifolia; Pelargonium graveolens; Valeriana officinalis*
congestion	*Ocimum basilicum* (uterine/prostate); *Pelargonium graveolens* (breast); *Pinus sylvestris* (ovarian, uterine)		
congestion, liver	*Citrus paradisi; Vetiveria zizanioides*	cramp, stomach	*Carum carvi; Citrus aurantium* var. *amara* per.; *Citrus reticulata* per.; *Matricaria recutita; Melissa officinalis; Mentha* x *piperita; Ocimum basilicum* (gastric); *Picea nigra; Satureia montana* (intestinal); *Syzygium aromaticum* (intestinal)
congestion, lung	*Pimpinella anisum*		
conjunctivitis	*Chamaemelum nobile; Eucalyptus radiata; Rosa damascena, R. centifolia*		
constipation	*Anethum graveolens* sem.; *Citrus aurantium* var. *amara* per.; *Citrus aurantium* var. *sinensis* per; *Citrus reticulata; Foeniculum vulgare; Mentha arvensis; Mentha spicata; Rosmarinus officinalis* ct. cineole, ct. camphor; *Satureia hortensis; Zingiber officinale*	cystitis	*Abies balsamea; Acorus calamus; Aloysia triphylla; Cinnamomum verum* fol.; *Cinnamomum verum* cort. (bacterial); *Coriander sativum; Eucalyptus citriodora; Eucalyptus globulus; Foeniculum vulgare; Inula graveolens; Juniperus communis* fruct.; *Lavandula angustifolia; Melaleuca leucadendron; Mentha* x *piperita; Mentha spicata; Ocimum basilicum* (coliform); *Ormenis mixta; Pimenta dioica; Pinus sylvestris; Rosmarinus officinalis* ct. cineole, ct. camphor; *Santalum album; Satureia montana; Syzygium aromaticum; Thymus satureioides; Thymus vulgaris* ct. geraniol, ct. linalool; *Thymus vulgaris* ct. thujanol-4
convulsions	*Nardostachys jatamansi*		
coughs	*Abies balsamea; Aniba rosaeodora; Cinnamomum verum* cort.; *Elettaria cardamomum; Eucalyptus globulus; Eucalyptus radiata; Eucalyptus smithii; Helichrysum angustifolium; Hyssopus officinalis; Illicium verum; Inula graveolens* (chronic); *Lavandula* x *intermedia; Melaleuca leucadendron; Melaleuca viridiflora; Myrtus communis* (chronic); *Origanum majorana; Pinus mugo* var. *pumilio; Piper nigrum; Ravensara aromatica; Rosmarinus officinalis* ct. cineole, ct. camphor; *Rosmarinus officinalis* ct. verbenone; *Salvia officinalis; Satureia montana; Tagetes minuta*	debility	*Aniba rosaeodora; Coriandrum sativum; Cupressus sempervirens; Juniperus communis* ram.; *Lavandula angustifolia; Lavandula* x *intermedia; Melaleuca alternifolia; Myristica fragrans; Ocimum basilicum; Origanum majorana; Pelargonium graveolens; Pinus sylvestris; Rosa*

Condition	Essential oils	Condition	Essential oils
	damascena, R. centifolia; Rosmarinus officinalis ct. cineole, ct. camphor; *Salvia officinalis* (nervous also); *Satureia hortensis; Satureia montana; Syzygium aromaticum; Thymus vulgaris* [population]; *Thymus satureioides*		*Mentha spicata; Myristica fragrans* (chronic); *Origanum majorana; Pelargonium graveolens; Rosmarinus officinalis* ct. cineole, ct. camphor (infection); *Santalum album; Satureia montana; Syzygium aromaticum; Zingiber officinale*
depression	*Abies balsamea; Aloysia triphylla; Aniba rosaeodora; Boswellia carteri; Chamaemelum nobile; Citrus aurantium* var. *amara* flos; *Citrus aurantium* var. *amara* fol.; *Citrus paradisi; Helichrysum angustifolium; Leptospermum scoparium; Melaleuca alternifolia; Melaleuca viridiflora* (post-viral); *Mentha spicata; Ocimum basilicum; Pimenta dioica; Pogostemon patchouli; Rosa damascena, R. centifolia; Satureia montana; Thymus vulgaris* [population]; *Thymus vulgaris* ct. thymol, ct. carvacrol; *Valeriana officinalis* (long-standing)	diarrhoea, infantile	*Chamaemelum nobile*
		digestion, painful	*Angelica archangelica* rad.; *Citrus limon; Citrus reticulata* (stomach); *Mentha x piperita; Pinus sylvestris* (gastric); *Rosmarinus officinalis* ct. cineole, ct. camphor; *Salvia officinalis; Satureia montana; Zingiber officinale*
		digestion, sluggish	*Achillea millefolium; Acorus calamus; Coriandrum sativum; Cymbopogon citratus; Elettaria cardamomum; Eucalyptus smithii; Hyssopus officinalis; Inula graveolens* (weak); *Laurus nobilis; Litsea cubeba; Mentha spicata; Myristica fragrans; Ocimum basilicum; Piper nigrum; Rosmarinus officinalis* ct. cineole, ct. camphor; *Salvia officinalis; Thymus vulgaris* [population]; *Zingiber officinale*
depression, nervous	*Cinnamomum verum* cort.; *Litsea cubeba; Nepeta cataria* var. *citriodora; Origanum majorana; Ormenis mixta; Rosmarinus officinalis* ct. verbenone		
dermatitis	*Helichrysum angustifolium; Inula graveolens; Litsea cubeba; Ormenis mixta; Thymus vulgaris* ct. thujanol-4	dysentery	*Acorus calamus; Cinnamomum verum* cort.; *Pimenta dioica*
diabetes	*Aloysia triphylla; Cananga odorata; Citrus aurantium* var. *amara* flos; *Citrus limon; Eucalyptus citriodora; Juniperus communis* fruct.; *Pelargonium graveolens; Ocimum basilicum; Pinus sylvestris* (pancreatic); *Salvia officinalis* (prediabetes); *Thymus vulgaris* ct. thujanol-4	dysmenorrhoea	*Achillea millefolium; Angelica archangelica* rad.; *Chamaemelum nobile; Foeniculum vulgare; Matricaria recutita; Melaleuca leucadendron; Myrtus communis; Pelargonium graveolens; Pimpinella anisum; Salvia officinalis; Salvia sclarea; Zingiber cassumunar*
diarrhoea	*Acorus calamus; Cinnamomum verum* cort.; *Citrus limon; Citrus aurantium* var. *sinensis* per. (chronic); *Melaleuca viridiflora;*	dyspepsia	*Aloysia triphylla; Anethum graveolens* sem.; *Angelica archangelica* rad.; *Carum carvi; Chamaemelum nobile; Citrus aurantium* var. *amara* per.; *Citrus bergamia; Citrus reticulata; Citrus*

Condition	Essential oils	Condition	Essential oils
	aurantium var. *sinensis* per.; *Coriandrum sativum; Cuminum cyminum; Elettaria cardamomum; Foeniculum vulgare; Hyssopus officinalis; Illicium verum; Leptospermum scoparium; Melissa officinalis; Mentha arvensis; Mentha* x *piperita; Mentha spicata; Origanum majorana; Pimenta dioica; Pimenta racemosa; Pimpinella anisum; Rosmarinus officinalis* ct. cineole, ct. camphor; *Salvia officinalis; Satureia hortensis*	fatigue	*Angelica archangelica* rad. (nervous); *Cinnamomum verum* cort.; *Cistus ladaniferus* (chronic); *Citrus aurantium* var. *amara* flos; *Citrus paradisi* (exhaustion); *Coriandrum sativum* (including mental); *Cymbopogon nardus; Eucalyptus radiata* (chronic); *Eucalyptus smithii; Juniperus communis* ram.; *Mentha spicata* (mental); *Pelargonium graveolens* (nervous); *Pimenta dioica; Pinus sylvestris; Rosmarinus officinalis* ct. cineole, ct. camphor; *Rosmarinus officinalis* ct. verbenone; *Salvia sclarea* (nervous); *Satureia montana* (mental, nervous); *Syzygium aromaticum; Syzygium aromaticum* (mental); *Thymus satureioides; Thymus vulgaris* [population]; *Thymus vulgaris* ct. geraniol, ct. linalool; *Zingiber officinale*
dyspnoea	*Hyssopus officinalis*		
earache	*Melaleuca leucadendron*		
eczema	*Cedrus atlantica; Chamaemelum nobile; Helichrysum angustifolium; Hyssopus officinalis; Juniperus communis* ram. (weeping); *Lavandula angustifolia; Matricaria recutita; Mentha arvensis; Mentha* x *piperita* (inflamed); *Ocimum basilicum* (dry); *Ormenis mixta; Picea nigra* (dry); *Pogostemon patchouli* (seborrhoeic); *Thymus vulgaris* ct. geraniol, ct. linalool (dry, weeping)	fever	*Achillea millefolium, Acorus calamus; Cinnamomum verum* cort. (tropical); *Cistus ladaniferus* (scarlet); *Citrus aurantifolia; Melaleuca viridiflora; Mentha* x *piperita; Mentha spicata; Pimenta racemosa; Piper nigrum; Salvia officinalis* (intermittent); *Valeriana officinalis*
emphysema	*Hyssopus officinalis; Thymus vulgaris* ct. thymol, ct. carvacrol	fever, glandular	*Ravensara aromatica*
enteritis	see gastroenteritis	flatulence	*Acorus calamus; Aloysia triphylla; Anethum graveolens* sem.; *Angelica archangelica* rad.; *Carum carvi; Chamaemelum nobile; Cinnamomum verum* cort.; *Citrus limon; Commiphora myrrha; Coriandrum sativum; Cuminum cyminum; Elettaria cardamomum; Foeniculum vulgare; Illicium verum; Lavandula angustifolia; Laurus nobilis; Mentha* x *piperita; Mentha spicata; Myristica*
enuresis	*Rosmarinus officinalis* ct. cineole,		
(bed wetting)	ct. camphor; *Thymus vulgaris* ct. thymol, ct. carvacrol		
epilepsy	*Nardostachys jatamansi; Ocimum basilicum; Origanum majorana; Rosmarinus officinalis* ct. cineole, ct. camphor; *Salvia sclarea*		
erethism, cardiovascular	*Citrus aurantium* var. *amara* flos; *Citrus reticulata; Melissa officinalis; Pimpinella anisum*		
excitability	*Citrus reticulata; Eucalyptus smithii*		
fainting	*Origanum majorana; Rosmarinus officinalis* ct. cineole, ct. camphor		

Condition	Essential oils
	fragrans; Ocimum basilicum; Origanum majorana; Pimenta dioica; Pimenta racemosa; Pimpinella anisum; Rosmarinus officinalis ct. cineole, ct. camphor; *Satureia hortensis; Satureia montana; Syzygium aromaticum; Thymus vulgaris* [population]; *Zingiber cassumunar; Zingiber officinale*
fluid retention (see water retention)	
food poisoning	*Inula graveolens*
freckles	*Citrus limon*
frigidity	*Cananga odorata; Myristica fragrans; Pimpinella anisum; Piper nigrum; Rosa damascena, R. centifolia*
gall bladder malfunction	*Inula graveolens; Rosmarinus officinalis* ct. cineole, ct. camphor; *Thymus satureioides*
gall bladder, inflamed	*Rosmarinus officinalis* ct. cineole, ct. camphor
gall stones	*Citrus limon; Melaleuca viridiflora; Nepeta cataria* var. *citriodora; Pinus mugo* var. *pumilio; Pinus sylvestris; Rosmarinus officinalis* ct. cineole, ct. camphor; *Thymus satureioides*
gastroenteritis/ gastritis	*Acorus calamus; Citrus limon; Coriandrum sativum; Foeniculum vulgare; Helichrysum angustifolium; Inula graveolens* (viral); *Lavandula* x *intermedia; Matricaria recutita; Melaleuca alternifolia* (viral); *Melaleuca leucadendron; Melaleuca viridiflora* (viral); *Mentha* x *piperita; Ocimum basilicum; Origanum majorana; Pelargonium graveolens; Pimpinella anisum; Pogostemon patchouli; Ravensara aromatica* (viral); *Rosmarinus officinalis* ct. cineole, ct. camphor; *Salvia officinalis* (viral); *Satureia montana; Syzygium aromaticum; Thymus vulgaris* ct. linalool, ct. geraniol (viral)

Condition	Essential oils
genital herpes	*Melaleuca viridiflora; Salvia officinalis*
genital infections	*Melaleuca alternifolia; Santalum album*
gingivitis	*Rosa damascena, R. centifolia; Salvia officinalis*
gout	*Acorus calamus; Chamaemelum nobile; Cinnamomum verum* fol.; *Citrus limon; Foeniculum vulgare; Juniperus communis* ram.; *Melaleuca leucadendron; Ocimum basilicum; Pinus sylvestris; Rosmarinus officinalis* ct. cineole, ct. camphor
haematoma	*Helichrysum angustifolium*
haemorrhage (uterine)	*Cistus ladaniferus; Pelargonium graveolens*
haemorrhoids	*Citrus aurantium* var. *amara* flos; *Cupressus sempervirens; Melaleuca alternifolia; Melaleuca leucadendron; Melaleuca viridiflora; Myrtus communis; Nardostachys jatamansi; Pelargonium graveolens; Pogostemon patchouli; Salvia sclarea; Santalum album*
hair, poor growth	*Cananga odorata; Carum carvi; Pimenta racemosa* (loss); *Salvia sclarea; Thymus vulgaris* [population]
halitosis	*Elettaria cardamomum*
hay fever	*Carum carvi; Helichrysum angustifolium; Hyssopus officinalis; Myrtus communis*
headaches	*Aniba rosaeodora* (stress related); *Chamaemelum nobile; Citrus limon; Citrus paradisi; Cuminum cyminum* (dyspeptic); *Elettaria cardamomum* (digestive); *Eucalyptus globulus* (congestive); *Eucalyptus smithii* (congestive); *Lavandula angustifolia; Melissa officinalis; Mentha* x *piperita; Rosmarinus officinalis* ct. cineole, ct. camphor
heart, tired	*Inula graveolens; Pimpinella anisum; Santalum album; Thymus vulgaris* ct. geraniol, ct. linalool

Condition	Essential oils	Condition	Essential oils
heart, weak	*Rosmarinus officinalis* ct. cineole, ct. camphor	hypotension	*Hyssopus officinalis*; *Mentha x piperita*; *Ocimum basilicum*; *Pimenta dioica*; *Pinus sylvestris*; *Rosmarinus officinalis* ct. cineole, ct. camphor (high dose); *Salvia officinalis*; *Satureia montana*; *Syzygium aromaticum*; *Thymus vulgaris* [population]
hepatitis	*Cuminum cyminum*; *Melaleuca viridiflora* (viral); *Mentha x piperita*; *Ocimum basilicum* (viral); *Pimenta dioica*; *Ravensara aromatica* (viral); *Rosmarinus officinalis* ct. cineole, ct. camphor; *Rosmarinus officinalis* ct. verbenone (viral); *Syzygium aromaticum*		
		hypothyroidism	*Myrtus communis*
		hysteria	*Litsea cubeba*; *Melissa officinalis*; *Nardostachys jatamansi*; *Rosmarinus officinalis* ct. cineole, ct. camphor
hepatobiliary deficiency	*Achillea millefolium*; *Anethum graveolens* sem.; *Cymbopogon citratus*; *Myrtus communis*; *Rosmarinus officinalis* ct. cineole, ct. camphor; *Salvia officinalis*; *Satureia hortensis*; *Thymus satureioides*; *Thymus vulgaris* ct. thujanol-4	immuno-deficiency	*Boswellia carteri*; *Cinnamomum verum* fol.; *Eucalyptus radiata*; *Melaleuca alternifolia* (see Appendix A(I)); *Melaleuca viridiflora*; *Origanum vulgare*; *Picea nigra*; *Pogostemon patchouli*; *Satureia montana*; *Syzygium aromaticum*; *Thymus satureioides*; *Thymus vulgaris* ct. linalool; *Thymus vulgaris* ct. thujanol-4; *Vetiveria zizanioides*
Herpes (unspecified)	*Citrus limon*; *Lavandula angustifolia*; *Mentha x piperita*: *Nepeta cataria* var. *citriodora*; *Syzygium aromaticum*		
Herpes simplex I	*Citrus bergamia*; *Melissa officinalis*	impetigo	*Pelargonium graveolens*; *Satureia montana*
Herpes simplex II (zoster, shingles)	*Eucalyptus citriodora*, *Mentha x piperita*, *Ravensara aromatica*	impotence	*Cananga odorata*; *Mentha x piperita*; *Myristica fragrans*; *Pimpinella anisum*; *Pinus sylvestris*; *Rosmarinus officinalis* ct. cineole, ct. camphor; *Santalum album*; *Syzygium aromaticum*; *Zingiber officinale*
hiccoughs	*Citrus reticulata* per., *Anethum graveolens* sem.		
high cholesterol	*Rosmarinus officinalis* ct. cineole, ct. camphor; *Salvia sclarea*		
hot flushes	*Mentha x piperita*; *Salvia officinalis*		
hyperpnoea	*Cananga odorata*; *Foeniculum vulgare*	indigestion	see dyspepsia
		infection, digestive tract	*Origanum vulgare*
hypertension	*Achillea millefolium*; *Aloysia triphylla*; *Anethum graveolens* sem.; *Cananga odorata*; *Citrus aurantium* var. *amara* flos; *Citrus limon*; *Eucalyptus citriodora*; *Inula graveolens*; *Lavandula angustifolia*; *Melaleuca viridiflora*; *Melissa officinalis*; *Origanum majorana*; *Rosmarinus officinalis* ct. cineole, ct. camphor (low dose)	infection, fungal	*Leptospermum scoparium*; *Melaleuca viridiflora*; *Salvia sclarea*
		infection, gum	*Syzygium aromaticum*
		infection, intestinal	*Cananga odorata*; *Melaleuca alternifolia*; *Ocimum basilicum*
		infection, respiratory	*Abies alba* fol.; *Aniba rosaeodora*; *Angelica archangelica* rad.; *Citrus aurantium* var. *amara* fol.; *Eucalyptus radiata*; *Inula graveolens* (lungs); *Melaleuca viridiflora*; *Origanum vulgare*;
hyperthyroidism	*Cuminum cyminum*; *Origanum majorana*; *Picea nigra*		

Condition	Essential oils	Condition	Essential oils
infection, urinary	*Pinus mugo* var. *pumilio*; *Pinus sylvestris*; *Satureia hortensis*; *Achillea millefolium*; *Angelica archangelica* rad.; *Cedrus atlantica*; *Cinnamomum verum* cort.; *Cistus ladaniferus*; *Foeniculum vulgare*; *Myrtus communis*; *Nepeta cataria* var. *citriodora*; *Origanum vulgare*; *Pinus sylvestris*; *Piper nigrum*; *Santalum album*		*Citrus reticulata*; *Citrus aurantium* var. *sinensis* per.; *Cuminum cyminum*; *Juniperus communis* fruct.; *Lavandula angustifolia*; *Litsea cubeba*; *Melissa officinalis*; *Myrtus communis*; *Ocimum basilicum* (nervous); *Origanum majorana*; *Ravensara aromatica*; *Thymus vulgaris* ct. geraniol, ct. linalool; *Valeriana officinalis*
infection, viral	*Cinnamomum verum* cort.; *Pimenta racemosa*; *Thymus mastichina*	irritability	*Chamaemelum nobile*; *Cupressus sempervirens*
inflamed eyelids	*Melaleuca viridiflora*	irritable bowel syndrome	*Mentha x piperita*; *Nepeta cataria* var. *citriodora*; *Salvia officinalis*
inflamed gums	*Chamaemelum nobile*	jaundice	*Mentha x piperita*; *Pelargonium graveolens*; *Rosmarinus officinalis* ct. cineole, ct. camphor; *Salvia officinalis*
influenza	*Cinnamomum verum* cort.; *Citrus paradisi*; *Commiphora myrrha*; *Coriandrum sativum*; *Cupressus sempervirens*; *Eucalyptus globulus*; *Eucalyptus radiata*; *Eucalyptus smithii*; *Helichrysum angustifolium*; *Hyssopus officinalis*; *Lavandula angustifolia*; *Laurus nobilis*; *Melaleuca leucadendron*; *Mentha spicata*; *Pimenta dioica*; *Pimenta racemosa*; *Pinus sylvestris*; *Ravensara aromatica*; *Rosmarinus officinalis* ct. cineole, ct. camphor; *Salvia officinalis*; *Syzygium aromaticum*; *Thymus vulgaris* ct. thujanol-4; *Thymus vulgaris* ct. thymol, ct. carvacrol	joints, painful	*Eucalyptus smithii*; *Juniperus communis* fruct.; *Leptospermum scoparium*; *Melaleuca leucadendron*; *Mentha arvensis*; *Pimenta racemosa*
		joints, stiff	*Thymus vulgaris* [population]
		kidneys, toxic	*Citrus paradisi*
		labour aid (facilitates delivery)	*Mentha x piperita*; *Myristica fragrans*; *Pimpinella anisum*; *Salvia officinalis*; *Thymus vulgaris* ct. geraniol, ct. linalool
		labour, problem	*Melaleuca viridiflora* (pain); *Syzygium aromaticum* (difficult, long)
insect bite	*Ocimum basilicum* (wasp stings); *Satureia montana*	laryngitis	*Commiphora myrrha*; *Eucalyptus globulus*; *Inula graveolens*; *Mentha arvensis*; *Mentha x piperita*; *Piper nigrum*
insect repellent	*Cymbopogon nardus* (mosquito); *Melaleuca leucadendron* (mosquito); *Ocimum basilicum* (house fly, mosquito); *Salvia officinalis* (gnat, mosquito); *Syzygium aromaticum* (mosquito, clothes moth)	leucorrhoea	*Cinnamomum verum* cort.; *Hyssopus officinalis*; *Lavandula angustifolia*; *Melaleuca viridiflora*; *Rosmarinus officinalis* ct. verbenone; *Salvia officinalis*; *Thymus vulgaris* [population]
insomnia	*Angelica archangelica* rad.; *Cananga odorata*; *Chamaemelum nobile*; *Citrus aurantium* var. *amara* flos; *Cistus ladaniferus*; *Citrus bergamia*; *Citrus limon*;	lichen	*Satureia montana*
		listlessness	*Lavandula x intermedia*
		liver, enlarged	*Rosmarinus officinalis* ct. cineole, ct. camphor

Condition	Essential oils	Condition	Essential oils
liver, sluggish	*Helichrysum angustifolium; Melissa officinalis; Ocimum basilicum; Ormenis mixta; Pelargonium graveolens; Piper nigrum*		*scoparium; Myristica fragrans; Origanum majorana; Pimenta racemosa; Pinus mugo* var. *pumilio; Rosmarinus officinalis* ct. cineole, ct. camphor
lumbago	*Santalum album; Thymus vulgaris* ct. thymol, ct. carvacrol	nail fungi (ungueal)	*Pelargonium graveolens; Tagetes minuta*
lymph, congestion	*Cedrus atlantica; Myrtus communis; Pelargonium graveolens; Pinus sylvestris*	nausea	*Citrus aurantifolia; Citrus limon; Elettaria cardamomum; Matricaria recutita; Mentha arvensis* (indigestion, pregnancy); *Mentha* x *piperita;*
lymph ganglion, inflammation	*Satureia montana*		*Mentha spicata; Salvia officinalis; Zingiber officinale*
malaria	*Aloysia triphylla; Laurus nobilis; Satureia montana*		
malignancy	*Salvia officinalis*	nephritis	*Eucalyptus dives*
melancholy	*Lavandula angustifolia*	nervous spasm	*Origanum majorana*
memory, loss	*Litsea cubeba; Rosmarinus officinalis* ct. cineole, ct. camphor; *Syzygium aromaticum*	nervous tension	*Citrus reticulata*
		nervousness	*Citrus aurantium* var. *amara* per.; *Citrus aurantium* var. *sinensis* per.; *Ocimum basilicum*
meningitis (viral)	*Salvia officinalis*		
menopause	*Illicium verum; Pimpinella anisum; Salvia sclarea*	neuralgia	*Achillea millefolium; Cymbopogon nardus; Melaleuca leucadendron; Mentha arvensis; Mentha* x *piperita; Myristica fragrans; Pelargonium graveolens; Rosmarinus officinalis* ct. cineole, ct. camphor; *Santalum album; Syzygium aromaticum*
menopause, problems	*Chamaemelum nobile; Foeniculum vulgare; Salvia officinalis*		
menorrhagia	*Cistus ladaniferus*		
mental instability	*Origanum majorana*		
mental strain	*Ocimum basilicum; Thymus vulgaris* ct. thymol, ct. carvacrol	neurasthenia	*Citrus aurantium* var. *amara* flos
migraine	*Chamaemelum nobile; Eucalyptus globulus* (congestive); *Lavandula angustifolia; Lavandula* x *intermedia* (chronic); *Mentha arvensis; Mentha* x *piperita; Ocimum basilicum; Origanum majorana; Pimpinella anisum* (nauseous); *Rosmarinus officinalis* ct. cineole, ct. camphor; *Thymus vulgaris* [population] (stimulant)	neuritis	*Achillea millefolium; Chamaemelum nobile; Laurus nobilis* (viral); *Litsea cubeba* (viral); *Mentha* x *piperita* (viral); *Pimenta dioica; Salvia officinalis* (viral)
		nightmares	*Citrus limon*
		obesity	*Citrus limon*
		oedema	*Foeniculum vulgare*
		oligomenorrhoea	*Achillea millefolium; Cinnamomum verum* cort.; *Foeniculum vulgare; Hyssopus officinalis; Illicium verum; Melaleuca viridiflora; Pimpinella anisum; Rosmarinus officinalis* ct. cineole, ct. camphor; *Salvia officinalis; Salvia sclarea; Vetiveria zizanioides*
milk, lack of	*Foeniculum vulgare*		
multiple sclerosis	*Aloysia triphylla; Cistus ladaniferus; Hyssopus officinalis; Pinus sylvestris; Rosmarinus officinalis* ct. cineole, ct. camphor		
muscles, aches and pains	*Eucalyptus smithii; Lavandula angustifolia; Leptospermum*	oliguria	*Pimpinella anisum; Salvia officinalis*

Condition	Essential oils
orchitis	*Cuminum cyminum*
oropharyngitis	*Cinnamomum verum* fol.
osteoarthritis	*Coriandrum sativum*; *Pelargonium graveolens*
otitis	*Eucalyptus dives*; *Eucalyptus radiata*; *Lavandula angustifolia*; *Melaleuca alternifolia*; *Rosmarinus officinalis* ct. cineole, ct. camphor; *Thymus vulgaris* ct. geraniol, ct. linalool; *Thymus vulgaris* ct. thujanol-4
ovarian insufficiency	*Nardostachys jatamansi*
ovaries, sluggish	*Salvia officinalis*
ovary problems	*Cupressus sempervirens*; *Foeniculum vulgare*; *Myrtus communis*
ovary, testicle problems	*Rosmarinus officinalis* ct. verbenone
overwork	*Aniba rosaeodora*
palpitations	*Citrus aurantium* var. *amara* per.; *Citrus aurantium* var. *sinensis* per.; *Foeniculum vulgare*; *Melissa officinalis*; *Mentha* x *piperita*; *Origanum majorana*; *Pimpinella anisum*; *Rosmarinus officinalis* ct. cineole, ct. camphor
pancreas, sluggish	*Juniperus communis* fruct.; *Ormenis mixta*; *Pelargonium graveolens*; *Piper nigrum*
pancreas, secretion insufficiency	*Vetiveria zizanioides*
parasites	*Abies balsamea*; *Cinnamomum verum* cort.; *Hyssopus officinalis*; *Laurus nobilis*; *Litsea cubeba*; *Melaleuca alternifolia*; *Melaleuca leucadendron*, *Melaleuca viridiflora*; *Mentha arvensis*; *Myrtus communis*; *Ocimum basilicum*; *Origanum vulgare*; *Ormenis mixta*; *Picea nigra*; *Pimenta dioica*; *Ruta graveolens*; *Satureia montana*; *Tagetes minuta*; *Thymus vulgaris* [population] (intestinal); *Thymus vulgaris* ct. linalool

Condition	Essential oils
	(intestinal); *Valeriana officinalis* (see Appendix A(I) for parasites affected)
pericarditis	*Eucalyptus citriodora*
periods, irregular	*Mentha* x *piperita*; *Salvia officinalis*
periods, scanty	*Lavandula angustifolia*; *Myristica fragrans*
perspiration (excessive)	*Cupressus sempervirens*; *Cymbopogon nardus*
phlebitis	*Citrus limon*; *Lavandula angustifolia*
pityriasis	*Lavandula angustifolia*; *Melaleuca leucadendron*
pleurisy	*Cinnamomum verum* cort.; *Eucalyptus globulus*; *Pinus mugo* var. *pumilio*
PMS	*Foeniculum vulgare*; *Matricaria recutita*; *Melaleuca alternifolia*, *Pimpinella anisum*
pneumonia	*Eucalyptus globulus*; *Hyssopus officinalis*; *Pinus sylvestris*
prostate, congestion	*Myrtus communis*
prostatitis	*Achillea millefolium*; *Melaleuca viridiflora*; *Myrtus communis*; *Picea nigra*; *Pinus sylvestris*
pruritus (itching)	*Cedrus atlantica*; *Mentha arvensis*; *Mentha* x *piperita*; *Ormenis mixta*; *Pelargonium graveolens*
psoriasis	*Aloysia triphylla*; *Citrus bergamia*; *Leptospermum scoparium*; *Melaleuca leucadendron*; *Melaleuca viridiflora*; *Nardostachys jatamansi*; *Thymus vulgaris* ct. geraniol, ct. linalool
pyelitis	*Pinus sylvestris*
pyorrhoea	*Abies sibirica*; *Cinnamomum verum* cort.; *Melaleuca alternifolia*
rheumatism (joints)	*Laurus nobilis*; *Thymus vulgaris* ct. thymol, ct. carvacrol
rheumatism	*Abies alba* fol.; *Achillea millefolium*; *Aloysia triphylla*; *Angelica archangelica* rad.; *Boswellia carteri*; *Chamaemelum*

Condition	Essential oils
	nobile (pain); *Cinnamomum verum* cort.; *Cinnamomum verum* fol.; *Citrus aurantifolia*; *Citrus limon*; *Coriandrum sativum* (pain); *Cuminum cyminum*; *Cymbopogon nardus*; *Cupressus sempervirens* (swelling); *Hyssopus officinalis*; *Juniperus communis* ram.; *Laurus nobilis*; *Lavandula angustifolia*; *Leptospermum scoparium*; *Matricaria recutita*; *Melaleuca leucadendron*; *Myristica fragrans*; *Nepeta cataria* var. *citriodora*; *Ormenis mixta*; *Pelargonium graveolens*; *Pimpinella anisum*; *Pinus mugo* var. *pumilio*; *Piper nigrum*; *Rosmarinus officinalis* ct. cineole, ct. camphor; *Salvia officinalis*; *Thymus vulgaris* [population]; *Thymus vulgaris* ct. linalool; *Thymus vulgaris* ct. thymol, ct. carvacrol; *Zingiber cassumunar*; *Zingiber officinale*
rhinitis	*Abies balsamea*; *Eucalyptus radiata*; *Helichrysum angustifolium*; *Juniperus communis* ram.; *Mentha arvensis*; *Origanum majorana*
rhinopharyngitis	*Cinnamomum verum* fol.; *Eucalyptus radiata*; *Hyssopus officinalis*; *Lavandula x intermedia*; *Melaleuca viridiflora*; *Mentha arvensis*; *Ravensara aromatica*; *Thymus vulgaris* ct. thujanol-4
ringworm	*Leptospermum scoparium*; *Mentha x piperita*
sadness	*Abies alba* fol.; *Coriandrum sativum*; *Origanum majorana*
salpingitis	*Cinnamomum verum* fol.; *Pimenta dioica*; *Syzygium aromaticum*
scalp, problem	*Carum carvi* (stimulant); *Cedrus atlantica* (stimulant)
scanty periods	*Laurus nobilis*; *Pimenta racemosa*
scars	*Achillea millefolium*; *Aniba rosaeodora*; *Boswellia carteri*;

Condition	Essential oils
	Helichrysum angustifolium; *Hyssopus officinalis*; *Lavandula angustifolia*; *Mentha spicata*; *Pogostemon patchouli*
sciatica	*Mentha arvensis*; *Mentha x piperita*; *Pimpinella anisum*; *Santalum album*; *Thymus vulgaris* ct. thymol, ct. carvacrol
scurvy	*Citrus aurantifolia*,
sexual problems	*Aniba rosaeodora* (debility); *Cinnamomum verum* cort. (debility); *Rosa damascena*, *R. centifolia* (debility); *Rosmarinus officinalis* ct. verbenone; *Thymus satureioides* (apathy); *Thymus vulgaris* ct. linalool
shock	*Chamaemelum nobile*
sickness, morning	*Matricaria recutita*; *Melissa officinalis*
sickness, travel	*Mentha x piperita*; *Mentha spicata*; *Ocimum basilicum*
sinusitis	*Abies balsamea*; *Cinnamomum verum* cort.; *Eucalyptus dives*; *Eucalyptus globulus*; *Helichrysum angustifolium*; *Hyssopus officinalis*; *Lavandula angustifolia*; *Melaleuca viridiflora*; *Mentha arvensis*; *Mentha x piperita*; *Myrtus communis*; *Origanum majorana*; *Pinus mugo* var. *pumilio*; *Pinus sylvestris*; *Ravensara aromatica*; *Rosmarinus officinalis* ct. cineole, ct. camphor; *Rosmarinus officinalis* ct. verbenone; *Salvia officinalis*; *Syzygium aromaticum*; *Thymus mastichina*; *Thymus satureioides* (chronic); *Thymus vulgaris* [population]; *Thymus vulgaris* ct. geraniol, ct. linalool; *Thymus vulgaris* ct. thujanol-4; *Thymus vulgaris* ct. thymol, ct. carvacrol
skin, blotchy	*Rosa damascena*, *R. centifolia*
skin, cracked	*Chamaemelum nobile* (nipples); *Pogostemon patchouli*
skin, cysts	*Ormenis mixta*
skin, dry	*Santalum album*

Condition	Essential oils	Condition	Essential oils
skin, greasy/oily	*Cedrus atlantica; Citrus limon; Juniperus communis* ram.; *Laurus nobilis; Myrtus communis*	tachycardia	*Aloysia triphylla; Cananga odorata; Inula graveolens; Lavandula angustifolia; Ocimum basilicum; Origanum majorana; Rosmarinus officinalis* ct. verbenone; *Valeriana officinalis*
skin, infected	*Leptospermum scoparium; Lavandula angustifolia; Melaleuca alternifolia*		
skin, inflamed	*Chamaemelum nobile; Cistus ladaniferus; Mentha x piperita; Ormenis mixta; Pogostemon patchouli*	tendonitis	*Thymus vulgaris* ct. thujanol-4
		throat, sore	*Citrus aurantium* var. *sinensis* per.; *Myrtus communis; Pinus mugo* var. *pumilio; Salvia officinalis; Satureia montana; Thymus vulgaris* ct. geraniol, ct. linalool
skin, irritated	*Angelica archangelica* rad.; *Chamaemelum nobile; Mentha × piperita*		
skin, problems – general	*Aniba rosaeodora; Rosa damascena, R. centifolia*	thrombosis	*Citrus limon; Helichrysum angustifolium*
skin, rash	*Mentha x piperita*	thyroid, imbalance	*Syzygium aromaticum*
skin, regeneration	*Helichrysum angustifolium*		
snake bites	*Cinnamomum verum* cort.	*Tinea pedis* (athlete's foot)	*Lavandula angustifolia; Lavandula x intermedia; Leptospermum scoparium; Pelargonium graveolens; Tagetes minuta*
spasm, bronchial	*Pimpinella anisum; Thymus vulgaris* ct. linalool		
spasm, respiratory	*Origanum majorana*		
		tonsillitis	*Pelargonium graveolens; Pimenta racemosa; Satureia montana; Thymus satureioides; Thymus vulgaris* ct. geraniol, ct. linalool
sprains	*Achillea millefolium; Lavandula angustifolia; Leptospermum scoparium; Myristica fragrans; Pimenta racemosa; Rosa damascena, R. centifolia*		
		toothache	*Cinnamomum verum* fol.; *Melaleuca leucadendron; Mentha arvensis; Myristica fragrans; Origanum majorana; Pimenta dioica; Piper nigrum; Salvia officinalis; Syzygium aromaticum; Zingiber officinale*
sterility	*Salvia officinalis*		
stomatitis	*Cinnamomum verum* fol.; *Laurus nobilis*		
stones	*Achillea millefolium* (kidney); *Aloysia triphylla* (kidney); *Foeniculum vulgare* (urinary); *Hyssopus officinalis* (urinary); *Juniperus communis* fruct. (bladder and kidney); *Juniperus communis* ram. (urinary)		
		tracheitis	*Inula graveolens; Pinus sylvestris*
		tremors	*Salvia officinalis*
		tuberculosis	*Citrus aurantium* var. *amara* flos; *Inula graveolens; Lavandula angustifolia; Pinus mugo* var. *pumilio; Pinus sylvestris; Satureia montana; Syzygium aromaticum; Thymus satureioides; Thymus vulgaris* ct. geraniol, ct. linalool; *Thymus vulgaris* ct. thymol, ct. carvacrol
stress	*Abies balsamea; Aloysia triphylla; Cananga odorata; Cymbopogon citratus; Leptospermum scoparium; Litsea cubeba*		
stretch marks	*Pelargonium graveolens*		
sunburn	*Ormenis mixta*		
sweating (hyperhidrosis)	*Cupressus sempervirens* (feet – odour); *Pinus sylvestris* (feet); *Salvia officinalis* (hands, armpits); *Salvia sclarea*	typhoid fever	*Cinnamomum verum* cort.
		ulcer	*Achillea millefolium* (varicose), *Angelica archangelica* rad. (stomach); *Boswellia carteri;*

Condition	Essential oils
	Cistus ladaniferus; Citrus aurantium var. *amara* per. (mouth); *Citrus limon* (stomach); *Commiphora myrrha* (mouth); *Helichrysum angustifolium; Laurus nobilis* (mouth); *Litsea cubeba* (duodenal); *Matricaria recutita* (duodenal); *Melaleuca viridiflora* (gastric and duodenal); *Mentha arvensis; Ocimum basilicum* (stomach); *Origanum majorana* (gastro/duodenal); *Pelargonium graveolens; Rosa damascena, R. centifolia* (mouth); *Syzygium aromaticum*
urethritis	*Melaleuca viridiflora; Pimenta dioica; Thymus vulgaris* ct. geraniol, ct. linalool; *Thymus vulgaris* ct. thujanol-4
urticaria	*Chamaemelum nobile; Mentha arvensis; Mentha* x *piperita; Vetiveria zizanioides*
vaginitis	*Cinnamomum verum* cort.; *Eucalyptus citriodora; Eucalyptus dives* (leucorrhoea); *Eucalyptus radiata; Inula graveolens; Melaleuca alternifolia; Melaleuca viridiflora* (vulva); *Rosmarinus officinalis* ct. verbenone; *Thymus vulgaris* ct. geraniol, ct. linalool
varicose ulcers	*Lavandula angustifolia; Pelargonium graveolens*
varicose veins	*Citrus aurantium* var. *amara* flos; *Citrus limon; Cupressus sempervirens; Melaleuca alternifolia; Melaleuca leucadendron; Melaleuca viridiflora; Myrtus communis; Nardostachys jatamansi; Pelargonium graveolens; Pogostemon patchouli; Salvia sclarea; Santalum album; Tagetes minuta*
vertigo	*Carum carvi; Citrus aurantium* var. *amara* per.; *Litsea cubeba;*

Condition	Essential oils
	Melissa officinalis; Mentha x *piperita; Ocimum basilicum; Origanum majorana; Pimpinella anisum; Rosmarinus officinalis* ct. cineole, ct. camphor; *Salvia officinalis*
verrucas, warts	*Citrus limon; Thymus vulgaris* ct. geraniol, ct. linalool, *Citrus aurantifolia*
viral attacks, repeated	*Thymus vulgaris* ct. geraniol, ct. linalool
vitiligo	*Citrus bergamia*
vomiting	*Mentha* x *piperita* (nervous); *Mentha spicata* (pregnant); *Pimpinella anisum* (nervous)
warts	*Cinnamomum verum* cort., *Citrus limon*
water retention	*Abies alba* fol.; *Cedrus atlantica; Citrus paradisi*
weak muscles	*Thymus satureioides* (uterus)
whooping cough	*Cupressus sempervirens; Helichrysum angustifolium; Inula graveolens; Origanum majorana; Ravensara aromatica; Rosmarinus officinalis* ct. cineole, ct. camphor
wounds/cuts	*Abies balsamea; Achillea millefolium; Aniba rosaeodora; Boswellia carteri; Cedrus atlantica; Chamaemelum nobile; Cistus ladaniferus; Citrus bergamia; Commiphora myrrha; Eucalyptus dives; Helichrysum angustifolium; Hyssopus officinalis; Lavandula angustifolia; Matricaria recutita* (infected); *Melaleuca viridiflora* (infected); *Mentha spicata; Pelargonium graveolens; Rosa damascena, R. centifolia; Rosmarinus officinalis* ct. cineole, ct. camphor; *Syzygium aromaticum; Tagetes minuta* (scratches, chronic lesions)
wrinkles	*Melaleuca viridiflora; Myrtus communis*

Appendix B

CONTENTS

1. Uterotonic oils which facilitate delivery

The percentage figure given for toxic components is the average or a typical range.

Cymbopogon martinii fol. [palmarosa]: alcohols 80–90% (geraniol).

Foeniculum vulgare var. *dulce* fruct. [sweet fennel]: phenolic ether 70%.

Mentha x *piperita* fol. [peppermint]: ketones 20–30%.

Myristica fragrans sem. [nutmeg]: terpenes 40%, myristicin 2–3%.

Pimenta racemosa fol. [bay]: phenol 90%. Difficult deliveries.

Pimpinella anisum fruct. [aniseed]: phenolic ether 90%.

Syzygium aromaticum flos [clove bud]: phenol 70–80%. Difficult deliveries.

Thymus vulgaris ct. geraniol, herb. [sweet thyme]: alcohol 60–80%.

2. Emmenagogic essential oils

The percentage figure given for toxic components is an average. See also Chapter 10.

Achillea millefolium flos [yarrow, milfoil]: combined ketone and oxide 30%. Not generally considered to be toxic.

Cinnamomum verum cort. [cinnamon]: phenolic ether 60%.

Foeniculum vulgare var. *dulce* fruct. [sweet fennel]: phenolic ether 60%. Also hormonelike, diuretic and lactogenic; facilitates delivery.

Melaleuca viridiflora fol. [niaouli]: oxide 50%. Contains the hormonelike sesquiterpenol viridiflorol.

Myristica fragrans sem. [nutmeg, mace]: phenolic ether 6%. Large dose produces narcosis, delirium and death – see also Appendix A(I). Also facilitates delivery.

Petroselinum sativum fruct. [parsley seed]: phenolic ether 55%.

Pimpinella anisum fruct. [aniseed]: phenolic ether 83%. Also hormonelike; facilitates delivery.

Salvia officinalis fol. [sage]: ketone 35%. Also hormonelike.

3. Disputed emmenagogic oils

Essential oils not yet mentioned, which some books suggest are emmenagogic and need care during pregnancy, although there is no research

to support or reject these suggestions.
See also Chapter 10.

Commiphora molmol (= *C. myrrha*) [myrrh]: hormonelike.

Juniperus communis fruct. [juniper berry]: diuretic.

Juniperus communis ram. [juniper]: no known toxic component.

Levisticum officinale rad. [lovage]: diuretic.

Matricaria recutita flos [German chamomile]: hormonelike.

Melaleuca leucadendron fol. [cajuput]: hormonelike.

Mentha x *piperita* fol. [peppermint]: hormonelike.

Ocimum basilicum fol. [basil].

Origanum majorana fol. [marjoram].

Rosa damascena, *R. centifolia* flos [rose otto]: hormonelike.

Rosmarinus officinalis ct. camphor [rosemary]

Salvia sclarea [clary]: hormonelike

Vetiveria zizanioides rad. [vetiver].

4. Toxic, neurotoxic and abortive oils not used in aromatherapy

This list comprises toxic, neurotoxic and abortive essential oils used by the medical profession in France. Whether or not they are known to aromatherapists, they are not normally used by them. The percentage figure given for toxic components is an average unless otherwise qualified. Common names are given where known.

Acorus calamus [calamus]: phenolic ether 75%.

Agathosma betulina [buchu]: ketone 60%.

Artemisia absinthium [wormwood]: ketone 35%. Also emmenagogic.

Artemisia afra: ketone 40%.

Artemisia annua: ketone 28%. Also hormonelike.

Artemisia arborescens: ketone 55%.

Artemisia herba alba: ketone 65%.

Artemisia pallens [davana]: ketone 40%.

Artemisia vulgaris [mugwort]. Also emmenagogic.

Brassica nigra [mustard]: allylisothiocyanate up to 99%.

Calamintha nepeta [wild basil]: ketone 65%.

Calamintha sylvatica [calamint]: ketone 65%.

Cedrus deodora [Himalayan cedarwood]: ketone 50%.

Chenopodium ambrosioides [wormseed]: oxide 60%.

Chrysanthemum balsamita: ketone 75%.

Cinnamomum camphora lig. [brown camphor, blue camphor]: safrole 60%.

Cochlearia armoracia [horseradish]: allyl isothiocyanate 90%.

Cupressus arizonica [blue cypress]: ketones >50%.

Curcuma longa [turmeric]: ketone 60%.

Foeniculum vulgare var. *amara* [bitter fennel]: anethole 60%.

Geranium macrorrhizum [Bulgarian geranium]: ketone 50%.

Gaultheria procumbens [wintergreen]: methyl salicylate 95%.

Illicium verum [star anise]: phenolic ether 80% – also hormonelike.

Juniperus oxycedrus [oil of cade, juniper tar]. Almost always a wood distillate and not an essential oil.

Juniperus sabina [savin]: podophyllotoxine content in the total extract.

Lantana camara [lantana]: ketone >50%. Also emmenagogic.

Lavandula stoechas [Spanish lavender]: ketone 75%.

Mentha longifolia [mint]: oxide 65%. Also hormonelike.

Myrica gale [bog myrtle]: ketone >50%.

Ocimum canum ct. camphor [dog basil]: ketone 60%.

Ocotea pretiosa [brazilian sassafras]: phenolic ether 85%.

Petroselinum sativum fruct. [parsley seed]: phenol ether (apiole).

Peumus boldus (= *Boldea fragrans*) [boldo]: oxide 30%.

Ruta graveolens [rue]: ketone 65%.

Santolina chamaecyparissus [lavender cotton, santolina]: ketone 35%.

Sassafras officinale [sassafras]: phenolic ether 85%.

Tanacetum vulgare [tansy]: ketone 75%.

Thuja occidentalis [thuja]: ketone 55%.

5. Neurotoxic and/or abortive oils occasionally used in aromatherapy

The following list comprises essential oils that are known and used by aromatherapists and are potentially neurotoxic and/or abortive (if used beyond the accepted maximum dosage).

Achillea millefolium [milfoil, yarrow]: ketone content variable. (See also Appendix A(I).)

Anethum graveolens sem. [dill]: ketone 50%.

Artemisia dracunculus [tarragon]: phenolic ether 65%. Held to be non-toxic by some.

Carum carvi [caraway]: ketone 50%. Usually held to be non-toxic. Also diuretic.

Cedrus atlantica [Atlas cedarwood]: ketone 20%. Considered toxic in France.

Cinnamomum camphora lig. [camphor]: ketone and oxide 70%. Camphor from the wood is usually a triple rectified oil and unsuitable for aromatherapy. The essential oil from the leaves contains mainly alcohols and has no known contraindications.

Eucalyptus dives, E. polybractea [broad leaved peppermint]: ketone 45%.

Hyssopus officinalis [hyssop]: ketone 50%. Not to be used on epileptics. See Appendix A(I).

Mentha pulegium [pennyroyal]: ketone 80%. Also emmenagogic.

Mentha spicata [spearmint]: ketone 60%.

Rosmarinus officinalis ct. verbenone [rosemary]: ketone 30%.

Tagetes glandulifera [taget, French marigold]: ketone 45%. Also phototoxic because of coumarin content; also emmenagogic.

6. Potential skin irritant oils

These phenolic or aldehydic essential oils generally have no special contraindications in pregnancy. The exceptions are *Cinnamomum cassia*, which contains *trans*-cinnamic aldehyde and *Cinnamomum verum* cort., which is also emmenagogic. Sensitivity reactions are three times more likely with oils which are degraded due to photo oxidation (Hausen, Reichling & Harkenthal 1999).

Cinnamomum cassia [cassia]: aldehyde 78-88%; phenol 5–6% typically. Very caustic on the skin.

Cinnamomum verum cort. [cinnamon bark]: aldehyde 40–76%. Neurotoxic.

Cinnamomum verum fol. [cinnamon leaf]: phenol 70–96%.

Cuminum cyminum fruct. [cumin]: aldehyde 20–50%.

Cymbopogon citratus fol. [lemongrass]: aldehyde 60–86%.

Origanum heracleoticum fol. [oregano]: phenol 51–63%.

Origanum vulgare fol. [oregano]: phenol 22–83%.

Syzygium aromaticum caul. [clove stem]: phenol 90–95%.

Syzygium aromaticum flos [clove bud]: phenol 60–90%.

Syzygium aromaticum fol. [clove leaf]: phenol 82–88%.

Thymus serpyllum herb. [wild or creeping thyme]: phenol 20–30%.

Thymus vulgaris ct. phenol herb. [red thyme]: phenol 50–60%.

7. Phototoxic oils

Some essential oils may render the skin hypersensitive to ultraviolet rays, producing the protective tanning reaction. Photosensitizing essential oils may contain up to approximately 2% furanocoumarins, generally found in the expressed citrus oils.

Angelica archangelica fruct., rad. [angelica root, seed].

Carum carvi fruct. [caraway]: low level phototoxicity.

Cinnamomum cassia fol. [cassia]: low level phototoxicity.

Cinnamomum verum cort. [cinnamon bark]: low level phototoxicity.

Citrus aurantifolia per. [lime].

Citrus aurantium var. *amara* per. [bitter orange].

Citrus bergamia per. [bergamot].

Citrus limon per. [lemon].

Cuminum cyminum fruct. [cumin].

Levisticum officinale fol. [lovage].

Aloysia triphylla (= *Lippia citriodora*) [lemon verbena]: low level phototoxicity.

Melissa officinalis fol. [melissa]: low level phototoxicity.

Ruta graveolens herb. [rue]. See also Appendix B.4.

Zingiber officinale rhiz. [ginger]: low level phototoxicity

Generally speaking the maximum concentration of essential oils in a carrier should not exceed 5% (equivalent to 10 drops of essential oils in 10 ml of carrier). Regarding phototoxicity and sensitization, even this quantity can be too much for a few oils, as the following information (extracted from the Code of Practice of IFRA) shows:

Angelica root oil [p]	0.8% max
Bergamot oil [p+s]	0.4% max
Cassia oil [s]	0.2% max

Cinnamon bark oil [s]	0.2% max
Costus root oil [s]	0.0% (i.e. do not use at all)
Cumin oil [p]	0.4% max
Fig leaf oil [p+s]	0.0% (i.e. do not use at all)
Lemon oil [p]	2.0% max
Lime oil [p]	0.7% max
Rue oil [p]	0.8% max
Savin oil	0.0% (i.e. do not use at all)
Verbena oil [p+s]	0.0% (i.e. do not use at all)

[p] = phototoxic, [s] = sensitizer. See also Appendix B.8.

8. Contact–sensitizing oils

Sensitization is a type of allergic reaction which can occur when a substance comes into contact with the body. A few essential oils applied to the skin may cause sensitization, perhaps only after repeated application (the amount used is not significant). The skin reaction appears as redness, irritation and perhaps vesiculation.

Cananga odorata flos [ylang ylang].
Cinnamomum cassia fol. [cassia].
Cinnamomum verum cort. [cinnamon bark oil].
Citrus bergamia per. [bergamot].
Costus speciosus rad. [costus root].
Ficus carica fol. [fig leaf].

Inula helenium rhiz. [elecampane].
Aloysia triphylla (= *Lippia citriodora*) [verbena].
Pimpinella anisum fruct. [aniseed].
Syzygium aromaticum caul. [clove stem].
Syzygium aromaticum flos [clove bud].

Cross-sensitization

With some essential oils an allergic reaction to one oil may lead to sensitivity to other material(s). Little is known of cross-sensitization reactions, but the risk is slight. Four examples are:

- Benzoin resinoid cross colophony (a resin) cross *Mentha* x *piperita* cross Peru balsam (not distilled) cross turpentine (a rectified oil).
- *Laurus nobilis* ram. et fol. cross *Costus speciosus* rad. cross *Cinnamomum verum* cort.
- Cross-reaction may occur with geranium cross lemongrass (citronella) (Keil 1947).
- There may be cross-sensitivity with tea tree oil (*Melaleuca alternifolia*) cross turpentine (Treudler & Richter 2000).

Some individuals show patch test reactions to *Achillea millefolium* [yarrow] and cross-sensitivity between this oil and other Asteraceae has been demonstrated (Duke 1985).

9. General properties of essential oils

See Table B1.

Table B1   General properties of essential oils

Properties

Latin name	Common name	Analgesic, antineuralgic	Antibacterial	Anticoagulant	Antidiabetic	Antiepileptic	Antifungal	Antihistaminic, antiallergic	Antiinfectious	Antiinflammatory	Antiirritant	Antilactogenic	Antimigraine	Antioxidant	Antiparasitic, larvicidal	Antipruritic	Antirheumatic	Antiseptic	Antisclerotic	Antispasmodic	Antisudorific	Antitussive	Antiviral	Arterial regenerative	Cardiotonic	Carminative	Cholagogic, choleretic	Cicatrizant, vulnerary	Circulatory stimulant	Decongestant	Deodorant	Depurative	Detoxicant, depurative	Digestive, stomachic, eupeptic	Diuretic	Emmenagogic
Abies alba (fol.)	European silver fir, white fir	×																×																		
Abies balsamea	Canada balsam		×															×				×						×								
Abies sibirica (fol.)	Siberian pine																			×		×														
Achillea millefolium	yarrow	×								×					×			×		×								×								
Acorus calamus	sweet flag, calamus									×										×						×	×			×				×	×	×
Aloysia triphylla	lemon verbena									×										×										×				×	×	
Anethum graveolens	dill		×						×	×										×						×	×							×		
Angelica archangelica (fruct.)	angelica seed																																			
Angelica archangelica (rad.)	angelica root																																			
Aniba rosaeodora (fol.)	rosewood		×				×		×	×					×			×		×			×					×								
Boswellia carteri (dist.)	frankincense	×							×					×														×								
Cananga odorata	ylang ylang				×													×		×																
Carum carvi (fruct.)	caraway		×					×							×					×						×	×								×	×
Cedrus atlantica (lig.)	Atlas cedarwood		×															×						×												
Chamaemelum nobile (flos)	Roman chamomile									×			×		×					×						×		×						×	×	×
Cinnamomum verum (cort.)	cinnamon bark		×				×		×	×					×			×		×			×			×								×		×
Cinnamomum verum (fol.)	cinnamon leaf		×				×		×	×					×					×			×			×								×		×
Cistus ladaniferus (ram., fol.)	labdanum		×	×					×									×					×					×								
Citrus aurantifolia (C. medica var. acida) (per.)	lime		×						×														×											×		
Citrus aurantium var. amara (flos)	neroli bigarade		×						×	×					×			×																		
Citrus aurantium var. amara (fol.)	petitgrain bigarade		×						×	×										×																
Citrus aurantium var. amara (per.)	orange bigarade			×																							×									
Citrus bergamia (per.)	bergamot		×	×			×		×	×					×			×	×	×			×			×								×		
Citrus limon (per.)	lemon		×	×	×		×											×	×	×			×											×	×	
Citrus paradisi (per.)	grapefruit								×									×		×								×						×	×	
Citrus reticulata (per.)	mandarin					×	×													×							×							×		
Citrus sinensis (per.)	sweet orange		×			×	×											×		×														×		
Commiphora myrrha var. molmol (res. dist.)	myrrh	×																×							×			×								
Coriandrum sativum (fruct.)	coriander	×	×							×										×					×	×								×		
Cuminum cyminum (fruct.)	cumin	×	×							×										×						×								×		?

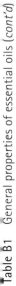

Table B1 General properties of essential oils (cont'd)

Properties

Latin name	Common name	Expectorant	Febrifuge, antipyrectic	Hepatic	Hormonelike	Hypertensor	Hypotensor	Immunostimulant	Insecticidal, parasiticidal	Insect repellent	Lactogenic	Laxative	Lipolytic	Litholytic	Lymph tonic	Mental stimulant	Mucolytic, anticatarrhal	Neurotonic, antidepressive, euphoric	Ophthalmic	Pancreatic stimulant	Phlebotonic	Photosensitizer, phototoxic	Psychoactive	Radioprotective	Reproductive stimulant	Respiratory tonic	Rubefacient	Scalp tonic	Sedative, calming, anxiolytic	Styptic, haemostatic, astringent	Sudorific	Tonic (general), energizing	Uterotonic	Vasodilator	Vermifuge, anthelmintic
Abies alba (fol.)	European silver fir, white fir	×															×											×					×			
Abies balsamea	Canada balsam																																			
Abies sibirica (fol.)	Siberian pine																																			
Achillea millefolium	yarrow	×	×				×							×																		×				
Acorus calamus	sweet flag, calamus																	×																	
Aloysia triphylla	lemon verbena		×		×									×														×	×						
Anethum graveolens	dill						×							×			×																		
Angelica archangelica (fruct.)	angelica seed																																		
Angelica archangelica (rad.)	angelica root																	×																	
Aniba rosaeodora (fol.)	rosewood																																		
Boswellia carteri (dist.)	frankincense	×						×									×	×												×			×		
Cananga odorata	ylang ylang						×								×										×			×	×				×		
Carum carvi (fruct.)	caraway												×				×																		
Cedrus atlantica (lig.)	Atlas cedarwood												×		×													×	×						
Chamaemelum nobile (flos)	Roman chamomile																	×	×										×			×			
Cinnamomum verum (cort.)	cinnamon bark								×																×					×		×			
Cinnamomum verum (fol.)	cinnamon leaf							×										×														×			
Cistus ladaniferus (ram., fol.)	labdanum							×																						×					
Citrus aurantifolia (C. medica var. acida) (per.)	lime		×																																
Citrus aurantium var. amara (flos)	neroli bigarade						×											×											×			×			
Citrus aurantium var. amara (fol.)	petitgrain bigarade																	×							×				×						
Citrus aurantium var. amara (per.)	orange bigarade																					×							×						
Citrus bergamia (per.)	bergamot																	×				×							×						
Citrus limon (per.)	lemon	×					×							×							×								×			×			
Citrus paradisi (per.)	grapefruit																				×								×			×			
Citrus reticulata (per.)	mandarin		×																	×									×						
Citrus sinensis (per.)	sweet orange																			×									×			×			
Commiphora myrrha var. molmol (res. dist.)	myrrh	×																												×		×			
Coriandrum sativum (fruct.)	coriander																	×					×									×			
Cuminum cyminum (fruct.)	cumin																												×			×			

Table B1   General properties of essential oils (*cont'd*)

Latin name	Common name	Analgesic, antineuralgic	Antibacterial	Anticoagulant	Antidiabetic	Antiepileptic	Antifungal	Antihistaminic, antiallergic	Antiinfectious	Antiinflammatory	Antiirritant	Antilactogenic	Antimigraine	Antioxidant	Antiparasitic, larvicidal	Antipruritic	Antirheumatic	Antiseptic	Antisclerotic	Antispasmodic	Antisudorific	Antitussive	Antiviral	Arterial regenerative	Cardiotonic	Carminative	Cholagogic, choleretic	Cicatrizant, vulnerary	Circulatory stimulant	Decongestant	Deodorant	Depurative	Detoxicant, depurative	Digestive, stomachic, eupeptic	Diuretic	Emmenagogic
Cupressus sempervirens (fol.)	cypress		×																	×	×	×									×				×	
Cymbopogon citratus, C. flexuosus	lemongrass	×	×				×		×	×											×	×												×		
Cymbopogon nardus and C. winterianus	citronella	×	×				×			×				×				×		×																
Elettaria cardamomum (fruct.)	cardamom	×								×								×		×						×								×	×	
Eucalyptus citriodora (fol.)	lemon scented gum	×	×				×		×	×										×														×		
Eucalyptus dives (fol.)	broad leaved peppermint	×			×		×		×							×						×													×	
Eucalyptus globulus (fol.)	Tasmanian blue gum	×	×				×		×	×			×									×						×		×						
Eucalyptus radiata (fol.)	narrow leaved peppermint								×	×							×					×														
Eucalyptus smithii (fol.)	gully gum, white iron bark	×															×		×			×								×				×		
Eucalyptus staigeriana	lemon scented ironbark								×	×																										
Foeniculum vulgare var. dulca (fruct.)	sweet fennel	×	×				×		×	×							×		×					×	×	×	×		×	×				×	×	×
Helichrysum angustifolium (flos)	everlasting		×	×	×		×	×	×	×												×		×		×		×						×		
Hyssopus officinalis (flos, fol.)	hyssop		×				×		×	×											×	×					×		×					×	×	×
Illicium verum	star anise		×				×																		×										×	×
Inula graveolens, I. helenium (flos, fol.)	elecampane								×	×										×		×	×		×									×		
Juniperus communis (fruct.)	juniper berry	×		×														×		×															×	
Juniperus communis (ram.)	juniper twig	×								×								×																	×	
Laurus nobilis	bay leaf	×	×						×						×			×		×			×											×		
Lavandula angustifolia (flos)	lavender	×	×				×		×	×			×							×					×	×		×								
Lavandula x intermedia "Super" (flos)	lavandin Super						×						×										×		×	×										
Leptospermum scoparium	manuka	×	×				×		×	×																								×		
Litsea cubeba (fruct.)	may chang						×			×								×		×			×											×		
Matricaria recutita (flos)	German chamomile							×		×																										×
Melaleuca alternifolia (fol.)	tea tree	×	×				×		×	×					×			×		×			×					×		×		×	×			
Melaleuca leucadendron (fol.)	cajuput	×					×		×	×								×		×												×	×			
Melaleuca viridiflora (fol.)	niaouli	×							×		×				×	×	×	×					×							×						
Melissa officinalis (fol.)	melissa		×						×		×	×								×			×				×							×		
Mentha x piperita (fol.)	peppermint	×	×				×		×	×		×								×			×			×	×			×				×		
Mentha spicata	spearmint						×					×						×		×						×	×	×	×					×		
Myristica fragrans (sem.)	nutmeg	×	×						×									×																×	×	×

Table B1 General properties of essential oils (*cont'd*)

Properties

Latin name	Common name	Vermifuge, anthelmintic	Vasodilator	Uterotonic	Tonic (general), energizing	Sudorific	Styptic, haemostatic, astringent	Sedative, calming, anxiolytic	Scalp tonic	Rubefacient	Respiratory tonic	Reproductive stimulant	Radioprotective	Psychoactive	Photosensitizer, phototoxic	Phlebotonic	Pancreatic stimulant	Ophthalmic	Neurotonic, antidepressive, euphoric	Mucolytic, anticatarrhal	Mental stimulant	Lymph tonic	Litholytic	Lipolytic	Laxative	Lactogenic	Insect repellent	Insecticidal, parasiticidal	Immunostimulant	Hypotensor	Hypertensor	Hormonelike	Hepatic	Febrifuge, antipyrectic	Expectorant
Cupressus sempervirens (fol.)	cypress						×	×								×			×													×			
Cymbopogon citratus, C. flexuosus	lemongrass		×		×	×		×																			×					×		×	
Cymbopogon nardus and C. winterianus	citronella	×			×																						×							×	
Elettaria cardamomum (fruct.)	cardamom																																		×
Eucalyptus citriodora (fol.)	lemon scented gum							×																											
Eucalyptus dives (fol.)	broad leaved peppermint																			×				×			×								×
Eucalyptus globulus (fol.)	Tasmanian blue gum							×												×															×
Eucalyptus radiata (fol.)	narrow leaved peppermint									×										×															×
Eucalyptus smithii (fol.)	gully gum, white iron bark																			×															×
Eucalyptus staigeriana	lemon scented ironbark																						×												
Foeniculum vulgare var. dulca (fruct.)	sweet fennel										×														×	×						×			
Helichrysum angustifolium (flos)	everlasting																		×	×													×		
Hyssopus officinalis (flos, fol.)	hyssop	×			×	×	×	×			×					×			×	×			×	×							×				×
Illicium verum	star anise	×			×																											×			×
Inula graveolens, I. helenium (flos, fol.)	elecampane																			×															×
Juniperus communis (fruct.)	juniper berry				×														×	×			×												
Juniperus communis (ram.)	juniper twig																		×	×			×												×
Laurus nobilis	bay leaf																			×										×					×
Lavandula angustifolia (flos)	lavender				×			×											×											×					
Lavandula x intermedia 'Super' (flos)	lavandin Super				×			×											×	×															×
Leptospermum scoparium	manuka				×		×				×																		×						
Litsea cubeba (fruct.)	may chang							×																				×					×		
Matricaria recutita (flos)	German chamomile																												×			×	×		
Melaleuca alternifolia (fol.)	tea tree																												×				×		×
Melaleuca leucadendron (fol.)	cajuput					×							×			×			×	×								×	×				×		×
Melaleuca viridiflora (fol.)	niaouli												×			×				×			×						×				×		×
Melissa officinalis (fol.)	melissa				×	×		×					×			×			×	×										×			×		×
Mentha x piperita (fol.)	peppermint		×		×														×	×													×		×
Mentha spicata	spearmint	×		×	×	×		×				×							×	×													×		×
Myristica fragrans (sem.)	nutmeg	×	×	×	×							×		×					×	×															×

Table B1 General properties of essential oils (cont'd)

Properties

Latin name	Common name	Analgesic, antineuralgic	Antibacterial	Anticoagulant	Antidiabetic	Antiepileptic	Antifungal	Antihistaminic, antiallergic	Antiinfectious	Antiinflammatory	Antiirritant	Antilactogenic	Antimigraine	Antioxidant	Antiparasitic, larvicidal	Antipruritic	Antirheumatic	Antiseptic	Antisclerotic	Antispasmodic	Antisudorific	Antitussive	Antiviral	Arterial regenerative	Cardiotonic	Carminative	Cholagogic, choleretic	Cicatrizant, vulnerary	Circulatory stimulant	Decongestant	Deodorant	Depurative	Detoxicant, depurative	Digestive, stomachic, eupepti	Diuretic	Emmenagogic
Myrtus communis	myrtle, red and orange																	×												×						
Nardostachys jatamansi (rad.)	spikenard					×	×			×															×											
Nepeta cataria var. citriodora (flos, fol.)	catnep					×	×			×																								×		
Ocimum basilicum (fol.)	basil	×	×			×	×		×	×			×					×		×			×		×	×										
Origanum heracleoticum, O. vulgare (herb.)	green oregano	×	×						×	×					×					×			×													
Origanum majorana (fol.)	sweet marjoram	×	×			×			×	×			×					×		×														×	×	
Ormenis mixta, O. multicaulis (flos)	Moroccan chamomile		×							×																		×		×						
Pelargonium graveolens (fol.)	geranium	×	×		×		×		×	×					×			×		×																
Picea nigra, P. mariana	black spruce		×				×		×	×					×			×		×																
Pimenta dioica	allspice	×	×				×											×								×										
Pimenta racemosa (fruct. fol.)	West Indian bay	×	×															×					×			×										×
Pimpinella anisum (fruct.)	aniseed	×											×							×			×		×	×								×	×	×
Pinus mugo var. pumilio	dwarf pine																													×					×	
Pinus sylvestris (fol.)	Scots pine	×	×		×																×									×						
Piper nigrum (fruct)	black pepper	×	×															×																×		
Pogostemon patchouli (fol.)	patchouli		×						×	×								×										×		×				×		
Ravensara aromatica (fol.)	ravensara		×				×		×	×													×					×					×			
Rosa centifolia, R. damascena (flos)	rose otto		×						×	×												×						×					×			
Rosmarinus officinalis ct. cineole, ct. camphor	rosemary	×	×				×		×	×				×						×		×	×		×	×	×	×					×	×	×	×
Rosmarinus officinalis ct. verbenone	rosemary verbenone		×						×					×						×		×			×	×	×	×					×	×		
Ruta graveolens	rue											×			×					×																
Salvia officinalis (fol.)	sage, Dalmatian sage	×	×				×		×	×										×	×		×				×	×	×					×	×	×
Salvia sclarea (flos, fol.)	clary		×				×		×											×	×									×	×					
Santalum album (lig.)	sandalwood		×				×		×																×		×			×			×		×	
Satureia hortensis (fol.)	summer or garden savory	×	×				×		×									×		×			×		×	×			×					×		
Satureia montana (fol.)	winter or mountain savory	×	×				×		×						×					×			×		×	×		×						×		
Syzygium aromaticum (flos)	clove bud	×	×				×		×	×								×		×			×			×		×						×		×
Tagetes glandulifera, T. minuta (flos)	French marigold														×													×	×						×	×
Thymus mastichina (herb.)	Spanish marjoram		×				×		×	×																										
Thymus satureioides	Moroccan thyme	×	×						×	×																										

Table B1 General properties of essential oils (cont'd)

Properties

Latin name	Common name	Expectorant	Febrifuge, antipyrectic	Hepatic	Hormonelike	Hypertensor	Hypotensor	Immunostimulant	Insecticidal, parasiticidal	Insect repellent	Lactogenic	Laxative	Lipolytic	Litholytic	Lymph tonic	Mental stimulant	Mucolytic, anticatarrhal	Neurotonic, antidepressive, euphoric	Ophthalmic	Pancreatic stimulant	Phlebotonic	Photosensitizer, phototoxic	Psychoactive	Radioprotective	Reproductive stimulant	Respiratory tonic	Rubefacient	Scalp tonic	Sedative, calming, anxiolytic	Styptic, haemostatic, astringent	Sudorific	Tonic (general), energizing	Uterotonic	Vasodilator	Vermifuge, anthelmintic
Myrtus communis	myrtle, red and orange	×			×												×												×	×					
Nardostachys jatamansi (rad.)	spikenard																												×						
Nepeta cataria var. citriodora (flos, fol.)	catnep																												×						
Ocimum basilicum (fol.)	basil			×		×			×					×				×			×								×						×
Origanum heracleoticum, O. vulgare (herb.)	green oregano			×				×										×														×			
Origanum majorana (fol.)	sweet marjoram	×			×		×											×								×			×			×		×	
Ormenis mixta, O. multicaulis (flos)	Moroccan chamomile			×				×																	×										
Pelargonium graveolens (fol.)	geranium				×			×		×					×			×			×								×	×					
Picea nigra, P. mariana	black spruce																																		
Pimenta dioica	allspice					×												×															×		
Pimenta racemosa (fruct. fol.)	West Indian bay																								×	×		×			×	×			
Pimpinella anisum (fruct.)	aniseed				×						×												×		×	×			×				×		
Pinus mugo var. pumilio	dwarf pine													×													×								
Pinus sylvestris (fol.)	Scots pine	×				×								×				×									×								
Piper nigrum (fruct.)	black pepper	×	×														×								×										
Pogostemon patchouli (fol.)	patchouli		×					×		×								×			×		×		×				×						
Ravensara aromatica (fol.)	ravensara	×															×	×																	
Rosa centifolia, R. damascena (flos)	rose otto																	×							×					×					
Rosmarinus officinalis ct. cineole, ct. camphor	rosemary												×	×		×	×	×							×										
Rosmarinus officinalis ct. verbenone	rosemary verbenone	×		×	×											×	×	×							×										
Ruta graveolens	rue															×	×	×																	
Salvia officinalis (fol.)	sage, Dalmation sage	×			×	×										×	×	×												×					
Salvia sclarea (flos, fol.)	clary				×												×	×			×							×							
Santalum album (lig.)	sandalwood																				×								×						
Satureia hortensis (fol.)	summer or garden savory	×				×		×								×		×							×							×			
Satureia montana (fol.)	winter or mountain savory	×				×		×								×		×							×							×			
Syzygium aromaticum (flos)	clove bud					×										×	×	×							×					×					
Tagetes glandulifera, T. minuta (flos)	French marigold																					×							×						×
Thymus mastichina (herb.)	Spanish marjoram																	×							×								×		
Thymus satureioides	Moroccan thyme							×										×														×	×		×

Table B1   General properties of essential oils (cont'd)

Properties

Latin name	Common name	Analgesic, antineuralgic	Antibacterial	Anticoagulant	Antidiabetic	Antiepileptic	Antifungal	Antihistaminic, antiallergic	Antiinfectious	Antiinflammatory	Antiirritant	Antilactogenic	Antimigraine	Antioxidant	Antiparasitic, larvicidal	Antipruritic	Antirheumatic	Antiseptic	Antisclerotic	Antispasmodic	Antisudorific	Antitussive	Antiviral	Arterial regenerative	Cardiotonic	Carminative	Cholagogic, choleretic	Cicatrizant, vulnerary	Circulatory stimulant	Decongestant	Deodorant	Depurative	Detoxicant, depurative	Digestive, stomachic, eupeptic	Diuretic	Emmenagogic
Thymus vulgaris 'Population'	thyme population		×				×							×	×			×		×						×		×	×					×	×	
Thymus vulgaris ct. geraniol (herb.)	sweet thyme		×				×			×								×					×		×		×									
Thymus vulgaris ct. linalool (herb.)	sweet thyme		×				×		×	×								×		×			×												×	
Thymus vulgaris ct. thujanol-4 (herb.)	thujanol thyme		×						×	×										×			×													
Thymus vulgaris ct. thymol, ct. carvacrol (herb.)	thyme		×				×								×													×						×	×	×
Valeriana officinalis	valerian									×										×																
Valeriana wallichi	Indian valerian								×																											
Vetiveria zizanioides (rad.)	vetiver																											×	×							×
Zingiber cassumunar	phrai, plai									×				×															×							
Zingiber officinale (rhiz.)	ginger	×																								×								×		

fol(ium) = leaf
flos = flower
caul(is) = stem
cort(ex) = bark
sem(en) = seed
rad(ix) = root
ram(unculus) = twig
per(icardum) = peel

Table B1   General properties of essential oils (*cont'd*)

Properties

Latin name	Common name	Expectorant	Febrifuge, antipyretic	Hepatic	Hormonelike	Hypertensor	Hypotensor	Immunostimulant	Insecticidal, parasiticidal	Insect repellent	Lactogenic	Laxative	Lipolytic	Litholytic	Lymph tonic	Mental stimulant	Mucolytic, anticatarrhal	Neurotonic, antidepressive, euphoric	Ophthalmic	Pancreatic stimulant	Phlebotonic	Photosensitizer, phototoxic	Psychoactive	Radioprotective	Reproductive stimulant	Respiratory tonic	Rubefacient	Scalp tonic	Sedative, calming, anxiolytic	Styptic, haemostatic, astringent	Sudorific	Tonic (general), energizing	Uterotonic	Vasodilator	Vermifuge, anthelmintic
Thymus vulgaris 'Population'	thyme population	×				×			×							×		×										×			×	×			×
Thymus vulgaris ct. geraniol (herb.)	sweet thyme																	×															×		
Thymus vulgaris ct. linalool (herb.)	sweet thyme				×			×										×															×		×
Thymus vulgaris ct. thujanol-4 (herb.)	thujanol thyme			×	×			×									×	×																	
Thymus vulgaris ct. thymol, ct. carvacrol (herb.)	thyme	×				×										×	×	×																	×
Valeriana officinalis	valerian		×																				?						×						×
Valeriana wallichii	Indian valerian																	×											×						
Vetiveria zizanioides (rad.)	vetiver			×				×													×														
Zingiber cassumunar	phrai, plai	×																																	
Zingiber officinale (rhiz)	ginger															×	×								?							×			

fol(ium) = leaf
flos = flower
caul(is) = stem
cort(ex) = bark
sem(en) = seed
rad(ix) = root
ram(unculus) = twig
per(icardum) = peel

Appendix C
Occupational Health and Safety

Although used only in very small amounts by aromatherapists to utilize their healing properties, essential oils are complex chemical compounds. When used knowledgeably and with due caution, they do not present a threat to health, although there are can be certain hazards – usually associated with incorrect use. This section considers the difference between 'hazard' and 'risk', and goes on to discuss the workplace regulatory requirements which must be observed when essential oils are being used.

A hazard is anything that has the potential to cause harm. Essential oils have the potential to cause harm and could thus be labelled as hazardous, because they:

- are flammable
- should be kept away from the eyes
- may be irritants
- may be sensitizers
- should be avoided or used with caution in certain circumstances
- should not, in general, be taken internally without specific training.

However, many substances have the potential to cause harm if used in excess – or incorrectly: although not named as hazardous, a surfeit of oranges or the ingestion of under ripe or 'green' potatoes can cause health problems; too much alcohol can impair the liver; too many aspirins can damage the lining of the stomach. None of these are labelled as hazardous – it is simply a question of correct, controlled and informed use; their overuse is almost always by personal choice. The use of essential oils may be regarded in the same light – sensible use will normally avoid problems.

If something is hazardous it does not necessarily mean a problem exists, but rather that caution is necessary – especially for the uninformed. *The likelihood that a hazard will lead to actual harm is the risk of it happening.* So, in order to obtain a clear picture of what could go wrong and how serious an accident could be, an assessment of risk must be carried out. The Management of Health and Safety at Work regulations (HMSO 1992) require employers to carry out such assessments, so that all workplace hazards can be identified, along with associated risks and actions necessary to eliminate or reduce risks of accidents and injuries.

Essential oil risk

Essential oils are complicated chemicals; although natural, they should nevertheless be a part of workplace risk assessment. Having said that, if they are used in correct amounts, with knowledge and all known precautions adhered to, then they are relatively safe. However, until training in aromatherapy is of a consistently high standard at every training school, there are several oils which may be hazardous and are therefore best used with caution in certain conditions, e.g. epilepsy and pregnancy. The latter is a moot point as any caution required is mainly in the first trimester, becoming less necessary as the pregnancy progresses. This means that the most important time to be heedful could be before the person concerned even knows she is pregnant! Nevertheless, it is important to be seen to be judicious, especially as many people without qualifications use essential oils without considering any risk that may be involved.

The molecular make-up of chemicals influences local or systemic toxicological effects and their elimination from the body. Some are known to be harmless and others harmful to varying degrees. For the vast majority there remains ambiguity over their effects and some are still a complete mystery (Fowler & Wall 1997).

Risk assessment (COSHH)

If a material has the potential to harm a person it is considered to be a hazardous substance and the Control of Substances Hazardous to Health (COSHH) regulations of 1999 (Health and Safety Commission 1999) apply. COSHH is a risk assessment process – the regulations do not set out specific requirements for specific circumstances; their aim is rather to assess, monitor and reduce the presence of possibly hazardous substances to the lowest possible level of risk, thereby preventing anyone who may come into contact with the materials from being harmed in any way. These demands are met by carrying out a specific risk assessment process, requiring employers to identify and control exposure to hazardous substances to prevent injury or ill-health to their employees and others.

Seven measures are specified under this regulation – the only one which may affect certain essential oils being chemicals or preparations classified as hazardous to health under CHIP 3 (Chemicals [Hazard Information and Packaging for supply] – see Box C.1). COSHH requires that:

- any hazardous substances in the workplace are identified
- any possible risks to health are considered
- a decision on precautions needed is made (prevention and adequate control)
- employees are properly informed, trained and supervised.

The legal obligation is that the assessment be suitable and sufficient – simpler and lower risk situations will require less consideration than will more serious and complex risks. The aim is to reach reliable conclusions based on informed judgement.

For most single essential oils, their presentation, the amount used and the frequency of use,

together with the correct packaging (e.g. integral drop dispensers), means that any possible harmful effects are minimized. A simple assessment for each essential oil in use, drawing attention to this, will meet the requirements of COSHH. The assessment must include not only the effects of essential oils on patients and clients but also on anyone else exposed to them, where cognitive function could be affected, thus altering the person's behaviour and reaction time, resulting in suppression of the cerebral inhibiting systems (Boyle 1993); the relaxation effects are now well established (Birchall 1990, Buchbauer et al 1991, Hardy 1991, Karamat et al 1992) so there may be the masking of warning signals, perhaps due to smell habituation or insensitivity to slow changes (Boyle 1987).

Assessment is not a one-off exercise; the regulations demand the situation is reviewed on a regular basis, the Approved Code of Practice (HSE 1997a) recommending an interval of no longer than 5 years. However, the assessment must be reviewed if anything changes – for example, if a new essential oil is in use.

Safety data sheets

Suppliers and manufacturers of essential oils to aromatherapists are required to provide safety data sheets – for each batch of the same botanically specified oil, identify hazards associated with the chemicals and package them safely. The regulations apply only to the supply and storage of bulk quantities of material – retailers do not have to provide a safety data sheet for domestic use of essential oils, but sufficient information must be given on the label to make recipients aware of any health and safety hazards. However, if a therapist intends to use the oils at work, a data sheet can be requested.

Although it is not certain if essential oils as used in aromatherapy come under the CHIP 3 hazard assessment regulations, the CHIP 3 safety data sheets can be an important source of the information needed when completing COSHH risk assessments. However, a safety data sheet alone is not sufficient as a COSHH assessment, and very few essential oils have been categorized by CHIP 3.

CHIP 3 does not specify exactly what should go into a safety data sheet; it gives headings under

---

Box C.1   CHIP 3 (Chemicals [Hazard Information and Packaging for supply])

Hazard assessment (CHIP)

As it is not certain that essential oils as used by aromatherapists come under CHIP 3, this is included for information only.

CHIP is a classification system that applies to the supply of chemicals – and new CHIP 3 regulations came into force in 2002.

CHIP 3 is concerned with the supply of chemicals (including essential oils) which may be hazardous, interpreting the word 'supply' as being anything 'to be sold, offered for sale, given as samples, importing or transferring chemicals from one person to the other'. The aim is to ensure that people supplied with chemicals receive the information needed to protect themselves, others and the environment. In the regulations, CHIP 3 defines a chemical as a single substance or preparation (mixture of substances) and as essential oils are not single substances, they are classified under 'preparations'.

The 2002 CHIP 3 implements four new EC directives, introducing a number of new features, including the fact that:

■ Preparations now have to be classified and labelled in relation to their environmental effects.
■ A warning must appear on labels of preparations which contain small quantities of sensitizing substances.
■ Safety data sheets must be available on request for preparations not classified as dangerous.

In summary, the basic requirement of CHIP 3 is for suppliers to identify whether the chemical they supply is hazardous – and label it accordingly. Essential oils used in an aromatherapy treatment where a full consultation has taken place do not come under CHIP regulations – neither do mixtures of essential oils (these are regulated by the Cosmetic Products Safety Regulations). However, a *single* essential oil could be regarded as subject to CHIP 3, e.g. tea tree has been classified in such a way (HSE 1997b) that the CHIP 3 regulations apply. As with COSHH (below), the CHIP 3 regulations are designed to protect people from the ill effects of chemicals.

---

which information has to be provided and says that this information has to be sufficient. In this context 'sufficient' means adopting a common-sense approach and giving enough information to ensure that both people at work and the environment can be properly protected.

Accordingly, any safety data sheet supplied should address the following issues:

■ Name and location of supplier.
■ Product identification.
■ Composition/ingredients.
■ First aid measures.
■ Fire fighting measures.
■ Accidental release and disposal precautions.
■ Handling and storage.
■ Health hazards.
■ Physical and chemical properties.
■ Other appropriate information.

Suppliers are responsible for the accuracy of the safety data sheet, and any doubts or worries should be addressed to them. A particular concern with essential oils is the variability in quality as there are no regulations about this (Trevelyan 1993). Adulteration and mislabelling are not uncommon, and clearly this will influence the accuracy of any related data sheets. This is yet another reason for ensuring that only genuine essential oils are used therapeutically; in other words, as they come from the still, with nothing added and nothing taken away.

DISPENSING AND STORAGE PRECAUTIONS

Labelling

As essential oils are freely available in most countries, the supplier needs to ensure that they are properly labelled, with proper cautions regarding children, eyes, pregnancy and skin. It is a legal requirement that essential oil containers carry appropriate printed cautions, although these vary in different countries. In France the sale of a few oils has been restricted since 1986 to the pharmacies; they include: mugwort, wormwood, cedarwood, hyssop, sage, tansy and thuja (botanical names not given): other governments also have quite strict laws (see Aromatherapy worldwide Ch. 17). Generally, self-regulation by an industry is to be preferred to governmental regulation and accordingly any oil which may be harmful when used injudiciously should not be offered for sale to anyone lacking adequate aromatherapy training. This would still leave a wide range of safe oils accessible for use by the general public.

Flammability

Care should be exercised when handling essential oils because they are volatile and are highly inflammable. Flash points for essential oils (Table 3.3) range typically between 32°C for frankincense and about 110°C for Atlas cedarwood, though the majority are in the range 43–70°C. They should be stored carefully in a cool, dark area, and working areas for mixing should contain no naked flame; static electricity should be guarded against. Smoking should not be permitted and the area should be well ventilated. It may be necessary to warn the building insurer if oils are to be stocked in bulk.

COST B4

European Cooperation in the field of Science and Technology (COST) aims to coordinate national research projects at a European level.

The European Research Action COST B4 was launched in 1993, in order to harmonize the research into the therapeutic significance of unconventional medicine and the associated cultural, psychological, legislative and economic aspects; this to be used as a basis for evaluating its possible usefulness or risks in public health. By 1995 14 countries had signed the Memorandum of Understanding, in which the signatory countries agree to cooperate in research into the above aspects.

Following its first meeting in October 1993, the Management Committee of the Action prepared a brochure of their current research projects including details of those involved. This was circulated in summer 1994 and has been updated annually during the 5-year programme, with the final report being due in July 1999. Several studies involving the use of aromatherapy appear in the COST B4 responses to the questionnaire; these included projects on dementia, Parkinson's disease (see Ch. 9), learning disabilities and cancer.

COST B4 includes projects from the USA and Israel, although not linked to the listed research centres in these two countries, but 'any of their institutes interested in this cooperation can apply to participate' (Riek 1994). The advantage of this approach lies in a quick and easy information exchange between the scientists involved, and in the distribution of tasks for the research work involved in the action.

The first COST B4 workshop took place in 1994, with delegates from 19 countries. The presentations included an overview of research currently taking place in the COST countries, which was followed by others covering several different modes of research. Conditions such as pain and complementary therapies such as homoeopathy were covered, plus practical considerations such as the interface between orthodox and complementary medicine and research issues such as methodology.

Delegates reported that the structure of the workshop and of the seminars in particular, was useful for information exchange and for networking. It is hoped that more specialized working groups will tackle specific research issues in considerably greater depth (Vickers 1995).

A future aim is to make a bridge between conventional and unconventional medicines, creating an open forum for official medicine of the various unconventional approaches to disease, illness and care.

SUMMARY

This Appendix has shown the great steps that have been taken towards self-regulation of aromatherapy in the UK and the current legislation situation directed by the European Union. It has also shown how policy and practice guidelines can be put into practice and it is to be hoped that more health provision agencies will follow the lead already made in the UK where appropriate.

It is to be hoped that aromatherapists will find the safety regulations for essential oils in the workplace (COSHH and CHIP 3) and the European research project started in 1993 (COST B4) both interesting and useful.

Appendix D
Essential oil: Definition for aromatherapeutic purposes

Essential oils

There are only two plant extracts which should be given this name for aromatherapy purposes.

1. Essential oils: these are plant extracts which have been achieved by steam distillation of plant material from a single botanical source; nothing is involved in this process save water, heat and the plant material. The essential oil is separated from the condensed steam and nothing is added and nothing is taken away.

2. Expressed oils: these are the product of citrus fruits, and they are achieved by simple pressing (expression) of the citrus peel, without heat or aid of solvents. Nothing is added and nothing is taken away.

Care is needed in the way essential oils are sold to protect both the lay public and aromatherapists. The oils for therapeutic use must be whole and unadulterated, accurately identified and labelled, and must have been correctly stored.

N.B. Not all plants yield an essential oil and some yield so little that the oil would be too expensive; oils such as hyacinth, lilac, honeysuckle and jasmine do not exist in a distilled form; their fragrance is extracted by other means and it is incorrect for anyone to name extracts from these plants as essential oils in the context of aromatherapeutic use.

Aromatherapy oils

This term is widely used in the marketplace, but is a vague, almost meaningless term, which does not adequately describe the product. Products labelled thus usually consist of a 2% maximum dilution of essential oil(s) in a fixed oil. Often these inexpensive products are sold in small bottles having an integral dropper, which is misleading as droppers are not necessary for diluted oils and their presence can give the impression (sometimes intentional) that they are essential oils – they are often sold at the pure essential oil price, thus yielding an excessive profit. Oils sold under this heading usually contain standardized oils of low quality, more suited to industries other than complementary medicine.

Other ways of extracting plant components follow; none should be classed as essential oils for aromatherapy purposes.

Absolutes

These are aromatic liquids extracted from the plant material using solvents such as hexane, butane, etc., which is then followed by alcohol extraction. It is a complex process, yielding a liquid substance called an absolute, which is totally soluble in alcohol and important in the perfume industry.

Macerated oils

Macerated oils are made by putting plant material into a fixed vegetable oil, when those plant molecules soluble in the oil are taken up by the vegetable oil used. Examples are calendula and hypericum (St John's wort). These should not be sold in small bottles as essential oils.

Ignorance is bliss?

Much of the misnaming of oils for aromatherapy comes through ignorance on the part of the suppliers. Occasionally a supplier sells an expensive fixed oil, such as evening primrose, as an essential oil, putting it into a small bottle with an integral dropper and within an essential oil price range. Unfortunately, aromatherapy is a popular bandwagon to jump on, and the very word aromatherapy has selling power, which is used by the unscrupulous, sometimes at the expense of the unwary honest dealer. Standardized oils are cheap and easy to obtain, unlike the genuine essential oils necessary for aromatherapy.

References to Appendices

Abdel Waheb S M A, Aboutabl E A, El-Zalabani S M, Fouad H A, De Pooter H L, El-Fallaha B 1987 The essential oil of olibanum. Planta Medica 53(4): 382–384

Abdullin K K 1962 Bactericidal effects of essential oils. Uchenye Zapiski Kazarskogo Veterinarnago Instituta 84: 75 In: Chemical Abstracts 1964 60: 11843b

Abraham M et al 1979 Inhibiting effects of jasmine flowers on lactation. Indian Journal of Medicine Research 69: 88–92

Abrissart J-L 1997 Aromathérapie essentielle. Trédaniel, Paris

Achterrath-Tuckerman U, Kunde R, Flaskamp O, Theimer I, Theimer K 1980 Pharmacological investigations with compounds of chamomile. V. Investigations on the spasmolytic effect of compounds of chamomile. Planta Medica 39: 38–50

Adam K, Sivropoulou A, Kokkini S, Lanaras T, Arsenakis M 1998 Antifungal activities of *Origanum vulgare* subsp. *hirtum*, *Mentha spicata*, *Lavandula angustifolia* and *Salvia fructicosa* essential oils against human pathogenic fungi. Journal of Agricultural Food Chemistry 46: 1739–1745

Adler V E, Jacobson M 1982 Journal of Environmental Science and Health A17: 667

Åkesson H O, Wålinder J 1965 Nutmeg intoxication. Lancet i: 1271

Aktug S E, Karapinar M 1986 Sensitivity of some common food-poisoning bacteria to thyme, mint and bay leaves. International Journal Food Microbiology 3: 349–354

Albert-Puleo M 1980 Fennel and anise as estrogenic agents. Journal of Ethnopharmacology 2: 337–344

Alexandrovich I, Rakovitskaya O, Kolmo E, Siderova T, Shushunov S 2003 The effect of fennel (*Foeniculum vulgare*) seed oil emulsion in infantile colic: a randomised, placebo controlled study. Alternative Therapies 9(4): 58–61

Al-Hader A A, Hasan Z A, Aqel M B 1994 Hyperglycemic and insulin release inhibitory effects of *Rosmarinus officinalis*. Journal of Ethnopharmacology 43: 217–221

Alimkhodzhaeva N Z, Khazanovich R L 1972 Mater. In: Chemical Abstracts 1975 82: 167491r

Al-Zuhair H, El-Sayeh B, Ameen H A, Al-Shoora H 1996 Pharmacological studies of cardamom oil in animals. Lipids 30(12): 1105–1110

Anderson J W 1923 Geranium dermatitis. Archives of Dermatology and Syphilology 7: 510

Anon 1974 Federal Register 39(185): 34215

Anon 1977 Federal Register 42(146): 38613

Anon 1994 Journal of Family Practice June 3: 6

Ansari M A, Vasudevan P, Tandon M, Razdan R K 2000 Larvicidal and mosquito repellent action of peppermint (*Mentha piperita*) oil. Bioresource Technology 71: 267–271

Anthony A et al 1987 Metabolism of estragole in rat and mouse and influence of dose size on excretion of the proximate carcinogen 1-hydroxyestragole. Food and Chemical Toxicology 25: 799–806

Appaiah K M, Nag U C, Kapur O P, Nagaraja K V 1983 Antifungal activity of orange and lime oils. Journal of Food Science Technology 20(5): 250–252

Arctander S 1960 Perfume and flavor materials of natural origin. Self published, Elizabeth, New Jersey

Aruna K, Sivaramakrishnan V M 1996 Anticarcinogenic effects of the essential oils from cumin, poppy and basil. Phytotherapy Research 10(7): 577–580

Asre S 1994 Chemical composition and antimicrobial activity of some essential oils. MSc Thesis, Macquarie University, Sydney

Atal C K, Bradu B L 1976 Analysis of oil yield in lemongrass (*Cymbopogon* spp). Indian Journal of Pharmacy 38(2): 61–63

Atanasova-Shopova S, Rousinov K S 1970 On certain central neurotropic effects of lavender essential oil. Bulletin of the Institute of Physiology 13: 69–77

Audicana M, Bernaola G 1994 Occupational contact dermatitis from citrus fruits: lemon essential oils. Contact Dermatitis 31: 183–185

Aureli P, Constantini A, Zolea S 1992 Antimicrobial activity of some plant essential oils against *Listeria monocytogenes*. Journal of Food Protection 55(5): 344–348

Aurore G S, Abaul J, Bourgeois P, Luc J 1998 Antibacterial and antifungal activities of the essential oils of *Pimenta racemosa* var. *racemosa* P. Miller (I.W. Moore) (Myrtaceae). Journal of Essential Oil Research 10: 161–164

Averbeck D, Averbeck S, Dubertret L, Young A R, Morliere P 1990 Genotoxicity of bergapten and bergamot oil in *Saccharomyces cervisiae*. Journal of Photochemistry and Photobiology B7: 209–229

Aydin S, Beis R, Özturk Y, Husnu K, Baser C 1998 Nepetalactone: a new opioid analgesic from *Nepeta caesarea* Boiss. Journal of Pharmacy and Pharmacology 50: 813–817

Badei A Z M 1992a Antimycotic effect of cardamom essential oil against mycotoxigenic moulds in relation to its chemical composition. Chemische Mikrobiologie Techologie Lebensmittel 14:177–182

Badei A Z M 1992b Antimycotic effect of cardamom essential oil components on toxigenic moulds. Egyptian Journal Food Science 20(3): 441–452

Bagci E, Digrak M 1996 Antimicrobial activity of essential oils of some *Abies* (fir) species from Turkey. Flavor and Fragrance Journal 11(4): 251–256

Baratta M T, Dorman D, Deans S G 1998 Chemical composition, antimicrobial and antioxidative activity of laurel, sage, rosemary, oregano and coriander essential oils. Journal of Essential Oil Research 10(6): 618–627

Bartram T 1995 Encyclopedia of herbal medicine. Grace, Christchurch

Bassett I B, Pannowitz D L, Barnetson R St C 1990 A comparative study of tea tree oil versus benzoyl peroxide in the treatment of acne. Medical Journal of Australia 153: 455–458

Baxter R M, Fan M C, Kandel S I 1962 Cis-trans-isomers of asarone, their liquid gas chromatographic behaviour and that of certain other propenylphenol ethers. Canadian Journal of Chemistry 40: 154–157

Beckstrom–Sternberg S M, Duke J A 1996 CRC Handbook of medicinal mints. CRC Press, Boca Raton

Belaiche P 1979 Traité de phytothérapie et d'aromathérapie. Maloine, Paris

Bennett A, Stamford I F, Tavares I A, Jacobs S, Capasso F, Mascolo N, Autore G, Romano V, Di Carlo G 1988 The biological activity of eugenol, a major constituent of nutmeg (*Myristica fragrans*): studies on prostaglandins, the intestines and other tissues. Phytotherapy Research 23: 124–130

Benouda A, Hasser M, Benjilali B 1988 The antiseptic properties of essential oils in vitro tested against pathogenic germs found in hospitals. fitoterapia 59(27): 115–119

Betts T 1994 Sniffing the breeze. Aromatherapy Quarterly 40: 19–22

Bhatnagae M, Kapur K K, Jalees S, Sharma S K 1993 Laboratory evaluation of insecticidal properties of *Ocimum basilicum* Linnaeus and *O. sanctum* Linnaeus plant essential oils and their major constituents against vector mosquito species. Journal of Entomology Research 17(1): 21–26

Birchall A 1990 A whiff of happiness. New Scientist 127 (1731): 45–47

Bisset N G (ed) 1994 Herbal drugs and phytopharmaceuticals. Medpharm, Stuttgart

Boland D J, Brophy J J, House A P N 1991 Eucalyptus leaf oils. Inkata, Melbourne

Bourrel C, Perrineau F, Michel G, Bessière J M 1993 Catnip (*Nepeta cataria* L.) essential oil: analysis of chemical constituents, bacteriostatic and fungistatic properties. Journal of Essential Oil Research 5: 159–167

Bourrel C, Vilarem G, Perineau F 1993 Chemical analysis, bacteriostatic and fungistatic properties of the essential oil of elecampane (*Inula helenium* L.) Journal of Essential Oil Research 5: 411–417

Boyanova L, Neshev G 1999 Inhibitory effect of rose oil products on *Helicobacter pylori* growth *in vitro*: preliminary report. Journal of Medical Microbiology 48: 705–706

Boyd E M, Pearson G L 1946 On the expectorant action of volatile oils. American Journal of Medical Science 211: 602–610

Boyd E M, Sheppard P 1970 Nutmeg oil and camphene as inhaled expectorants. Archives of Otolaryngology 92(4): 372–378

Boyle R J 1993 Human reliability. Risk assessment and control. Version 2. Occupational Health and Safety Unit, Portsmouth University Enterprises Ltd, Section 9–13

Brandt W 1988 Spasmolytische Wirker Ätherische Öle. Zeitschrift für Phytotherapie 9: 33–39

Bruneton J 1995 Pharmacognosy, phytochemistry, medicinal plants. Intercept, Andover

Buchanan R L 1978 Toxicity of spices containing methylenedioxybenzene derivatives: a review. Journal of Food Safety 1: 275

Buchbauer G, Jirovetz L, Jäger W, Dietrich H, Plank C, Karamat E 1991 Aromatherapy: evidence of sedative effects of the essential oil of lavender. Zeitschrift Natürforschaft 46c: 1067–1072

Buchbauer G, Jäger W, Jirovetz L, Ilmeberger J, Dietrich H 1993 Fragrance compounds and essential oils with sedative effects upon inhalation. Journal of Pharmaceutical Science 86(6): 660–664

Buck D S, Nidorf D M, Addino J G 1994 Comparison of two topical preparations for the treatment of onychomycosis: *Melaleuca alternifolia* (tea tree) oil and clotrimazole. Journal of Family Practice 38(6): 601–605

Buckle J 1993 Does it matter which lavender essential oil is used? Nursing Times 89(20): 32–35

Buckle J 1997 Clinical aromatherapy in nursing. Arnold, London

Buil P, Garnero J, Guichard G 1975 Composition chimique de l'huile essentielle de verveine de Provence. Rivista Italica 57: 455–466

Bullerman L B, Lieu F Y, Seier S A 1977 Inhibition of growth and aflatoxin production by cinnamon and clove oils, cinnamic aldehyde and eugenol. Journal of Food Science 42(4): 1107–1109

Bunny S (ed) 1984 Illustrated book of herbs. Octopus, London

Burkhill J H 1966 A dictionary of the economic products of the Malay Peninsula. Art Printing Works, Kuala Lumpur

Bye R A Jr 1986 Medicinal plants of the Sierra Madre. Economic Botany 40(1): 103–124

Caldwell J 1991 Basil and methyl chavicol – statement on new data. International Journal of Aromatherapy 3(1): 6

Carson C F, Riley T V 1993 Toxicity of the essential of *Melaleuca alternifolia* or tea tree oil. Clinical Toxicology 33: 193–194

Carson C F, Riley T V 1994 The antimicrobial activity of tea tree oil. Medical Journal ofAustralia 160: 236

Carson C F, Hammer K A, Riley T V 1995 Broth microdilution method for determining the susceptibility of *Escherichia coli* and *Staphylococcus aureus* to the essential oil of *Melaleuca alternifolia* (tea tree oil). Microbios 82(332): 181–185

Carson C F, Cookson B D, Farrelly H D, Riley T V 1995 Susceptibility of methicillin-resistant *Staphylococcus aureus* to the essential oil of *Melaleuca alternifolia*. Journal of Antimicrobial Chemotherapy 35: 421–424

Carter G T 1976 Dissertation Abstracts International B37: 766

Chandhoke N, Ghatak B J R 1969 Studies on *Tagetes minuta*: some pharmacological actions of the essential oil. Indian Journal of Medical Research 57: 864–876

Chandler R F, Hawkes D 1984 Aniseed – a spice, a flavour, a drug. Canadian Pharmaceutical Journal 117: 28–29

Chandler R F, Hooper S N, Harvey M J 1982 Ethnobotany and phytochemistry of yarrow, Achillea millefolium, Compositae. Economic Botany 36: 203–223

Charai M, Mosaddak M, Faid M 1996 Chemical composition and antimicrobial activities of two aromatic plants: *Origanum majorana* L. and *O. compactum* Benth. Journal of Essential Oil Research 8: 657–664

Chinou I B, Roussis V, Perdetzoglou D, Loukis A 1996 Chemical and biological studies on two *Helichrysum* species of Greek origin. Planta Medica 62: 377–379

Claus E P 1961 Pharmacognosy, 4th edn. Lea & Febiger, Philadelphia

Cooke A, Cooke M D 1994 An investigation into the antimicrobial properties of manuka and kanuka oils. Cawthron Institute Report no 263 Nelson, New Zealand

Corbier B, Teisseire P 1974 Contribution to the knowledge of neroli oil from Grasse. Recherches 19: 289–290

Council of Scientific and Industrial Research 1984–1976 The wealth of India, 11 vols. New Delhi

Craig J O 1953 Poisoning by the volatile oils in childhood. Archives of Disease in Childhood 28: 475–483

Cuong N D et al 1994 Antibacterial properties of Vietnamese cajuput oil. Journal of Essential Oil Research 6: 63–67

D'Auria F D et al 2001 In vitro activity of tea tree oil against Candida albicans mycelial conversion and other pathogenic fungi. Journal of Chemotherapy 13(4): 377–383

Dale H H 1909 Nutmeg. Society of Experimental Biology, New York 23, p. 69

Deans S G, Ritchie G 1987 International Journal of Food Microbiology 5: 165–180

Deans S G, Svoboda K P 1990 The antimicrobial properties of marjoram (Origanum majorana L.) volatile oil. Flavor and Fragrance Journal 5(3): 187–190

Deans S G, Noble R C, Hiltunen R, Wuryani W, Penzes L 1995 Antimicrobial and antioxidant properties of Syzygium aromaticum (L.) Merr. & Perry: impact upon bacteria, fungi and fatty acid levels in ageing mice. Flavor and Fragrance Journal 10(5): 323–328

Debelmas A M, Rochat J 1967 Etude pharmacologique des huiles essentielles. Activité antispasmodique étudiée sur une cinquantaine d'échantillons différents. Plantes Médicinales et Phytotherapie 1: 23–27

Deshpande R S, Ripnis H P 1977 Insecticidal activity of Ocimum basilicum Linn. Pesticides. 11(15): 11

Deshpande R S et al 1974 Bulletin of Grain Technology 12: 232 through Chemical Abstracts 1976 84: 55270c

Dew M J, Evans B K, Rhodes J 1984 Peppermint oil for the irritable bowel syndrome: a multicentre trial. British Journal of Clinical Practice 38(11–12): 394–398

Dikshit A, Husain A 1984 Antifungal action of some essential oils against animal pathogens. Fitoterapia 55(3): 171-176

Dobrynin V N et al 1976 Antimicrobial substances of Salvia officinalis. Khimiia Prirodnykh Soedinenii 5: 686 In: Chemical Abstracts 1977 86: 117603r

Domokos J D, Hethelyi E, Palinkas J, Szirmal S 1997 Essential oil of rosemary (Rosmarinus officinalis L.) of Hungarian origin. Journal of Essential Oil Research 9: 41–45

Draize J H 1959 Dermal toxicity. In: Appraisal of the safety of chemicals in foods, drugs and cosmetics. Association of Food and Drug Officials of the United States, Austin, p. 52

Drinkwater N R et al 1976 Hepatocarcinogenicity of estragole (1-allyl-4-methoxybenzene) and 1-hydroxyestragole in the mouse and mutagenicity of 1-acetoxyestragole in bacteria. Journal of the National Cancer Institute 57: 1323–1331

Dube S, Upadhyay D, Tripathi S C 1988 Antifungal, physicochemical and insect repelling activity of the essential oil of Ocimum basilicum. Canadian Journal of Botany 67: 2085–2087

Dubey N K, Kishore N, Singh S K 1983 Antifungal properties of the volatile traction of Melaleuca leucadendron. Tropical Agriciculture 60(3): 227

Duke J A 1985 Handbook of medicinal herbs. CRC Press, Boca Raton

Duke J A, Ayensu E S 1985 Medicinal plants of China. Reference Publications, Algonac, Michigan

Duke J A, Wain K K 1981 Medicinal plants of the world. Computer Index, 3 vol, p. 1654

Duraffourd P 1982 En forme tous les jours. La Vie Claire, Périgny

Duthie H L 1981 The effect of peppermint oil on colonic motility in man. British Journal of Surgery 68: 820

Dwivedi C, Abu-Ghazaleh A1997 Chemopreventive effects of sandalwood oil on skin papillomas in mice. European Journal of Cancer Prevention 6(4): 399–401

El Tahir K E H, Shoeb H, Al-Shora H 1997 Exploration of some pharmacological activities of cardamom seed (Elettaria cardamomum) volatile oil. Saudi Pharmaceutical Journal 5(2,3): 96–102

Elegbede J A, Maltzman T H, Verma A K, Tanner M A, Elson C E, Gould M N 1986 Mouse skin tumour promoting activity of orange peel oil and d-limonene: a re-evaluation. Carcinogenesis 7(12): 2047–2049

Emboden W A Jr 1972 Narcotic plants. Macmillan, New York

Epstein W L 1973 Report to RIFM. 30 October

Faoagali J, George N, Leditschke J F 1997 Does tea tree oil have a place in the topical treatment of burns? Burns 23(4): 349–351

Farnsworth N R 1975 Potential value of plants as sources of new antifertility agents I. Journal of Pharmaceutical Sciences 64: 535–598

Feinblatt H M 1960 Cajuput type oil for the treatment of furunculosis. Journal Natural Medical Association 1: 32–34

Foggie W E 1911 Eucalyptus oil poisoning. British Medical Journal 1: 359–360

Food and Drug Administration 1978 Health foods business, June

Forbes P D, Urbach F, Davies R E 1977 Photo toxicity testing of fragrance raw materials. Food and Cosmetics Toxicology 15: 55–60

Force M, Sparks W S, Ronzio R A 2000 Inhibition of enteric parasites by emulsified oil of oregano in vivo. Phytotherapy Research 14: 213–214

Ford R A, Api A M, Letizia C S 1992a Petitgrain bigarade oil. Food and Chemical Toxicology 30 (suppl): 101S

Ford R A, Api A M, Letizia C S 1992b Mandarin oil. Food and Chemical Toxicology 30 (suppl): 69S

Ford R A, Letizia C S, Api A M 1988 Tea tree oil. Food and Chemical Toxicology 26(4): 407

Foster S 1991 Chamomile, Matricaria recutita and Chamaemelum nobile. Botanical Series no 307, American Botanical Council, Austin

Foster S 1993a Chamomile. The Herb Companion December/January: 64–68

Foster S 1993b Herbal renaissance. Gibbs Smith, Layton, p. 79

Fowler P, Wall M 1997 COSHH and CHIPS: ensuring the safety of aromatherapy. Complementary Therapies in Medicine 5: 112–115

Franchomme P, Pénoël D 1990 L'Aromathérapie exactement. Jollois, Limoges

Franchomme P, Pénoël D 2001 L'Aromathérapie exactement. Jollois, Limoges

Fujii T, Furukawa S, Suzuki S 1972 Studies on compounded perfumes for toilet goods: on the non-irritative compounded perfumes for soaps. Yukugaku 21(12): 904–908

Gabrielli G, Loggini F, Cioni P L, Gianiccini B, Mancuso E 1988 Activity of lavandino essential oil against non-tubercular opportunistic rapid growth mycobacteria. Pharmacological Research Communications 20(suppl. 5): 37–40

Garg S C 1974 Antifungal effects of Boswellia serrata leaf oil. Indian Journal of Pharmacy 36: 46

Garg S C, Dengre S L 1986 Antibacterial activity of essential oil of Tagetes erecta Linn. Hindustan Antibiotics Bulletin 28(1–4): 27–29

Garg S C, Dengre S L 1988 Antifungal activity of the essential oil of Myrtus communis var. microphylla. Herba Hungarica 27(2,3): 2–3

Gattefossé R-M 1937 Aromathérapie. Girardot, Paris. (English transl 1993 Daniel, Saffron Walden)

Gauthier R, Agoumi A, Gourai M 1989 The activity of extracts of Myrtus communis against Pediculus humanis capitis. Plantes Médicinales Phytotherapie 23(2): 95–108

Ghelardini C, Galeotti N, Salvatore G, Mazzanti G 1999 Local anaesthetic activity of the essential oil of Lavandula angustifolia. Planta Medica 65: 700–703

Ghfir B, Fonvieille J L, Dargent R 1997 Influence of essential oil of Hyssopus officinalis on the chemical composition of the walls of *Aspergillus fumigatus* (Fresenius). Mycopathologia 138(1): 7–12s

Ghfir B, Fonvieille J L, Koulali Y, Ecalle R, Dargent R 1994 Effect of essential oil of *Hyssopus officinalis* on the lipid composition of *Aspergillus fumigatus*. Mycopathologia 126(8): 163–167

Gobel H, Schmidt G, Soyka D 1994 Effect of peppermint and eucalyptus oil preparations on neurophysiological and experimental algesimetric headache parameters. Cephalalgia 14: 228–234

Gogoi P, Baruah P, Nath S C 1997 Antifungal activity of the essential oil of *Litsea cubeba* Pers. Journal of Essential Oil Research 9: 213–215

Goodman L, Golman A 1942 The pharmacological basis of therapeutics. Macmillan, New York

Grieve M 1980 A modern herbal. Penguin, Harmondsworth

Grieve M 1998 A modern herbal. Tiger Books International, London

Griggs B 1997 New green pharmacy. Vermilion, London

Grochulski V A, Borkowski B 1972 Influence of chamomile oil on experimental glomerulonephritis in rabbits. Planta Medica 21: 289–292

Grube D D 1977 photosensitising effects of 8-methoxypsoralen on the skin of hairless mice. II. Strain and spectral differences for tumorigenesis. Photochemistry and Photobiology 25: 269–276

Guarrera P M, Leporatti M L, Foddai S, Moretto D, Mercantini R 1995 Antimycotic activity of essential oil of *Lippia citriodora* Kunt. (*Aloysia triphylla* Britton). Rivista Ital EPPOS 15: 23–25

Guenther E 1949 The essential oils, 6 vols. Van Nostrand, New York

Guillemain J, Rousseau A, Delaveau P 1989 Neurodepressive effects of the essential oil of *Lavandula angustifolia* Mill. Ann Pharm Fr 47(6): 337–343

Gui–Yuan Y, Wei W 1994 Clinical studies on treatment of coronary heart disease with *Valeriana officinalis* var. *latifolia*. Chung Kuo CHICH Tsa Chih 14(9): 540–542

Habersang S, Leuschner O, Theimer I, Theimer K 1979 Pharmacological studies of chamomile constituents. IV. Studies on the toxicity of (–)-α-bisabolol. Planta Medica 35: 118–124

Hajji F, Fkih-Tetouani S 1993 Antimicrobial activity of twenty one Eucalyptus essential oils. fitoterapia 64(1): 71–77

Hammer K A, Carson C F, Riley T V 1996 Susceptibility of transient and commensal skin flora to the essential oil of *Melaleuca alternifolia* (tea tree oil). Australian Journal of Infection Control 24(3): 186–189

Hammer K A, Carson C F, Riley T V 1998 *In vitro* activity of essential oils, in particular *Melaleuca alternifolia* (tea tree) oil and tea tree oil products against *Candida* ssp. Journal of Antimicrobial Chemotherapy 42(5): 591–595

Harborne J B, Baxter H (eds) 1993 Phytochemical dictionary, a handbook of bioactive compounds from plants. Taylor & Francis, London

Harry R G 1948 Cosmetic materials, vol. 2. Hill, London

Hartwell J L 1967–1971 Plants used against cancer: a survey. Lloydia 30

Hausen B M, Busker E, Carle R 1984 The sensitising capacity of Compositae plants. VII. Experimental investigations with extracts and compounds of *Chamomilla recutita* (L.) Rauschert and *Anthemis cotula* (L.). Planta Medica 229–234

Hausen B M, Reichling J, Harkenthal M 1999 Degradation products of monoterpenes are the sensitizing agents in tea tree oil. American Journal of Contact Dermatitis 10: 68–70

Hay R K M 1993 Physiology. In: Hay & Waterman (eds) Volatile oil crops. Longman, Harlow, pp. 23–43

Health and Safety Commission 1999 The control of substances hazardous to health regulations. HMSO, London

Hendricks H, Bos R, Woerdenbag H, Kaster A 1985 Central nervous depressant activity of valeric acid in the mouse. Planta Medica 51: 28–31

Hendricks H, Bos R, Allersma D P, Malingre Th M, Koster A Sj 1981 Pharmacological screening of valerenal and some other components of the essential oil of *Valeriana officinalis*. Planta Medica 42: 62–67

Herb Society 1994 Herbalism (newsletter) March: 17

Herrmann E C, Kucera L S 1967 Proceedings of the Society of Experimental Biology and Medicine 124: 865

Hethelyi E, Danos B, Tetenyi P, Juhasz G 1987 Phytochemical studies on the essential oil in *T. Minuta* and *T. tenuifolia*. Herba Hung. 26(2–3): 145–158

Hitokoto H, Morozumi S, Wauke T, Sakai S, Veno I 1980 Inhibitory effects of spices on growth and toxin production of toxigenic fungi. Applied and Environmental Microbiology 39: 818–822

Hmamouch M, Tantaoui-Elaraki A, Es-Safi N, Agoumi A 1990 A report on the antibacterial and antifungal properties of eucalyptus essential oils. Plantes Médicinales Phytothérapie 24(4): 278–289

HMSO 1992 Management of Health and Safety at Work Regulations. HMSO, London

Hodgson I, Stewart J, Fyfe L 1998 Inhibition of bacteria and yeast by oil of fennel and paraben: development of synergistic antimicrobial combinations. Journal of Essential oil Research 10: 293–297

Holmes E M 1916 Perfume Record 8: 78

Homburger F, Boger E 1968 The carcinogenicity of essential oils, flavors and spices: a review. Cancer Research 28: 2372–2374

HSE 1997 General COSHH ACOP, carcinogens ACOP and biological agents ACOP (1996 edn). Control of Substances Hazardous to Health Regulations

Huang T C, Liu P K, Chang C F, Chou C, Tseng H L 1981 Study of antiasthmatic constituents in Ocimum basilicum Benth. Yao Hsueh T'ung Pao 16(4): 56

IFRA 1992 Code of practice. International Fragrance Association, Geneva

Isaac O 1979 Pharmakologische Untersuchungen von Kamillen-Inhaltsstoffen I. Zur Pharmakologie des (–)-α-bisabolol und der Bisabololoxide (Übersicht). Planta Medica 35: 118–124

Jacobs M R, Hornfeldt C S 1994 Melaleuca oil poisoning. Clinical Toxicology 32: 461–464

Jäger W, Buchbauer G, Jirovetz L, Dietrich H, Plank C 1992 Evidence of the sedative effects of neroli oil, citronellal and phenyl ethyl acetate on mice. Journal of Essential Oil Research 4: 387–394

Jäger W, Buchbauer G, Jirovetz L, Fritzer M 1992 Percutaneous absorption of lavender oil from a massage oil. Journal Society Cosmetic Chemist 43(1): 49–51

Jakovlev V et al 1979 Pharmacological investigations with compounds of chamomile. II. New investigations on the antiphlogistic effects of (–)-α-bisabolol and bisabolol oxides. Planta Medica 35: 125–140

Jalsenjak V, Peljnjak S, Kustrak D 1987 Microcapsules of sage oil: essential oils content and antimicrobial activity. Pharmazie 42(6): 419–420

Janssens J et al 1990 Nutmeg oil: identification and quantification of its most active constituents as inhibitors of platelet aggregation. Journal of Ethnopharmacology 29: 179–188

Jedlickova Z, Mottl O, Sery V 1992 Antibacterial properties of the Vietnamese cajuput oil and Ocimum oil in combination with antibacterial agents. Journal of Hygiene, Epidemiology, Microbiology and Immunology 36(3): 303–309

Jitoe A, Masuda T et al 1994 Novel antioxidants, cassumunin A, B and C from *Zingiber cassumunar*. Tetrahedron Letters 35(7): 981–984

Joubert L, Gattefossé M 1968 Mezhdunar Kongr Efirnym Maslam (Mater.) 4th 1: 99 *through* Chem Abstr 1973 78: 119653r

Juven B J, Kanner J, Schved F, Weisslowicz H 1993 Factors that interact with the antibacterial action of thyme essential oil and its active constituents. Journal of Applied Bacteriology 76: 626–631

Kaddu S, Helmut K, Wolf P 2001 Accidental bullous phototoxic reactions to bergamot aromatherapy oil. Journal of the American Academy of Dermatology 45: 458–461

Kaiser R, Lamparsky D 1976a Inhaltsstoffe verbenaöls. I Mitteilung, Natürliches Vorkommen der Photocitrale und einiger ihrer Derivate. Helvetica Chimica Acta 59: 1797–1802

Kaiser R, Lamparsky D 1976b Inhaltsstoffe verbenaöls. II Mitteilung, Caryophyllan-2-6-β-oxide, eine neue Sesquiterpeverbindung aus dem Öl von *Lippia citriodora* Kunth. Helvetica Chimica Acta 59: 1803–1808

Karamat E, Ilmberger J, Buchbauer G, Rößlhuber J, Rupp C 1992 Excitatory and sedative effects of essential oils on human reaction time performance. Chemical Senses 17: 847

Keil H 1947 Contact dermatitis due to oil of citronella. Journal of Investigative Dermatology 8: 327–334

Keller K, Stahl E 1983 Zusammersatzung des Ätherischen Öle von Beta-asaronfreiem Kalmus. Planta Medica 47: 71–74

Keville K 1991 The illustrated herb encyclopedia. Grange Books, London, p. 129

Khan M T, Potter M, Birch I 1996 Podiatric treatment of hyperkeratotic plantar lesions with marigold *Tagetes erecta*. Phytotherapy Research 10(3): 211–214

Kim H-M, Cho S-H 1999 Lavender oil inhibits immediate type reaction in mice and rats. Journal of Pharmacy and Pharmacology 51(2): 221–226

Kirkness W R 1910 Poisoning by oil of eucalyptus. British Medical Journal 1: 261

Kirov M, Vankov S 1988 Rose oil and girosital. Medico Biologic Information 3: 3–7

Kirov M, Burkova T, Kapurdov V, Spasovski M 1988 Rose oil. Lipotropic effect in modelled fatty dystrophy of the liver. (Morphological and enzymohistochemical study). Medico Biologic Information 3: 18–22

Kivanc M, Akgul A 1986 Antibacterial activity of essential oils from Turkish spices and citrus. Flavor and Fragrance Journal 1: 175–179

Kline R M, Kline J J, Di Palma J, Barbero G J 2001 Enteric-coated, pH-dependent peppermint oil capsules for the treatment of irritable bowel syndrome in children. Journal of Paediatrics 138: 125–128

Koh K J, Pearce A L, Marshman G, Finlay-Jones J J, Hart P H 2002 Tea tree oil reduces histamine-induced skin inflammation. British Journal of Dermatology 147: 1212–1217

Kosta Y et al 2004 Repellency of citronella for head lice: double blind randomised trial of efficacy and safety. IMAJ 6: 756–759

Kovar K A, Gropper B, Friess D, Svendsen A 1987 Blood levels of 1,8-cineole and locomotor activity of mice after inhalation and oral administration of rosemary oil. Planta Medica 53(4): 315–318

Krall B, Kraus W 1993 Efficacy and tolerance of *Mentha arvensis aetheroleum*. 24th International Symposium Essential Oils

Kriegelstein J, Grusla D 1988 Deutsche Apotheker Zeitung 128: 2041–2046

Kubota M, Ikemoto T, Komaki R, Iniu M 1992 Paper given to the 12th International Congress on Flavours, Fragrances and Essential Oils. Vienna, Austria

Kudrzycka-Bieloszabska F W, Glowniak K 1966 Pharmacodynamic properties of *Oleum chamomillae* and *Oleum millefolii*. Dissertationes Pharmaceuticae et Pharmacologicae 18: 449–454

Kumar A, Sharma V D, Sing A K, Singh K 1988 Antibacterial properties of different Eucalyptus oils. fitoterapia 59(2): 141–144

Lavy G 1987 Nutmeg intoxication in pregnancy. Journal of Reproductive Medicine 32: 63–69

Lawless J 1995 The illustrated encyclopedia of essential oils. Element, Dorset, p. 177

Lawrence B M 1977 Progress in essential oils. Perfumer & Flavorist February/March 2(1): 3

Lawrence B M 1979a Essential oils 1976–1978. Allured, Carol Stream, p. 20

Lawrence B M 1979b Essential oils 1976–1978. Allured, Wheaton, p. 23

Lawrence B M 1981 Essential oils 1979–1980. Allured, Wheaton

Lawrence B M 1984 Progress in essential oils. Perfumer & Flavorist August/September 9(4): 37

Lawrence B M 1989 Progress in essential oils. Perfumer & Flavorist 14(6): 87

Lawrence B M 1989 Progress in essential oils. Perfumer & Flavorist 14(3): 71

Lawrence B M 1991 Progress in essential oils. Perfumer & Flavorist 16(1): 49

Leach E H, Lloyd J P F 1956 Experimental ocular hypertension in animals. Transactions of the Ophthalmological Societies of the United Kingdom 76: 453–460

Lee K-G, Shibamoto T 2001 Inhibition of malonaldehyde formation from blood plasma oxidation by aroma extracts and aroma components isolated from clove and eucalyptus. Food and Chemical Toxicology 39: 1199–1204

Lehrner J, Eckersberger C, Walla P, Potsch G, Deecke L 2000 Ambient odour of orange in a dental office reduces anxiety and improves mood in female patients. Physiology and Behaviour 71: 83–86

Leicester R J, Hunt R H 1982 Peppermint oil to reduce colonic spasm during endoscopy. Lancet 30th October: 989

Lens-Lisbonne C, Cremieux A, Maillard C, Balansard C 1987 Methods of evaluating the antibacterial properties of essential oils: applied to thyme and cinnamon. Journal de Pharmacie de Belgique 42(5): 297–302

Leung A Y 1980 Encyclopedia of common natural ingredients used in foods, drugs and cosmetics. Wiley, New York, p. 409

Leung A Y, Foster S 1996 Encyclopedia of common natural ingredients used in food, drugs and cosmetics. Wiley, New York

Lewis W H, Elvin-Lewis M P H 1977 Medical botany. Plants affecting man's health. Wiley-Interscience, New York

Lin T S 1983 Variation in content and composition of essential oil from *Litsea cubeba* collected in different months. Bulletin of the Taiwan Forestry Research Institute, No. 398. 9 pp.

Lis-Balchin M, Hart S 1998 An investigation of the essential oils of manuka (*Leptospermum scoparium*) and kanuka (*Kunzea ericoides*) Myrtacease on guinea pig smooth muscle. Journal of Pharmacy and Pharmacology Jul; 50(7): 809–811

Lis-Balchin M, Hart S 1999 Studies on the mode of action of the essential oil of lavender (*Lavandula angustifolia* P. Miller). Phytotherapy Research 13: 540–542

Lis-Balchin M, Deans S, Hart S 1994 Paper given to the 25th International Symposium on Essential Oils, Grasse

Lis-Balchin M, Deans S G, Hart S 1997 A study of the variability of commercial peppermint oils using antimicrobial and pharmacological parameters. Medical Science Research 25(3): 151–152

Lis-Balchin M, Hart S, Roth G 1997 The spasmolytic activity of the essential oils of scented *Pelargoniums* (Geranaceae). Phytotherapy Research 11: 583–584

List P H, Hörhammer L 1969–1979 Hager's Handbuch der Pharmazeutischen Praxis. Springer-Verlag, Berlin

List P H, Hörhammer L (eds) 1979 Hagers Handbuch der Pharmazeutischen Praxis, 4th edn, vol. 6B Springer-Verlag, Berlin

Loveman A B 1938 Stomatitis venenata: report of a case of sensitivity of the mucous membranes and the skin to oil of anise. Archiva Dermatologica 38: 906

Low D, Rawal B D, Griffin W J 1974 Antibacterial action of the essential oils of some Australian Myrtaceae with special references to the activity of chromatographic fractions of oil of *Eucalyptus citriodora*. Planta Medica 26: 184–189

Löwenfeld W 1932 Ekzematose überempfindlichkeit gegen Eukalyptusöl. Dermatologie Wochenschrift 95: 1281

Ludvigson H W, Rottman T R 1989 Effect of ambient odours of lavender and cloves on cognition, memory and mood. Chemical Senses 14(4): 525–536

Mabey R (ed) 1988 The complete new herbal. Elm Tree Books, London

Manley C H 1993 Critical revue. In: Food Science and Nutrition 39(1): 57–62

Mann C, Staba E J 1986 The chemistry, pharmacology and commercial formulations of chamomile. In: Craker L E, Simon J E (eds) Herbs, spices and medicinal plants: recent advances in botany, horticulture, and pharmacology, vol 1. Oryx Press, Arizona, pp. 235–280

Manohar V, Ingram C, Gray J, Talpur N A, Echar B W, Bagchi D, Preuss H G 2001 Antifungal activities of origanum oil against *Candida albicans*. Molecular and Cellular Biochemistry 228: 111–117

Maradufu A R, Lubega R, Dorn F 1978 Isolation of (5E)-Ocimerme, a mosquito lavicide from *Tagetes minuta*. Lloydia 41: 181–183

Martijena I D, Gargia D A, Marin R H, Perillo M, Zygadlo J P 1998 Anxiogenic-like and antidepressant-like effects of the essential oil from *Tagetes minuta*. fitoterapia 69(2): 155–160

Martinez Nadal N G, Montolvo A E, Seda M 1973 Antimicrobial properties of bay and other phenolic essential oils. Cosmetiques et Parfumerie 88(10): 37–38

Maruzzella J C et al 1960 Antibacterial activity of essential oil vapours. Journal of the American Pharmaceutical Association 49: 692–694

Maruzzella J C, Henry P A 1958 The *in vitro* antibacterial activity of essential oil combinations. Journal of the American Pharmaceutical Association 47: 294–296

Maruzzella J C, Liguori L 1958 The *in vitro* antifungal activity of essential oils. Journal of the American Pharmaceutical Association 47 (4): 250–254

Maruzzella J C, Sicurella N A 1960 Antibacterial activity of essential oil vapours. Journal of the American Pharmaceutical Association 49: 692–694

Marzulli F N, Maibach H I 1970 Perfume photo toxicity. Journal of the Society of Cosmetic Chemists 2: 695

Masakova N, Tserevatuy B S, Trofimenko S L, Remmer G S 1979 The chemical composition of volatile oil in lemon balm as an indicator of therapeutic use. Planta Medica 36: 274

Mastura M, Nor Azah M A, Khozirah S, Mawardi R, Manal A A 1999 Anticandidal and antidermatophytic activity of *Cinnamomum* species essential oils. Cytobios 98: 17–23

Masuda T, Jitoe A 1994 Antioxidative and anti-inflammatory compounds from tropical gingers: isolation, structure determination and activities of cassumunarins A, B and C new complex curcuminoids from *Zingiber cassumunar*. Journal of Agriculture and Food Chemistry 42(9): 1850–1856

Masuda T, Jitoe A et al 1995 Isolation and structure determination of cassumunarins A, B and C: new anti-inflammatory antioxidants from a tropical ginger *Zingiber cassumunar*. Journal of the American Oil Chemists' Society 72(9): 1053–1057

Mathur A C, Saxena B P 1975 Introduction of sterility in male houseflies by vapour of *Acorus calamus* L. oil. Die Natürwissenschafter 12: 576

May B, Kuntz H-D, Kieser M, Köhler S 1996 Efficacy of a fixed peppermint oil/caraway oil combination in non-ulcer dyspepsia. Arzneimittel Forschung/Drug Research 46(II): 1149–1153

Mayo W L 1992 Australian tea tree oil: a summary of medicinal, pharmacological and alternative health research and writings. International Journal of Alternative and Complementary Medicine Dec 13–16

Mazzanti G, Battinelli L, Salvatore G 1998 Antimicrobial properties of the linalool rich essential oil of *Hyssopus officinalis* L. var. *decumbens*. Flavor and Fragrance Journal 13: 289–294

McGeorge B C, Steele M C 1991 Allergic contact dermatitis of the nipple from Roman chamomile ointment. Contact Dermatitis 24(2): 139–140

McPherson J 1925 The toxicology of eucalyptus oil. Medical Journal of Australia 2: 108–110

Melegari M, Albasini A, Provvisionato A, Bianchi A, Vampa G 1985 Research into the characteristic chemical and antibacterial properties of the essential oil of *Satureia montana*. Fitoterapia 56(2): 85–91

Melegari M, Albasini A, Pecorari G, Vampa G, Rinaldi M 1988 Chemical characteristics and pharmacological properties of the essential oil of *Anthemis nobilis*. Fitoterapia (Milan) 59(6): 449–455

Mezzadra G, Guarnieri B, Grupper C, Forlot P 1981 Effects of chronic field exposure of humans to bergapten. In: Cahn J, Forlot P, Grupper C, Meybeck A, Urbach A (eds) Psoralens in cosmetics and dermatology. Pergamon Press, Oxford, pp. 383–395

Micklefield G, Greving I, May B 2000 Effects of peppermint oil and caraway oil on gastroduodenal motility. Phytotherapy Research 14: 20–23

Micklefield G H, Jung O, Greving I, May B 2003 Effects of intraduodenal application of peppermint oil (WS® 1340) and caraway oil (WS® 1520) on gastroduodenal motility in healthy volunteers. Phytotherapy Research 17: 135–140

Millet Y 1979 Étude expérimental des propriétés toxiques convulsivantes des essences de sauge et d'hysope du commerce. Revue d'Electoencephalographie et de Neurophysiologie Clinique 1: 12–18

Millet Y, Jouglard J, Steinmetz M, Tognetti P, Joanny P, Arditti J 1981 Toxicity of some essential oils. Clinical and experimental study. Clinical Toxicology 18(12): 1485–1498

Mills S Y 1991 The essential book of herbal medicine. Penguin Arkana, Harmondsworth

Mills S Y 1993 The essential book of herbal medicine. Penguin Arkana, London

Mishra D, Samuel C O, Tripathi S C 1993 Synergistic antifungal efficacy of essential oils of *Apium graveolens* and *Cuminum cyminum*. Indian Perfumer 37(2): 134–140

Mishra D et al 1995 The fungitoxic effect of the essential oil of the herb Nardostachys jatamansi DC. Tropical Agriculture 72(1): 48–52

Mitchell J C, Rook A 1979 Botanical dermatology. Greenglass, Vancouver

Monges Ph, Joachim G, Bohor M, Petit L, Reynier J P 1994 Comparative *in vivo* study of the moisturising properties of three gels containing essential oils: mandarin, German chamomile, orange. Nouvelle Dermatologie 13(6): 470–475

Monograph 1990a *Angelicae fructis*. Bundesanzeiger no 101

Monograph 1990b *Angelicae radix*. Bundesanzeiger no 101

Monograph 1990c *Cymbopogon* species. Bundesanzeiger no 22

Moreno O M 1973 Report to RIFM, 21 September

Morris M, Donoghue A, Markovitz J, Osterhoudt K 2003 Ingestion of tea tree oil (Melaleuca oil) by 4 year old boy. Paediatric Emergency Care 19: 169–171

Morton J F 1981 Atlas of medicinal plants of Middle America. Thomas, Springfield

Moshonas M G, Shaw P E 1972 Analysis of flavor constituents from lemon and lime essence. Journal of Agriculture and Food Chemistry 20: 1029–1030

Moss M, Cook J, Wesness K, Duckett P 2003 Aromas of rosemary and lavender essential oils differentially affect cognition and mood in healthy adults. International Journal of Neuroscience 113: 15–38

Mulkens A et al 1985 Pharmaceutica Acta Helvetica 60(9–10): 276 In: Chemical Abstracts 1985 103: 211224j

Murakami A, Kuki W, Takahashi Y, Yonei H, Nakamura Y, Ohto Y, Ohigashi H, Koshimizu K 1997 Auraptene, a citrus coumarin, inhibits 12-0-tetradecanoylphorbol-13-acetate-induced tumor promotion in ICR mouse skin, possibly through suppression of superoxide generation in leucocytes. Japanese Journal Cancer Research 88: 443–452

Murdock D I, Allen W E 1960 Food Technology 14: 441

Murray F A 1921 Dermatitis caused by bitter orange. British Medical Journal 1: 739

Musajo L, Rodighiero G, Caporale G 1953 The photodynamic activity of the natural coumarins. Chimica Industria (Milan) 35: 13–15

Musajo L, Rodighiero G, Caporale G 1954 The photodynamic activity of the natural coumarins. Bulletin Société de Chimie et Biologie 36: 1213–1224

Nacino F M, Barretto C B, Cruz L J 1975 The effect of citrus oil on tumour production by DMBA. Kalikasan Philipp. Journal Biology 4: 240–247. In Chemical Abstracts 1976 84: 39528n

Naganuma M, Hirose S, Nakayama K, Someya T 1985 A study of the phototoxicity of lemon oil. Archives of Dermatological Research 278(1): 31–36

Nano G M, Sacco T, Frattini C 1974 Botanical and chemical research on *Anthemis nobilis* L. and some of its cultivars. Paper no 114, Sixth International Essential Oil Congress, San Francisco

Neale A 1893 Case of death following blue gum (*Eucalyptus globulus*) oil. Australasian Medical Gazette 12: 115–116

Nenoff P, Haustein U-F, Brandt W 1996 Antifungal activity of the essential oil of *Melaleuca alternifolia* (tea tree oil) against pathogenic fungi *in vitro*. Skin Pharmacology 9: 388–394

Nidiry E S J 1998 Structure-fungitoxicity relationships of the monoterpenoids of the essential oils of peppermint (*Mentha x piperita*) and scented geranium (*Pelargonium graveolens*). Journal of Essential Oil Research 10: 628–631

Novak D 1968 Archives de Roumaine Pathologie et Experimental Microbiologie 27: 721 In: Chemical Abstracts 1969 71: 58264w

Occhiuto F, Circosta C 1996 Antianginal and antiarrhythmic effects of bergamottine, a furocoumarin isolated from bergamot oil. Phytotherapy Research 10(6): 491–496

Occhutio F, Circosta C 1997 Investigations to characterise the antiarrhythmic action of bergamottin, a furocoumarin isolated from bergamot oil. Phytotherapy Research 11: 450–453

Occhiuto F et al 1995 Effects of the non-volatile residue from the essential oil of *Citrus bergamia* on the central nervous system. International Journal of Pharmacognosy 33(3): 198–203

Ognyanov I 1984 Bulgarian lavender and Bulgarian lavender oil. Perfumer and Flavorist 8(6): 29–41

Oishi K et al 1974 Nippon Suisan Gakkaishi 40: 1241 In: Chemical Abstracts 1975 82: 84722r

Okugawa H, Ueda R, Matsumoto K, Kato A 1995 Effect of α-santalol and β-santalol nom sandalwood on the central nervous system in mice. Phytomedicine 2(2): 119–126

Onawunmi G O, Oguniana E O 1981 Antibacterial constituents in the essential oil of *Cymbopogon citratus*. Ethnopharmacology 24: 64–68

Opdyke D L J 1973a Monographs on fragrance raw materials. Food and Cosmetics Toxicology 11

Opdyke D L J 1973b Caraway oil. Food and Cosmetics Toxicology 11: 1051

Opdyke D L J 1973c Bergamot oil, expressed. Food and Cosmetics Toxicology 11: 1031

Opdyke D L J 1973d Coriander oil (*Coriandrum sativum* L.). Food and Cosmetics Toxicology 11: 1077

Opdyke D L J 1973e Basil oil, sweet. Food and Cosmetics Toxicology 11: 867

Opdyke D L J 1973f Anise oil (*Pimpinella anisum* L.). Food and Cosmetics Toxicology 11: 865

Opdyke D L J 1974a Monographs on fragrance raw materials. Food and Cosmetics Toxicology 12: 403

Opdyke D L J 1974b Monographs on fragrance raw materials. Food and Cosmetics Toxicology 12: 735

Opdyke D L J 1974c Monographs on fragrance raw materials. Food and Cosmetics Toxicology 12: 733

Opdyke D L J 1974d Ylang ylang oil. Food and Cosmetics Toxicology 12. Special issue I Monographs on fragrance raw materials: 1049

Opdyke D L J 1974e Chamomile oil, Roman. Food and Cosmetics Toxicology 12. Special issue III Monographs on fragrance raw materials: 709

Opdyke D L J 1974f Chamomile flower, Hungarian, oil (*Matricaria chamomilla* L.). Food and Cosmetics Toxicology 12. Special issue I Monographs on fragrance raw materials: 851

Opdyke D L J 1974g Bitter orange oil (*Citrus aurantium* L.). Food and Cosmetics Toxicology 12: 735

Opdyke D L J 1974h Lemon oil, expressed. Food and Cosmetics Toxicology 12: 725

Opdyke D L J 1974i Lemon oil, distilled. Food and Cosmetics Toxicology 12: 727

Opdyke D L J 1974j Fennel oil. Food and Cosmetics Toxicology 12. Special issue I Monographs on fragrance raw materials: 879

Opdyke D L J 1974k Geranium oil, bourbon. Food and Cosmetics Toxicology 12. Special issue I Monographs on fragrance raw materials: 883

Opdyke D L J 1974l Rose oil (*Rosa damascena* Mill.). Food and Cosmetics Toxicology 12. Special issue I Monographs on fragrance raw materials: 979, 981

Opdyke D L J 1974m Rosemary oil (*Rosmarinus officinalis* L.). Food and Cosmetics Toxicology 12. Special issue I Monographs on fragrance raw materials: 977

Opdyke D L J 1974n Sage Dalmatian oil (*Salvia officinalis* L.). Food and Cosmetics Toxicology 12. Special issue I Monographs on fragrance raw materials: 987

Opdyke D L J 1974o Sandalwood oil, East Indian. Food and Cosmetics Toxicology 12. Special issue I monographs on fragrance raw materials: 989

Opdyke D L J 1974p Thyme oil, red. In: Food and Cosmetics Toxicology 12. Special issue I Monographs on fragrance raw materials: 1003

Opdyke D L J 1974q Vetiver oil (*Vetiveria zizanioides* Stapf.). Food and Cosmetics Toxicology 12. Special issue I Monographs on fragrance raw materials: 1013

Opdyke D L J 1974r Ginger oil. Food and Cosmetics Toxicology 12. Special issue I Monographs on fragrance raw materials: 901

Opdyke D L J 1974s Monographs on fragrance raw materials. Food and Cosmetics Toxicology 12: 731

Opdyke D L J 1974t Monographs on fragrance raw materials. Food and Cosmetics Toxicology 12: 729

Opdyke D L J 1974u Estragon oil. Monographs on fragrance raw materials. Food and Cosmetics Toxicology 12: 709–710

Opdyke D L J 1974v Monographs on fragrance raw materials. Food and Cosmetics Toxicology 12: 723

Opdyke D L J 1975a Monographs on fragrance raw materials. Food and Cosmetics Toxicology 13

Opdyke D L J 1975b Monographs on fragrance raw materials. Food and Cosmetics Toxicology 13 (suppl): 713

Opdyke D L J 1975c Linalool. In: Food and Cosmetics Toxicology 13. Special issue II Monographs on fragrance raw materials: 827

Opdyke D L J 1975d Eucalyptus oil (*Eucalyptus globulus* Labille). Food and Cosmetics Toxicology 13: 107

Opdyke D L J 1975e Rose oil (*Rosa damascena* Mill.). Food and Cosmetics Toxicology 13. Special issue II Monographs on fragrance raw materials: 913

Opdyke D L J 1975f Rose absolute, French. Food and Cosmetics Toxicology 13. Special issue II Monographs on fragrance raw materials: 911

Opdyke D L J 1975g Clove bud oil (*Eugenia* ssp.) Food and Cosmetics Toxicology 13. Special issue II Monographs on fragrance raw materials: 761

Opdyke D L J 1976a Monographs on fragrance raw materials. Food and Cosmetics Toxicology 14: 197

Opdyke D L J 1976b Monographs on fragrance raw materials. Food and Cosmetics Toxicology 14: 457

Opdyke D L J 1976c Monographs on fragrance raw materials. Food and Cosmetics Toxicology 14: 307

Opdyke D L J 1976d Monographs on fragrance raw materials. Food and Cosmetics Toxicology 14: 337

Opdyke D L J 1976e Monographs on fragrance raw materials. Food and Cosmetics Toxicology14(suppl.): 813

Opdyke D L J 1976f Monographs on fragrance raw materials. Food and Cosmetics Toxicology 14: 335

Opdyke D L J 1976g Cedarwood oil Atlas. Food and Cosmetics Toxicology 14. Special issue III Monographs on fragrance raw materials: 709

Opdyke D L j 1976h Neroli oil, Tunisian. Food and Cosmetics Toxicology 14. Special issue III Monographs on fragrance raw materials: 813

Opdyke D L J 1976i Myrrh oil (*Commiphora* ssp.). Food and Cosmetics Toxicology 14: 621

Opdyke D L J 1976j Juniper oil (*Juniperus communis* L.). Food and Cosmetics Toxicology 14: 333

Opdyke D L J 1976k Lavender oil (*Lavandula officinalis* Chaix). Food and Cosmetics Toxicology 14: 451

Opdyke D L J 1976l Lavandin oil (*Lavandula hybrida*). Food and Cosmetics Toxicology 14: 447

Opdyke D L J 1976m Cajeput oil (*Melaleuca leucadendron* L.). Food and Cosmetics Toxicology 14. Special issue III Monographs on fragrance raw materials: 701

Opdyke D L J 1976n Nutmeg oil, East Indian. Food and Cosmetics Toxicology 14: 631

Opdyke D L J 1976o Marjoram oil, sweet (*Origanum majorana*). Food and Cosmetics Toxicology 14: 469

Opdyke D L J 1976p Pinus sylvestris oil. Food and Cosmetics Toxicology 14. Special issue III Monographs on fragrance raw materials: 845

Opdyke D L J 1976q Savory summer oil (*Satureia hortensis* L.). In: Food and Cosmetics Toxicology 14. Special issue III Monographs on fragrance raw materials: 859

Opdyke D L J 1976r Marjoram oil, Spanish (*Thymus mastichina*). In: Food and Cosmetics Toxicology 14: 467

Opdyke D L J 1978a Bois de rose, Brazilian. Food and Cosmetics Toxicology 16 suppl 1. Special issue IV Monographs on fragrance raw materials: 653

Opdyke D L J 1978b Olibanum absolute. In: Food and Cosmetics Toxicology 16 suppl 1. Special issue IV Monographs on fragrance raw materials: 835

Opdyke D L J 1978c Cypress oil. Food and Cosmetics Toxicology 16. Special issue IV Monographs on fragrance raw materials: 699

Opdyke D L J 1978d Hyssop oil (*Hyssopus officinalis* L.). Food and Cosmetics Toxicology 16. Special issue IV Monographs on fragrance raw materials: 783

Opdyke D L J 1978e Pepper, black, oil (*Piper nigrum* L.) Food and Cosmetics Toxicology 16. Special issue IV Monographs on fragrance raw materials: 651

Opdyke D L J 1982a Monographs on fragrance raw materials. Food and Cosmetics Toxicology 20

Opdyke D L J 1982b Tagetes oil (*Tagetes erecta* L.; *T. patula* L.; or *T. glandulifera* Schrank). Food and Cosmetics Toxicology 20. Special issue VI Monographs on fragrance raw materials: 829

Opdyke D L J 1992 Monographs on fragrance raw materials. Food and Cosmetics Toxicology 30

Opdyke D L J, Letizia C 1982a Patchouli oil. Food and Chemical Toxicology 20 (suppl): 791

Opdyke D L J, Letizia C 1982b Clary oil. Food and Chemical Toxicology 20 (suppl): 823

Oser B L et al 1965 Food and Cosmetics Toxicology 3: 563

Ostad S N, Soodi M, Shariffzadeh M, Khorshidi N, Marzban H 2001 The effect of fennel essential oil on uterine contraction as a model for dysmenorrhoea, pharmacology and toxicology study. Journal of Ethnopharmacology 76: 299–304

Ozaki Y, Kawahara N, Harada M 1991 Anti-inflammatory effect of *Zingiber cassumunar* Roxb. and its active principles. Chemical and Pharmacological Bulletin (Tokyo) Sep: 39(9): 2353–2356

Pandit V A, Shelef L A 1994 Sensitivity of *Listeria monocytogenes* to rosemary (*Rosmarinus officinalis* L.). Food Microbiology 11: 57–63

Patakova D, Chladek M 1974 The antibacterial activity of thyme and wild oils. Pharmazie 29: 140

Patel S, Wiggins J 1980 Eucalyptus oil poisoning. Archives of Disease in Childhood 5: 405–406

Pathak M A, Fitzpatrick T B 1959 Relation of molecular configuration to the furocoumarins which increase the cutaneous responses following long wave ultraviolet radiation. Journal of Investigative Dermatology 32: 255–262

Pellecuer J, Allegrini J, Simeon de Buochberg M, Passet J 1975 The place of *Satureia montana* L. (Lamiaceae) essential oil in the therapeutic arsenal. Plantes Médicinales Phytothérapie 9(2): 99–106

Penfold A R, Willis J L 1961 The eucalypts. Leonard Hill, London

Pénoël D 1991 Médecine aromatique, médecine planetaire. Jollois, Limoges

Pénoël D 1993 A special eucalyptus (*E. smithii*). The Aromatherapist 1(2): (insert)

Perry L M 1980 Medicinal plants of East and Southeast Asia. MIT Press, Cambridge MA, p. 620

Perry N B et al 1997a Essential oils from New Zealand Manuka and Kanuka: chemotaxonomy of *Kunzea*. Phytochemistry 45: 606–612

Perry N B et al 1997b Essential oils from New Zealand Manuka and Kanuka: chemotaxonomy of *Leptospermum*. Phytochemistry 44: 1485–1494

Perucci S, Macchioni G, Cioni P C, Flamini G, Morelli I, Taccini F 1996 The activity of volatile compounds from *Lavandula angustifolia* against *Psoroptes cuniculi*. Phytotherapy Research 10(1): 5–8

Peterson H R, Hall A 1946 Dermal irritating properties of perfume materials. Drug and Cosmetic Industry, 58 (January): 113

Phillips H F 1989 What thyme is it? A guide to the thyme taxa cultivated in the United States. In: Simon J E (ed) Proceedings of the fourth national herb growing and marketing conference. International Herb Growers and Marketers Association, Silver Spring, USA

Phillips H F 1991 The best of thymes. The Herb Companion April/May: 22–29

Piccaglia R, Deans S G, Marotti M, Eaglesham E 1993 Biological activity of essential oils of lavender, sage, winter savory and thyme of Italian origin. Programme Abstracts. 24th International Symposium of Essential Oils

Piromrat K, Tuchinda M et al 1986 Antihistaminic effect of plai (*Zingiber cassumunar* Roxb.) on histamine skin test in asthmatic children. Siriraj Hospital Gazette 38(4): 251–256

Pizsolitto A C 1975 Rev. Fac. Farm. Odontol. Araraquara 9: 55 In: Chemical Abstracts 1977 86: 12226s

Pongprayoon U, Soontornsaratune P, Jarakasem S, Sematong T, Wasuwat S, Claeson P 1996 Topical anti–inflammatory activity of the major lipophilic constituents of the rhizome of *Zingiber cassumunar*. Part 1: the essential oil. Phytomedicine 3(4): 319–322

Poretta A, Casolari A 1966 Industria Conserve (Parma) 41: 287 In: Chemical Abstracts 1967 66: 84879s

Porter N G, Wilkins A L 1998 Chemical, physical and antimicrobial properties of essential oils of *Leptospermum scoparium* and *Kunzea ericoides*. Phytochemistry 50(3): 407–415

Prager M J, Miskiewicz M A 1979 Gas chromatographic-mass spectrometric analysis, identification and detection of adulteration of lavender, lavandin and spike lavender oils. Journal of the American Organization of Analytical Chemists 62: 1231–1238

Prakash S et al 1972 Indian Oil Soap Journal 37: 230 Chemical Abstracts 1973 79: 727y

Prakash V 1990 Leafy spices. CRC Press, Boca Raton

Price S 2000 Aromatherapy workbook. Thorsons, London, pp. 45, 72

Ramadan F M et al 1972a Chemische Mikrobiologische Technologische Lebensmittel 1: 96

Ramadan F M et al 1972b Chemische Mikrobiologische Technologische Lebensmittel 2: 51

Ramadan F M et al 1972c Chemische Mikrobiologische Technologische Lebensmittel 1: 96

Raman A, Weir U, Bloomfield S F 1995 Antimicrobial effects of tea tree oil, and its major components on *Staphylococcus aureus*, *Staph. epidermidis* and *Propionibacterium acnes*. Letters of Applied Microbiology 21(4): 242–245

Ramaswami S K et al 1988. In Lawrence B M et al Flavors and fragrances: a world perspective. Elsevier, Amsterdam p. 951

Rao B G V N, Joseph P L 1971 Die Wirksamt einiger Ätherischer Öle gegenüber phytopathogenen Fungi. Riechstoffe Aromatische 21: 405

Razdan T K, Wanchoo R K, Dhar K L 1986 Parfum Kosmet 67(1): 52–53

Recio M C et al 1989 Antimicrobial activity of selected plants employed in the Spanish Mediterranean area. Part II. Phytotherapy Research 3: 77

Rees W D, Evans B K, Rhodes J 1979 Treating irritable bowel syndrome with peppermint oil. British Medical Journal 2(6194): 835–836

Reichling J, Becker H, Drager P-D 1978 Herbicides in chamomile cultivation. Acta Horticultiva 73: 331–338

Reynolds J E F (ed) 1972 Martindale: the extra pharmacopoeia, 26th edn. Pharmaceutical Press, London

Reynolds J E F (ed) 1989 Martindale: the extra pharmacopoeia, 29th edn. Pharmaceutical Press, London

Reynolds J E F (ed) 1993 Martindale: the extra pharmacopoeia, 30th edn. Pharmaceutical Press, London

Riek 1994 COST B4 Unconventional medicine in Europe. Responses to the COST B4 questionnaire. European Commission, Luxembourg

Rodriguez E, Towers G H N, Mitchell J C 1976 Biological activities of sesquiterpenes lactones. Phytochemistry 15: 1573–1580

Rook M J 1979 Botanical dermatology: plant and plant products injurious to the skin. Greengrass, Vancouver

Rose F J C, Field W E H 1965 Food and Cosmetics Toxicology 3: 311

Rose J E, Behm F M 1994 Inhalation of vapor from black pepper extract reduces smoking withdrawal symptoms. Drug and Alcohol Dependence 34: 225–229

Rossi T, Melegari M, Bianchi A, Albasini A, Vampa G 1988 Sedative, antiinflammatory and antidiuretic effects in rats by essential oils of varieties of *Anthemis nobilis*: a comprehensive study. Pharmacological Research Communications 20(5): 71–74

Röst L C M, Bos R 1979 Biosystematic investigation with Acorus. 3. Communication. Constituents of essential oils. Planta Medica 36: 350–361

Roulier G 1990 Les huiles essentielles pour votre santé. Dangles, St-Jean-de-Braye

Rouvière A, Meyer M-C 1983 La santé par les huiles essentielles. M.A. editions, Paris, p. 30

Rovesti P, Colombo E 1973 Contact Dermatitis 2: 196–200

Saeed S A, Gilani A H 1994 Antithrombotic activity of clove oil. Journal of the Pakistan Medical Association 44(5): 112–115

Saksena N, Tripathi H H S 1985 Plant volatiles in relation to fungistasis. Fitoterapia 56(4): 243–244

Salamon I 1992 Chamomile production in Czecho-Slovakia. Focus on Herbs 10: 1–8

Saleh M M, Hashem F A, Grace M H 1996 Volatile oil of Egyptian sweet fennel (*Foeniculum vulgare* var. *dulce* Alef.) and its effects on isolated smooth muscles. Pharmacy and Pharmacology Letters 6(1): 5–7

Sangster S A et al 1987 The metabolic disposition of (methoxy-C) labelled trans-anethole, estragole and p-propylanisole in human volunteers. Xenobiotica 17: 1223–1232

Sanyal A, Varma K C 1969 *In vitro* antibacterial and antifungal activity of *Mertha aversis* var. *piparescens* oil obtained from different sources. Indian Journal of Microbiology 9(1): 23–24

Satchell A C, Saurajen A, Bell C, Barnetson R StC 2002 Treatment of interdigital *Tinea pedis* with 25% and 50% tea tree oil solution: a randomised, placebo-controlled, blinded study. Australasian Journal of Dermatology 43: 175–178

Saxena B P et al 1977 A new insect chemosterilant isolated from *Acorus calamus* L. Nature 270: 512–513

SCCP (Scientific Committee on Consumer Products) 2004 Opinion on tea tree oil. European Commission Report SCCP/0843/04

Schilcher H, Leuschner F 1997 Studies of potential nephrotoxic effects of juniper essential oil. Arzneimittel Forschung 47(7): 855–858

Schnaubelt K 1998 Advanced aromatherapy. Healing Arts Press, Rochester, Vermont

Schnitzler P, Schon K, Reichling J 2001 Antiviral activity of Australian tea tree oil and eucalyptus oil against *Herpes simplex* virus in cell culture. Pharmazie 56: 343–347

Schwarz L 1934 Skin hazards in American industry. Part 1. US Publication Health Bulletin no 215

Schwarz L, Peck S M 1946 Cosmetics and dermatitis. Hoeber, New York

Schwarz L, Tulipan L, Peck S M 1947 Occupational diseases of the skin. Lea & Febiger, Philadelphia

Secondini O 1990 Handbook of perfumes and flavors. Chemical Publishing, New York

Seth G, Kokate C K, Varma K C 1976 Effect of essential oil of *Cymbopogon citratus* Stapf. on the central nervous system. Indian Journal Experimental Biology 14(3): 370–371

Sewell J S 1925 Poisoning by eucalyptus oil. British Medical Journal 1: 922

Shafran I, Maurer W, Thomas F B 1977 Prostaglandins and Crohn's disease. New England Journal of Medicine 296: 694

Sharma J N, Ishak F I, Yusof A P M, Srivastava K C 1997 Effects of eugenol and ginger oil on adjuvant arthritis and kallikreins in rats. Asia Pacific Journal of Pharmacology 12(1–2): 9–14

Sharma V D, Prasad G, Singh A K, Battacharya A K, Singh K, Gupta K C 1985 Antimicrobial activity of essential oil of *Illicium verum* Hook. Indian Journal of Microbiology 25(3,4): 221–222

Sherry E, Boeck H, Warnke P H 2001 Topical application of a new formulation of eucalyptus oil phytochemical clears methicillin-resistant *Staphylococcus aureus* infection. American Journal of Infection Control 29: 346

Shrivastav P, George K, Balasubramaniam N, Padmini Jasper M, Thomas M, Kanagasabhapathy A S 1988 Suppression of puerperal lactation using jasmine flowers (*Jasminum sambac*). Australian and New Zealand Journal of Obstetrics and Gynaecology 28: 68–71

Shu C K, Waradt J P, Taylor W I 1975 Improved methods for bergapten determination by high performance liquid chromatography. Journal of Chromatography 106: 271–282

Shukla H S, Tripathi S C 1987a Antifungal substance in the essential oil of anise (*Pimpinella anisum* L.). Agricultural Biological Chemistry 51(7): 1991–1993

Shukla H S, Tripathi S C 1987b Studies on physico-chemical, phytotoxic and fungitoxic properties of essential oil of *Foeniculum vulgare* Mill. Beiträge zur Biologie der Pflanzen 62: 149–158

Sigmund C J, McNally E F 1969 The action of a carminative on the lower oesophageal sphincter. Gastroenterology 56: 13–18

Silva J, Abebe W, Sousa S M, Duarte V G, Machado M I L, Matos F J A 2003 Analgesia and antiinflammatory effects of essential oils of Eucalyptus. Journal of Ethnopharmacology 89(2–3): 277–283

Silyanovska K et al 1969 Parfümerie and Kosmetik 50: 293

Simeon de Bouchberg M et al 1976 Rivista Italiano Esseny, Profumi, Piante Offic. Aromi, Safoni, Cosmet Aerosol 58: 527 In: Chemical Abstracts 1977 86: 84201c

Simpson E 1993 Essential oils and the ageing process. Aroma 93 Symposium, Brighton

Singatwadia A, Katewa S S 2001 *In vitro* studies on antifungal activity of essential oil of *Cymbopogon martinii* and *Cymbopogon citratus*. Indian Perfumer 45(1): 53–55

Singh G, Upadhyay R K 1991 Fungitoxic activity of cumaldehyde, main constituent of the *Cuminum cyminum* oil. fitoterapia 62(1): 86

Singh A K, Dikshit A, Dixit S N 1983 Fungitoxic properties of essential oil of *Mentha arvensis* var. *piparescens*. Perfumer & Flavorist 8: 55–58

Singh S P, Negli S, Chand L, Singh A K 1992 Antibacterial and antifungal activities of Mentha arvensis essential oil. Fitoterapia 63(1): 76–78

Singh G, Upadhyay R K, Narayanan C S, Padmkumari K P, Rao G P 1993 Chemical and fungitoxic investigations on the essential oil of *Citrus sinensis* (L.) Pers. Journal of Plant Disease and Protectection 100(1): 69–74

Singh H B, Srivastava M, Singh A B, Srivastava A K 1995 Cinnamon bark oil, a potent fungitoxicant against fungi causing respiratory tract mycoses. Allergy 50(12): 995–999

Sivropoulou A, Papanikolaou E, Nikolaou C, Kokkini S, Lanaras T, Arsenakis M 1996 Antimicrobial and cytotoxic activities of Origanum essential oils. Journal of Agricultural Food Chemistry 44(5): 1202–1205

Sparavigna A, Viscardi G, Galbiati G 1993 Evaluation of the antimicrobial effectiveness of a detergent with a base of thyme and sage essential oils. Giornale Italanio di Dermatologia e Venereologia 128(9): 95–98

Sparks M J W, O'Sullivan P, Herrington A A, Morcos S K 1995 Does peppermint oil relieve spasm during barium enema? British Journal of Radiology 68(812): 841–843

Stanic G, Samarzija I 1993 Diuretic activity of *Satureia montana* subsp. *montana* extracts and oil in rats. Phytotherapy Research 7(5): 363–366

Stiles J C, Sparks M S, Ronzio B S, Ronzio R A 1995 The inhibition of Candida albicans by oregano. Journal of Applied Nutrition 47(4): 96–102

Storp F 1996 Harze in der Parfümerie. Drom, Baierbrunn p. 38

Stuart M (ed) 1982 Herbs and herbalism. Van Nostrand. Reinhold, New York p. 57

Stuart M ed 1987 Encyclopedia of herbs and herbalism. Black Cat, London

Subba M S et al 1967 Antimicrobial action of citrus oils. Journal of Food Science 32: 225–227

Suleimanova A B, Fedotov V P, Gladyshev V V, Koryakovsky V A 1995 Experimental assessment of fungicidal activity of 3% ointment with wild rosemary ether oil in external therapy of *T. rubrum*-induced mycosis of the soles. Vestnik Dermatologii e Venerologii 0(1): 17–18

Svoboda K P, Deans S G 1990 A study of the variability of rosemary and sage and their volatile oils on the British market: their antioxidant properties. Flavor and Fragrance Journal 7: 81–87

Swales N J, Caldwell J 1992 Cytotoxicity and depletion of glutathione (GSH) by cinnamaldehyde in rat hepatocytes. Human and Experimental Toxicology 10: 488–489

Swanson A B et al 1981 The side-chain epoxidation and hydroxylation of the hepatocarcinogens safrole and estragole and some related compounds by rat and mouse liver microsomes. Biochemica Biophysica Acta 673: 504

Szelenyi I, Thiemer O I K 1979 Pharmacological investigations with compounds of chamomile. III. Experimental studies of the ulcer protective effect of chamomile. Planta Medica 35: 218–227

Taddei I, Giachetti D, Taddei E, Mantovani P 1988 Spasmolytic activity of peppermint, sage and rosemary essences and their major constituents. Fitoterapia 59(6): 463–468

Takechi M, Tanaka Y 1981 Purification and characterization of antiviral substance eugeniin from the bud of *Syzygium aromaticum*. Planta Medica 42(1): 69

Tasev T, Toleva P, Balabanova V 1969 The neuro-psychic effect of Bulgarian rose, lavender and geranium. Folia Medica 11(5): 307–317

Taylor B D, Luscombe D K, Duthie H L 1983 Inhibitory effect of peppermint oil on gastrointestinal smooth muscle. Gut 24: 992

Taylor J M et al 1967 Toxicity of oil of calamus (Jammu variety). Toxicology and Applied Pharmacology 10: 405

Terhune S J et al 1974 International Congress of Essential Oils (Pap.) 6: 153

Tester-Dalderup C B M 1980 Drugs used in bronchial asthma and cough. In: Dukes M N G (ed) Meyler's side effects of drugs, 9th edn. Excerpta Medica, Amsterdam

Thailand Institute of Scientific and Technological Research, Chatuchak

Thulin M, Claeson P 1991 The botanical origin of scented myrrh (bisabolol or habak hadi).

Tierra M 1980 The way of herbs. Unity Press, Santa Cruz CA

Tisserand R, Balacs T 1995a Essential oil safety. Churchill Livingstone, New York, pp. 98–99

Tisserand R, Balacs T 1995b Essential oil safety; a guide for health care professionals. Churchill Livingstone, Edinburgh, pp. 186, 210

Tiwari R, Dixit V, Dixit S N 1994 Studies on fungitoxic properties of essential oil of *Cinnamomum zeylanicum* Breyn. Indian Perfumer 38(3): 98–104

Tong M M, Altman P M, Barnetson R StC 1992 Tea tree oil in the treatment of *Tinea pedi*s. Australasian Journal of Dermatology 33(3): 145–149

Torii S, Fakuda H, Kanemoto H, Miyanchi R, Hamanzu Y, Kavasaki M 1988 Contingent negative variation and the psychological effects of odour. In: Van Toller S, Dodd G H (eds) 1988 Perfumery. The psychology and biology of fragrance. Chapman & Hall, London, pp. 107–120

Tovey E, McDonald L G 1997 A simple washing procedure with

eucalyptus oil for controlling house dust mites and their allergens in clothing and bedding. Journal of Allergy and Clinical Immunology 100(4): 464–466

Trease G E, Evans W C 1983 Pharmacognosy, 13th edn. Baillière Tindall, Eastbourne

Trevelyan J 1993 Aromatherapy. Nursing Times 89(25): 38–40

Trigg J K 1996 Evaluation of a Eucalyptus based repellent against *Anopheles* ssp. in Tanzania. Journal of the American Mosquito Control Association 12(2): 243–246

Trigg J K, Hill N 1996 Laboratory evaluation of a eucalyptus based repellent against four biting arthropods. Phytotherapy Research 10(4): 313–316

Tsoukatou M, Roussis V, Chinou I, Petrakis P, Ortiz A 1999 Chemical composition of the essential oils and headspace samples of two *Helichrysum* species occurring in Spain. Journal of Essential Oil Research 11: 511–516

Tubaro A, Zilli C, Redaelli C, Della Loggia R 1984 Evaluation of antiinflammatory activity of a chamomile extract topical application. Planta Medica 50(4): 359

Tucker A O 1986 Frankincense and myrrh. Economical Botany 40(4): 425–433

Tulipan L 1938 Cosmetic irritants. Archiva Dermatologica 38: 906

Tyler V E 1982 The honest herbal: a sensible guide to the use of herbs and related remedies. Stickley, Philadelphia, p. 263

Tyler V E 1992 Phytomedicines in Western Europe: their potential impact on herbal medicine in the United States. Lecture delivered at the annual meeting of the American Chemical Society, San Francisco, April

Tyler V E 1993 The honest herbal: a sensible guide to the use of herbs and related remedies, 3rd edn. Stickley, Philadelphia

Uehleke H, Brinkschulte-Freitas M 1979 Oral toxicity of an essential oil from myrtle and adaptive liver stimulation. Toxicology 12(3): 335–332

Umezu T 1999 Anticonflict effects of plant derived essential oils. Pharmacology, Biochemistry and Behaviour 64(1): 35–40

Urbach F, Forbes P D 1973 Report to RIFM, 16 August

Uzdenikov B N 1970 Nauchi Trudove Tyumen. Sel. Khoz. Inst. 7: 116 through Chemical Abstracts 1972 77: 8429x

Valnet J 1980 The practice of aromatherapy. Daniel, Saffron Walden

Van Den Broucke C O, Lernli J A 1981 Pharmacological and chemical investigation of thyme liquid extracts. Planta Medica 41: 129–135

Verma M M 1981 Dissertation Abstracts Int. B 41(12 pt 1): 4514

Vichkanova S A et al 1977 through Chemical Abstracts 1977 87: 162117s

Vickers A 1995 COST Action B4 Unconventional medicine. First annual report 1993–94. European Commission, Luxembourg

Vömel A, Reichling J, Becker H, Dräger P D 1977 Herbicides in the cultivation of *Matricaria chamomilla*. 1st communication: influence of herbicides on flower and weed production. Planta Medica 31: 378–379

Von Skramlik E V 1959 Über die Giftigkeit und Verträglichkeit von Ätherischen Ölen. Pharmazie 14: 435–445

Wagner H, Bladt S, Zgainski E M 1984 Plant drug analysis. Springer-Verlag, Berlin, p. 13

Wagner H, Proksh A 1985 An immunostimulating active principle from *Eckinaceae purpurae*. Farnsworth N, Hikino N H, Wagner H (eds) Economic and medicinal plant research. Vol. 1 Academic Press, New York, p. 113

Wagner H, Sprinkmeyer L 1973 Die pharmakologische Wirking von Melissengeist (Pharmacological effect of balm spirit). Deutsche Apotheke Zeitung 113: 1159–1166

Wagner H, Wierer M, Bauer R 1986 *In vitro*-Hemmung der Prostaglandin-Biosynthe durch Ätherische Öle und phenolische Verbindungen. Planta Medica 4: 185–186

Watt J M, Breyer-Brandwijk M G 1962 The medicinal and poisonous plants of Southern and Eastern Africa, 2nd edn. Churchill Livingstone, New York

Weiss E A 1997 Essential oil crops. CAB International, Oxford

Weiss R F 1988a Herbal medicine. Arcanum, Gothenburg

Weiss R F 1988b Herbal medicine. Beaconsfield Publishers, Beaconsfield

Winter R 1984 A consumer's dictionary of cosmetic ingredients. Crown, New York

Winter R 1999 A consumer's dictionary of cosmetic ingredients, 5th edn. Three Rivers, New York

Woeber K, Krombach M 1969 Zur Frage der Sensibilisierung durch Ätherische Öle (Vorläufige Mitteilung). Berufsdermatosen 17: 320

Wren R C (ed) 1988 Potter's new cyclopedia of botanical drugs and preparations, 8th edn. Daniel, Saffron Walden

Yadav P, Dubey N K 1994 Screening some essential oils against ringworm fungi. Indian Journal of Pharmaceutical Sciences 56(6): 227–230

Yagyu T 1994 Neurophysiological findings on the effects of fragrance: lavender and jasmine. Integrative Psychology 10: 64–67

Yamada K, Mimaki Y, Sashida Y 1994 Anticonvulsive effects of inhaling lavender oil vapour. Biological and Pharmaceutical Bulletin (Tokyo) 17(2): 359–360

Yang D, Michel D, Mandin D, Andriamboavonjy H, Poitry P, Chaumont J-P 1996 Antifungal and antibacterial properties, *in vitro*, of three Patchouli essential oils of different origins. Acta Botanica Gallica 143(1): 29–35

Young A R, Walker S L, Kinley J S, Plastow S R, Averbeck D, Morliere P, Dubertret L 1990 Phototumorigenesis studies of 5MOP in bergamot oil: evaluation and modification of risk in human use in an albino mouse skin model. Journal of Photochemistry and Photobiology B 7: 231–250

Zajdela F, Bisagni E 1981 5MOP, the melanogenic additive in suntan preparations is tumerogenic in mice exposed to 365 nm UV radiation. Carcinogenesis 2: 121–127

Zakarya D, Fkih-Tetouani S, Hajji F 1993 Chemical composition – antimicrobial activity relationships of Eucalyptus essential oils. Plantes Médicinales Phytothérapie 26(4): 319–331

Zangouras A et al 1981 Dose-dependent conversion of estragole in the rat and mouse to carcinogenic metabolite 1-hydroxyestragole. Biochemical Pharmacology 30: 1383–1386

Zaynoun S T, Johnson B E, Frain-Bell W 1977 A study of bergamot and its importance as a phototoxic agent. II. Factors which affect the phototoxic reaction induced by bergamot oil and psoralen derivatives. Contact Dermatitis 3: 225–239

Zheng G Q, Kenney P M, Lam L K T 1992a Anethofuran, carvone and limonene: potential cancer chemopreventative agents from dill weed oil and caraway oil. Planta Medica 58: 338–341

Zheng G, Kenney P M, Lam L K T 1992b Sesquiterpenes from clove (*Eugenia caryophyllata*) as potential anticarcinogenic agents. Journal of Natural Products 55(7): 999–1003

Zheng G, McKenney P M, Lam L K T 1992c Myristicin: a potential cancer chemopreventative agent from parsley leaf oil. Agricultural Food Chemistry 40: 107–110

Zheng G-G, Kenney P M, Lam L K T 1992d Anethofuran, carvone and limonene: potential cancer chemopreventative agents from dill weed oil and caraway oil. Planta Medica 58(4): 339–341

Zheng G, McKenney P M, Zhang J, Lam L K T 1992 Inhibition of benzo[a]pyrene-induced tumorigenesis by myristicin, a volatile aroma constituent of parsley leaf oil. Carcinogenesis 13(10): 1921–1923

Zola A, LeVanda J P 1975 Quelques huiles essentielles en provenance de la Corse. Rivista Italica 57: 467–472

Zondek B et al 1938 Phenol methyl esters as estrogenic agents. Biochemical Journal 32: 641–645

Sources to Appendices

Abdel-Malek S, Bastien J W, Mahler W F, Jia Q, Reinecke M G, Robinson W E, Shu Y, Zalles-Asin J 1996 Drug leads from the Kallawaya herbalists of Bolivia. Journal of Ethnopharmacology 50: 157–166

Adames M, Mendoza E, Ospina de Nigrinis L S 1983 Study of the essential oil of *Eucalyptus citriodora*. Bailey. Revista Colombiana Ciencias Quimica Farmacia 4(1): 95–113

Agnel R, Teisseire P 1984 Essential oil of French lavender: its composition and its adulteration. Perfumer and Flavorist 9(2): 53–56

Alberto-Puleo M 1980 Fennel and anise as estrogenic agents. Journal of Ethnopharmacology 2(4): 337–344

Al-Hader A A et al 1994 Hyperglycemic and insulin release inhibitory effects of *Rosmarinus officinalis*. Journal of Ethnopharmacology 43: 217–221

Anon 1994 Herbal licensing post. Pharmaceutical Journal 253: 746

Aschner B 1986 Lehrbuch der Konstitutionstherapie. Hippokrates, Stuttgart

Bardeau F 1976 La médicine aromatique. Robert Laffont, Paris

Bartram T 1995 Encyclopedia of herbal medicine. Grace, Christchurch

Battaglia S 1997 The complete guide to aromatherapy. Perfect Potion, Virginia, Queensland p. 200–201

Becker H, Förster W 1984 Biologie, Chemie und Pharmakologie pflanzlicher Sedativa. Zeitschrift für Phytotherapie (Stuttgart) 5: 817–823

Benigni R, Capra C, Cattorini P E 1962 Piante medicinali: chimica farmacologia e terapia. Inverni and Della Beffa, Milan

Bernadet M 1983 La phyto-aromathérapie pratique. Dangles, St-Jean-de-Braye

Beylier M F 1979 Bacteriostatic activity of some Australian essential oils. Perfumer and Flavorist 4(2): 23–25

Bown D 1995 The Royal Horticulture Society encyclopedia of herbs and their uses. Dorling Kindersley, London pp. 159, 312

Boyd E M, Pearson G L 1946 On the expectorant action of volatile oils. American Journal of Medical Science 211: 602–610

Briozzo J, Nunez L, Chirife J, Herszage L, D'Aquino M 1989 Journal of Applied Bacteriology 66(1): 69–75

British Herbal Pharmacopoeia 1983 British Herbal Medicine Association, Cowling

Bruneton J 1995 Pharmacognosy, phytochemistry, medicinal plants. Intercept, Andover

Brunke E J et al 1996 The chemistry of sandalwood fragrance. Actes des 15èmes Journées Internationales Huiles Essentielles, pp. 48–83

Budavari S (ed) 1996 The Merck index: encyclopedia of chemicals, drugs and biologicals, 12th edn. Merck, Whitehouse Station, New Jersey

Buil P, Garnero J, Guichard G 1975 Composition chimique de l'huile essentielle de verveine de Provence. Rivista Italica 57: 455–466

Caldwell J et al 1990 Comparative studies on the metabolisation of food: case examples in the safety evaluation of the allylbenzene natural flavours. Nutritional Biochemistry 1: 402–409

Carson C F, Riley T V 1993 Antimicrobial activity of the essential oil of *Melaleuca alternifolia*. Letters in Applied Microbiology 16: 49–55

Carson C F, Hammer K A, Riley T V 1995 Broth microdilution method for determining the susceptibility of *Escherischia coli* and *Staphylococcus aureus* to the essential oil of *Melaleuca alternifolia* (tea tree oil). Microbios 82(332): 181–185

Chan V S W, Caldwell J 1992 Comparative induction of unscheduled DNA synthesis in cultured rat hepatocytes allylbenzenes and their 1'-hydroxy metabolites. Food and Chemical Toxicology 30(10): 831–836

Chandler R F, Hooper S N, Harvey M J 1982 Ethnobotany and phytochemistry of yarrow, *Achillea millefolium*, Compositae. Economic Botany 36(2): 203–223

Chen Y-D, Yang L, Li S-X, Jiang Z-R 1983 Study on the chemical components of essential oil from the leaves of *Eucalyptus* spp. Chemical Industries Forest Products 3(2): 14–31

Clarke S 2002 Essential chemistry for safe aromatherapy. Churchill Livingstone, Edinburgh

De Vincenzi M, Dessi M R 1991 Botanical flavouring substances used in foods: proposal of classification. Fitoterapia 62(1): 39–63

Deans S G, Svoboda K P 1990 The antimicrobial properties of marjoram (*Origanum majorana* L.) Volatile oil. Flavor and Fragrance Journal 5(3): 187–190

Deans S G, Svoboda K P et al 1992 Essential oil profiles of several temperate and tropical aromatic plants: their antimicrobial and antioxidant properties. Acta Horticulturae 306: 229–232

Denny E F K 1981 The history of lavender oil: disturbing inferences for the future of essential oils. Perfumer & Flavorist 6: 23–25

Do Vgich N A 1971 Antimicrobial effect of essential oils. Mikrobiolohichnyi Zhurnal (Kiev) 33: 253–259

Duke J A 1982 Herbs as a small farm enterprise and the value of aromatic plants as economic intercrops. Research for small farms. In: Kerr H W, Knutson L (eds) Proceedings of a Special Symposium. USDA Miscellaneous Publications no. 1422, p. 76

Duke J A 1987 CRC handbook of medicinal herbs. CRC Press, Boca Raton, Florida

Duraffourd P 1987 Les huiles essentielles et la santé. La Maison de Bien-Etre, Montreuil-sous-Bois

Engen T 1982 The perception of odors. Academic Press, New York

Formacek K, Kubeczka K H 1982 Essential oils analysis by capillary chromatography and carbon-13 NMR spectroscopy. John Wiley, New York

Forster H B, Niklas H, Lutz S 1980 Planta Medica 40(4): 309

Franchomme P, Pénoël D 1985 Aromatherapy: advanced therapy for infectious illnesses (1). Phytoguide no 1, International Phytomedical Foundation, La Courtête

Garnero J, Buil P, Tabacchi R 1976 Composition chimique de l'huile essentielle de verveine-les alcools sesquiterpences. Rivista Italica 58: 486–493

Gottlieb O R, Fineberg M, Guimasraes M L, Taveira Magalhaes M, Maravalhas N 1964 Notes on Brazilian rosewood. Perfume and Essential Oil Records 55: 253–257

Grieve M 1980 A moderm herbal. Penguin, Harmondsworth

Grieve M 1998 A modern herbal. Tiger Books International, London

Guba R 1994 'New' essential oils. Journal of International Federation of Aromatherapists (Australia) Issue 12

Gümbel D 1986 Principles of holistic skin therapy with herbal essences. Haug, Heidelberg

Harkiss K J 1993 Eight peak index of essential oils, version 2.2. Self published, Bingley

Hay R K M 1993 Physiology. In: Hay & Waterman (eds): Volatile oil crops. Longman, Harlow pp. 23–43

Hoffman W 1979 Lavendel-Inhaltsstoffe und ausgewählte Synthesen. Seifen-Öle-Fette-Wachse 105: 287–291

Hunt R S, von Rudloff 1974 Chemosystematic studies in the genus Abies. 1. Leaf and twig oil analysis of alpine and balsam firs. Canadian Journal of Botany 52: 477–487

Kaul V K, Nigam S S 1977 Antibacterial and antifungal studies of some essential oils. Journal of Research in Indian Medicine, Yoga and Homoeopathy 12: 132–135

Knobloch K, Pauli A, Iberl B, Weigand H, Weiss N 1989 Antibacterial and antifungal properties of essential oil components. Journal of Essential Oil Research 1: 119–128

Krall B, Drause W 1994 Mint oil relieves injury pain. Cited in Journal of International Federation of Aromatherapists (Australia) Issue 12

Kresánek J 1982 Healing plants. Byeway Books

Lahariya A K, Rao J T 1979 In vitro antimicrobial studies of the essential oil of Cyperus scariosus and Ocimum basilicum. Indian Drugs 16: 150–152

Landis R 1998 Herbal defence. Harper Collins, London

Lautié R, Passebecq A 1979 Aromatherapy. Thorsons, Wellingborough

Law D 1982 The concise herbal encyclopedia. Bartholomew, Edinburgh

Lawless J 1992 The encyclopaedia of essential oils. Element, Shaftesbury

Lawrence B M 1979 Essential oils 1976–1978. Allured, Wheaton

Lawrence B M 1981 Essential oils 1979–1980. Allured, Wheaton

Lawrence B M 1987/1988 Progress in essential oils. Perfumer & Flavorist 12(6): 59

Lawrence B M 1989 Essential oils 1981–1987. Allured, Wheaton, pp. 187–188

Lawrence B M 1993 Essential oils 1988–1991. Allured, Wheaton

Lin T S 1981 Study on the variation of yield and composition of essential oil from Litsea cubeba. Bulletin of the Taiwan Forestry Research Institute, No. 355. 14 pp.

Mailhebiau P 1989 La nouvelle aromathérapie. Vie Nouvelle, Toulouse

Manitto P, Monti D, Colombo E 1972 Two new beta-diketones from Helichrysum italicum. Phytochemistry 11: 2112–2114

Masada Y 1976 Analysis of essential oils by gas chromatography and mass spectrometry. John Wiley, New York

May B et al 1996 Efficacy of a fixed peppermint oil/caraway oil combination in non-ulcer dyspepsia. Arzneimittel-Forschung/Drug Research 46(11): 1149–1153

Merck Index 1983 An encyclopedia of chemicals and drugs, 10th edn. Merck, Rahway NJ

Miller E C et al 1983 Structure-activity studies of the carcinogenicities in the mouse and rat of some naturally occurring and synthetic alkenylbenzene derivatives related to safrole and estragole. Cancer Research 43: 1124–1134

Miranda M, Perez Zayas J 1985 Influencia de la epoca de recoleccion sobre el rendimiento de aceite esencial la composicion quimica del Eucalyptus citriodora Hook. que crece in Cuba. Revista Cubana Farmacia 19: 121–127

Miranda M, Perez Zayas J, Rosado A 1983 Estudio de la composition quimica del aceite esencial de Eucalyptus citriodora Hook. Revista Ciencias Quimica 14: 211–221

Miranda Martinez M, Perez Guimeras J L, Magraner Hernandez J et al 1992 Antibacterial activity of essential oil components. International Journal of Food Microbiology 16: 337–342

Montejo L 1986 Estudio preliminar de los aceites esenciales de esperie de eucalyptus introducidas en la region de topes de Collantes. Revista Cubana Farmacia 20: 159–168

Mosley J 1979 Jane Mosley's Derbyhire remedies (1669–1712). Derbyshire Museum Service, Derby

Mwangi J W, Guantai A N, Muriuki G 1981 Eucalyptus citriodora – essential oil content and chemical varieties in Kenya. East African Agriculture and Forestry Journal 46(4): 89–96

Nigam I C, Levi L 1963 Essential oils and their constituents XIX. Detection of new trace components in oil of rosewood. Perfume and Essential Oil Record 54: 814–816

Nishimura H, Kaku K, Nakamura T, Fukazawa Y, Mizutani J 1982 Allelopathic substances (±)-p-menthan-3,8-diols isolated from Eucalyptus citriodora Hook. Agricultural, Biological and Chemical 46: 319–320

Opdyke D L J (ed) 1979 Monographs on fragrance raw materials. Pergamon Press, Oxford

Pénoël D 1994 A staple essential oil: presentation of a new eucalyptus oil – Eucalyptus staigeriana – for aromatherapists. The Aromatherapist 1(3): 22–27

Pénoël D, Pénoël R-M 1992 Pratique aromatique familiale. Osmobiose, Aoste

Perry L M 1980 Medicinal plants of East and Southeast Asia. MIT Press, Cambridge

Peyron L, Roubaud M 1971 L'essence d'imortelle del'Estorel. Parfumerie, Cosmetiques et Savons 1: 129–138

Price S 2000 The aromatherapy workbook. Thorsons, London

Renz-Rathfelder S 1986 Vom Duft der Pflanzen. Palmengarten, Frankfurt

Reynolds J E F (ed) 1993 Martindale: the extra pharmacopoeia, 30th edn. Pharmaceutical Press, London

San Martin R, Granger R, Adzet T, Passer J, Tevlade-Arbousset M G 1973 Chemical polymorphism in two Mediterranean labiates, Satureia montana L. and Satureia obovata Lag. Plantes Médicinales et Phytothérapie 7: 95

Schnaubelt K 1995 Neue Aromatherapie. vgs, Köln

Shaw A C 1953 The essential oil of Abies balsamea (L.) Mill. Canadian Journal of Chemistry 31: 193–199

Stanic G, Samarzija I 1993 Diuretic activity of Satureia montana ssp. montana extracts and oil in rats. Phytotherapy Research 7(5): 363

Starý F 1998 The natural guide to medicinal herbs and plants. Tiger Books International, Twickenham

Stevenson C J 1994 The psychophysiological effects of aromatherapy massage following cardiac surgery. Complementary Therapies in Medicine 2: 27–35

Stewart M 1987 The encyclopedia of herbs and herbalism. Black Cat, London

Sugimoto S, Kato T 1983 Composition of eucalyptus oils. Kanzei Chuo Bunsekisho Ho 2: 31–34

Tantaoui-Elaraki A, Beraoud L 1994 Journal of Environmental Pathology, Toxicology and Oncology 13(1): 67–72

Tong M M, Altman P M, Barnetson R S 1992 Tea tree oil in the treatment of *Tinea pedis*. Australian Journal of Dermatology 33(3): 145–149

Tucker A O, Tucker S S 1988 Catnip and the catnip response. Economic Botany 42(2): 214–231

Viaud H 1983 Huiles essentielles: hydrolats. Présence, Sisteron

Wagner H, Bladt S, Zgainski E M 1983 Plant drug analysis. Springer-Verlag, Berlin

Weiss E A 1997 Essential oil crops. CAB International, Wallingford

Williams D G 1996 The chemistry of essential oils. Micelle Press, Weymouth

Yamada K, Mimaki Y, Sashida Y 1994 Anticonvulsive effects of inhaling lavender oil vapour. Biological and Pharmaceutical Bulletin 17(2): 359–360

Glossary

abortifacient: inducing an abortion; causing expulsion of the foetus

adaptogenic: having a positive general effect on the body irrespective of disease condition, especially under stress

alcohols: group of hydrocarbon compounds frequently found in volatile oils

aldehydes: class of organic compounds standing between alcohols and acids

allelopathy: a plant exerting an adverse influence over another to protect its environment by the production of a chemical inhibitor, usually a terpenoid or a phenol

allopathy: system of medicine which uses drugs with effects opposite to the symptoms produced by the disease (in contrast to homoeopathy)

amenorrhoea: absence of menstruation outside pregnancy in premenopausal women

analeptic: a restorative remedy (in former times smelling salts) for states of weakness that are frequently accompanied by dizziness and fainting

anaphrodisiac: of a drug, diminishing sexual drive

anodyne: relieving pain; analgesic

anthelmintic: destructive of intestinal worms; see vermifugal

antiphlogistic: see antipyretic

antipyretic: counteracting inflammation or fever

antithermic: cooling; antipyretic

antitussive: relieving or preventing coughing

anxiolytic: relieving anxiety and tension

aperient: mildly laxative

aperitive: stimulating the appetite

aromatic: organic chemical compound derived from benzene; also called aromatic compound

astringent: causing contraction of living tissues (often mucous membranes), reducing haemorrhages, secretions, diarrhoea, etc.

balneotherapy: treatment by medicinal baths

bitters: botanical drugs with bitter-tasting constituents used to stimulate the gastrointestinal tract; also used as antiinflammatory agents and as relaxants

calmative: mildly sedative

cardiotonic: having a tonic effect on the heart

carminative: relieving flatulence

cathartic: strongly laxative

chemotype: visually identical plants with significantly different chemical components, resulting in different therapeutic properties; abbreviated to ct., as in *Thymus vulgaris* ct. alcohol

cholagogic: stimulating gall bladder contraction to promote the flow of bile

choleretic: stimulating the production of bile in the liver

cicatrizant: promoting formation of scar tissue and healing

cohobation: the operation of repeatedly using the water used in the distillation process of the same or fresh plant material; thus no water is discarded and water soluble molecules from the plant material are not lost

coumarin: a chemical compound, $C_9H_6O_2$, with a high boiling point (290°C) found within the lactones; hardly volatile with steam thus found mainly in expressed oils and sparingly in some distilled essential oils; characteristic smell of new-mown hay

cultivar: cultivated variety: a plant produced by horticulture or agriculture not normally occurring naturally; labelled by adding a 'name' to the species, as in *Lavandula angustifolia* 'Maillette'

depurative: purifying or cleansing

diaphoretic: causing or increasing perspiration; sudorific

digestive: aiding digestion

dysmenorrhoea: painful or difficult menstruation

dyspepsia: disturbed digestion

emmenagogic: inducing or regularizing menstruation; euphemism for abortifacient

enuresis: bedwetting

erethism: abnormal irritability or sensitivity

essential oil: plant volatile oil obtained by distillation

eubiotic: brings about conditions favourable to life and healing

eupeptic: aiding digestion

febrifuge: agent which reduces temperature; antipyretic

fixed oil: non-volatile oil; plant oils consist of esters of fatty acids, usually triacylglycerides

forma: lowest botanical rank in general use, denoting trivial differences within a species

fruit: the ripe seeds and their surrounding structures, which can be fleshy or dry

galactagogic: promoting the secretion of milk; lactogenic

genus: important botanical classification of related but distinct species given a common name; genera (pl.) are in turn grouped into families; the first word of the binomial botanical name denotes the genus

glycoside: sugar derivative found in certain plants (e.g. digoxin, used to treat heart failure)

haemoptysis: blood spitting, a symptom possibly indicating serious disease

haemostatic: checking blood flow; styptic

hallucinogen: agent affecting any or all of the senses, producing a wide range of distorted perceptions and reactions

herb: non-woody soft leafy plant; plant used in medicine and cooking

homoeopathy: system of medicine using tiny amounts of drugs which in a healthy body would produce symptoms similar to those of the disease (as distinct from allopathy)

hybrid: natural or artificially produced plant resulting from the fertilization of one species by another; indicated by 'x', as in *Mentha* x *piperita*

hyperhidrosis: excessive sweating

hyper-menorrhoea: profuse or prolonged menses

hypertensor: increasing blood pressure; pressor

hypotensor: reducing blood pressure; antihypertensive

immuno-stimulant: stimulating the immune system

lactogenic: promoting the secretion of milk; galactagogue

laxative: loosening the bowel contents, promoting evacuation

lipid:	a fat or fat-like substance insoluble in water and soluble in organic solvents
lipolytic:	breaking down fat
lipophilic:	having strong affinity for lipids
litholytic:	breaking down stones
maceration:	the extraction of substances from a plant by steeping in a fixed oil
MbOCA:	symbol for methylenebis(ortho-chloroaniline); a curing agent for polyurethane and epoxy resins; believed to be carcinogenic
MDA:	methylenedioxyamphetamine; has hallucinogenic effects; subject to abuse and dependence
menorrhagia:	excessive periods
metrorrhagia:	uterine haemorrhage occurring outside menstrual periods
narcotic:	inducing insensibility (sleep) and relieving pain in small dosage, toxic in high dosage
oestrogenic:	simulating the action of female hormones
officinalis:	used in medicine; recognized in the pharmacopoeia
oligomenorrhoea:	a condition of infrequent menstruation
organic:	grown without the use of chemical fertilizers, pesticides, etc.
organoleptic:	concerned with testing the effects of a substance on the senses, particularly taste and smell
parenteral:	by means other than the gastrointestinal tract; the introduction of substances into an organism by an intravenous, cutaneous, intramuscular or intramedullary pathway
percutaneous:	applied through the skin
pharmaco-kinetics:	study of absorption, distribution, metabolism and elimination of drugs
photo-sensitization:	abnormally increased sensitivity of the skin to ultraviolet radiation or natural sunlight; can follow ingestion of or contact with various substances
photosynthesis:	use of light energy to drive chemical reactions in a plant, which is a photosynthetic organism, whereby carbon dioxide is reduced to carbohydrates and water to free oxygen
phytotherapy:	treatment of disease by the use of plants and plant extracts; herbalism
polymenorrhoea:	unusually short menstrual cycles
probiotic:	favouring the beneficial bacteria in the body, while inhibiting harmful microbes; literally 'for life' as distinct from antibiotic 'against life'
prophylactic:	preventing disease
psoralens:	polycyclic molecules whose structure gives them the ability to absorb ultraviolet photons
psycho-pharmaceutical:	pertaining to drugs affecting the mind or mood
psychotropic:	of a drug, affecting the brain and influencing behaviour
purgative:	strongly laxative
rhizome:	underground stem bearing roots, scales and nodes
rubefacient:	increasing local blood circulation causing redness of the skin
spasmolytic:	relieving convulsions, spasmodic pains and cramp
stomachic:	agent which stimulates the secretory activity of the stomach
styptic:	arresting haemorrhage by means of an astringent quality; haemostatic
subspecies:	subdivision of a species, often denoting a geographic variation; structure or colour are peculiar to subspecies and are more definite than characteristics identifying varieties; subspecies can interbreed; abbreviated to subsp.
sudorific:	inducing sweating
synergy:	increased effect of two or more medicinal substances working together
taxonomy:	an ordered, scientific classification of living things
thymoleptic:	antiseptic

tonic: producing or restoring normal vigour or tension (tone)

trichome: hairlike structure on the epidermis of a plant

variety: indicates a botanical rank between subspecies and forma; abbreviated to var., as in *Citrus aurantium* var. *amara*

vermifugal: expelling intestinal worms; see anthelmintic

vesicant: producing blisters (therapeutically, to induce counterirritant serosity)

vulnerary: agent promoting healing of wounds

Useful addresses

Training schools
Penny Price Academy of Aromatherapy
41 Leicester Road
Hinckley
Leics LE10 1LW
Tel: 01455 25 10 20
Fax: 01455 25 10 65
Email: info@penny-price.com
Website: www.penny-price.com

Sandra Day School of Health Studies
Ashley House
185a Drake Street
Rochdale OL11 1EF
Email: course@sandraday.com
Website: www.sandraday.com

The Institute of Traditional Herbal Medicine &
Aromatherapy (ITHMA)
Oaklands
Postmans Lane
Little Baddow
Chelmsford CM3 4SF
Email: gm@aromatherapy-studies.com

Products
Penny Price Aromatherapy
41 Leicester Road
Hinckley
Leics LE10 1LW
Tel: 01455 25 10 20
Fax: 01455 25 10 65
Email: info@penny-price.com
Website: www.penny-price.com

Sandra Day School of Health Studies
Ashley House
185a Drake Street
Rochdale OL11 1EF
Email: course@sandraday.com
Website: www.sandraday.com

Essentially Oils
8–10 Mount Farm
Churchill
Chipping Norton
Oxfordshire OX7 6NP
Email: sales@essentiallyoils.com
Website: www.essentiallyoils.com

Associations
IAM (Institute of Aromatic Medicine)
4 Woodland Road
Hinckley
Leics LE10 1JG
Email: aromed@hotmail.com

IFA (International Federation of Aromatherapy)
61/63 Churchfield Road
London W3 6AY
Tel: 0208 992 9605
Tel/Fax: 0208 992 5095
Email: office@ifaroma.org

IFPA (International Federation of Professional
Aromatherapists)
82 Ashby Road
Hinckley
Leicestershire LE10 1 SN

Tel: 01455 637 987
Fax: 01455 890 956
Email: admin@ifparoma.org
Website: www.ifparoma.org

Aromatherapy Consortium (AC)
Tel: 0870 7743477
Email: aromatherapy-regulation.org.uk
Website: www.aromatherapy-regulation.org.uk

Aromatherapy Trades Council (ATC)
PO Box 387
Ipswich, Suffolk IP2 9AN
Email: info@a-t-c.org.uk
Tel/Fax: 01473 603630
Website: www.a-t-c.org.uk

Other interesting websites
Alzheimer's society:
www.alzheimers.org.uk

Aromatherapy Global Online Research Archives
homepage:
www.nature-helps.com/agora/agora.html

Aromatherapy Today – a lightweight journal for
the interested therapist:
www.aromatherapytoday.com

Chemical components – information includes
structures:
www.chemfinder.cambridgesoft.com
Cochrane Library:
www.cochrane.org

Essential Oil Resource Consultants (Bob & Rhi
Harris) – providers of research, information and
education in the field of essential oils:
www.essentialorc.com

European Union:
www.europa.eu.int

Her Majesty's Stationery Office:
www.legislation.hmso.gov.uk/si/si2004/2004215
2.htm

In Essence – Journal of the International
Federation of Professional Aromatherapists:
www.aromatherapy-studies.com/ifpa-
journal.html

International Fragrance Association (IFRA)
homepage – latest guidelines for components in
fragrance products:
www.ifraorg.org

Medicines & Healthcare Products Regulatory
Agency (MHRA)
www.mhra.gov.uk

National Occupational Standards with Skills for
Health:
www.skillsforhealth.org.uk

Phytochemical and Ethnobotanical Databases
(Dr Jim Duke):
www.ars-grin.gov/duke/

Riverhead – publisher, and designer of great
websites:
www.riverhead.co.uk

Search Medline and Pub Med Central –
providing access to biomedical journal articles:
www.ncbi.nlm.nih.gov/Literature/index.html

The Aromatherapy Global Online Research
Archives – homepage
www.nature-helps.com/agora/agora.htm

The International Journal of Clinical
Aromatherapy:
ww.ijca.net/information.htm

The International Journal of Aromatherapy –
peer reviewed scientific aromatherapy journal:
www.intl.elsevierhealth.com/journals/ijar

Index